W9-BIL-230

Occupational Therapy for Physical Dysfunction

Second Edition

Occupational Therapy for Physical Dysfunction
Second Edition

Edited by

CATHERINE ANNE TROMBLY, M.A., OTR, F.A.O.T.A.

Associate Professor, Department of Occupational Therapy
Sargent College of Allied Health Professions
Boston University, Boston, Massachusetts

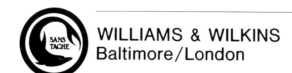

WILLIAMS & WILKINS
Baltimore/London

Copyright ©, 1983
Williams & Wilkins
428 E. Preston Street
Baltimore, Md. 21202, U.S.A.

All rights reserved. This book is protected by copyright. No part of this book may be
reproduced in any form or by any means, including photocopying, or utilized by any
information storage and retrieval system without written permission from the copyright owner.

Made in the United States of America

Published July 1977
  Reprinted 1978
  Reprinted 1979
. Reprinted 1980
  Reprinted 1981
  Reprinted 1982

Library of Congress Cataloging in Publication Data

Main entry under title:

Occupational therapy for physical dysfunction

  Rev. ed. of: Occupational therapy for physical dysfunction / Catherine Anne
Trombly, Anna Deanne Scott. c1977.
    Includes bibliographical references and index.
    1. Occupational therapy. 2. Physically handicapped—Rehabilitation. I. Trombly,
Catherine Anne. II. Trombly, Catherine Anne. Occupational therapy for physical
dysfunction. [DNLM: 1. Handicapped. 2. Occupational therapy. WB 555 T849o]
RM735.033 1982   615.8'515   81-21925
ISBN 0-683-08387-2   AACR2

Composed and printed at the
Waverly Press, Inc.
Mt. Royal and Guilford Aves.
Baltimore, Md. 21202, U.S.A.

Dedication

This book is dedicated to my mother
(in memoriam), my father, and Christopher.

Preface

The purpose of this book is threefold: to compile evaluation and treatment procedures, to present the theoretical bases of these treatment procedures, and to challenge the clinician to research the effectiveness of his/her practice.

Accordingly, the book presents a compilation of evaluation and therapeutic procedures used in the practice of occupational therapy with physically disabled adults. Although a comprehensive compilation was attempted, it is not possible to include every procedure used in the practice of occupational therapy. Each therapist brings his or her own knowledge, perceptions, and unique creativity to his/her practice. Knowledge of the information in this textbook and development of skill in the procedures cited here will enable the beginning therapist to offer quality care to clients. Even the beginning therapist should not use this as a cookbook, however, without regard to the individuality of each patient and his or her unique response to any therapeutic procedure. The book, therefore, presents material in such a way as to help the student therapist begin to develop a process of thinking about the therapeutic process and its application. The book is organized into three approaches to treatment. For each approach, information from the basic sciences which form the theoretical bases for therapeutic procedures is presented in order that the student therapist may understand the rationale for therapeutic procedures and thereby gain flexibility in application of the procedures. Innovative treatment can be developed and treatment planning can be imaginative when the "whys" are known. Further, goal setting is the key to effective treatment. Within each approach, methods of identifying and implementing the goals are clearly stated. The reader is referred to the references listed at the end of each chapter for greater depth of knowledge, or specific directions for certain procedures, or for other points of view on specific issues.

Research on the effectiveness of therapeutic procedures is included. The research is sparse, although there has been a small increase since the last edition. Much more research is needed to identify what the minimally effective therapeutic dosages are, what the long-term effects of treatment are, and whether the effects of treatment are as expected on certain types of patients. All effectiveness research must eventually tell us what treatment, administered in what way, over what period of time improves the *function* of what type of patient. Clinicians are the source of this information. I look forward to including your studies in the next edition of this textbook!

Ideas for the present revision have been generated not only from our own experiences with using this book as a textbook, but also from clinicians, students, and educators who very kindly sent us constructive criticism. This revision is characterized by more examples in an attempt to help the student therapist translate theory into practice. Chapters on Closed Head Injuries and Biofeedback as an Adjunct to Therapy have been added as a reflection of increased involvement by OTR's with these issues. Published information was used primarily. In a few instances where important information was only available from workshops, theses, or verbal communication with experts, this is indicated.

We have assumed that student therapists who use this book have prerequisite knowledge of anatomy, physiology, neuroanatomy, neurophysiology, kinesiology, and orthopedic and neurological clinical conditions, and also prerequisite skills in use of tools and basic construction procedures used in splint-making.

To simplify both the writing and reading of this textbook, we have arbitrarily assigned the feminine gender to the therapist and masculine to the patient. It is not meant to assign value to either group of people.

Catherine A. Trombly

Acknowledgments

Many people contributed to the production of the second edition of this textbook and their time, effort, and expertise are gratefully acknowledged. Constructive criticism and detailed suggestions for improvement were received from Frederic J. Kottke, M.D., Anita Bundy, M.S., OTR, Lillian Hoyle Parent, M.A., OTR, Virgil Mathiowetz, M.S., OTR, and Shelly Earley, M.O.T.

The photography for this edition was done by Anne G. Fisher, M.S., OTR. Mark Erickson posed for many of the new photographs, as well as Gail Bliss, M.O.T., Anita Bundy, M.S., OTR, and Deborah Yarett Slater, M.S., OTR. Alice Follows, M.S., OTR, Chief Occupational Therapist at University Hospitals of Boston University Medical Center arranged for photographing of hand splints. Deborah Yarett Slater, M.S., OTR directed the efforts of the occupational therapy staff at University Hospitals in the construction of hand splints especially for the purpose of photographing them for this edition. Gayle M. Thompson, M.Ed, OTR, Assistant Professor at Boston University, made suggestions and arrangments for the photographing of activities. Margaret Hayes, OTR, Director of Occupational Therapy at the Veteran's Administration Medical Center, West Roxbury, Mass. arranged for the photography of a powered hand splint.

Many photographs from the first edition also appear in this edition. Photography for that edition was done by Judy La Drew. Sam Fitzpatrick posed for those photographs.

The production of this edition has been further facilitated by the efforts of Nancy Talbot, M.Ed., Chairperson of the Occupational Therapy Department at Boston University, Maureen Hayes, Ed.D., Chairperson of the Occupational Therapy Department of Tufts University, and Lee Ann Quintana, M.S., OTR.

Specific help has also been offered by others to some of the contributing authors, and they are cited at the end of the particular chapter.

Contributors

Anne G. Fisher, M.S., OTR
Doctoral candidate, Sargent College of Allied Health Professions, Boston University, Boston, Massachusetts.

Beverly J. Myers, B.S., OTR
Staff Occupational Therapist, South Metropolitan Association for Low-Incidence Handicapped, Harvey, Illinois and Midwest Consultant for Fred Sammons, Inc.

Lillian Hoyle Parent, M.A., OTR, F.A.O.T.A.
Associate Professor, Department of Occupational Therapy, College of Associated Health Professions, University of Illinois-Medical Center, Chicago, Illinois.

Cynthia A. Philips, M.A., OTR
Hand Therapist, New England Baptist Hospital and Hand Surgical Associates, Brookline, Massachusetts.

Anna Deane Scott, M.Ed., OTR
Associate Professor, Department of Occupational Therapy, Sargent College of Allied Health Professions, Boston University, Boston, Massachusetts.

Catherine Anne Trombly, M.A., OTR, F.A.O.T.A.
Associate Professor, Department of Occupational Therapy, Sargent College of Allied Health Professions, Boston University, Boston, Masachusetts.

Hilda P. Versluys, M.Ed., OTR
Assistant Clinical Professor, Department of Occupational Therapy, Sargent College of Allied Health Professions, Boston University, Boston, Massachusetts.

Patricia L. Weber, M.S., OTR
Staff Occupational Therapist, Children's Hospital, New Orleans, Louisiana

Contents

PART ONE

Framework for Therapy

PART TWO

Neurodevelopmental Approach

PART THREE

Biomechanical Approach

PART FOUR

Activity

PART FIVE

Biofeedback

PART SIX

Orthotics

PART ONE

Framework for Therapy

The two introductory chapters of this book present ideas that underlie the practice of occupational therapy with the adult physically disabled. The first one identifies the reasoning processes that the author uses in making evaluation and treatment planning decisions. By identifying these processes I hope to assist the student occupational therapist to organize and utilize the information of the remainder of the book. With experience, the student therapist may develop his/her own organizational framework.

The second chapter specifically addresses the psychological needs and adjustments of a person who has become physically disabled. Hilda Versluys, M.Ed., OTR, has applied sound principles of psychiatric occupational therapy to the treatment of the unique emotional needs of the physically disabled. The emotional adjustment of the patient must be the foremost consideration when implementing planned therapy so that the patient may achieve his highest potential. The therapist must remain cognizant that the patient will be motivated by his primary concerns: his membership in his family and society.

The remainder of this book is organized according to my view that there are three treatment approaches from which the therapist may choose in attempting to assist the physically disabled person in reaching as high a level of independent functioning and life satisfaction as is possible for that person. These approaches are: neurodevelopmental, biomechanical, and rehabilitative.

The neurodevelopmental approach aims at facilitating change in the sensorimotor integration of the central nervous system of persons who have been born with a dysfunctional central nervous system or who have suffered trauma or disease to their central nervous system. If we respond negatively to the key question, "Does this person have an intact, fully matured central nervous system (CNS)?", then we would likely select neurophysiologically and/or developmentally based methods of treatment in an effort to effect an essential change in the organization of the central nervous system and thereby improve overall functioning of the disabled person. Techniques developed as part of the neurodevelopmental approach are also appropriate for patients with an intact central nervous system in that this approach capitalizes on and enhances the functioning of the central nervous system.

The biomechanical approach deals with increasing strength, endurance, and range of joint motion in patients who have an intact central nervous system but who have dysfunction in the peripheral nervous system or the musculoskeletal, integumentary, or cardiopulmonary systems. If we respond affirmatively to the key question, "Does this person have an intact, fully matured central nervous system?", then we would focus our attention on biomechanically oriented theories of treatment related to the specific problems of the disabled person. This approach is not appropriate, however, for the person with central nervous system dysfunction.

The rehabilitative approach aims at making the person as independent as possible in spite of residual disability that has resulted for any reason. If a person must live with a disability which decreases his independent functioning, then the occupational therapist will concentrate on helping him find ways to compensate for his losses by adapted techniques and/or equipment.

The book is further organized to present evaluation procedures, treatment principles, and techniques within each approach to treatment. Specific diagnoses are used to illustrate the application of treatment principles and techniques, as well as to point out unique treatment problems which these commonly seen diagnoses present. Whatever the treatment approach, activity is the medium of occupational therapy. Examples of therapeutic selection and adaptation of activity are presented throughout.

Knowledge and understanding are continually changing as a result of ongoing research. Consequently this compilation can only report currently acknowledged concepts with the expectation that they will change.

chapter

1

The Treatment Planning Process

Catherine A. Trombly, M.A., OTR

Treatment planning is problem solving applied to patient care. Methodology is similar to that used by scientists and businessmen to solve problems in their spheres of endeavor. Every member of the treatment team utilizes this problem-solving process.

The team members must collaborate to plan an overall, nonconflicting, program for the patient that enhances all of the patient's capabilities but does not overstress him. The composition of the team varies depending upon the particular problem and needs of the patient. In a rehabilitation center a core team of physician, nurse, occupational therapist, physical therapist, speech therapist, social worker, psychologist, and rehabilitation counselor are occasionally joined by the orthotist, prosthetist, rehabilitation nurse, teacher, and medical or surgical specialists, such as rheumatologists, cardiologists, etc. Each member is responsible for developing a treatment plan related to his or her own unique area of expertise.

The occupational therapy treatment planning process is the same whether it is applied to persons with physical, psychosocial, or cognitive-perceptual-motor disabilities. It is the process of *identifying the problem(s), establishing the goal(s),* and *determining the approaches, principles, and methods* by which *this person* with *these problems* can reach *those goals.* The process can be further clarified by Figure 1.1.

DATA GATHERING

Important information that will influence the development of the occupational therapy treatment program can be obtained from the following sources:

1. The *medical record* should yield information concerning the person's diagnosis(es), date of onset, medical and surgical histories, precautions, medications, age, pertinent social and vocational history, discharge plan, as well as reports of the nursing staff about the disabled person's daily physical and psychological functioning.

2. *Observation of the disabled person* as he attempts to perform functional activities will allow the therapist to determine the person's present functional level as well as his sense of safety and judgment. These observations will also give the therapist a clue as to what is limiting the patient's functional performance so that appropriate evaluations may be selected to evaluate the limitations more objectively. For example, the disabled person may be unable to feed himself. By watching the person try to do this, the therapist observes that the patient can lift a heavy mug but cannot approach his mouth. The therapist concludes that the patient seems to have adequate strength but range of motion seems to be the limiting factor. The therapist will check out this observation by doing a

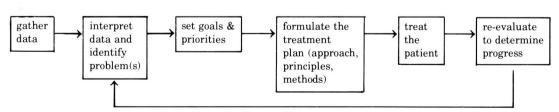

Figure 1.1 Treatment planning process.

cursory strength evaluation and, not finding a limitation here, a more detailed range of motion evaluation.

3. *Measurement* of the disabled person's *performance* to determine baseline performance. The therapist, having observed the patient and knowing the implications of the diagnosis, makes a judgment about which areas to evaluate and which evaluation procedures to use to elicit the necessary measurements or information regarding the strengths and limitations of the person. Specifics of measurement are described in succeeding chapters of this book.

4. *Interview of the disabled person* should yield knowledge of his goals, feelings, readiness to participate in or to take responsibility for treatment, expectations of therapy, cognitive abilities such as memory, ability to sequence and organize information, orientation to time, place, and person, comprehension of directions, his perception of what he can do for himself, and his interests.

5. *Reports of other professionals* who are simultaneously gathering data in regard to the person relative to their particular service should be available from the medical record, be reported at team conferences, or be shared in other less formal ways. These reports will influence the development of the occupational therapy treatment plan.

6. *Interview of family members* should result in gaining knowledge of their goals for the disabled family member and their views about how the disability has affected the person, as well as how it has affected each of them and the family unit. Brain injury may cause changes in personality characteristics. The family is the source of information about the patient's premorbid personality.

7. It may be necessary for the therapist to *read resource material* regarding the classical symptoms, course, and prognosis of the person's disease(s) or to review the precautions and effects of the patient's medication before planning treatment.

INTERPRETING THE DATA AND IDENTIFYING THE PROBLEM(S)

A profile of strengths and limitations will emerge from results of evaluations and other data-gathering processes. In order to identify the problem(s) toward which the therapeutic plan will be directed, it is necessary to select the significant information. Significant information refers to that data and those scores which reflect limitations that decrease physical functioning, that limit the likelihood of return of function, and/or that lead to deformity or maladaptive personal-social functioning.

Equally significant information that influences problem identification are the patient's goals for himself, his feelings, and his values.

Once the problems are identified, a problem list is developed and recorded.

SETTING GOALS AND PRIORITIES

Once the problems are identified, the goals of the treatment program are listed. Because it is impossible to accomplish all goals at once, the goals are prioritized. There are two bases for establishing the particular order of priority. One is the client's (and his family's) view of what is most important. The other is the therapist's knowledge that some abilities must precede accomplishment of others. To help in setting priorities, therapists identify long-term goals and short-term goals.

Long-term goals specify the end product of therapy. They describe the expected level of functioning the patient will achieve by the termination of the therapy program. An example of this is: "although requiring a wheelchair for locomotion, the patient will be independent in self-care." Long-term goals are educated guesses which may need modification as the patient's progress is observed.

To achieve long-term goals, the therapist plans a series of short-term goals which are the mini-goals, the building blocks that lead to one or more long-term goals. Short-term goals imply sequencing and priority. The sequencing is started from the point at which the patient is functioning successfully and stopped at the point where the long-term goal is achieved.

Several sequences of short-term goals may be ongoing concurrently. For example, in order to reach the long-term goal mentioned above, the patient must learn to (a) operate the wheelchair and (b) do self-care activities. If the person's disability is weakness, then one sequence of short-term goals will be to progress the person from one plateau of strength to the next. Concurrently, short-term goals related to self-care will be sequenced so that the person is taught to do those activities for which he has sufficient strength at any given time to assure successful experiences at each stage. In terms of priority, we see that activity to increase strength must precede each self-care task that requires greater strength and that certain aspects of self-care must be mastered before others which depend on a prior skill or are of a developmentally higher nature.

Labeling a goal "long-term" or "short-term" simply informs others that the goal is being aimed for eventually or is being worked on immediately. The labeling is not what is important in treatment planning; the establishment of a laddering of goals that the patient can successfully accomplish and by which he can succeedingly approach his final level of functioning is the essence of treatment planning.

Long-term goals must be established in collaboration with the person receiving therapy and other members of the rehabilitation team. Short-term goals are established by each professional and are specifically related to the expertise of that discipline. It is very important that the patient understand the relationship of each short-term goal to the long-term goals and how the activity implements the short-term goal.

FORMULATE THE TREATMENT PLAN FOR EACH SHORT-TERM GOAL

In order to formulate the plan for a treatment program, the therapist must identify the treatment approach or approaches that are appropriate for the patient (see Fig. 1.3). Some patients may require one or more of the treatment approaches. Selection of the appropriate treatment approach at any given time depends upon the nature of the presenting problem, its causes, the state of recovery, and established priorities. For example, if the patient has a weak upper extremity secondary to a cerebrovascular accident, the therapist must choose from among three major therapeutic approaches: neurodevelopmental, biomechanical, or rehabilitative. A rehabilitative approach would be chosen if weakness were long-standing and apparently unlikely to improve. The therapist's reason for choosing this approach would be that teaching methods of compensation for the loss of the use of this extremity could help the patient be as independent as possible.

If recovery was hoped for, a biomechanical approach with its direct strengthening techniques involving maximal resistance might appeal to the therapist. However, this would be rejected in favor of the neurodevelopmental approach in answer to the key question, "Does this patient have an intact fully matured central nervous system?" This is because the patient who has suffered a cerebral vascular accident may lack voluntary control of his musculature, or his muscle tone may be altered due to lack of influence of the higher centers of the central nervous system: he would be unable to selectively strengthen certain muscles because he is probably only able to move in developmentally lower patterns of motion.

After identifying the treatment approach, the therapist must identify the underlying principle of treatment to use for each of the problems. For example, using the above example, the neurodevelopmental approach having been chosen, the choice of principle within that approach depends on what is applicable to the patient at his particular stage of recovery. Our hypothetical therapist may select sensory stimulation to facilitate weak movements and simple functional tasks as a means of establishing voluntary control over the movement.

The method of implementing the principle must be determined. The treatment principles and methods for each approach are described in the remainder of this book.

Day[1] diagrammed a model for treatment planning as shown in Figure 1.2 and 1.3.

TREAT THE PATIENT

The planned activity is presented to the person in such a way that he can concentrate on the process and goal of the activity and not the specific movements or muscle contractions desired. The activity should be one, whether adapted or not, that automatically calls forth the correct response.

The therapist observes the performance of the activity to determine whether the patient is just able to do the activity, or whether it is either too easy or too difficult. If the selected activity is not exactly right to challenge the patient's existing capabilities, grading or adaptation is necessary.

Fatigue of the person and safe use of the tools are monitored throughout the treatment period. Termination of the treatment period, rest, or further instruction may be necessary.

REEVALUATION

Periodically, depending upon the course of the illness and the changes observed in the patient's performance or as a requirement of third party payers, the therapist remeasures the parameters of performance. These data are interpreted and compared with prior evaluation data to note changes. The problem list, goals, and treatment are adjusted to meet the person's rate of progress or new level of performance. The progress is recorded in the patient's medical record.

ONE EXAMPLE OF THE TREATMENT PLANNING PROCESS

Data Gathering

1. The medical record yielded the following information that will be used to plan treatment: quadriplegia secondary to fracture dislocation of C_{6-7}; incomplete lesion; C_6 functional level; no medical complications; cervical fusion and laminectomy performed on the day of the accident; multiple lacerations of both hands; currently in traction with tongs.

2. Observation of the patient led the therapist to conclude that there is slight movement in right toe; no motion in left lower extremity; sensory loss below T_4; is able to do teeth care, other light hygiene and feeding when sidelying but is dependent in all else due to positioning requirements for cervical traction.

3. Measurement of the performance is too complicated to record here. A summary exists under significant information noted below.

4. Interview with the patient produced this information: He is 24 years old; is a high school graduate; is now a computer operator; lives with his parents in a second floor apartment; has four siblings all married and living away from home; his interests are sports and camping. He plans to return to work eventually and continue to live with his parents when accessible housing is located.

5. Reports of other professionals yielded the following: The patient has a very supportive family and many friends. He does not know the implication of spinal cord injury and expects to walk out of the hospital. Health is good.

6. Interview of the family (parents) informed the therapist that temporarily, the patient will live with a married brother and sister-in-law, but will eventually live with the parents. The family does not yet know the implications of spinal cord injury.

7. The therapist had forgotten the effects of Dantrium and Decadron; when the Physician's Desk Reference[2] was consulted, it was learned that Decadron is a corticosteroid; the patient is on a low dosage so no adverse effects should occur (muscle weakness would be an adverse reaction). Dantrium is used to control spasticity of upper motor neuron (UMN) origin. The adverse reactions that may occur during dosage regulation are weakness and drowsiness. Another adverse reaction that may occur is photosensitivity; therefore, the patient should not be exposed to strong sunlight. Persons taking Dantrium should not operate machinery or motor vehicles.

Interpreting the Data and Identifying the Problems

The significant information is: There is normal sensation of the upper extremities (UEs). PROM (passive range of motion) of the UEs is WNL (within normal limits). Muscles of the left shoulder, elbow, and forearm are adequate for function, being graded G to N (good to normal). The right upper extremity, including the wrist, is graded G to N. The left extensor carpi radialis (longus and brevis) is normal; the extensor carpi ulnaris is F+ (fair plus), and the wrist flexors grade F. The right finger muscles are stronger than the left; they grade P+ (poor plus) to G−, whereas the left finger muscles grade 0 except for T (trace) for the extensor digitorum and the flexor digitorum profundus 3,4. Thumbs: the left = 0; right grades range from 0 in the opponens and long flexor to F in the extensor pollicis longus. There are some muscles of the lower extremities that grade T.

The problems are:

1. Weakness of the left wrist.
2. Weakness of the fingers and thumbs bilaterally.
3. Spotty weakness (G) of proximal musculature.
4. Prevention of contractures at joints where muscles grade less than F.
5. Need for protection of the tenodesis function of the left wrist and hand.
6. ADL (activities of daily living) dependency.
7. Denial of meaning and/or permanency of the disability.

Setting Goals and Priorities

The long-term goal for this patient is to return to work as a computer operator and to be w/c (wheelchair)-independent in his parent's home when they locate accessible housing.

Intermediate long-term goal is to maximize functional level of independence within the limits of disability and includes the following:

a. Teach patient correct positioning so that he can supervise his positioning by all personnel.
b. Passive ranging twice daily to all joints with subfunctional muscles; special precautions to preserve left tenodesis.
c. Strengthen weak muscles in the right hand.
d. Strengthen weak muscles in the left hand.
e. Strengthen spotty weakness in proximal musculature.
f. Assess need and order required rehabilitation equipment to increase independence.

g. Home evaluation and family teaching.
h. Homemaking and vocational evaluation and training.
i. Driver evaluation and training.
j. Training in recreation for the w/c-bound.
k. Community reintegration.

The short-term goals, in order from beginning to end, to achieve intermediate long-term goal c are:

1. Increase strength of finger extensors from P+ to F−.
2. Increase strength of finger extensors from F− to F.
3. Increase strength of finger extensors to normal or as much as possible.
4. Increase strength of finger flexors from F to F+.
5. Increase strength of finger flexors from F+ to G−.
6. Increase strength of finger flexors to normal or as much as possible.
7. Increase strength of thumb extensors from F to F+.
8. Increase strength of thumb extensors from F+ to G−, etc.

Formulating the Treatment Plan for Each Short-Term Goal

Short-term goal 1 is to increase strength of the finger extensors of the right hand from P+ to F−. The approach to be used is biomechanical. The principle to be used is increasing resistance in a gravity-eliminated plane.

The method to be used is as follows: Patient is sidelying (due to cervical traction). The right arm is supported on a table with the forearm in midposition. A strap is placed around the fingers at the level of the proximal phalanges. A nylon fishline is attached to the strap, runs over a pulley attached to the edge of the table, and is attached at the other end to a 7-gm (½ oz.) weight. This amount of weight had been determined to be the weight that could be lifted 10 times through range.

This process is repeated for each short-term goal. The flow chart in Figure 1.4 has been devised to assist the student occupational therapist to sort out a patient's physical problems and to select appropriate treatment approaches and principles. The chart does not include the detail of the therapeutic process (methods), which is the substance of this book, nor is it meant to take the place of the knowledge and professional judgment of an experienced therapist.

Treat the Patient

The patient lifts the weight through full range 10 times. Following a rest period, finger extension is used functionally by requiring the patient to extend his fingers to pick up larger and larger lightweight objects. This would combine treatment of the flexors and extensors which is desirable.

Reevaluation

Reevaluation would be carried out for each of the problems which are being addressed in therapy. In the case of the goal under consideration in this example, muscle strength would be remeasured, and progress, or lack of it, would be recorded. Treatment would be modified based on these results.

FLOW CHART FOR PLANNING TREATMENT

The chart (Fig. 1.4) represents a series of choices which the therapist makes as a response to each question in working through each of the patient's problems. Because a patient may have several problems, it may be necessary to break into the chart at any of the questions designated by a letter (*A*, *B*, *C*, or *D*).

The chart reflects the author's bias that although neurodevelopmental principles may be effective for orthopedic patients, the biomechanical principles which focus primarily on force and motion of muscles and joints rather than nervous system function, *per se*, are not necessarily the best choice for developmentally immature patients nor those with a motor disorder of central nervous system origin. Biomechanical principles are appropriately applied to patients with orthopedic or cardiovascular disorders or patients who have regained motor control following a central nervous system lesion.

References

1. Day, D. A systems diagram for teaching treatment planning. *Am. J. Occup. Ther.*, 27(5): 239–243, 1973.
2. *Physician's Desk Reference* (34th ed). Oradell, N.J.: Medical Economics Co., 1980.

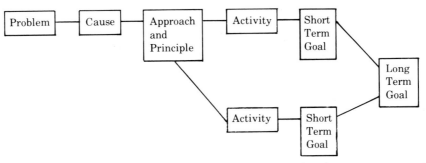

Figure 1.2   Day's model for treatment planning.

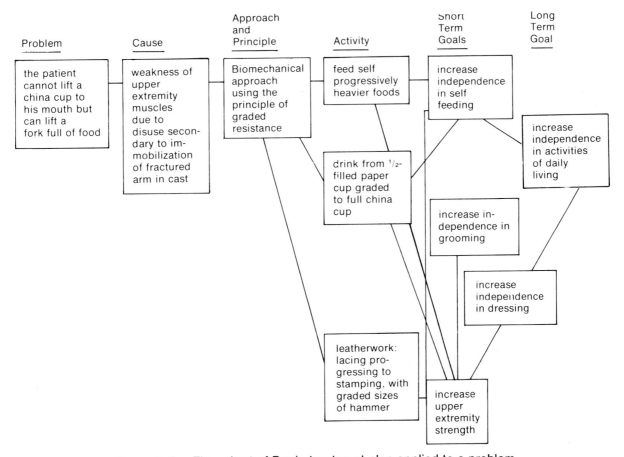

Figure 1.3   Flow chart of Day's treatment plan applied to a problem.

* START HERE

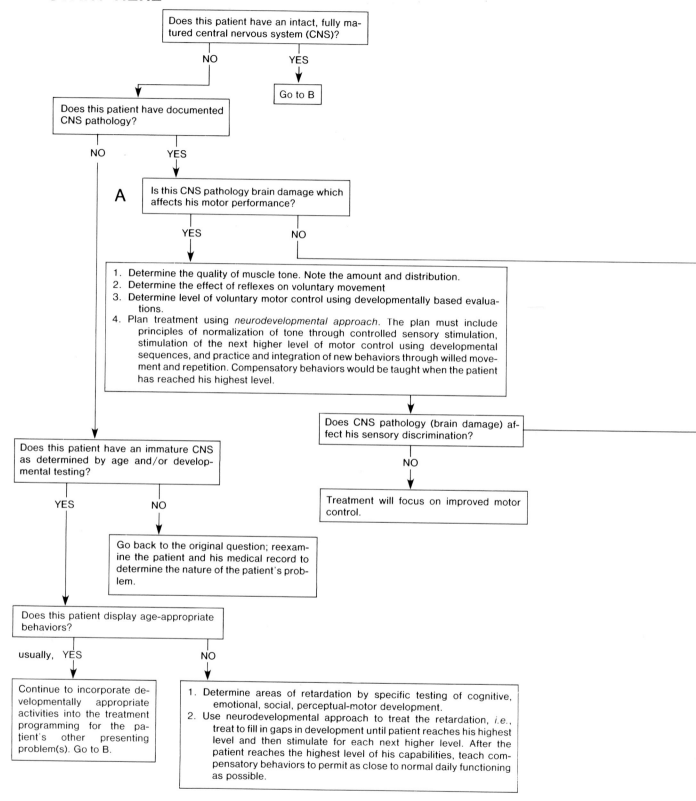

Figure 1.4 Treatment planning for patients with physical disabilities.

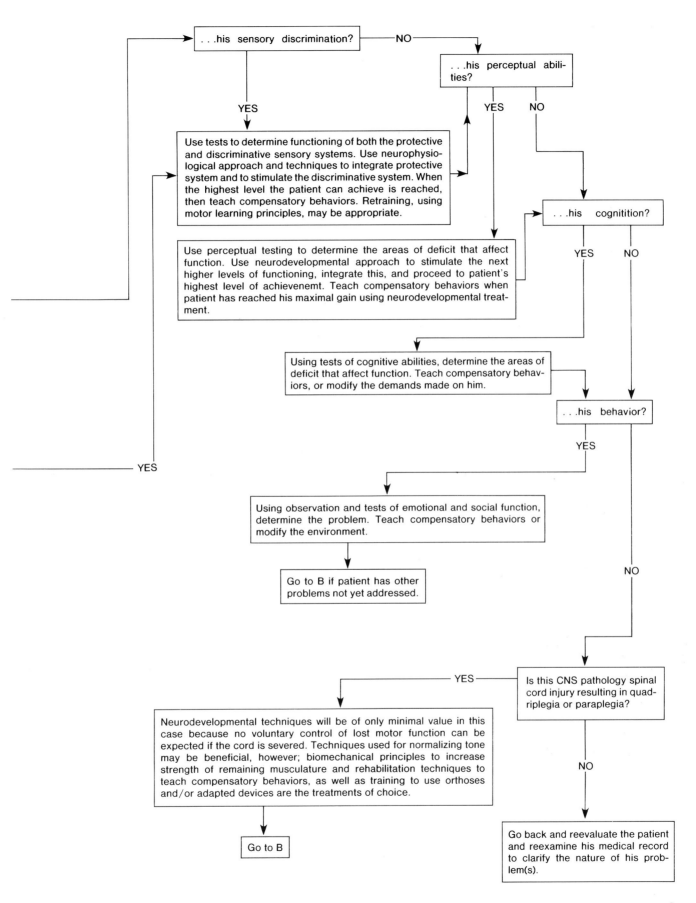

... his sensory discrimination? ——NO——

... his perceptual abilities?

YES   NO

YES

Use tests to determine functioning of both the protective and discriminative sensory systems. Use neurophysiological approach and techniques to integrate protective system and to stimulate the discriminative system. When the highest level the patient can achieve is reached, then teach compensatory behaviors. Retraining, using motor learning principles, may be appropriate.

... his cognitition?

YES   NO

Use perceptual testing to determine the areas of deficit that affect function. Use neurodevelopmental approach to stimulate the next higher levels of functioning, integrate this, and proceed to patient's highest level of achievenemt. Teach compensatory behaviors when patient has reached his maximal gain using neurodevelopmental treatment.

Using tests of cognitive abilities, determine the areas of deficit that affect function. Teach compensatory behaviors, or modify the demands made on him.

... his behavior?

YES

YES

Using observation and tests of emotional and social function, determine the problem. Teach compensatory behaviors or modify the environment.

Go to B if patient has other problems not yet addressed.

NO

——YES—— Is this CNS pathology spinal cord injury resulting in quadriplegia or paraplegia?

Neurodevelopmental techniques will be of only minimal value in this case because no voluntary control of lost motor function can be expected if the cord is severed. Techniques used for normalizing tone may be beneficial, however; biomechanical principles to increase strength of remaining musculature and rehabilitation techniques to teach compensatory behaviors, as well as training to use orthoses and/or adapted devices are the treatments of choice.

NO

Go to B

Go back and reevaluate the patient and reexamine his medical record to clarify the nature of his problem(s).

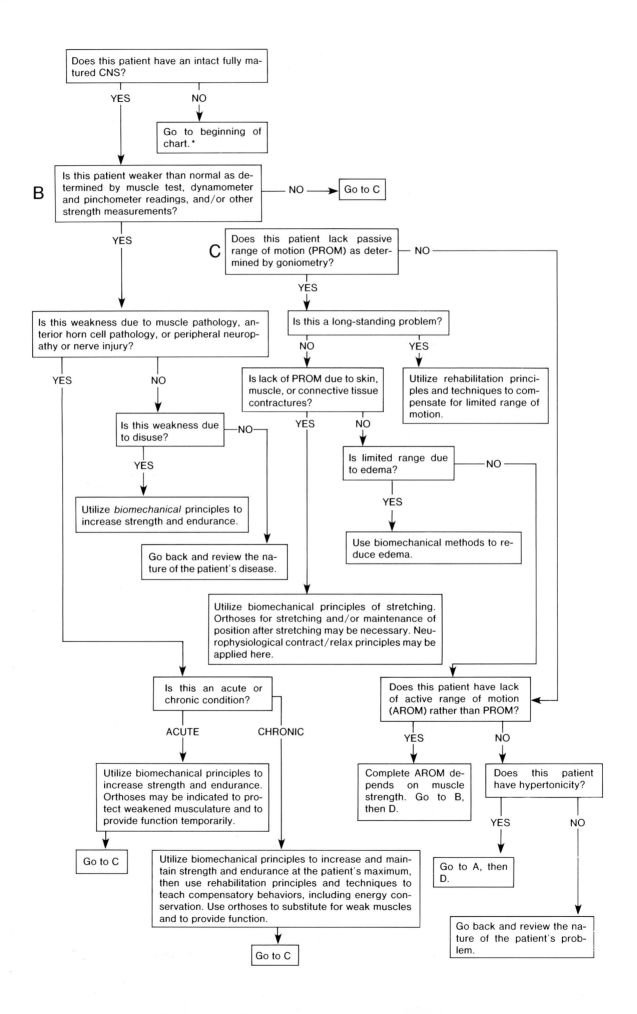

Does this patient have an intact fully matured CNS?

YES | NO

NO → Go to beginning of chart.*

B Is this patient weaker than normal as determined by muscle test, dynamometer and pinchometer readings, and/or other strength measurements?

NO → Go to C

YES

C Does this patient lack passive range of motion (PROM) as determined by goniometry?

NO

YES

Does this patient lack passive range of motion (PROM) as determined by goniometry?

Is this a long-standing problem?

NO | YES

Is this weakness due to muscle pathology, anterior horn cell pathology, or peripheral neuropathy or nerve injury?

YES | NO

Is lack of PROM due to skin, muscle, or connective tissue contractures?

YES | NO

Utilize rehabilitation principles and techniques to compensate for limited range of motion.

Is this weakness due to disuse?

NO

YES

Is limited range due to edema?

NO

YES

Utilize *biomechanical* principles to increase strength and endurance.

Go back and review the nature of the patient's disease.

Use biomechanical methods to reduce edema.

Utilize biomechanical principles of stretching. Orthoses for stretching and/or maintenance of position after stretching may be necessary. Neurophysiological contract/relax principles may be applied here.

Is this an acute or chronic condition?

ACUTE | CHRONIC

Does this patient have lack of active range of motion (AROM) rather than PROM?

YES | NO

Utilize biomechanical principles to increase strength and endurance. Orthoses may be indicated to protect weakened musculature and to provide function temporarily.

Complete AROM depends on muscle strength. Go to B, then D.

Does this patient have hypertonicity?

YES | NO

Go to C

Utilize biomechanical principles to increase and maintain strength and endurance at the patient's maximum, then use rehabilitation principles and techniques to teach compensatory behaviors, including energy conservation. Use orthoses to substitute for weak muscles and to provide function.

Go to A, then D.

Go back and review the nature of the patient's problem.

Go to C

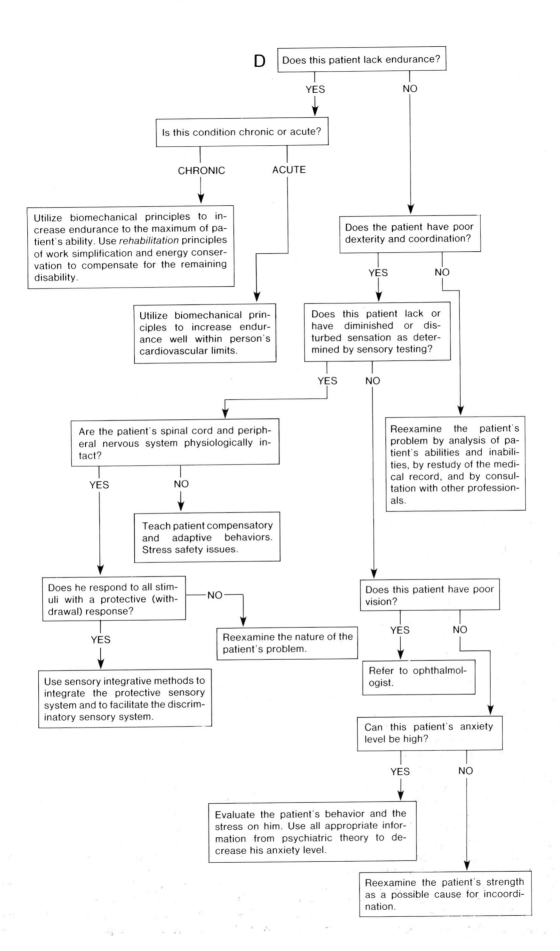

D Does this patient lack endurance?

YES → Is this condition chronic or acute?

CHRONIC → Utilize biomechanical principles to increase endurance to the maximum of patient's ability. Use *rehabilitation* principles of work simplification and energy conservation to compensate for the remaining disability.

ACUTE → Utilize biomechanical principles to increase endurance well within person's cardiovascular limits.

NO → Does the patient have poor dexterity and coordination?

YES → Does this patient lack or have diminished or disturbed sensation as determined by sensory testing?

NO → Reexamine the patient's problem by analysis of patient's abilities and inabilities, by restudy of the medical record, and by consultation with other professionals.

YES → Are the patient's spinal cord and peripheral nervous system physiologically intact?

NO → Teach patient compensatory and adaptive behaviors. Stress safety issues.

Are the patient's spinal cord and peripheral nervous system physiologically intact?

YES → Does he respond to all stimuli with a protective (withdrawal) response?

NO → Teach patient compensatory and adaptive behaviors. Stress safety issues.

Does he respond to all stimuli with a protective (withdrawal) response?

NO → Reexamine the nature of the patient's problem.

YES → Use sensory integrative methods to integrate the protective sensory system and to facilitate the discriminatory sensory system.

Does this patient have poor vision?

YES → Refer to ophthalmologist.

NO → Can this patient's anxiety level be high?

Can this patient's anxiety level be high?

YES → Evaluate the patient's behavior and the stress on him. Use all appropriate information from psychiatric theory to decrease his anxiety level.

NO → Reexamine the patient's strength as a possible cause for incoordination.

chapter

2

Psychosocial Adjustment to Physical Disability

Hilda P. Versluys, M.Ed., OTR

This chapter is concerned with the multiple factors which influence the direction of the rehabilitation effort. Physical disability and serious illness pose a major threat to an individual and may precipitate a life crisis. Before the illness the patient could love and work, was unrestricted and could move about freely. He had outlets for physical tension, aggression, and creativity.[1, 2]

Now physical trauma or the onset of chronic illness may leave the patient with multiple disabilities which disrupt family life and future plans, alter his body image, terminate work roles, reduce self-esteem, security, and independence. In addition, opportunities for social contacts are reduced, psychological integrity is threatened, and the patient may lose control over intimate physical functions.

In the hospital the patient may be treated in an impersonal restrictive environment which is efficient in meeting medical needs but encourages feelings of helplessness and dependency. The patient may begin to identify with the role of disabled or ill person. Faced with integrating new and threatening realities and dealing with frightening implications about the future, the patient is in danger of being overwhelmed. Thus the patient may now develop both adaptive and maladaptive defenses to shield him from reality and provide time to make adjustments. Upon discharge the patient may fail to cope with the realities of community living and require frequent hospitalizations.[2-6]

Despite excellent treatment programs and personal dedication, occupational therapists may encounter blocks to rehabilitation. Patients may demonstrate severe regressions, fail to move out of denial or mourn-

ing, seem unable to accept life style changes, and fail to make the most of their assets. Therapists may feel a sense of failure and frustration concerning the lack of rehabilitation progress. Therapists need to review the factors influencing rehabilitation progress, namely, the premorbid personality, developmental level, symbolic meaning of the loss, and intrapsychic coping strategies. In addition to acceptance of the slow motion effect of rehabilitation the therapist must establish realistic treatment objectives for the specific patient and target short-term goals so that small increments of success can be recognized.

Siller[7] maintains that adjustment to physical dysfunction and chronic illness is of long duration and continues after the patient is discharged. It is important to remember that many patients make successful life-style adjustments despite personal losses and the disruption of their lives.[7]

Strain,[5] a medical liaison psychiatrist, found that despite medical and technological advances staff often failed to consider the total impact of psychological and social issues on the patient. Thus excellent medical treatment and rehabilitation programs have not been sufficient to motivate patients to reach and retain the maximal level of functioning available to them or to use skills and energy productively. Physical rehabilitation may increase physical function but has not provided training in the social and personal role skills necessary for successful, permanent return to independent community living.[3, 4] The therapist's understanding, intervention, and treatment of the psychological and social dysfunctions of the patient lay the groundwork for the future. It is hoped that a consideration of the influencing factors in rehabilitation will be useful in encouraging occupational therapists to realize the importance of their contribution and to define their role in the treatment of psychosocial aspects of physical disability and illness.

PSYCHOLOGICAL CONSIDERATIONS

The patient's effort to adjust to illness, disability, and hospitalization are accompanied by psychological stressors. The patient finds that his body is not indestructable, that he can be suddenly vulnerable to death, physical loss, and pain. In addition, skills, community status, and the personal qualities that make him an individual are not recognized in the hospital. The patient cannot always influence the environment, he is expected to comply with the medical regime and to invest trust in the staff who make important decisions concerning his health, life, and future. The patient is separated from family, friends, and familiar environment. He is at risk concerning loss of developmentally achieved physical functions, such as motor ability, bowel control, and physical strength and developmentally achieved psychological functions, such as autonomy and security. The patient may experience a breakdown in cognitive functioning, *i.e.*, confusion, disorientation, inability to reality test and to think logically.[2, 3, 5, 6] The patient's dependent position reawakens infantile conflicts and fears of abandonment and destruction. This may cause regression and irrational, anxious behavior. Injury or fears of mutilation may result in castration anxiety. Although such fears may be symbolic they also may be experienced in reality through amputations due to injury, cancer, or diabetes. Intimate medical procedures and lack of privacy not only cause embarrassment but may stimulate sexual fantasies which are threatening to the patient and may produce extreme emotional arousal.[2, 5, 6]

Stewart and Rossier,[6] in a discussion of accommodation to disability, state that the psychological impact of paralysis is influenced by the patient's age and position in the life cycle. At adolescence the patient is concerned with developmental tasks related to formation of identity, sexuality, life-style, and career choice. There is a concern with peer group acceptance, body image, and social interaction. Since the personality is incompletely formed, integration of the paralysis is difficult and often disruptive. The middle-aged patient is already facing issues of multiple loss, *i.e.*, parents, friends, physical decline, and questions concerning the meaning of life and the shortening of available time. Stewart and Rossier[6] state that the paralysis may amplify the preexisting sense of decline and deterioration. Quigley[8] states that patients forget their intact skills and abilities and become preoccupied with their premorbid real or fantasized successes and satisfactions, making adaptation to their present situation more difficult. The following statements illustrate the variety of nonproductive and often unconscious beliefs that affect the patient's reactions to their

disability: (1) The injury may be seen as confirmation of lack of self-worth and helps the patient become reconciled to a negative self-image.[9] (2) The injury and deformity may relieve the patient of guilt for some real or imagined past act and lead to a sense of well-being.[10] (3) The patient may have difficulty adjusting his original body image and developing a compromise one. He may never accept the disability.[10] (4) Physical illness and disability may satisfy security and dependency needs without stigmatizing the patient since the sick role is accepted by society. The patient allows others to care for him and shows little self-motivation.[11] (5) The patient may wish to maintain security and financial support, *i.e.* insurance, family assistance. (6) When confronted with destructive changes in health and physical status, the patients often need to find a reason and search their own past behaviors. They locate and focus on personal mistakes or what they consider to be sinful thoughts or actions.[5, 9, 12, 13]

In addition, patients' personal values and criteria for self-definition are lost. They feel shame when standards for presentation of self are lowered, *i.e.*, demonstrating anxiety, crying, acting out, or losing their temper. The patient struggling with these personal agendas is in no position to benefit from rehabilitation.

The Premorbid Personality

An examination of the premorbid personality of the patient provides perspective for understanding the patient's way of coping with the stress of his predicament and assists the staff in planning interventions and treatment programs. Treatment success is more certain when the dysfunction does not interfere with the patient's ability to sustain a valued self-image and life-style and when the patient is assured of continued membership in valued groups.[1] Too great a variance between the premorbid life-style and present functional possibilities may reduce options acceptable to the patient. For example, some patients are cognitively orientated and enjoy intellectual and creative activities. Their interests and education more easily translate into career and avocation possibilities consistent with physical dysfunction. Motorically orientated people value strength, stamina, motor expression, and functions based on expression of these skills. This may make transition to passive, functionally restrictive roles more difficult.[1] These are generalizations, and much depends on the patient's range of interests, skills, past experiences, intelligence, and adaptability.

Personality style is also influential. The perfectionist has internalized high standards for maintenance of self-esteem. The criteria by which he judges himself may be inflexible. Slow and less-than-perfect achievement and a reduction in the ability to maintain valued standards will be especially threatening. This includes the upkeep of a home or level of function vocationally.

The authoritative personality needs to be in control. They want things done a certain way and have rigid perceptions about rules, values, and the way people should live and behave. They tend to be judgmental, concerned with status, limited in the ability to develop insight or to empathize with others. Adaptation to disability requires compromise and acceptance, which is difficult for the authoritative personality.

The sociopathic and impulsive personality cannot tolerate the restrictions of hospitalization and the rules and procedures of medical treatment, such as casts, turning frames, or even splints. They fail to exercise good medical judgment and often exacerbate their dysfunctions by failure to comply with self-care procedures. Acting out behaviors are disruptive on the ward and in treatment.

The passive-aggressive personality is defensive and aggressive, expressing hostility passively through stubborness, procrastination, obstructiveness, and intended inefficiency. They work poorly with others and may have a demoralizing influence on the staff and in therapy groups.[7, 14-16]

The paranoid personality is hypersensitive, jealous, envious, and self-important. Such a patient is alert in collecting clues through staff behaviors or medical procedures which he interprets as a plan to harm him. Such a patient is unwarrantedly suspicious of the intentions of others.[16]

Stewart and Rossier[6] have cited the work of Kahana and Bibring on personality patterns requiring special attention after disability. Some patients have a deep fear of being abandoned and left helpless and thus require continual reassurances that the staff is concerned and their condition understood. Others rely heavily on information from the staff to decrease their anxiety and benefit from clear explanation of their conditions and treatment plans. Narcissistic patients feel superior and are threatened by a reduction of this image. They need to know that they are still acceptable. Some patients have a history of withdrawal and poor interpersonal skills and will find the closeness of the rehabilitation environment anxiety-provoking. They require special consideration and gradual inclusion into rehabilitation groups.[6]

Compulsive work achievement, over-independence, and high productivity are qualities valued in our society and are also compensatory ways of dealing with intrapersonal conflicts and low self-esteem. Diminished ability to use these techniques due to aging or disability may lead to feelings of worthlessness, helplessness, and terminate in intractable depression.[17] Some individuals may have always had unrealistically high goals for themselves. Their pace not only wards off depression but they derive satisfaction from being the strong person who gives to others. A reduction in their ability to fill caretaking roles or the need to accept help is intolerable. They may see everything as lost and continue to define their worth in terms of the original abilities.

Neurosis

For the patient, the primary purpose of neurotic illness is to reduce tension and conflict and to obtain secondary gains. Such gains may include attention, sympathy, care, and security. Disability exacerbates underlying pathology.[16] The following material demonstrates the relationship between physical and emotional pathology.

Olshansky mentions traumatic or compensation neurosis which develops after an accident and may present with signs of depression, irritability, hypochondria, acceptance of the role of invalid, or conversion hysteria. Patients are predisposed to these neurotic solutions by anxiety, fear about the future, castration fears, the wish to escape work roles and family responsibility, or the desire for compensation.[18]

Hodge,[19] in a discussion of developing psychological problems after a whiplash injury, states that patients have unconscious pathology and conflicts and develop individual and related patterns of handling stress. Such a patient finds in an injury a release for neurotic hostility and dependency needs. The symptoms of the injury become necessary to maintain the rewarding secondary gains. The symptom complex attracts attention and interest, allows dependency, and gains protection and support. The ego will struggle to maintain the rewarding symptoms.

Some patients present a pseudodisability and fail to demonstrate improvement even when function has returned. Such behavior may indicate latent dependency needs, avoidance of responsibility, or the expression of anger through retaliation. The patient may keep information concerning physical gains from the family, thus evading responsibilities and prolonging attention and service.

Hypochondriacal neurosis is demonstrated by preoccupation with health, heightened awareness of body sensations, the transformation of psychological anxiety into physical sensations, and the fear of disease in various organs. Common sites for this intense focus are the abdominal viscera, chest, head, and neck. The hypochondriacal patient is worried, anxious, and vigilant in locating physiological and physical symptoms which are then exaggerated. The patient focuses on these concerns to the exclusion of personal development in other areas. The hypochondriac's health concerns dominate his life and relationships with family and friends. In addition, the medical symptoms provide both primary and secondary gains. Such patients need supportive relationships but resist being deprived of their role of invalid and the physical rationale for the psychological discomfort.[14, 15]

Conversion hysteria is characterized by bodily symptoms that resemble those of physical disease (paralysis, blindness, deafness, anesthesia, and pain). Such physical symptoms allow the patient a defense against anxiety while maintaining self-respect and obtaining the secondary gains of illness. In conversion hysteria anxiety and conflicts are not consciously expressed but displaced or converted into functional symptoms in organs or body parts innervated by the sensorimotor systems. The location may be symbolic of the underlying conflicts.[14]

Freedman et al.[16] report a shift in the presentation of conversion hysteria symptoms, with less frequent presentations of paralysis, anesthesia, and convulsions and more clinical observation of pain and simulation of body disease.

It is difficult for hypochondriacal and conversion hysterical patients to relinquish symptoms and to deal or understand their unconscious anxiety, conflicts, and dependency needs. Such patients resist losing the role of invalid and the secondary gains it provides. Treatment requires a team approach, realistic treatment objectives, supportive therapy, and programming to assist the patient in meeting some of his unconscious needs. Assisting the patient to safely express and identify dependency needs and anger by utilizing activities and expressive media may provide an outlet and assist in some reduction of symptoms.

Patients with physical illness or disability may have a history of functional psychosis, psychosomatic illness, antisocial, impulsive, or inadequate personalities. Such premorbid states influence treatment objectives and discharge/community integration planning.

The more advanced a person's psychological and social development and integration of previous conflicts, the more capable he will be of coping with crisis in an adaptive way.[1] Therefore, a psychologically healthy patient with a severe physical disability may make a better adjustment and have a more independent life than a patient with a slight disability whose emotional pathology interferes with successful rehabilitation.[20]

Stages of Accommodation

Occupational therapists need to understand the dynamics behind the behavior of their patients during the initial stages of recovery and the accommodation process which follows the onset of physical disability and illness. All patients have emotional reactions to disability, and these reactions are expected and normal. Normal reactions include anxiety, denial, depression, grief, mourning, and regression. Despite commonalities, movement through the stages of accommodation also follow an individual schedule. The therapist's concern is that the patient will become fixed in this process and that defenses will become techniques of resistance rather than ways to survive and progress.

McDaniel cites Cohn's description of five stages in the adjustment process as shock, expectancy of recovery, mourning, defense, and final adjustment and Find's four stages as shock, defensive retreat, acknowledgement, and adaptation.[21]

An understanding of the normal adjustment process allows the therapist to be aware of the patient's psychological needs at each stage and to identify the point at which therapeutic intervention may be required. For example: (1) a patient's depression may be exacerbated by the isolation and restriction of being on a turning frame, inactivity, lack of social stimulation, disinterest of the family, or the inability to meet usual role responsibilities; (2) a patient may regress in treatment because he is concerned that continued success may mean discharge before he is emotionally ready to handle separation from the hospital.

An understanding of accommodation dynamics will enable the therapist to: (1) encourage and support the patient when accommodation proceeds normally; (2) understand that the patient has diminished cognitive skills during the initial stages; (3) identify the development of maladaptive coping mechanisms, such as overcompensation and projection; (4) determine when depression or denial are excessive in duration or intensity; (5) know not to take the patient's outbursts personally but to look for sources of anxiety and stress in the patient's perception of his medical condition, in the therapeutic relationship, in the family, on the ward, with staff, or in areas of role loss; (6) determine when the patient is overwhelmed by the demands of therapy and "needs to get a feeling of himself in the new terms at his own pace."[7]

Safilios-Rothschild[9] cites three modes of accommodation to physical disability including both adaptive and maladaptive responses. There are (1) those patients who never resolve the physical changes and the limitations imposed. Such patients desperately attempt to remain normal, pretend that they are, and act surprised and grieved when they cannot do everything the nondisabled does. They tend to refuse the company of other disabled people, preferring to develop a group of normal friends. This group of patients remains unaccepting, frustrated, and constantly setting up situations they cannot carry out. They are committed to preventing the breakdown of their denial. (2) There are patients who are able to accept the fact that they are still worthwhile and build a life on their unchanged assets, both physical and nonphysical. Such patients eventually accept the limitations of the disease and make the most of their lives. (3) There are patients who seem eager to accept the limitations, even those that could be overcome. The more opportunity the patient has to hide the disability and its limitation the more he may avoid integrating changes in self-concept and body image.[9]

The patient's feelings about his disability may be a very private matter and should be respected. Patients are entitled to their individual ways of managing the adjustment process. However, some rehabilitation systems and staff members also tend to deny the meaning of the disability to the patient, and the opportunity, time, and catalyst for dealing with feeling issues are not provided. The patient may enter the community with his loss, anguish, and anger unexpressed and unresolved. This may reduce his chances of maximizing assets and remaining independent in the community.

DEFENSES AND EMOTIONAL REACTIONS

Due to the significance of disability or illness we would expect to see clinically observable emotional or defensive reactions. Defense mechanisms can be useful in helping the patient through a difficult period after severe trauma. According to Siller,[7] in some cases the affects are displaced, delayed or disguised so that the superficial clinical picture suggests their absence while careful observation generally reveals their operation.

An effort should be made to understand the patient's perceptions of his medical situation since an entrenched defense commitment will impede aspects of rehabilitation. Therapists should be aware that behaviors indicative of severe neurosis or psychotic states, such as delusions or hallucinations, may be transitory stress reactions and situational in patients who have sound original coping skills.

Defenses and emotional reactions frequently seen in reaction to traumatic injury and chronic illness are depression, denial, regression, repression, compensation, overcompensation, projection, introjection, intellectualization, and reaction formation.

Moos and Tsu[22] refer to mental and behavioral coping skills as techniques used to deal with severe physical illness. They use the word "skill" to underline the positive aspects of these techniques stating that they are not inherently adaptive or maladaptive. Such coping skills may be positive in one situation and not in another.

Severe behavioral reactions may be very reversible with correct intervention, time, support, change in environment, family involvement, psychosocial treatment.

Treatment and intervention suggestions for emotional reactions to disability and illness are included in the treatment section at the end of the chapter.

Denial

Denial is an unconscious emergency defense useful as a transient form of adaptation to physical trauma. Denial eases the burden of reality, defends against the shock reaction to loss and the threat of dissolution of the ego by eruption of an overwhelmingly painful affect.[12]

For example, too sudden awareness of the extent of the loss could be so overwhelming as to terminate in psychosis or disintegration of the personality. Thus, denial directly after a traumatic injury allows the patient time to begin integration of the painful facts of loss and dysfunction at a pace he can accept. At times denial appears to be necessary as a safety valve; when the patient is stressed or becoming depressed he may again use denial as a protective device. Denial runs on a variable continuum. It is always present in cases of severe disability and varies in intensity and use by the patient. At one level denial can be adaptive in that it protects the patient from overwhelming depression caused by full recognition of the extent and permanence of the disability. The patient is motivated and directs energy to the development of compensatory skills within the limits set by the disability. Denial can also be excessive, resulting in refusal to recognize reality situations. This total incomprehension of the facts, the pathological denial of reality, involves severe distortions and a complete repression of memory concerning the accident. The patient not only lacks investment for rehabilitation but fails to be responsible for medical care or precautions.[13]

In extreme and pathological denial, the patient admits to past illnesses but denies the present medical situation, projects the ownership of the illness, minimizes the disability, and denies major incapacities, stressing less threatening aspects or inconveniences. The patient simply avoids painful and anxiety-producing reality by denying that it exists. Studies show that the patient who continually denies is somewhat compulsive and perfectionistic and regards illness as an imperfection or weakness. Patients may hold on to a hope that when they are home their condition will improve. Placed in the reality situation of the community they may begin gradually to give up denial and accept their physical dysfunction.

It should be noted that the patients who express a cheery, optimistic, instant acceptance of their dysfunction are suspect, and their psychological condition should be evaluated. Such a patient may require psychiatric treatment to help him express the sadness and meaning of his loss.

Another type of patient may appear well motivated in the initial stages of treatment until he reaches a plateau in functional progress. At this point he will find it difficult to accept the permanence of the disability, may become dependent or insist that a cure is possible. Prognosis is far better when the patient faces the reality of the situation, becomes depressed, and mourns for a period of time than in cases of extreme denial.[21] As patients begin to give up their denial they feel the awful facts and enter a phase of depression and mourning.[8]

Depression

Depression is an appropriate response to disability and is related to multiple and simultaneous losses.[2] It varies in intensity and duration with the meaning of the loss, premorbid personality, location and degree of disability or illness. Quigley[8] describes reactive depression as depression with a focus following a disabling loss. When the early defenses against the pain of acceptance are relinquished the impact of the loss is felt and confronted. Depression is also a response to the loss of self-esteem and perceived helplessness. Depression is normal at the beginning of the adjustment process and then periodically as the patient becomes discouraged, overwhelmed, is isolated, fails to progress in treatment, or remembers the losses in the form of an anniversary reaction.[1, 8]

Once the patient's concept of himself has changed permanently and he sees himself in a disabled, dependent, and helpless role, he may continue to function at a low level. The depressed patient has little energy or interest in treatment or the future, tires quickly, is unable to make the mental effort to plan ahead, is pessimistic about the future, dwells on somatic complaints, and ruminates about losses and the past.[21]

Somatic symptoms often represent masked depression and depression may be overt and spotted at a glance or it may be hidden, masked by the presence of somatic symptoms and even somatic disease.[23] Examples of somatic symptoms include inexplicable pain, weakness, or a dermatologic condition.

The therapist should understand the difference between reactive depression and neurotic or psychotic depression which would indicate premorbid personality problems, exacerbated by physical and personal issues. Normal depression and grieving would be primarily focused on the loss of function, an organ or limb, and the concomitant losses of life-style and personal roles.[3]

Grief and Mourning

Grief and mourning are considered necessary stages in the response to loss and prerequisite in the reconstruction of self-concept, a compromise body image and acquisition of new coping mechanisms.[21] The patient has lost the recognition of self and those skills and roles he has spent a lifetime developing. The whole personality tries to adjust to a radically altered course of life.[7] Simos[24] states that grieving can be an overwhelming and total experience and may require a moratorium from routine living. The clinician must understand the process rather than become impatient and misinterpret the patient's lack of progress as deliberate.

Tucker[2] sees mourning for lost physical capacity as an incomplete process since it needs to be reworked with each new experience which stimulates an awareness of the handicap and what the patient can no longer do or have.

Wright describes mourning as: (1) a sudden and massive constriction of the life space in which the unimpaired capacities are ignored; (2) preoccupation with the loss; (3) a mood of helplessness and worthlessness; (4) perceptions are dominated by premorbid comparisons; (5) personal values influence the severity of this stage of adjustment; (6) gradual abatement of mourning is followed by reconstruction of self-concept and body image.[21] Wright[12] also states, "There is good reason to believe that the period of mourning can be a healing period during which the wound is first anesthetized and then gradually closed, leaving the least scarring. Mourning clearly is not a stage through which one passes and then leaves behind. It is experienced intermittently after the deepest pangs are mitigated."

The duration of the depression-mourning period may be anywhere from 6 months to 1 year and may vary in its intensity during this time.[10] Provided the time span is reasonable, it should be allowed to run its course. Intervention can be made in both depression and mourning if in the judgment of the rehabilitation team their intensity or longevity is injurious to the patient.

Regression

Freedman et al.[16] state that regression is an emotional and physical retreat from adult standards of independence and self-determination to a more infantile level of weakness, passivity, and dependence on others. Hospitalization and medical treatment normally promote a degree of regression.

In a regressive state the patient returns to an earlier and less mature level of function and adaptation.[25] Injury, isolation, hospitalization, and other stressful situations can cause regressive behavior, such as acting out in a childish manner, persistently dependent behaviors, low motivation and passivity.

Strain[5] states that some patients are able to regress adaptively in the service of their recovery and accept nursing care, while others regress maladaptively by denying problems and acting in ways that will exacerbate their medical conditions.

Factors influencing regression may be incontinence, being ill, helpless and forced into a dependent role; pushing the patient too fast in treatment and missing the signs that he is becoming overwhelmed; the patient's anger about what has happened to his body and the control of the medical regime. During regression, the original battles in the developmental continuum may emerge and become again issues of conflict and crisis. The patient may again fear abandonment, destruction, and physical attack.[25]

Anxiety

Anxiety is a vague and unspecific apprehension which occurs as a response to threats to personal security, to biological integrity, or to self-esteem. Patients with a poor history of anxiety management will have problems in illness and disability where there are frequent encounters with stressful conditions. Anxiety results in somatic preoccupation, sensitivity to pain, and a decrease in response to treatment adaptation and learning.[21] Anxiety is a common problem relating to trauma, illness, and medical care. The patient may develop overwhelming anxiety as a response to what is perceived as catastrophic and be immobilized cognitively, emotionally, and physically. The resulting behavior is not always easy for the therapist to interpret. The patient may act in an unreliable, confusing manner and react to irrelevant cues; be unable to concentrate; be fearful, euphoric, or tense; misinterpret or develop false expectations concerning his dysfunction and treatment.[21] The staff may find that patients have completely missed the point in therapeutic discussions concerning their disability and treatment. (This may also be due to denial.) The patient is not deliberately trying to confuse or sabotage but is probably attempting to deal with considerable anxiety or fear. Certainly these are the possibilities the therapist should check before going on to look for other causes. The patient's interest and energy may be directed inward, and there may be little energy available for rehabilitation. A patient is reacting to an often unspecified danger and feels a vague, uneasy sense of dread, nervousness, and apprehension.[26] In a mild form, anxiety causes discomfort for the patient and in a more severe form, it interferes with rehabilitation. Once anxiety has been aroused it is slow to die down, and the effect spreads to all aspects of the patient's experience.[21]

McDaniel feels that the level of anxiety is significant in the rehabilitation process. Very high arousal levels of anxiety or very low or absent arousal levels suggest poor results in patient responses to treatment. A high arousal level of anxiety interferes with adaptation and learning, reduces motivation, and increases sensitivity to pain and somatic preoccupation. A very low or absent level of anxiety does not support motivation.[21]

Some patients respond to the anxiety connected to threats of disability by a flight into activity (overactivity) and try to achieve what is now impossible. In addition, patients and families may make radical changes in their life, i.e., selling their house, buying a boat, taking an expensive vacation. Such a flight supports denial and temporarily eases anxiety but at the same time absorbs the economic, emotional, and energy resources needed for the rehabilitation effort.[27]

A patient may be too anxious to understand what is causing the uncomfortable feelings; he may consider it weak to be afraid and since adults have been taught to conceal fears, the patient may have little experience in verbalizing feelings. Men often feel that the expression of feelings and concerns is not manly. The patient needs help in recognizing why he feels as he does, in formulating statements concerning the source of the anxiety, in verbalizing feelings, and in judging the realistic boundaries of his source of anxiety.

Anger

Another reaction to disability is anger, which may be described as hostility, hate, resentment, rage, or fury. Anger may be expressed in an outward manner or may be internalized and involve complex intellectual, emotional, and physical responses.

Anger is a response to feelings of helplessness, misperception, a fear of losing control, anxiety, and/or the threat of abandonment.

Anger may be described as follows: (1) outward anger is expressed through controlling maneuvers, attack, sarcasm, glaring, or physical hitting, (2) inward anger is expressed by somatizing, depression, or suicide and is used when the outward expression of anger is felt to be dangerous or inappropriate.[26] Patients do not always recognize or admit that they are angry, and unexpressed anger not only impedes treatment but may cause the development of physiological problems. Therapists may recognize anger in attempts to sabotage treatment, in withdrawal, depression, verbal attacks on staff, and acting out behavior.

The cause of the patient's behavior should be identified not only for the patient's welfare but because these behaviors cause the patient to be rejected by the staff and impede treatment.

Wallen, as cited by McDaniel, found that among orthopedically disabled adults who were considered rehabilitated, the mildly disabled directed guilt and hostility outward where it could be recognized and remedied, whereas the more severely disabled internalized these feelings.[21] Such internalized and repressed feelings result in maladaptive behaviors, such as passive-aggressive, manipulative, and sabotaging, and in clinically observable tension and anxiety. To maintain social contacts, the more severely disabled

will tend to internalize their hostile, negative, and angry feelings. Therapists should be conscious of this and encourage both verbal and nonverbal expressions of feelings, indicate that it is important to express such feelings, normal to have them under the circumstances, and teach productive expressions of affect. The reality is that severely injured patients may find this threatening and in order to verbalize strong feelings would need reliable, proven, and strong support systems and relationships.

Compensation

Wright[12] defines compensation as a way to make up for a shortcoming in order to redeem oneself. At times compensation may be used by the physically disabled to fill psychological needs and to provide self-satisfaction. However, a disabled person may be granted respect for his accomplishments by the nondisabled who may view these successful activities as compensation. Overlooked is the reality that these accomplishments may be due to special talents, aptitudes, or interests, or to a high level of maturity, creativity, or adaptive skill. The disability may influence the direction of the achievements by realistically ruling out areas of limitation; however, this does not make it compensatory, since all people make decisions guided by a consideration of their own reality.[12]

Repression

By using repression the ego keeps threatening impulses, feelings, fantasies, and memories from being conscious.[25] Patients attempt to deal with negative feelings concerning the accident, the nondisabled, the rehabilitation staff and/or their families by repressing the feelings rather than risking the loss of support and care that they need. Complete repression is not possible, and feelings surface to cause interpersonal problems and misunderstandings.

Daydreaming and Fantasy

Daydreaming and fantasy allow the patient to escape periodically from reality, to maintain ego integrity, to ward off severe depression, and to tolerate the medical situation. Most people escape into daydreams. However, fantasy becomes maladaptive when it is used by the patient as a method of problem solving.

Overcompensation

Overcompensation in one area can lead to higher constructive achievement or may be an expression of neurotic drives. The danger for rehabilitation is that the patient's personal growth and development of a breadth of skills may be sacrificed for compulsive development in just one skill area.[12] As therapists we should attempt to guide the patient so that an unreasonable amount of time and energy will not be devoted to being successful in just one area due to feelings of inadequacy. Therapists need to help patients find other ways to get attention for achievement and to feel acceptable.

Dependency

Dependency is a major problem for rehabilitation staff. The acutely ill patient is placed in a position where he is cared for and where decisions are made for him. Such a situation feeds into a patient's sense of helplessness, reinforces latent dependency needs and the underlying desire to be cared for by a strong parent figure. Regressive behaviors may lead to permanent dependent and patient roles.

The patient with psychological problems may use his new patient status as a legitimate means of extracting the last ounce of attention and energy from his caretakers, as a means of avoiding personal responsibility, and as a weapon to demand love.[28]

In severe disability certain components of the dependent role are legitimate and necessary. Kutner[28] discusses the need for the traumatically disabled patient to accept some aspect of a dependent role if he is to be successfully rehabilitated.

Feldman[1] describes positive and negative dependency. Depending on the degree of disability a patient needs to be pragmatic and accept care. Patients need to be encouraged in acceptance of positive dependency and permitted to practice those skills and attitudes which will allow receiving help to achieve maximal independence. Feldman states that the patient must learn to ask for help and not feel helpless or inadequate because of his need.

Unfortunately independent behavior and determination to influence decisions on medical care are seen by staff as interfering, difficult behavior. Such behavior may in the beginning be accentuated by an overlay of defenses and emotional responses to disability and illness. The patient may be labeled a troublemaker and discouraged in his attempt to retain control over his situation.[3]

INFLUENCING FACTORS IN REHABILITATION

Crisis Periods in Hospitalization

Therapists should be aware of crisis and stress points in rehabilitation, such as admission, the initial stages of accommodation, the breakdown of denial when the patient becomes aware of the permanence of the disability or illness, when questions concerning ambulation arise, when the time comes to order adaptive equipment, and when the patient plateaus and is put on a maintenance schedule in physical or occupational therapy. Other stressful situations develop due to family disputes, staff tension, or a death on the ward. The therapist should plan treatment and supportive intervention to meet the patient's special needs during crisis periods.

Discharge

The time of discharge may be very threatening to the patient who may feel he does not have the capacity to deal with the move to the community. Kutner[3] says,

"One of the most deceptive aspects of rehabilitation is the condition of the patient at the time of discharge." Patients come to depend on the security of the hospital environment and support of the staff. They fear the loss of protection and reliable care. It is also easier to deny the severity of the handicapping condition in the hospital where mobility is easier and sophisticated equipment, such as electric wheelchairs, mask the patient's real level of function. In addition, personal needs, such as bathing and feeding, are provided for. In social situations the patient is not "unlike" the others.

Patients not emotionally prepared to deal with separation from the hospital may put obstacles in the way of discharge, such as accidental injuries and relapses which require continued hospitalization. They may fall and break a limb, spike a high and unexplained fever, may regress in functional gains, complain of somatic pain, and thus sabotage treatment toward the day of discharge.

Culture

Cultural attitudes and values acquired from childhood are influencing factors in the process and outcome of rehabilitation. Cultural education within the family affects such matters as how pain is perceived and expressed, what is considered physically attractive, what aspects of the body are most prized and thus will represent the greatest loss, what physical and mental disabilities are the most acceptable, and what degree of deviation from the norm will be allowed without social rejection. Within each culture there may be considerable variation in the intensity of feelings toward specific handicaps.[9] Cultural education may not prepare its members to be flexible in the consideration of a new life of leisure time. Cultural role expectations for work, family, and sexual roles may be narrowly defined. Thus options for compensatory role change or treatment for role disorders may be culturally limited. For example, patients and their families may assume that there is only one way to fill family membership roles.[29]

Culture influences the way in which patients view their health, their acceptance of medical care, their respect and trust of the staff. Szapocznik et al.[30] describe American rehabilitation philosophies as stressing humanism, the importance of the individual, being independent, having plans and working toward them, being clean and on time. Cross-culturally these may not be valued goals. Sanchez[31] states that cultural background influences patient's attitudes toward types of therapy, use of modalities, treatment activities, work, and education.

Some cultural values encourage the patient to feel that they are being punished for something sinful and that to feel good is wrong. Because group activities are often enjoyable the patient may feel guilty and withdraw. Therapist awareness of certain cultural attitudes and values will prevent labeling certain patient behaviors as neurotic or nonmotivated.

The therapist concerned with rehabilitation may find a distrust toward staff and hesitance in following medical recommendations. The opinions of friends and family may carry more weight than that of the physician, and their advice may influence important health decision.[9]

In social and cultural backgrounds where illness is a sanctioned role patients may use delayed recovery as a defense mechanism and there will be a high degree of psychosomatic illness. Some cultural values do not allow for the expression of strong feelings, such as anger or aggression, which may exacerbate the psychosomatic process.[11]

Culture also influences a patient's understanding of his personal worth, what he is entitled to, his privileges as a human being and as a disabled person. Illness and disability may be seen as providing sanction to stop working and to be cared for by the family. Some patients consider this the right they have earned, even though the degree of disability still allows employment. Other patients, especially in their middle years, may see the disability as a threat to their status both professionally and economically and are anxious to retain aspects of valued vocational roles and to return to work quickly. In American society, people often exclusively define themselves by their work roles.[9]

Our culture places a strong emphasis on production, personal success, and being physically or personally attractive. These goals are so emphasized that not moving toward achieving them causes depression, self-blame, self-hatred, and blocked motivation. The problem is one of self-definition, and if personal worth is defined in terms of lost self-image after disability and no compromise change takes place, the patient will never feel worthwhile.[32]

The reality is that all patients will not attain the rehabilitation goals we set nor can all patients economically maintain themselves in the community. If the focus is on making the disabled employable we may do so at the risk of underdeveloping other equally important social, problem-solving, and personal skills. This is something that therapists must learn to live with and society must examine its value structure in regard to the work ethic for all.

Sanchez[31] suggests that the therapist be sensitive to cultural differences and attempt to understand the basic values and assumptions of the patient's culture, both on a conscious and unconscious level. He suggests that occupational therapy treatment principles be adjusted to consider the cultural orientation of the ethnic population.

Religion

Religious beliefs, taboos, and traditions contribute to a patient's feelings about his role in the injury or illness, his own worth, and his interest in rehabilitation. For example, the disability may be seen as punishment for a known sin or as evidence that a sin was committed. The family may reinforce this perception and the patient may decide to accept the punishment and is not motivated in rehabilitation. Religious attitudes concerning the human body, illness, disability,

sin and the soul come down through antiquity and are deeply ingrained, often operating on an unconscious level.[12] Such statements as, "God will punish you if you're bad," "God asks us to bear our suffering," or "The sins of the father shall be visited upon the sons until the 10th generation," are influential. Diamond[33] states that attitudes held by ancient people are reproduced today in modern man without much change. The Hebrews felt that illness marked a person as a sinner who was being punished. The ancient Greeks looked on illness not as a sign of sin but of inferiority, and the early Christians saw sickness and pain as a way to grace or salvation through suffering.

Wright[12] finds that physical disability may be worn with pride, and the patient may feel especially selected by God for trial by physical suffering. The disability may give a purpose to life. Such patients appear peaceful, uplifted and almost superior. They often dedicate their lives to help others.[12]

Patients may believe in spiritualism, medicine men, folk healers, prayer ceremonies, laying on of hands, signs, and the power of symbolic artifacts. Staff and institutions need to be sensitive to the meaning of the patient's religious beliefs and to incorporate those beliefs and ceremonies into treatment programming whenever possible.

The Disadvantaged Patient

Attention should be focused on the special problems of the socially disadvantaged patient whose handicap is compounded by developmental disability and lack of those social and interpersonal skills required for survival in the community. If patients are to be self-confident, independent members of society they need to learn all possible age-appropriate tasks, for example, how to handle impulses and drives, to fill needs appropriately, to focus aggressive energy, to problem solve, to plan and work toward goals.[35]

Treating a developmentally disabled population requires reasonable goals based on possible and practical skill acquisition and the actual postdischarge needs of patients.[35] Value judgments about social and cultural attitudes inherent in the patient's expected environment can cause the therapist frustration and the patient pain and confusion. Staff goals may be irrelevant in terms of the rehabilitant's particular values, needs, family, social life, vocational prospects, and personality structure.[9]

The disadvantaged patient may function very well in the hospital environment demonstrating unexpected talents and skills which may fail to carry over into the community. This higher level of function is facilitated by the climate of the hospital, positive therapist and peer relationships, and enabling group experiences, all of which meet basic needs for security, belonging, etc. Failure to transfer these skills into the community may be due, in part, to inadequate bridging of skill training, social isolation, poor self-image, lack of family support, lack of know-how in locating and attracting helping agencies, unawareness of resources available, poor communication skills, and inability to structure the use of time. Follow-up programming and the coordination of hospital and community services are imperative.

After discharge such patients tend to become depressed, apathetic, cannot exercise control over their environment, neglect self-care, become ill, and are continuously readmitted. Occupational therapists should be flexible and creative in sequencing the priorities of treatment for their patients and in choosing, adapting, and experimenting with treatment methods, techniques, and modalities to meet different learning styles and individual patient needs. Concern with follow-up community programming is essential for skill maintenance.

Body Image

Simon states that "Neurologically speaking, the body image consists of past experiences of the body and current sensation as organized in neuronal and biochemical structures of the brain, mainly integrated in the parietotemporal areas of the cerebral cortex."[10] The lost part of function is thus represented by hundreds of separate memories which the patient has to gradually relinquish.

The body image is also a product of relevant early experiences and has its primary source in the relationships and attitudes of significant people in the patient's early life. We can gain an understanding of the unconscious and conscious issues of body image for the patient by tracing personal values and self-concept back to their primary source in the cultural education and attitudes of the family.[10] Development of a positive and realistic body image is important in the development of a healthy ego and sense of self-worth. It includes the patient's personal investment in aspects of his body, his values and fantasies and those of other significant people in his life.[10] Body image is part of the self-concept of a patient and does not easily yield to changes of time or incident. The acknowledgement of a flawed body image and reaction to the loss of function or organ loss through surgery causes emotional reactions and the readjustment can take as long as 2 years.[36] In addition, patients need to integrate orthotic devices into the self-image, a difficult task which may result in rejection of the equipment.[6]

Individual reactions to disability and possible successes of integration of a compromise body image depend, in part, on the type, nature, location of the injury, premorbid concept of the body, and psychological defenses chosen to maintain self-esteem. Ideally, after the sadness, depression, and a period of mourning has past, the lost image is given up intrapsychically and a compromise image is formed. At this point energy is released and becomes available for the development in other areas.[10]

Recreational and sport activities may be helpful in the reorganization of body image.

The Hospital Environment

The hospital environment has great impact upon the admitted patient. It is alien, impersonal, monotonous, and confining with unfamiliar rules and norms of behavior with which the patient is expected to comply. The patient is expected to yield gracefully all ordinary personal roles, activities, and usual control over his actions to those in authority who do not know his skills, needs, or see him as an individual. Relationships with the staff may not be experienced at an adult level and are often authoritative and parental, encouraging regression and dependency behavior, which is opposite to the goals of treatment.[4]

The environmental influence within the institution becomes critical as the acute stage of the illness subsides. The patient cannot influence his environment; there is little opportunity for decision making, exercise of initiative, or continuing a role of responsibility for oneself.

The description of therapeutic models to reduce the negative impact of hospitalization and prepare the patient for successful discharge are included in the treatment section at the end of the chapter.

Community Attitudes

The patient who progresses favorably in the psychological accommodation to disability and restoration of physical function still faces a formidable hurdle. He must experience, understand, and overcome the response of his society to its handicapped members. Patients may experience staring, rejections, intimate personal questions concerning the disability and degree of dysfunction, or intrusive assistance which they do not require.

There is a tendency for both society and professionals to consider patients incapable of decision making, thinking or planning independently, and of understanding communications. Wright uses the term "spread" to show how deficiencies in one area are thought to affect other abilities such as mental and social skills. Also attributed to the handicapped are personal maladjustment and incompetence, although there may be no evidence of these qualities.[28] Unfortunately, the patient exposed consistently to some of those feelings will internalize the message and experience the same spread phenomenon, believing that all abilities have been swept away by a localized disability.

Origins of prejudicial and fearful attitudes toward the disabled may stem from a variety of sources and are complex, largely unconscious, and firmly entrenched. The reaction of the able-bodied to those with disability may be related to the visibility of the disability, the type and location of the injury, and the personal meaning of the injury to the able-bodied. Past and early experiences, cultural conditioning, and personality style are found to influence attitudes toward the disabled and the degree of uneasiness, rejection, and aversion felt by the nondisabled. Other explanations of prejudicial attitudes are found in "the dislike of the unlike" and authoritarian hostile attitudes toward minorities and those markedly different from self.[28]

Healthy acceptance of the disabled is related to qualities in the nondisabled, such as positive self-image, sound, stable interpersonal relationships, personal confidence, and security in their own concepts of body image and self-worth.[21]

There is a tendency to deny the extent of the injury and its functional loss by the nondisabled viewer. This denial is a self-protective technique employed to avoid feelings of sadness, horror, and fear of threat to self. Thus, prejudice is found to be modified by cosmetic appearances, the severity and visability of the disability, and the degree of competence and social ability shown by the disabled.[21] Modern adaptive devices such as electric wheelchairs somewhat mask the extent of helplessness of the disabled, allowing the viewer to feel more comfortable and enter into a relationship of social interaction. The less confident and inexperienced patient will find it a devastating experience to face the community and to handle those constant vibrations of rejection. The successfully rehabilitated and more experienced patient may shrink from the experience but has developed the social skills and the confidence to handle the community, to maintain his sense of worth, and to manipulate social situations.

Staff Attitudes

An examination of staff attitudes and behaviors reveals concern and loyalty to the patient and concept of good rehabilitation. The demanding nature of the treatment of the physically disabled and ill patient requires a long-term commitment, dedication to service, and a high tolerance for stress and frustration. What is less obvious are some of the unconscious needs and attitudes of staff which may impede the very process to which the team is committed. Such things as excessive need to nurture and have others be dependent, paternalistic attitudes, strong need for lines of social division between patients and staff, the need to control people and information, and strong value judgments concerning goals for patients are problem areas.[37]

Staff are asked to assume responsibility for patients and at the same time deal with conflicts concerning their own unresolved dependency needs and longing for care and affection. Transference and countertransference heighten staff anxiety. Emotionally stressed patients often display anger, anxiety, complain, demand attention, and project feelings in ways that alienate staff.

Stewart states that constant exposure to physical disability can be emotionally overwhelming and threatening to the therapist's own sense of intactness. Staff may go through identical stages of adaptation, may deny the extent of the dysfunction and become depressed and mourn.[6]

Staff working with the severely physically disabled may have unconscious fears of becoming disabled, of being helpless, or of regressing to an infantile state and being overwhelmed.[10] Staff may feel guilty over personal health and thus self-protective in denying the extent of the patient's disability and his feeling concerning his losses. They may, without conscious intent, encourage unrealistic rehabilitation goals based on the need to feel successful professionally and to be liked by patients and their families. Lamb[38] states that when patients do not improve, therapists may feel failure, guilt, and inadequacy and then reject the patient.

Leviton[37] states that medical professionals are often taught to value emotional neutrality and that the behavior important for this value is maintaining a distance from the patient. The fear is that too much closeness will develop, that patient and professionals will not keep a balance in their relationship, and that tight emotional control is part of the role of the professional.[37] Involvement with patients in distress who are depressed and anxious can be exhausting. Thus, emotional neutrality becomes a psychological protection for staff. The concern for and use of the therapeutic relationship stressed in the mental health setting is apt to be of low priority in rehabilitation centers.

Stereotyping of the physically disabled was found also to be prevalent among the professional staff at rehabilitation agencies. It was noted that an attitudinal sample of physicians showed considerable degree of pessimism about success in rehabilitation.[28] If professionals even unconsciously tend toward stereotyping and labeling patients as impossible to rehabilitate they may fail to evaluate the total person and underview long-term rehabilitation potential.

The patient needs to be treated by a professional who demonstrates respect, empathy, and a humanistic philosophy. Siller[7] sees the therapist as an assist to the patient so that the principal investment is from the patient.

In addition, the staff therapeutic role differs during each phase of rehabilitation. At one point the patient requires support and to be appropriately dependent and needs to have his regression understood and supported. Later the therapist-patient relationship should encourage autonomy and personal decision making.

Environmental Deprivation

The restricted environment and treatment procedures of the physically disabled may cause social and sensory deprivation. The immobilization of the patient through, for example, traction, turning frames, or body casts in combination with the decrease in stimulation of other senses can produce disorientation and even psychotic behavior. Such observable behaviors include depression, panic, irritability, regression and even psychotic behaviors, such as hallucinations or delusions.[21] Patients who have severe personality problems, i.e., impulsive or immature will have difficulty tolerating the restrictions of immobility and hospitalization and may present a management problem for the staff.

Parent[39] states that "The nature of the illness or the treatment of some medical and surgical conditions may result in a drastic reduction of the amount of everyday stimulation such as that found in work and social activities." Examples of causative diagnosis and treatment procedures include the following: (1) a cerebral vascular accident (CVA) may reduce the ability to perceive tactile, auditory, or visual stimulation; (2) burn patients who remain in sterile isolation to prevent infection, renal patient on dialysis, cancer patients receiving chemotherapy, spinal cord-injured (SCI) patients on turning frames, and orthopedic patients in traction experience the isolation of their particular form of treatment; (3) treatment procedures that prevent vision or hearing (sensory loss), such as bandaging, intensive care, sterile rooms; and (4) a foreign language.

Restriction of Energy

The therapist may find the patient is unable to concentrate on decisions and planning concerning treatment and the future. The theory of Shontz et al.[40] on restriction of energy due to intensive threat (traumatic injury or illness) explains that the patient is blocked by the disability from engaging in the behaviors which exchange and release energy. At this stage personal values change and body functions become more important to the patient. The effort to overcome the threat sacrifices high level activities, such as psychosocial functioning, abstract thinking, reality testing, problem solving, and planning until a level of adjustment occurs and energy is again available.[40]

This theory is important to the occupational therapist because it explains why the patient is not as realistic as the therapist would like him to be and is less concerned with gaining hand function or planning a future education and more concerned with the priorities of bowel training and the ability to walk.

Motivation

Rabinowitz[41] states that a set of crucial psychological unknowns surround the patient's ability to make constructive use of the rehabilitation services. Enabling are: (1) therapist-patient development of acceptable, graduated, practical recovery goals; (2) democratic therapeutic relationships; (3) an opportunity for the patient to visibly observe his progress; (4) adequate frustration tolerance.[41]

McDaniel[21] describes the patient's subjective estimates concerning the possibility of rehabilitation success. A patient's motivation to work toward a treatment objective depends on the value he places on the attainment of the goals and then his assessment of personal costs, such as pain, effort, money, time, and his estimation of chances of success. McDaniel[21] states that past, present, or continuous failure in training will have a damaging effect on the patient's future motivation. Patients who see reasonable improvement due to intense effort will be more motivated.

Other factors influencing the patient's motivation are family attitudes toward the disability, family maintenance of the patient's role, the patient's understanding of his disability, and meaningful future goals.

Patients may rebel against the hospital setting which provides little opportunity for autonomy and self-directed behaviors. Some patients work hard to beat the system and use their energy and creativeness in a way destructive to their own future. Such a patient's energy is not channeled to meet rehabilitation objectives. For example, a patient who feels he can find an efficient way to put on his socks that will bear the stamp of his own planning will be neutralized by a therapist who feels there is only one proper way to put on socks. A patient who refused activity of daily living (ADL) treatment but wants to work in an occupational therapy, task-orientated group planning social events for the hospital will rebel if the staff insists on the priority of ADL treatment. This patient will quickly learn how to get dressed when he finds it is important in his social tasks.

The value and meaning to the patient of specific rehabilitation goals influence his motivation to work and achieve these goals. We should not underestimate the patient's resources of intelligence and strength. If given a chance he may be able to formulate a sounder plan for himself than might occur to us as professionals.

Planned group and individual experiences where the patient can explore, learn to alter his environment, have fun, socialize, begin to feel good about himself, and be more in control of his own affairs will generate motivation. White considered these experiences, the drive for learning and the feelings of competency achieved through these explorations, the prelude to motivation.[32, 33]

Age Tasks

Age tasks complicate rehabilitation and compound the adjustment process. The patient who has just had a stroke (CVA) or spinal cord injury (SCI) may also be dealing with the stresses of adolescence or the middle years. During the adolescent period there are enough personal adjustments, turmoil, identity crises, and final issues concerning leaving the dependency of childhood without the double blow of injury and disability.[6] At middle age patients are concerned about the aging process, recognition of physical decline, trauma of personal reappraisal, vocational dissatisfaction, the development and education of their children, care of aging parents, and awareness of death.[43] These stresses are increased by the presence of physical and sensory losses. Occupational therapists should understand the adjustment and tasks of each stage of human development for consideration in evaluation and treatment planning.

The Family

The family's ability to cope with the crisis of having an injured member and their willingness to retain their family membership roles is crucial in the success of rehabilitation. The enabling family provides support useful to the patient and meets crises through interfamily problem solving. Such families maintain the patient's valued role, involve the patient in family discussions and decision making, and assist in compliance to medical procedures.[44, 45]

One type of solution to a family crisis resulting from physical disability is alienation.[28] Families may also prevent maximal rehabilitation by overprotection, neglect, avoidance of discharge planning, and punitive action toward the patient. Such families may precipitate more problems than they solve. They have difficulty making a steady commitment, avoid future planning, fill the patient's roles on a permanent basis, and are noncompliant medically. In addition, long-standing resentments, interfamily control issues, dependent, neurotic, or psychotic family constellations may absorb staff time and endanger the patient's emotional equilibrium. Families that project their problems onto the staff and patient may become ill themselves, demanding attention.[4, 27, 44, 46]

Versluys[44] states that the patient can be placed in the position of dealing with his own personal adjustment and also supporting the family in their denial and anxiety. Litman, as cited by Safilios-Rothschild, found that the existence of close family ties and the willingness of others to take care of the disabled often discouraged possible independence.[9] For example, the mother whose family is reared may be tempted to encourage dependence in a handicapped adolescent.

The way in which the family views the assets and strengths of the disabled is very important. When others make all the decisions, do the planning for the patient, feel that the disabled patient's life is over or irrevocably damaged, or are very threatened by the handicapping condition, the disabled will rapidly lose self-esteem and confidence required for independence.

Safilios-Rothschild[9] states that the single disabled tends to be more independent in daily living functions than the married disabled due to the necessity of developing all skills and problem-solving abilities to find ways of maximal independence. Another investigation shows that married women with children, even if seriously disabled, are usually taken back by the family unit and can maintain a part of their usual role functions. Even in cases of severe disability, the role of the homemaker in planning and organizing can be utilized by the family, with active tasks carried out by others. The frequency of wives deserting husbands who are severely disabled is greater, especially when there is inability to perform a sexual and economic role.[9, 44]

Other family reactions include anxiety in dealing with patient's behaviors, i.e. depression, hostility, or delirium, and powerlessness about their ability to influence the patient's recovery; distress at having to trust strangers to care for the patient; and disappointment at results the medical staff considers very good.[44, 47] During the plateau stage patient and family both face realities and stresses. Christopherson[48] states ". . . all hope for a complete recovery is gone, economic and emotional resources have worn thin and future decisions must be made concerning placement."

The prospect of caring for the disabled causes fears and anxieties in the family and can lead to instinctive withdrawal. It is particularly difficult when wives must seek employment; the economic conditions of the family deteriorate; the spouse needs to assume greater responsibility for home management; children take over household duties; plans for the children's education are affected; and living accommodations must be changed.[9]

It is unrealistic to expect families to deal with these problems unaided. The family is also traumatized and needs information, attention, and support. Families vary in their ability to assess the patient's situation, to accept responsibility, and to make compromises in their plans. Not all families have the resources, maturity, or stability to care daily for the severely disabled. Families who are made to feel guilty about their perceived inadequacies may be driven away from any involvement with the patient.[44]

Families may find that they are in the way on the wards or in the treatment areas. Busy therapists may have little time or patience with questions, anxieties, and fears. They may find the family intrusive and express rejection. Staff can be very critical of the disabled patient's family, finding some families not interested enough or other families showing the patient too much attention. They note neurotic tendencies and call attention to refusal to make necessary home adjustment and to order equipment on time. In other words, the staff, while caring for the patient and understanding this process of accommodation, has a tendency to expect the family to show instant ability to cope with the problems and adjustments of having a disabled family member.[44]

Professionals can help by identifying family stress and planning interventions, such as informal problem solving, providing medical information and progress reports, encouraging expression of feelings, creating opportunities to ask questions, and assisting the family in keeping a focus on the real boundaries of the crisis, thus preventing the spread of anxiety.

DISEASE- AND ILLNESS-SPECIFIC REACTIONS

It has been suggested that certain types of premorbid personality are associated with specific physical and neurological illnesses. For example, the commonalities of emotional reactions and behaviors seen in multiple sclerosis (MS) or rheumatoid arthritis (RA) suggest this. Strain[5] cautions against the assumption that a particular neurotic conflict influences a disease course. It can be shown that certain personality constellations are more prone to certain illnesses and there is some evidence that life stresses increase the probability of falling ill with a number of diseases.

Two groups of researchers feel that personality characteristics described as "rheumatoid arthritis personality" are secondary responses to the disease course of remissions and exacerbations and the pain and crippling of an anxiety-producing disease process.[49, 50]

Siller,[7] in reference to spinal cord patients states that ". . . there is no direct relationship between types of physical condition and personality structure. The physical injury represents another stress situation to which the patient brings a repertoire of response patterns characteristic of him.[7]

Shontz[51] feels that no one can understand the meaning of an illness to a patient unless he understands all aspects of the patient's life that are affected by it.

Thus, the patient, in addition to individual emotional reactions to disability/illness, hospitalization, and treatment, copes with disease-specific stresses related to his illness, for example, the breathing and choking of chronic obstructive pulmonary disease, technical failure for renal dialysis patients, fear of amputations in diabetic patients, the mobility problems of physically disabled patients, and the pain and physical appearance of burn patients.

The following is a consideration of disease-specific stressors, adjustment problems, and treatment issues.

Rheumatoid Arthritis (RA)

The disabling and painful symptoms of RA plus the decrease in functional ability and the resulting deformed physical appearance cause patients to be very anxious, fearful, depressed, and ashamed.

Zeitlin[50] states that "The weight of research suggests a multicausal hypothesis in which genetic, autoimmune, infectious, and psychological factors interact to varying degrees to create a, "pre-disposition matrix."

Spergel et al.[49] state that RA patients are not homeogeneous in terms of personality and that it is dangerous to consider all patients with RA as psychologically similar. Evidence begins to point to a chronic disease personality.[49] It is possible that psychological factors play a precipitating role for some but not all patients who have RA. Secondary responses to the course of the disease are overreaction to illness, masochism, rigidity, conformity, perfectionism, and difficulty dealing with hostility and aggression. In addition, RA patients are seen to be very sensitive, vulnerable to stress, have diminished body image related to crippling deformity, difficulty in flexible management of their lives and in seeing alternative ways of problem solving.[50]

The patient behaviors mentioned above plus a tendency to be demanding, negative, regressive, and anxious make the development of a therapeutic relationship sometimes difficult. However, the patient needs support, and a relationship should be developed that is trusting, warm, and patient. It is assistive if the therapists indicate that they understand the pain and frustration of having arthritis and at the same time remind the patient of what he can do. The RA patient needs structure for management of the disease, help in accepting chronicity, identification and reduction of stress areas, improved communication, and encouragement of expression of feelings, in addition to occupational therapy treatment for physical dysfunction.

Multiple Sclerosis (MS)

Multiple sclerosis is characterized by a progressive course of uncertain remissions and exacerbations. The patient progressively experiences gait and locomotor problems, spasticity, impaired sensation, incontinence, blurred or double vision, and difficulty in communication, i.e., halting or slurred speech.[52, 53]

MS requires a rearrangement of life priorities and most adult roles. The uncertain clinical picture, i.e., waiting for the next exacerbation of the disease with the probability of increased disability causes great anxiety. The patient may be hostile, irritable, resentful, and demanding of those around him.[52, 54]

MS patients fear total dependency, loss of intellect, and of family and vocational roles. Baretz and Stephenson[52] state that unrealistic optimism or euphoria may be masked depression, while the inappropriate emotional reactions, instability and impaired judgment, are due to organic changes in the brain. Schneitzer[54] states that emotional reactions to disability in MS usually take one of two forms: the denial of illness with euphoria or reactive depression with anxiety states and other psychoneuroses.

Schneitzer describes the need to minimize the effects of the disease through a total rehabilitation program, for example, to maintain function and independence, enable control over significant life issues for as long as possible, provide attention to psychological needs. The MS patient needs support in acceptance of the disability and in negotiating varying levels of function while dealing with long-term progressive disease. Treatment suggestions include: (1) group therapy in hospital or community to provide peer support, to problem solve, to encourage social involvement, and to assist the patient and family in dealing with the uncertain progressive disease; (2) architectural and home design with an eye to the patient's present and future needs; (3) assisting the patient in reassessing life priorities and role changes[52]; (4) support during exacerbations, depression, and mourning; (5) innovative ideas for job maintenance or volunteer opportunities; (6) adaptation of recreational and other equipment for special interests and; (7) clothing design. The above suggestions for rehabilitation are applicable to other physical disabilities/illnesses.

Pulton[53] states that although the relationship between MS and stress is unclear it does influence temporary exacerbations. The occupational therapist can help the patient identify and problem solve to reduce areas of stress.

Burns

Brodland and Andreasen[47] state that "Patients who have been severely burned experience intense and varied trauma involving catastrophic injury, severe pain, possible cosmetic or functional deformities and a threat to their sense of identity and worth." Treatment is long, often in isolation, and includes immobilization and painful surgical procedures. This creates great anxiety, depression, fear, and regression. The patient may feel abandoned while waiting for skin grafts and restricted and isolated during autografts.[47] There are continued emotional reactions after trauma, such as nightmares, crying spells, emotional lability, and phobias related to fire.

Patients must incorporate a distorted appearance such as scarring and deformity into their body image. Malick[55] states that fear of mutilation and disfigurement is a major concern and increases as a patient faces discharge. Andreasen and Norris[56] state that children may not recognize their parents, creating interfamily crisis. Molinaro[57] speaks of the social problems encountered by burn children after their reentry into the community. Interpersonal relationships are influenced by extreme sensitivity and fear of rejection, which may limit social contacts and cause revision in vocational and educational planning, with withdrawal and entrenched regressions. People with facial scarring and deformities may seek or receive jobs where they are not visible to others, limiting the use of their abilities and vocational potential. The patient, both during treatment and transition into the community, needs supportive staff relationships, interpretation of treatment procedures, opportunities to express feelings related to the accident and the future, realistic helpful appraisal of problems, assistance with on-going normal activities and social and transitional problems.[55]

Myocardial Infarction (MI)

Residual results of MI may be more emotional than physical. Contributing to this are misconceptions about heart attacks, the catastrophic results it signals to the patient, *i.e.*, death, loss of sexual potency, and invalidism.[58]

Cassem and Hackett[59] state that inactivity and bed rest are a disease in itself. In addition to deep vein thrombosis, postural hypotension, muscle atrophy, the extended inactivity contributes to entrenched emotional reactions and cardiac neurosis. They feel that combating these problems requires early remedial activity programming, early ambulation and discharge, and assertive community-focused follow-up.[59]

During the initial part of recovery in the CCU the patient may use denial as a defense and in the beginning, as long as the patient follows medical directions, denial is useful in reduction of anxiety and in keeping the patient calm. Denial is maladaptive when the patient denies the cardiac symptoms or projects the pain, claiming indigestion, muscle strain, or nerves. In addition, the patient may insist on leaving the hospital or overcompensate through intense physical activity. Bed rest and inactivity, myths and misconceptions about heart disease, fear of helplessness, and restriction in pleasurable habits and life-style contribute to anxiety, depression, and a feeling of "being all washed up" and "falling apart."[59, 61]

Cassem and Hackett consider depression a serious complication of MI both in the hospital and upon discharge. They state that depression may be missed in the early stage, and the patient may appear quiet and withdrawn or the depression may present somatically. In addition, the patient is not prepared for the extreme weakness felt on leaving the hospital. Predischarge, the physician may discuss the cardiac condition and medications but neglect clear guidelines for activity, rest, life-style, sexual information, and handling of stress. The resulting confusion may lead to misperceptions at home of somatic signs, anxiety about the condition, and delayed convalescence, plus the possibility of becoming a cardiac cripple.[59, 64] Strain[5] states that there is a fear of casual relationships between activity, death, and heart attacks. Thus 20% of patients who could return to work do not despite the medical ability to do so. Bilodeau and Hackett[62] state that to counteract the restrictions upon discharge, the patient needs someone who can provide clear guidance and follow the patient in the community through a telephone follow-up program.

Emotional rehabilitation can include: (1) taking a detailed activity history, close to admission, which also provides information on the patient's habits and life-style; (2) activity programming that starts the 3rd day of hospitalization on the CCU and demonstrates that the patient is not considered to be a hopeless invalid; (3) a sequenced activity plan for discharge including clear guidelines for all activities including rest, sexual activity, and handling of stress.[62, 63]

It is important to talk with the family and patient together. This reduces the chance that the family will overprotect the patient or that the patient can manipulate for secondary gains.

There are a number of interesting articles on rehabilitation programming for post-MI patients. Zohman, as cited by Strain, describes vocational rehabilitation programming involving social and recreational activities, psychological group counseling, exercise programming, and on-the-job training.[5] Baile and Engel[64] describe a treatment strategy for noncompliant patients tailored to individual needs and using patient-selected activities of interest. Patients were encouraged to choose their own goals; attention was on doing rather than restriction; supportive and therapeutic relationships provided positive reinforcement.

Spinal Cord Injury (SCI)

SCI patients not only lose physical functions but may have continuing physical problems, such as urinary tract infections, decubitus ulcer, and weight gain. To maintain health status and avoid hospitalization require consistent monitoring of health, discipline, and motivation on the part of the patient.[65]

The SCI patient is vulnerable to feelings of shame and guilt. Incontinence is not only regressive, but the patient is always anxious that accidents will cause social embarrassment. The need to ask for help with personal hygiene may curtail social involvement. The tendency for skin breakdown requires a daily check by patient or family, and the patient who is prone to decubiti may be frequently on bedrest, which is restrictive and requires time out from social plans and work. In addition, decubitus ulcers are ugly and arouse feelings of disgust. Dependency-independence issues, maintaining self-esteem while accepting the need for help, dealing with a standing public from a seated position, using all available energy and time to deal with minimal tasks of living are difficult hurdles to overcome.[6, 7, 65]

Paralyzed patients feel vulnerable to attack and have lost the ability to defend themselves. They fear being trapped in case of fire and face the daily frustration of inaccessibility to meet their needs, *i.e.*, bathroom, library, restaurant. They are at a disadvantage when insisting on their rights and during interpersonal arguments. The severely disabled patient tends to internalize their hostile, negative, and angry feelings because expression may prevent them from getting the care they need and damage social contacts. Such social contacts and friendships are precious and for a variety of reasons not always available.[66] This continual repression may find some outlet through passive-aggressive behavior and in intolerable emotional stress, resulting in verbal explosions, depression, or breakdowns.[21]

Severe limitation of function and mobility restrict the SCI patient from physically expressing feelings of affection or from relieving tension through action or moving away from unpleasant interpersonal situations. In addition, the careful advance planning necessary for shopping and social experiences prevent the pleasures of acting on impulse.[7]

Successful community reintegration includes the ability to be mobile and to gain access to educational, vocational and social environments. The SCI patient is often confronted with barriers that have supposedly been cleared for accessibility; i.e., curbs, forgotten or overlooked steps or rises, ledges, and snow piled or plowed in handicapped parking areas that prevents access to cars may be frequent irritants. Patients are embarrassed at causing inconveniences to friends, having to be carried into buildings, scraping paint off doorways by their wheelchairs, and having the furniture moved for them.

After discharge, patients may become depressed and feel they do not have the strength and skills to deal with the frustrations and restrictions of community living. Cogswell[66] states that upon reentry to the community paraplegic patients demonstrate a reduction in social contacts and use of community settings. She suggests rehabilitation programming focused on post-discharge planning and anticipatory guidance for community living.[66]

Treatment suggestions include social skill training, rebuilding links to the community with increasing involvement before discharge, exploration and adaptation of recreational and avocational interests, review of options for family, work, social roles, problem solving for travel, and provision of modalities and activities that will allow identification and expression of feelings. For satisfactory transfer of learning to occur, patients need to practice new skills in the community and to participate in follow-up programming to reinforce and integrate.

Cerebral Vascular Accident (CVA)

Diller[67] states that after traumatic onset, the patient may be left with both obvious and subtle residual neurological deficits which require physical, social, and psychological rehabilitation. Some changes in function and cognition are not easily observable and may lead staff and family to feel that lack of progress is due to lack of effort on the patient's part.[67] Goldberg et al.[68] state that the patient not only experiences deficits in cognition, memory, speech, and sensation but must also cope with dependency conflicts, anger,

and the loss associated with the sudden and traumatic impairment caused by stroke. The severity and permanence of brain tissue damage may prevent the patient's return to adult responsibilities and pleasures.[68]

Identification of potential in rehabilitation is usually based on a positive premorbid personality, good coping skills, problem solving ability, intelligence, and education. With CVA the location and size of the lesion (brain tissue damage) influences the patient's ability to retain and to utilize such attributes.[67] The CVA patient's denial can be both psychological and organic. An example of organic denial would be an unawareness of the inability to read or neglect of the affected side. Compounding this type of denial are problems in cognitive processing, inability to retain facts, and perceptual problems. Psychological denial may be seen in the patient's belief in a complete recovery and his interpretation of the slightest change or spasm as evidence that complete return may be expected. The patient may alternate between denial and depression, while refusing to learn new skills, denying the need to be involved in his own treatment, and looking for total recovery. Such patients may want to do things no longer possible, such as drive a car or go back to work. The patient may continue to work obsessively toward goals that are no longer feasible.[67]

Patients with neurological damage may not be able to shift their thinking from the disability and losses and to focus on positive gains or remaining skills. They compare their present abilities to premorbid functioning and refuse to accept less. Such patients may continuously ruminate over the loss of mastery and become involved with grieving over all losses. The resulting depression does not benefit from ventilation or discussion, since the brain-damaged patient tends to perseverate his affect and becomes increasingly preoccupied with somatic losses and problems.[67]

Social interaction is threatening for patients with residual neurological and physical deficits. Embarrassment at the new body image, feelings that others will think less of him after the stroke, and the inability to hold food in the mouth contribute to these feelings.[69] In addition, the CVA patient may be confused by a change in environment, has problems with cognitive organization and abstract concepts, feels easily fragmented and confused, may have a visual and auditory loss, and cannot take in the whole gestalt of a situation.[67] Due to sensory loss, the patient may misperceive the actions and communications of others, leading to suspicions and paranoid tendencies.

Diller[67] states that the left hemiplegic tends to deny the disability and the right hemiplegic is more anxious. Anxiety is a common reaction to a traumatic injury, the fear of a second stroke, and somatic preoccupation. The anxious patient often reacts as if he were facing a series of catastrophies.[67]

Therapists need to distinguish between behaviors due to stress reactions and those caused by neurologic barriers. It is important to understand the meaning of the stroke to the patient. For example, does the patient recognize that it is a medical condition or attribute the trauma to an act of God or the result of a moral slip? How will this influence attitudes toward rehabilitation?

Treatment suggestions include: (1) a good relationship with a kind but firm therapist who provides a consistent, stress-free structure in which the patient can learn; (2) treatment activities designed to meet special learning needs, *i.e.*, problems of sensation, perception; (3) clarity and repetition for reinforcement; (4) feedback to benchmark even small gains.

Brinkmann and Hoskins[70] describe the value of a physical conditioning program for hemiplegic patients in developing positive attitudes toward self and increasing the ability to tolerate the physical and physiological stresses of functional activities. Such a program was demonstrated to increase morale and feelings of control and participation in their own recovery. An increased level of physical fitness lead to improvement in self-concept.[70]

EVALUATION

The occupational therapy assessment of psychosocial dysfunction in the physically disabled or ill patient should be broad enough to provide information on the patient's past and present developmental level, usual behaviors and coping skills, functional performance skills, cognitive function, social interactive skills, recreation and leisure time interests, activity of daily living performance, including the use of time and the requirements of the patient's home and community environment.

Assessment should be further expanded to include information on the premorbid personality, aptitudes, educational background, personal goals, cultural and religious values, family dynamics, the patient and family view of health and medical/psychiatric treatment, and those adult role skills necessary to preserve the patient's self-esteem and identity.

Assessment of function or dysfunction in the psychosocial, adaptive, and or performance skill areas can be drawn from theoretical frames of reference, such as Mosey's[34] behavioral/aquisitional, developmental/adaptive skill levels and Reilly's occupational behavior model.[71]

The occupational therapist can also design structured observations by setting up a specific situation for the patient in which skills and behaviors can be observed.[72]

Assessment techniques may include projective testing, observation of group and social interactions, avocational and recreational questionnaires, play history, occupational and role inventories, life skill batteries, and structured interviews.

Tests requiring functional skills can be adjusted so that the severely handicapped patient can participate. For example, the therapist can check a list or write in answers based on the patient's verbal instructions. Departures from the usual testing methods should be documented.

Rather than expose the patient to overlap in assessment, the occupational therapist can utilize information from team meetings, charting, and discussions with other staff. Such information should be validated, and when in doubt the patient should be retested.[72]

The information gained from assessments and interviews will assist the occupational therapist in development of treatment objectives and in determining the areas in which the patient needs special attention,[73] for example, the practice of social skills to improve communication, interaction with attendants and new friends; medical information for the patient and family; career and educational counseling; development of new avocational activities; or problem solving to retain valued roles.

The occupational therapy assessment data form a baseline for the development of realistic treatment goals keyed to the patient's developmental level and personality structure, the requirements of the expected environment, and vocational and personal needs. Whenever possible these goals are integrated with treatment for physical dysfunction.[73] The occupational therapist also needs to discriminate between transient dysfunction in cognition, skills, and behavior and more permanent problems caused by entrenched maladaptive emotional reactions or defenses.

A patient may have never reached the developmental level where he had full use of adaptive, performance skills. However, many patients have had mature adaptive skills which atrophied due to severe injury, illness, isolation, hospitalization, and a continued lack of opportunity to use functional skills as usual. Focus of the assessment may also be on determining where the patient was functioning, his chances of regaining these former skills and roles, identifying treatment goals for retraining, and the substitution of new competencies.

Human beings are complex and highly individual in their reactions to physical disability, and there may be strengths and weaknesses not observable during the initial reaction phase. The therapist should be flexible and continually reassess on the basis of new input.

TREATMENT

Principles to Guide Program Development

The pressure of front line responsibility in the treatment of physical disability or illness can be overwhelming. Therapists may see their efforts diminished by the formidable constellation of physical, cognitive, psychological, and social problems. It is therefore useful to review occupational therapy beliefs and principles generic in the development of treatment objectives and programs that focus on our population of concern. Such a belief code forms an effective overlay to the treatment of physical dysfunction enabling a holistic and inclusive approach.

Mosey states that the, "legitimate tools" of occupational therapy are use of self, the nonhuman environment, the teaching-learning process, purposeful activities, activity groups, and activity analysis and synthesis.[73] Fidler and Fidler[74] state that "doing" enables the development and integration of the sensory, motor, cognitive, and psychological systems, serves as a socialization agent, and verifies one's efficacy as a competent contributing member of society.[74] Physically disabled patients have difficulty learning new skills through vicarious experiences. Formal teaching or discussion groups fail in the initial phase of rehabilitation because the patient threatened by the destruction of his physical self does not have the ego strength and energy to participate and benefit. At this stage, patients cannot integrate the verbal material due to cognitive disorientation and a reduction in psychic energy needed to maintain defenses and deal with accommodation. Didactic or vicarious teaching independent of an experiential component is not facilitating. Purposeful activities provide evidence to the patient of his capabilities. Action and involvement is reinforcing.

Therapeutic activities assist the patient in adjusting to physical dysfunction and in the reestablishment of a satisfactory life-style. Activities should be within the patient's capabilities and elicit a sense of accomplishment and satisfaction. The patient becomes actively engaged in self-directed activities and tasks which match his interests and abilities and thus are motivational.[75, 76]

A wide variety of activities presented both individually or in a group context provide the patient with an opportunity to communicate, to socialize, to develop physical and task competencies, and to develop the skills of negotiation, organization, and long range planning which he will need upon discharge.[3] Through selected activities the patient can learn to satisfy his own mental health needs and meet environmental demands.

Activities leading to expressive behavior will channel some of the patient's energy through mental modes of expression. The severely disabled patient may have no release for energy except in dreams and rebellions. Facilitation activities may include: literature, poetry and writing groups, play readings, putting on plays and musicals, planning groups for trips, recreational and leisure-time activities.

For the patient who can never leave the hospital or take up full-time participation in a former way of life, it is equally important to provide opportunities to find new social roles, to be part of a cohesive group experience, and to have on-going and satisfying interests. Occupational therapists believe that activities should be developmentally sequenced, age-appropriate, and culturally relevant.

Activity analysis is a key part of the occupational therapy evaluation and treatment process. It is the responsibility of the occupational therapist to analyze, choose, and design activities relevant to the patient's special needs.[73] The facilitation of adaptive responses is central to the occupational therapy view of rehabilitation. King states that ". . . occupational therapy is unique in its utilization of the demands of the real life environment." An adaptive response cannot truly be said to have occurred until the individual consistently carries it out in the course of ordinary activites. Thus, the occupational therapist is responsible for utilizing tasks and goal-oriented activities within a structured environment to elicit specific adaptive responses and stimulate acquisition of new habits and skills.[77] Techniques and skills of ADL, travel, or work must be practiced and reinforced in the environment where they will be used.[72]

Anderson[78] and Mosey[73] outline the value of the teaching-learning process in which the patient is viewed not in the role of invalid but as an adult learner. The Anderson model[78] equates treatment and education and sees the therapist as responsible for assisting the patient in learning those skills needed for the performance of their own health care, their new vocation, or in making adaptations to their home, farm, or business. The therapist's responsibilities under this model include: (1) assignment of learning tasks toward the development of new role and task skills; (2) development of a teaching methodology consistent with patient's learning style and previous knowledge; (3) concern with sequencing and timing of the learning tasks; (4) concern with the appropriateness of the learning goals for each patient; (5) identifying learning readiness and assessing ways to teach; and (6) identification and transmission of the information to the patient and family relative to the tasks the patient needs to perform.[78] Mosey[72] states that the patient will learn more easily if new material is presented in conjunction with something he does well.

Play and recreation help to balance life, are a legitimate use of time, and an important treatment modality. The important contribution of play and recreation to physical remediation, adjustment, development of a compromise body image, an increase in self-esteem, decrease in depression and apathy, and the ability and opportunity to socialize needs to be stressed. Play allows the exploration of new behaviors and ways of relating in the handicapped state. Recreational experiences for the patient and family smoothes awkwardness and has a cementing effect. Recreational activities assist the patient toward management of their physical selves, in the use of new equipment (braces, wheelchair), and in exploration of the community. It should be strongly stated that having fun, enjoying others, and being part of a team or group activity is helpful in regaining confidence and in the enjoyment of life. In the author's opinion the adaptation of recreational and sports equipment, provision of opportunities for play, and sports and social activities can fulfill multiple treatment goals and is as important as other treatment objectives for physical dysfunction. It may be a priority.

Rogers and Figone[76] state that the development of avocational potential is a legitimate terminal objective and especially useful to those patients who will be unable to assume vocational roles. They state that substitution of passive social interests for active strenuous interests merits as much attention as replacement of wrist extensors with tenodesis action or mechanical devices."[76]

Patients should be encouraged to meet their personal mental health needs within their present physical and medical conditions. Exploration of avocational interests, methods of adaptation, and new physical techniques will assist the patient toward the development of all his potential.

Rogers and Figone[79] state that an area of concern for patients is the transportation of skills learned in the hospital into the community. In their study, patients expressed the desire to have more opportunities to participate in skill training focused on doing in the community and for opportunities to practice these skills before discharge.[79] Realistic preparation for discharge should include bridging activities and skill training which reflects the patient's real needs. Broad programming will provide opportunities for patients to learn these community survival skills, i.e., mobility and travel skills, preparation to meet their own social needs for friendships, and community interaction. A patient thus equipped will be more likely to maintain maximal independence in the community and to avoid multiple readmissions.

Rogers and Figone[79] state that rehabilitation of quadriplegics is as much a psychosocial process as a physical one and that a primary focus in treatment is the reshaping of life goals.

This author found, in an informal study, that patients who had been injured for 5 years or more and were discharged felt that early socialization experiences soon after hospitalization would have been motivational in preparation and in interesting them in physical rehabilitation tasks.

Geis[32] sees the issue of personal worth as major in the rehabilitation of disabled persons and a central psychodynamic issue for all patients. Patients value themselves when they feel capable of giving satisfaction to the self and to others.[32] The therapist who wishes to help the client maintain feelings of self-worth should intervene by showing the patient, through action and discussion, that there are many ways to achieve satisfactions, to contribute, and to please the self and others.

In addition, occupational therapists' believe: (1) that social isolation is the enemy of interactive skills, self-esteem, and personal identity; (2) that a patient is entitled to therapeutic relationships, treatment objectives, and programming whether he has a short or long time to live and despite his skill level, intelligence, values, and culture; (3) in learning the demographics of the patient's history; (4) in empathetic understanding of the everyday facts of life as the patient will experience them; (5) that reality must be substituted for fantasy concerning the world the patient will be discharged to; (6) that each individual has a special way of learning which must be understood; (7) that peer role models should be included to maximize and facilitate learning; (8) in continual reassessment of the validity of treatment objectives and level of treatment

delivery, and (9) that a therapeutic goal is to create opportunities for the patient to take responsibility.

Patients are not always psychologically prepared for rehabilitation nor are they each ready at a consistent time to benefit from treatment programming.

A treatment priority is to enable the patient to feel more helpful, less helpless and depressed, and more in control of his own affairs.

Facilitating Psychological Adjustment

Moos and Tsu[22] state that the human system requires social and psychological equilibrium as well as physiological homeostasis. In a variety of crisis situations the individual will try to restore balance using previous coping strategies and problem-solving techniques. Coping strategies include all mechanisms, conscious and unconscious, used for adapting to environmental demands. Eventually a balance will be negotiated. A healthy resolution will lead to human growth and a maladaptive one to psychological deterioration, i.e., permanent regression or dead-end depression. Without a good adjustment the patient's life will be impoverished.[8, 22]

The patient utilizes defense responses to minimize the medical/physical situation. Eventually the patient must reassess the effectiveness of this protection. The result of the reappraisal can be effective use of coping mechanisms, or negative responses, including anxiety, entrenched defenses, and little motivation for rehabilitation. Shontz[51] states that while the therapist can not impose adaptation he can assist in its emergence.

Occupational therapists need to anticipate the development of maladaptive coping strategies, intervene appropriately at a point where the patient can benefit, and seek consultation and supervision when the problems are too severe, persistent, and long-standing.

The following material suggests intervention techniques.

Denial

Denial is useful as a temporary solution but becomes a problem when it persists as the major way of dealing with accommodation to disability.[7] The therapist can be supportive, assist in identifying remaining skills, provide opportunities for the patient to demonstrate these skills, and outline hopeful but realistic possibilities for the future within the patient's capabilities.

While the patient may not appear to hear this approach, it has demonstrated value. Encourage patient involvement in therapeutic and social groups but watch the timing and the theme of the group. Bringing a newly disabled patient into a group of disabled old timers may be too threatening and would depend on an appraisal of the patient's emotional situation.

As long as denial is not so excessive as to prevent rehabilitation progress in the learning of new skills and the patient is able to attend to all life tasks possible for him as a handicapped person, denial should not be a concern to the therapist. The therapist must guard against joining the patient in denial but should not be surprised at the patient's need to rely on this safety valve.

The therapist should allow the patient to give up areas of denial gradually. When a patient denies the need for treatment stating that he will walk again, the therapist can suggest that during this period of waiting the patient can learn activities of daily living skills for use now. Often this is enough to encourage rehabilitation activity and the patient is relieved that his dream has not been destroyed. Time and experience in the community may make the patient more realistic, but he may wish to hold onto the hope of functional return some day.

Depression

The type of severity of depression must be identified and, if it is of long duration, intervention techniques may be considered. For example, the occupational therapist should: (1) encourage the patient to ventilate his sadness and loss and what it means to him; (2) express an understanding of the appropriateness of such feelings; (3) assist the patient in evaluation of his problems, identifying what the objective losses actually are, i.e., the realistic boundaries of the losses; (4) arrange interactive and activity experiences for discovery of remaining assets and strengths; (5) help the patient examine alternative ways of gaining satisfaction in living; (6) decrease feelings of helplessness by reminding the patient that you are working for him and assist him in taking control of his own rehabilitation and learning in areas he can influence. An appreciation of the importance of the patient-therapist relationship is crucial in the treatment of depression.

Ventilation of feelings and the awareness that someone understands often helps the patient feel more hopeful and frees energy to work on other tasks. As Siller[7] states, "The goal of rehabilitation never changes—it is always directed toward promoting ego integrity and feelings of self worth." When depression is severe and/or continues for a long time it is a danger signal requiring psychiatric intervention.

Grief and Mourning

Because our culture values adequacy and strength, patients are sometimes criticized for the expression of their grieving reactions to what are frequently multiple losses. Demanding high levels of controlled social behaviors is asking the patient to behave as if nothing of significance had happened. Blocking of mourning or incomplete or partial grieving can lead to future difficulties.[8, 24]

Quigley[8] states that help comes through a steady understanding and accepting relationship. The therapist should not expect steady progress since regressions will occur intermittently.[8] Communicate the message that you value the patient and that his feelings are normal. Patients often need to repeatedly verbalize feelings of loss, discussing how it was before the accident, surgery, or illness. Simos[24] states that one must be able to tolerate another's pain with em-

pathy without prematurely cutting it off to relieve one's own discomfort.

Regression

The therapist should skillfully observe the onset or presence of regression in the patient. Regressive behaviors that are dependent, childish, or sabotaging should be recognized as a defense used by a patient who is overwhelmed, frightened, and anxious. Remedial efforts include reassurance, support, realistic restructuring of treatment objectives, and a focus on attainable short-term goals. Regression may occur in a patient who becomes fatigued, aware of the enormity of the rehabilitation task, overwhelmed with the realities of his medical situation, or whose therapist is too assertive and eager for results. Such a patient should be allowed to regress in the service of recovery, should be protected, and should be given an opportunity for rest and change. The therapist should maintain a therapeutic relationship that is caring, realistically hopeful, and supportive. The therapist may indicate that everyone needs to stop and catch his breath.

Freedman et al.[16] indicate that management of the regressed medical patient requires a tolerant and gentle but insistent push program by all staff. If the patient continues to be regressed, psychiatric consultation and/or intervention is necessary.

Dependency

There are times during rehabilitation and when patients are adjusting to community living that they need the therapist's support and assistance. The interest and concern of the therapist aids the patient in being more efficacious.

The occupational therapist needs to discriminate between types of dependency needs of the patient. Those patients with latent dependency needs require a consistent staff approach and a spread of relationships. Other patients are initially dependent due to trauma, regression, feelings of helplessness, and confusion. Patients may also present behaviors of pseudoindependence while hiding anxiety and fear. The pseudoindependent patient needs to understand that we all have dependency needs, fears, and concerns about ourselves and that there are times and situations when it is appropriate and necessary to be dependent in some areas. Treatment strategies for dependency can include careful weaning from a parent/child relationship, problem solving to maintain responsibility in personal and family roles, opportunities to be in control of life issues and to feel capable. Weaning the patient from the role of invalid so that he has to take increased personal responsibility may be difficult unless the passive role is quickly discouraged and the patient is encouraged to collaborate in the treatment and decision-making process from the beginning. Such responsibilities can be sequenced, and the patient must be given every opportunity to make choices, exercise his own decision-making skills, and be autonomous.

Feldman[1] in his description of positive and negative dependency identifies the new skills the disabled patients need to learn to receive the assistance necessary for maximal independence. They are: (1) the ability to deal with personal feelings concerning accepting the necessary help; (2) skillful and acceptable ways of asking for help without diminishing self-esteem; (3) communication and social skills; and (4) the ability to organize others tactfully.

The therapist can assist the patient in identifying appropriate independent and dependent roles and help the patient to communicate his needs effectively, to problem solve for maximal independence, and to receive satisfactions in all facets of his life. For example, the patient can be helped to recognize that help with time-consuming ADL skills will free energy for self-actualization in other areas.

Siller[7] states that somewhere in between treating the patient like a plant and expecting him to forge ahead without support, there is a middle ground.

Anxiety and Anger

The therapist should expect that strong emotions, such as anxiety and hostility, exist for the disabled patient and that while these issues remain unresolved and unexpressed the patient may not be successfully motivated for rehabilitation. Patients should be encouraged to express fears, anxieties, and worries about disability and loss. Help the patient to feel it is acceptable to verbally blow up; create situations where this can safely happen; and, with the patient, design outlets for feelings, through expressive modes. White and Sweet, as cited in McDaniel, state that the best analgesic is achieved when the patient's attention is turned from somatic preoccupation through activity and change.[21] This provides us with the rationale for therapeutic intervention, such as activity and task-oriented group work.

The therapist can help the patient be realistic about actual threats to self, can show that some of the anxiety is not warranted, nor are the problems as encompassing as the patient thought. Sharing of feelings may allow the patient to begin to adjust and consider alternatives and possibilities for his life. The therapist should never minimize the patient's problems.

Culture and ethnic groups may have a different understanding of feelings and the appropriateness of their expression. Therefore, patients need help in identification, labeling, accepting, and understanding the reasons for the feeling generated by physical illness, disability, and hospitalization. They need support and guidance in dealing with them.

Therapeutic Environment and Relationship

The development of a therapeutic environment is a major treatment consideration. Reilly[80] contends that occupational therapy is a milieu or culture which must be built and functioning before rehabilitation for psychosocial problems can occur and treatment objectives can be met. Pierce and Dickerson[81] state that the occupational therapy clinic is a culture and that the cultural ideal is a place where experience is shared and yet where one feels he is not missing something or not living up to the standards of others. It is clean, pleasant, relaxing, and dynamic.

Elements of a therapeutic environment include a consistent approach and acceptance of each patient within the limits of his capabilities. It is a place where no one feels left out or rejected, where experience can be safely shared, and where the staff behaves appropriately and models behavior that is facilitating and lacks pathological interactions (i.e., demands for perfection, indulgence, dominance). The clinic culture is a place where the patient can make choices, play, feel in control, release feelings, receive support, and also be in treatment.

Kutner's[3] concept of milieu therapy is borrowed from the mental health field. In this model the therapeutic environment or milieu is utilized as a training ground for patients to utilize their social, political skills and to test their ability to deal with the simple and complex problems they would experience in society. The focus is on maintenance of social skills and adult roles to improve and ease the adjustment process and to encourage motivation for the retention of physical function and psychosocial gains on return to the community. Such an environment frees the patient to explore and learn at his own pace at a level consistent with is development, aptitudes, interests, and past experiences.

People grow when they have a good relationship and a climate that is secure and supportive. Trust should be established as a priority, and there should be no violation of this trust or infringment on the rights of the individual for consideration and respect. Essentially it is the personality of the therapist that sets the climate, the therapist's way of relating, of caring, of being genuine and trustworthy.

The therapeutic relationship develops with the patient's awareness that the occupational therapist is willing and able to tolerate painful feelings without moving away. When the concepts of therapeutic relationship and human relating skills are utilized to the fullest in the treatment of the physically disabled the results have been gratifying both for staff and patients.

The period of initial adjustment directly after hospitalization can be a productive time for the development of a supportive therapeutic relationship. When the patient is ready to leave the isolation of his room for treatment, trust will have been established and the therapist will understand the patient's historical, psychological, and medical status. The attitudes of staff as reflected in the patient are crucial in his adjustment. If the staff can accept the patient with the deformity, show respect, and recognize individuality there will be a positive effect on his self-concept and self-respect. Good social feedback from the nondisabled encourages maintenance of identity and self-respect. The patient who is accepted as he is by the staff can more easily accept himself.

Rogers and Figone[79] state that patients found the

following qualities of therapists significant in their rehabilitation. They valued a consistent relationship with the same therapist who was aware of their current medical status, who was flexible in letting them experiment with rehabilitation tasks, and who demonstrated understanding.

Mosey[73] states that the use of self is one of the legitimate tools of occupational therapy. She defines the conscious use of self as planned interactions with another person in order to alleviate anxiety or fear, give reassurance, obtain and provide information, or assist the patient in gaining understanding of self and others.

Working with patients for acceptance and change is less dependent on use of specific techniques than upon perception, comprehension, warmth, sincerity, and responsiveness. Therapists need to be clear about what they are communicating verbally and nonverbally. The therapist should be sensitive to self in therapy, personally capable in life skill functions, and have developed mature skills of human interaction. Therapists need to develop therapeutic skills of listening, responding, and communicating, and should be aware of personal responses to stress.[82]

These statements are not intended to convey the idea that understanding of theory, frames of reference, specific treatment methods, models, and techniques are not important. The professional therapist has an obligation to be fully prepared in all phases of the physical, medical, and psychological sciences.

Guidance For Discharge

The ultimate objective of rehabilitation is to enable the patient to live successfully and independently, to be reintegrated into his family and community, and there to fill contributory and self-satisfying roles through paid or voluntary activity. It is the therapist's goal to anticipate and to prevent discharge failure and personal or interfamily crises. Prevention through better preparation of the patient for discharge includes: (1) a focus on independent living issues early in the treatment process; (2) the design of experiential tasks to develop social interaction skills with opportunities to practice within the hospital and community; (3) the willingness of both the therapist and patient for a realistic appraisal of the problems and emotional adjustment of community living; (4) identification and intervention in maladaptive emotional reactions and defenses; (5) reduction of the need to cling to secondary gains by providing access to other satisfactions; and (6) persistent follow-up with psychological support.

Postdischarge stress will continue for 3 months to a year or longer, and during this period the patient may withdraw and be vulnerable to depression.[83] Follow-up of home- and community-based treatment problems are crucial in the final success of rehabilitation objectives. Community reintegration programs are not well developed at the present time.

Kutner[28] feels that much can be learned from psychiatric literature on the concept of "therapeutic community" as a treatment model. He feels that in the field of physical rehabilitation this model has not been adequately put to use and that there should be a concern for carryover of treatment from the institution to the community so that the negative impact of transition can be minimized. Within the "therapeutic community" model considerable attention has been given to the rolelessness of the institutionalized patient.

The "pacemaker" model proposed by Keith includes two stages of therapy. The first is medical and deals with the acute crisis. The second is concerned with the acquisition of independent living skills, increased personal problem solving, and responsibility for self, including those skills required for successful living in the community. In the pacemker model the second stage of therapy is usually removed from the medical setting.[28]

Environmental Deprivation

The occupational therapist needs to identify patients at risk and plan intervention and addition of stimulation. This might include programming to maintain intellectual function, sensory stimulation project, such as objects to view and music, or manipulation of the environment. Whenever possible the patient should be transported to observe or become involved in social or task-oriented groups and to resume normal patterns of human interaction

Group Work

Treatment objectives for patients are often more effectively met through group work. It is the responsibility of the occupational therapist to design flexible and specialized treatment groups able to meet the individual and changing needs of a patient population with psychosocial dysfunction secondary to physical disability and illness.

Miller et al.[83] states that self-esteem is positively influenced by group participation and there is a strong positive relationship between group work, patient self-concept, and response to treatment. Versluys states that after evaluating the degree of physical and adult role dysfunction the treatment emphasis includes guiding the patient in reexperiencing early developmental tasks through the learning lab of group experiences.[29] In a study by Mumford[84] a significant increase in interpersonal skills was noted when activities were used in group work as compared to strictly verbal discussion groups. Shatin, Brown and Loezeaux report that patients receiving recreational and rehabilitation activities in group therapy and also having increased contact with staff showed more gains and interest in rehabilitation than those patients whose treatment did not include these factors.[21] Mann et al.[85] state that group work provides an opportunity to observe the patient's psychosocial functioning, including important personal qualities, such as initiative, creativeness, persistence, and originality.[85]

Group interaction provides a support base allowing patients to cope more effectively with disability and depression through externalization of emotions, to modify severe defensive reaction through shared feelings, to influence adjustment through a sense of universality, to provide an effective way to dispense information concening disability and illness, and to encourage the development of new interhospital friendships which may have continuity in the community.[29, 85]

In addition, a cohesive group sustains the patient while he experiences and masters skills necessary for physical and psychological survival in the community. The first stage of treatment can be focused on adjustment problems and the second stage on acquisition of skills needed for success in the community and maintenance of psychological health. Interactive and experiential groups provide the patient with a training ground to encourage the development of social and political skills by which he may influence the environment. Group experiences facilitate the development of new roles, provide the patient with an opportunity to test behaviors in the disabled condition, to find he can become productive and contributing, and to take initiative and the responsibility for meeting his own needs. Through group interaction, patients are exposed to a variety of social roles, obtain peer feedback, and benefit from group problem solving around common issues of concern. Through planning, playing, choosing, helping, and sharing they find there are many ways of being acceptable and successful.[3,32,35]

The supportive elements of the group cannot be overstated. It is much easier to face uncertainty, an operation, personal loss, and family or community problems when you are involved with a group of caring people.

Patient-led groups multiply motivation and provide support clarification and educational functions. The inclusion of rehabilitated patients as models and leaders motivates the patient toward maximal use of his remaining functions and toward exploration of alternatives for the future, and can provide a liaison function for patients during the transition period before discharge.

Therapist and group feedback provides the patient with consensual validation, modifies perceptual distortions, and reduces defensive resistance to remediation. Therapists must facilitate and monitor the patient's interaction and performance. Tasks need to be assigned, and feedback that reinforces the direction and pace of new learning must be provided.[3,21,29]

Patients' reactions to being part of a group vary, and some patients initially need to watch from the sidelines and become gradually involved for the following reasons: (1) being in a group with physically disabled patients means that one is like them, and this is very threatening for newly injured patients; (2) some people never developed good social interpersonal skills and are uncomfortable with others; (3) some people distrust and are suspicious of the intentions of others; (4) some cultural values encourage the patient to feel that the disability is their punishment and since group activities are often seen as enjoyable, such a patient may withdraw.

Therapeutic modalities such as literature or expressive modalities can be structured to stimulate group interaction. For example, in a poetry group the patient is stimulated by the media to focus on his own feelings and needs, especially if the environment and relationship make him feel safe and supported. The same patient might have withdrawn in a formally organized discussion group concerning his feelings about the disability.

Group work also encompasses "curative factors" which are an integral part of the therapeutic adjustment and change process. Yalom[86] described 10 such factors, all of which are useful in meeting the psychosocial and adjustment needs of the physically disabled; examples include the *installation of hope*, that is, the patient can note that others have been successful in coping with disability, have succeeded in becoming independent and in building a productive and satisfying life and *universality*, through which the disabled can realize that others also have problems with the rehabilitation process.[86] This chapter does not allow a more complete coverage of the curative factors but Yalom's work is useful for the therapist who wishes to treat patients in groups. Therapists should not consider this form of treatment without both a knowledge of group theory and practice and specialized training/supervision.

The following are examples of experiential treatment groups. Family task-oriented groups can provide activities and experiences which help in the interactions between patients and their families. The occupational therapist who is training the patient in living skills and treating the physical dysfunction is in a major position to teach, clarify, and counsel the family. The family can be involved in the treatment process, in task-oriented social groups, in discussion groups, in community trips, dinner parties, art and music groups, and recreational activities. This provides an opportunity for the patient and the family to relate to each other again in a comfortable social situation and to see how the staff acts toward the patient and what they expect in the way of independent activities.

Transitional groups, held both in the hospital and community, facilitate community reintegration through programming that focuses on problem solving, activity, task skills, and social experiences that will aid in the patient's success in community living. Bridging activities may include shopping first with a group from the hospital and then with family, friends, or alone; attending concerts and other community activities before discharge; job interviewing; and educational activities. Therapists should design hospital/community experiences and activities that provide practice opportunities.

Leisure time or recreational groups explore new avocational interests, adaptation of the leisure or sport activities, an opportunity to practice, and patient organization of sport rallies or art shows.

The mental health field has pioneered transitional group models that have a history of success. Such transitional groups start in the hospital before discharge and continue in the community (pre- and post-discharge). The postdischarge transitional group can be held in a convenient community location or on a rotating basis in patients' homes. Postdischarge transitional programming is assistive in providing peer support and the opportunity for problem solving and social contacts which prevent exacerbation of physical or emotional problems.

SUMMARY

Lamb[38] states that patients vary greatly in their potential for rehabilitation. The therapist must accept this or feel continually frustrated, have unrealistic expectations, and a sense of failure. Rehabilitation potential can, however, be increased by involving the patient in a partnership of choice with the therapist in the development of treatment objectives. If the patient's goals are initially too ambitious the therapist should remember that these are not necessarily the final choice. Patients, like the rest of us, are capable of experiencing failure and of reassessing and thinking through the need to change direction. The therapist can guide treatment by sequencing achievable short-term goals to support the patient's long-term objectives.

The occupational therapist's role is to focus on the assets and the strengths and skills of the patient. Helping the patient to reach one goal at a time keeps him from being overwhelmed with the enormity of his task. The therapist should be clear on when to support, when to give more responsibility for self, when to be the patient's advocate, and when to encourage him to solve his own problems and initiate his own planning.

The occupational therapist can assist the patient in his accommodation to disability by provision of experiences where the patient will feel more in control of his life and more aware of his competencies toward the development of mastery over the environment. Integration and permanence of the new skills and attitudes will depend on the presence and quality of transitional and community treatment and follow-up programs.

References

1. Feldman, D. J. Chronic disabling illness: A holistic view. *J. Chronic Dis.*, 27: 287–291, 1974.
2. Tucker, S. J. The psychology of spinal cord injury: Patient-staff interaction. *Rehabil. Lit.* 41(5–6): 114–160, 1980.
3. Kutner, b. Milieu therapy. *J. Rehabil.*, 34(2): 14–17, 1968.
4. Kutner B., and Weissman, R. Role disorders in extended hospitalization. *Hosp. Admin.*, 12(1):14–17, 1967.
5. Strain, J. J. *Psychological Care of the Medically Ill: A Primer in Liaison Psychiatry.* New York: Appleton-Century-Crofts, 1975.
6. Stewart, T. D., and Rossier, A. B. Psychological consideration in the adjustment to spinal cord injury. *Rehabil. Lit.*, 39(3): 75–80, 1978.
7. Siller, J. Psychological situation of the disabled with spinal cord injuries. *Rehabil. Lit.*, 30(10): 290–296, 1969.
8. Quigley, J. L. Understanding depression—helping with grief. *Rehabil. Gazette*, 19: 2–6, 1976.
9. Safilios-Rothschild, C. *The Sociology and Social Psychology of Disability and Rehabilitation.* New York: Random House, 1970.
10. Simon, J. I. Emotional aspects of physical disability. *Am. J. Occup. Ther.*, 25(8): 408–410, 1971.
11. Chernewski, E. The social determinants of mental illness and psychosomatic disease. *Am. J. Occup. Ther.*, 25(5): 193–195, 1961.
12. Wright, B. A. *Physical Disability—A Psychological Approach.* New York: Harper & Row, 1961.
13. Kiely, W. F. Coping with severe illness. *Adv. Psychosom. Med.*, 8: 110–117, 1972.
14. Kolb, L. D. *Modern Clinical Psychiatry*, 8th ed. Philadelphia: W. B. Saunders, 1968.
15. Shapiro, D. *Neurotic Styles.* New York: Basic Books Inc., 1965.
16. Freedman, A. M., Kaplan, H. I., and Sadock, B. J. *Modern Synopsis of Comprehensive Textbook of Psychiatry/II.* Baltimore: Williams & Wilkins, 1976.
17. McCranie, E. J. Neurotic problems in middle age. *Psychosomatics*, 19(2): 106–112, 1978.
18. Olshansky, S. S. The challenge of traumatic neurosis to rehabilitation. *Am. J. Occup. Ther.*, 4(1): 12–13, 1950.
19. Hodge, J. R. The whiplash neurosis. *Psychosomatics*, 12(4): 42–44, 1971.
20. Shontz, F. D. Physical disability and personality. In *Rehabilitation Psychology*, edited by W. Neff. Washington, D.C.: American Psychological Association, 1971.
21. McDaniel, J. S. *Physical Disability and Human Behavior.* New York: Pergamon Press, 1969.
22. Moos, R. H., and Tsu, V.D. The crisis of physical illness: An overview. In *Coping with Physical Illness*, edited by R. H. Moos. New York: Plenum Medical Book, Co., 1977.
23. Dorfman, W. Depression: Its expression in physical illness. *Psychosomatics*, 19(11): 702–708, 1978.
24. Simos, B. G. Grief therapy to facilitate healthy restitution. *Social Casework*, 58(6): 337–342, 1977.
25. Solomon, P., and Patch, V. D. *The Handbook of Psychiatry.* Los Altos, Calif.: Lange Medical Publications, 1974.
26. Thomas, M. D., Baker, J. M., and Ester, N. J. Anger: A tool for development of self awareness. *Am. J. Nurs.*, 70(12): 2586–2590, 1970.
27. Kaplan, D. M., Smith, A., Grobstein, R., and Fischman, S. E. Family mediation of stress. In *Coping with Physical Illness*, edited by R. H. Moos. New York: Plenum Medical Book Co., 1977.
28. Kutner, B. The social psychology of disability. In *Rehabilitation Psychology*, edited by W. Neff. Washington, D.C.: American Psychological Association, 1971.
29. Versluys, H. P. The remediation of role disorders through focused group work. *Am. J. Occup. Ther.*, 34(9): 609–614, 1980.
30. Szapocznik, J., Scoppetta, M. A., and Aranalde, M. A. Cuban value structure: Treatment complications. *J. Consult. Clin. Psychol.*, 46(5): 961–970, 1978.
31. Sanchez, V. Relevance of cultural values: For occupational therapy programs. *Am. J. Occup. Ther.*, 28(1): 1–5, 1964.
32. Geis, H. J. The problem of personal worth in the physically disabled patient. *Rehabil. Lit.*, 33(2):34–39, 1972.
33. Diamond, H. Some psychiatric problems of the physically disabled. *Am. J. Occup. Ther.*, 10(3): 113–117, 1956.
34. Mosey, A. C. *Three Frames of Reference for Mental Health.* Thorofare, N.J.: Charles B. Slack, 1970.
35. Gordon, W. W. Race, ethnicity, social disadvantage and rehabilitation. In *Rehabilitation Psychology*, edited by W. Neff. Washington, D.C.: American Psychological Association, 1971.
36. Elberlik, K. Organ loss, grieving and itching. *Am. J. Psychother.*, 24(4): 523–533, 1980.
37. Leviton, G. The professional-client relationship. In *Rehabilitation Psychology*, edited by W. Neff. Washington, D.C.: American Psychological Association, 1971.
38. Lamb, H. R. Staff burnout in work with long-term patients.

Hosp. Community Psychiatry, 30(6): 396–398, 1979.

39. Parent, L. H. Effects of a low stimulus environment on behavior. *Am. J. Occup. Ther., 32*(1): 19–25, 1978.

40. Shontz, F. C., Fink, S. L., and Hallenbeck, C. E. Chronic physical illness as threat. *Arch. Phys. Med. Rehabil., 41*(4): 143–148, 1960.

41. Rabinowitz, H. S. Motivation for recovery: Four social-psychological aspects. *Arch. Phys. Med. Rehabil., 42*(12): 799–807, 1961.

42. White, R. H. Motivation reconsidered: The concept of competence. *Psychol. Rev., 69*(6): 297–333, 1967.

43. Irwin, T. Male Menopause, Crisis in the Middle Years, Public Affairs Pamphlet No. 526, Washington, D.C.: U.S. Government Printing Office.

44. Versluys, H. P. Physical rehabilitation and family dynamics. *Rehabil. Lit., 41*(3–4): 58–65, 1980.

45. Hill, R. Social stresses on the family, generic features of families under stress. *Social Casework, 39*: 139–150, 1958.

46. The Source Book: Rehabilitation of the Person with Spinal Cord Injury. Washington, D.C.: Superintendent of Documents, U.S. Govt. Printing Office, 1972.

47. Brodland, G. A., and Andreasen, J. J. C. Adjustment problems in the family of the burn patient. In *Coping With Physical Illness*, edited by R. H. Moos. New York: Plenum Medical Book Co., 1977.

48. Chistopherson, V. A. The patient and family. *Rehabil. Lit., 23*: 34–41, 1962.

49. Spergel, P., Ehrlich, G. F., and Glass, D. The rheumatoid arthritic personality: A psychodiagnostic myth. *Psychosomatics, 19*(2): 79–86, 1978.

50. Zeitlin, D. J. Psychological issues in the management of rheumatoid arthritis. *Psychosomatics, 17–18*(8): 7–14, 1977.

51. Shontz, F. C. *Psychological Aspects of Physical Illness and Disability*. New York: MacMillan Pub., 1975.

52. Baretz, R. M., and Stephenson, G. R. Emotional responses to multiple sclerosis. *Psychosomatics, 22*(2): 117–127, 1981.

53. Pulton, T. W. Multiple Sclerosis: A social-psychological perspective. *Phys. Ther., 57*(2): 170–173, 1977.

54. Schneitzer, L. Rehabilitation of patients with multiple sclerosis. *Arch. Phys. Med. Rehabil., 59*(9): 430–436, 1978.

55. Malick, M. H. Burns. In Willard and Spackman's Occupational Therapy, 5th ed., edited by H. L. Hopkins and H. D. Smith. Philadelphia: J. B. Lippincott, 1978.

56. Andreasen, N. J. D., and Norris, A. S. Long-term adjustment and adaptation mechanisms in severely burned adults. In *Coping With Physical Illness*, edited by R. H. Moos. New York: Plenum Medical Books Co., 1977.

57. Molinaro, J. R. The social fate of children disfigured by burns. *Am. J. Psychiatry, 13*: 979–990, 1978.

58. Carnes, G. D. Understanding the cardiac patient's behavior. *Am. J. Nurs., 71*(6): 1187–1188, 1971.

59. Cassem, N. H., and Hackett, T. P. Psychological rehabilitation of myocardial infarction patient in the acute phase. *Heart Lung, 2*(3): 382–388, 1973.

60. Cassem, N. H. Lecture, Cardiac Rehabilitation for Occupational therapy and Physical Therapy Seminar. Sargent College, Boston University, Boston, 1976.

61. Hackett, T. P. Lecture, Cardic Rehabilitation for Occupational Therapy and Physical Therapy Seminar. Sargent College, Boston University, Boston, 1976.

62. Bilodeau, C. B., and Hackett, T. P. Issues raised in a group setting by patients recovering from myocardial infarction. *Am.*

J. Psychiatry., I(July): 73–78, 1971.

63. Semmler, C., and Semmler, M. Counseling the coronary patient. *Am. J. Occup. Ther., 28*(10): 609–614, 1974.

64. Baile, W. F., and Engel, B. T. A behavioral strategy for promoting treatment compliance following myocardial infarction. *Psychosom. Med, 40*(5): 413–419, 1978.

65. Starch, P. L. Maslow's needs and the spinal cord injured client. *Assoc. Rehabil. Nurs.*, (September-October): 17–20, 1980.

66. Cogswell, B. E. Self socialization. The readjustment of paraplegics in the community. *J. Rehabil., 34*(3): 11–35, 40, 1968.

67. Diller, L. Hemiplegia. In *Rehabilitation Practices with the Physically Disabled*, edited by J. F. Barrett and E. S. Levine. New York: Columbia University Press, 1973.

68. Goldberg, R. L., Wise, T. H., and LeBuffe, F. P. The stroke unit: Psychological aspects of recovery. *Psychosomatics, 20*(5): 316–321, 1979.

69. Hyman, M. E. The stigma of stroke. *Geriatrics, May*: 132–141, 1971.

70. Brinkmann, J. R., and Hoskins, T. A. Physical conditioning and altered self-concept in rehabilitated hemiplegic patient. *Phys. Ther., 59*(7): 859–865, 1979.

71. Kielhofner, G. *The Evolution of Knowledge in Occupational Therapy—Understanding Adaptation of the Chronically Disabled* master's thesis, University of Southern California, Los Angeles, 1973.

72. Mosey, A. C. *Activities Therapy*. New York: Raven Press, 1973.

73. Mosey, A. C. A model for occupational therapy. *Occup. Ther. Mental Health, 1*(1): 11–31, 1980.

74. Fidler, G. S., and Fidler, J. W. Doing and becoming: Purposeful action and self actualization. *Am. J. Occup. Ther., 32*(5): 305–316, 1978.

75. Turk, D. C., Sobel, H. J., Follick, M. J., and Youkilil, H. D. A sequential criterion analysis for assessing coping with chronic illness. *J. Hum. Stress*, June: 35–39, 1980.

76. Rogers, J. D., and Figone, J. J. The avocational pursuits of rehabilitants with traumatic quadriplegia. *Am. J. Occup. Ther., 32*(9): 571–576, 1978.

77. King, L. J. Toward a science of adaptive responses. *Am. J. Occup. Ther., 32*(7): 429–437, 1978.

78. Anderson, T. P. Educational frame of reference: An additional model for rehabilitation medicine. *Arch. Phys. Med. Rehabil., 59*(5): 203–206, 1978.

79. Rogers, J. D., and Figone, J. J. Psychosocial parameters in treating the person with quadriplegia. *Am. J. Occup. Ther., 33*(7): 432–439, 1979.

80. Reilly, M. A psychiatric occupational therapy program as a teaching model. *Am. J. Occup. Ther., 20*(2): 61–67, 1966.

81. Pierce, C., and Dickerson, R. The occupational therapy shop as a culture. *Am. J. Occup. Ther., 16*(5): 231–235, 1962.

82. Carkhuff, R. R., and Berenson, B. G. *Beyond Counseling and Therapy*. New York: Holt, Rinehart and Winston, 1967.

83. Miller, D. K., Wolfe, M., and Spiegel, M. H. Therapeutic groups for patients with spinal cord injuries. *Arch. Phys. Med. Rehabil., 56*(3): 130–135, 1975.

84. Mumford, M. S. A comparison of interpersonal skills in verbal and activity groups. *Am. J. Occup. Ther., 28*(5): 281–283, 1974.

85. Mann, W., Godfrey, M. D., and Dowd, E. T. The use of group counseling procedures in the rehabilitation of spinal cord injured patients. *Am. J. Occup. Ther., 27*(2): 73–77, 1973.

86. Yalom, I. D. *The Theory and Practice of Group Psychotherapy*. New York: Basic Books, 1970.

PART TWO

Neurodevelopmental Approach

This section will include the evaluation and restorative treatment procedures used for patients with motor problems due to brain dysfunction. As a result of brain damage, a patient's movement patterns may lack control, may be immature, and/or may be unduly controlled by sensory stimulation. Treatment to promote development and voluntary control must be based on neurophysiological and developmental principles. Therefore, this section is entitled "neurodevelopmental."

Sensation and movement are closely allied in all persons. Therefore, the neurodevelopmental approach is applicable to patients with both orthopedic and neurological motor disorders. Its potential value depends on the integrity of neural transmission. In a patient with spinal cord transection, sensation is lost below the level of the lesion and movements below that level cannot be voluntarily controlled. Sensations from the periphery can only produce reflex responses at segmental levels of the spinal cord with no lasting effect on motor function. In complete peripheral nerve lesions, sensations do not even travel to the spinal cord and are ineffective in influencing motor response. In brain injury, however, spinal cord and peripheral neural pathways are intact, and sensory stimulation can be transmitted to the brain with a potential for influencing voluntary motor control. Sensory stimuli have an effect whether the stimuli are environmental or deliberately applied by the therapist.

The neurodevelopmental approach is in the process of evolution. New information in neurophysiology is being generated from research on primates and humans. Theories of motor learning are being reconsidered in light of the newer emphasis on theories of central control of movement. Occupational and physical therapy clinicians and graduate students are doing studies on the effectiveness of techniques used in clinical practice. As all this new information is reported and integrated, practices may change.

chapter

3

Evaluation and Treatment of Sensation

Anna Deane Scott, M.Ed., OTR

Sensory dysfunction may accompany any disease or trauma affecting the nervous system. The reception of stimuli or the transmission of sensory impulses may be interrupted at any point from the receptor, to the peripheral nerve, to the sensory tract in the spinal cord and brain stem, to the thalamus, or to the sensory cortex. Any patient who has suffered trauma or disease which might affect any part of the sensory system must be evaluated to determine the nature and extent of sensory dysfunction because of the close relationship of sensory input and motor output.

Sensory modalities, receptors, and pathways have been classified for descriptive and functional purposes. Modalities are divided into superficial, deep[1, 2] and combined,[1] or cortical.[2] Sensory receptors are classified as exteroceptors that receive stimuli from the external environment via the skin[1, 2] and proprioceptors that receive stimuli from muscles, tendons, ligaments, and joints.[2] Head's classification of sensory modalities divided tactile sensations into two systems. The protopathic system was for defense from harmful stimuli such as pain, strong temperature stimuli,[1] and any diffuse unpleasant light touch sensation, such as itching, tickling, or tingling.[3] The epicritic system, considered to be phylogenetically newer, was for discriminative perception of stimuli such as 2-point discrimination, small temperature changes,[1] localization of light touch stimuli, and object recognition.[3] Stereognosis is generally agreed to require cortical integrity.[1, 2] Sensations have also been classified according to whether the sensory modalities are projected via the spinothalamic or lemniscal systems.[3] The spinothalamic system projects pain and temperature stimuli, light touch, and light pressure; the lemniscal system projects stimuli of tactile discrimination, such as deep pressure, 2-point discrimination, vibration from perception, and kinesthesia (conscious proprioception).[1, 3] Since these two systems have some overlapping functions they are considered to be more interdependent as a result of developmental evolution than strictly distinct and separate.[3] The specificity of receptors has also been investigated. Receptors for each sensory modality are named in neurology texts including Meissner's and Merkel's corpuscles for touch, Pacinian corpuscles for pressure, Krause's end bulbs for cold, and Ruffini's end organs for warm.[1] Wynn Parry[4] summarizes other findings concerning receptors in which certain receptors are found to have a low threshold for particular stimuli. However, all receptors and fibers will fire in response to different types of stimuli, and the sensation is a result of the temporal pattern of impulses transmitted by the nerve. Johansson[5] and Johansson and Vallbo[6] describe the location of four different types of mechanoreceptive units in the glabrous, i.e., hairless, skin of the hand. Two units (PC and SA II) are evenly distributed and sensitive to vibration and stretch. The other two units (RA and SAI) are primarily located in the fingertips and are most suitable for tactile spatial analysis as required in 2-point discrimination. Further investigations may verify, clarify, or change current knowledge and thereby influence evaluation and treatment procedures.

EVALUATION

The results of a sensory evaluation are available to the therapist in the medical report if a neurological examination has been done. If the results of a recent sensory evaluation are not available, it is necessary for the occupational therapist to do a sensory evaluation in order to plan treatment. Methods currently used in clinical practice will be described.

A sensory evaluation involves presentation of stimuli appropriate to each sensory modality and an observation of the patient's responses.

Testing Procedure

The patient is oriented to the purpose and procedure of sensory evaluation. He should be comfortable and relaxed. The patient's vision must be occluded for each test procedure. This may be done by asking the patient to keep his eyes closed, by using a blindfold, or by shielding the patient's vision with a screen. Between each test procedure, the patient is allowed to open his eyes for the following reasons. Instructions for the next procedure must be given. Persons with cortical damage may become easily disoriented if their vision is occluded for a long time. People's attention may decrease due to lack of visual stimulation.

Stimuli are applied distally to proximally in order to determine the distribution of loss or impairment because sensory deficit is usually more severe distally. In peripheral nervous system deficit, return of function occurs proximally to distally.

Stimuli are applied in an unpredictable pattern with variation in timing to assure reliability and accuracy of response. Uninvolved areas of the body are tested both to assure that the patient understands the directions and to establish "normal."

Each treatment facility has a method of recording the results of the evaluation of sensation, and the method used often reflects the case load of a particular unit. Although the manner of recording varies, responses are usually scored as follows: _Intact_ indicates that the responses were quick and accurate. _Absent_ indicates that no response was obtained. _Impaired_ indicates a delay of response, a sensation inappropriate to the stimulus, or variable accuracy of response. Note is made if the patient reports causalgia, hyperaesthesia, paraesthesia, or other abnormal sensations.

In peripheral nerve lesions exact localization of sensory loss or impairment is often required as part of the evaluation of regeneration of the nerve. Recording may be done on a diagram of the involved extremity with color coding of different sensory modalities. Less exact recording may be sufficient in some instances and a description of the loss noted, for example, loss of touch, pain, and temperature in the distribution of the radial nerve distal to the midforearm. In spinal cord lesions the losses may be marked on a full body diagram with an anterior and posterior view or a note may include a description indicating losses below a particular dermatomal level or body part such as the nipple line or umbilicus. In cortical lesions the body part affected is usually described by indicating which modalities are impaired or absent in terms of the body part, for example, pain and temperature impaired in the upper arm and absent distal to the elbow (or other descriptive designations).

Reference to the sensory distribution of peripheral nerves and dermatomal charts is often helpful in both the evaluation process and the description of sensory impairment or loss (see Figs. 3.1 to 3.5).

Superficial or Exteroceptive Sensations

Light Touch. _Stimulus._ Lightly touch a small area of the patient's skin with cotton, a camel's hair brush, a tissue, or a fingertip.[2, 7] Use a gentle stroke rather than a light touch to intensify the stimulus if necessary due to limited attention.[2]

Response. The patient says "now," "yes," or gives other indication each time the stimulus is felt. Note any response that may indicate hypersensitivity or other unusual sensation. For nonverbal patients squeezing the therapist's finger or nodding may be used. For patients unable to communicate movement of the part, a change of facial expression or looking toward the part can be used as indicators of a response to touch.[2]

The stimulus-response is repeated so that those surfaces of the patient's skin which would correlate with the expected distribution of dysfunction according to the diagnosis are tested.

Pressure. _Stimulus._ The therapist uses a fingertip to apply a firm pressure to a small area of the patient's skin.[2] This pressure must be firm enough to indent the skin to stimulate the deep receptors.

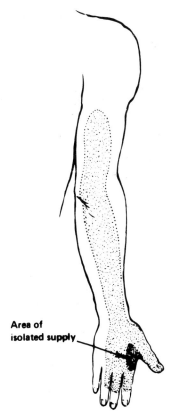

Figure 3.1 Sensory distribution, radial nerve. (Reproduced with permission from S. G. Chusid.[1])

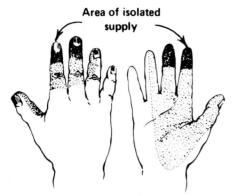

Figure 3.2 Sensory distribution, median nerve. (Reproduced with permission from S. G. Chusid.[1])

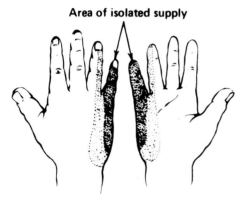

Figure 3.3 Sensory distribution, ulnar nerve. (Reproduced with permission from S. G. Chusid.[1])

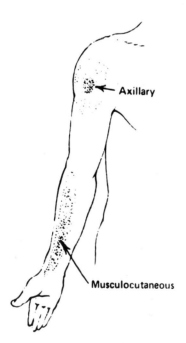

Figure 3.4 Sensory distribution, musculocutaneous and axillary nerves. (Reproduced with permission from S. G. Chusid.[1])

Response. The patient indicates each time the stimulus is felt. The stimulus-response is repeated so that those surfaces of the patient's skin which would correlate with the expected distribution of dysfunction according to the diagnosis are tested.

A pressure aesthesiometer can be used to determine, in grams or milligrams, the threshold of the response to pressure stimulation.[8] Nylon von Frey hairs may also be used.[9] With both of these tools the lighter filaments or hairs indicate the touch threshold, whereas those filaments which indent the skin before bending test pressure.

Pain. Stimulus. Using a pin which provides one sharp and one blunt end, the therapist applies mixed sharp and dull stimuli in random pattern of presentation to verify accuracy of responses.

Response. The patient says "sharp" or "dull." Scoring is based on the accuracy of responses to the sharp stimuli; dull stimuli are used so that the patient must discriminate between pain and touch stimuli.[2, 7] For nonverbal patients the responses described for touch may be used when applying the sharp stimulus.[2] Again, all surfaces are tested.

Temperature. If pain sensitivity is normal it is rare to find temperature impaired, and temperature testing can be eliminated.[2] If pain is impaired, temperature must be tested.

Stimulus. Before testing, be sure that the patient's skin is of normal temperature. Capped test tubes, one filled with hot water and one filled with cold water, are applied in random order to the patient's skin. Glass test tubes are generally used, but metal tubes are preferable if available because metal is a better temperature conductor. Very hot and very cold stimuli may be perceived as pain, so approximately 110°F (43°C) for hot and approximately 40°F (4°C) for cold are recommended.[2]

Response. After each presentation of a stimulus, the patient indicates if he felt "hot" or "cold." Again, appropriate skin surfaces are tested.

Deep or Proprioceptive Sensations

Proprioception is the unconscious awareness of information from muscles, tendons, ligaments, and joints, and conscious awareness occurs only when attention is focused.[3] Kinesthesia is the conscious awareness of joint position and movement as a result of stimulation of joint receptors.[3] Position sense as distinct from movement sense is the awareness of position at rest.[2] The common test for position sense is the distinction between "up" and "down."[7] This is actually a test of movement sense or kinesthesia[2, 3] and is described here under that heading. Bender[10] notes that movement and position sense are usually tested in the fingers and toes only and recommends testing the larger joints which may also be involved in gross defects. Kent[11] described tests of position sense in upper extremity motions of the shoulder, elbow, forearm, wrist, and fingers.

Position Sense. Stimulus. The therapist holds the

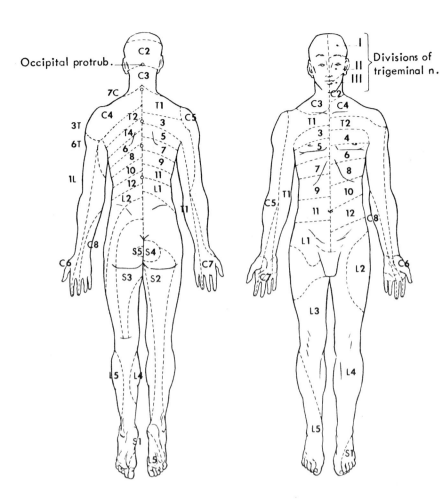

Figure 3.5 Sensory chart according to dermatomes. (Reproduced with permission from J. Gilroy and J. S. Meyer: *Medical Neurology*, 3rd ed. New York: MacMillan, 1979.)

part laterally to avoid tactile or pressure input and places the joints of one extremity into easily describable positions. In the upper extremity these could be arm out to the side with the palm down, arm in front with elbow bent, and hand toward face, etc. Test the hand separately. Paine and Oppé[2] suggest arranging the fingers of one hand.

Response. The patient imitates each position with the opposite extremity or describes the position. Note: When one side is involved this side is positioned and the noninvolved side copies the position. Errors are attributed to impairment or loss of position sense on the involved side, *i.e.*, the one positioned.

Other tests of position sense:[2]

a. Move a joint up and down rapidly several times and stop in the up or down position. The patient then says if it is "up" or "down."

b. Have the patient touch his two index fingers together in front of him or the therapist holds one of the patient's arms with the index finger pointed and the patient touches it with his other index finger.

Kinesthesia (movement sense). *Stimulus.* Again, holding the part laterally to reduce tactile input, the therapist moves a joint up or down. Large and small ranges of motion are tested on representative large and small joints. In the upper extremity the shoulder,

elbow, forearm, wrist, index, and little fingers are often tested.

Response. After each stimulus, the patient indicates whether the joint was moved "up" or "down." The ability to distinguish large ranges but not small ones is an impairment of kinesthesia.

Combined or Cortical Sensations

Tactile Localization. Stimulus. The therapist touches the patient's skin with the fingertip. The stimulus is applied to distal and proximal areas.

Response. The patient places a finger on the spot touched after each stimulus. Accuracy is normally greatest in the hand and less precise proximally.[7] Note: Localization of touch, pressure, and pain stimuli are often tested. Localization may be tested separately or included with tests of recognition by having the patient indicate the location of the stimulus after indicating that is was felt. Eyes may be opened for localization. Measurements in millimeters or centimeters are taken so change can be recorded on reevaluation. Note if the limitation is large enough to be functionally significant. Werner and Omer[8] describe a more exact test of point localization in which the patient must place the end of a dowel on each spot touched by an aesthesiometer.

Evaluation and Treatment of Sensation **41**

Stereognosis. *Stimulus.* An easily recognizable object is placed in the involved hand. The object is to be identified by touch. Assistance in manipulation of the object may be required in the presence of paralysis.[11] Items commonly used include a coin, key, safety pin, pencil, or pen. A button, coin, and bottle cap are stimuli of approximately the same size requiring fine discrimination.[2] Presenting the items without previously showing them to the patient is a more difficult and critical test; but if the patient is unable to respond to this method of presentation, show the items and have the patient name them before testing.[2]

Response. The patient names the object or selects it from an array of objects placed in front of him if a nonverbal response is required. Astereognosis is the term used to designate an absence of stereognosis. Note: If touch is intact, stereognosis may be impaired. However, if stereognosis is intact, touch need not be tested.

Two-point Discrimination. *Stimulus.* Two points are applied simultaneously to an area of the skin. The distance between the two points is decreased on sequential presentations to determine how close together the points can be brought until the stimulus is perceived as one point. One point is applied in random order occasionally. Two-point discrimination is most refined in the fingertips where there are more receptors than in more proximal areas of the body. Normal two-point discrimination is 3 to 5 mm on the tips of the fingers and 7 to 10 mm near the base of the hand.[12] See Table 3.1. The stimulus is applied with a calibrated compass,[7, 8] a Boley gauge,[8] or a 2-point aesthesiometer.

Response. The patient says whether he felt "one" or "two" points, or for nonverbal patients holding up one or two fingers can indicate the response.

Other tests which may be performed but usually are not done unless stereognosis and two-point discrimination are impaired[2] include:

1. Weight discrimination—the patient determines the weight difference of blocks which are the same size, but different weights.[2, 7]

2. Size discrimination—the patient determines the size difference of blocks which are the same weight and shape, but different sizes.[2]
3. Texture discrimination—the patient is asked to identify various textures of fabrics.[2, 7]
4. Graphesthesia—the patient is asked to identify a number[2, 7] or letter[7] drawn in his palm (facing toward the patient). The blunt end of a pen is used to draw on the skin.[2]

Bilateral Simultaneous Stimulation. *Stimulus.* The therapist touches the patient simultaneously on both hands or other homologous parts.

Response. The patient says where he was touched. In right hemisphere damage[10] of the parietal lobe[2] the stimulus on the left may not be perceived by this test, although responses were intact when the extremity was tested individually.[10]

If two simultaneous stimuli are applied on the same side the more proximal one may be perceived with extinction of the distal stimulus.[2] Ayres[3] notes that recognition of the more proximal stimulus is most necessary for survival, *i.e.*, a person can live longer without a hand than without his face.

Patient participation in sensory testing is recognized as a variable influencing results. Wolf *et al.*[13] had patients read a statement encouraging their attention and accurate responses. Active participation was increased and there was some evidence of improved sensory reception, but further investigation with more subjects is needed.

There have been efforts to establish objective methods of sensory evaluation. Renfrew[14] devised a depth sense aesthesiometer. He states that two-point discrimination tests space sense on a plan parallel to the skin and suggests use of the depth sense aesthesiometer to test space sense in the fingertip on a plane at right angles to the skin. He found loss of depth sense in patients with intact two-point discrimination, and in some patients depth sense loss was the only sensory sign in the upper extremities. Electronic devices to measure sensation are being developed and may become more common in clinical use as well as for

Table 3.1
NORMAL THRESHOLDS FOR THE VOLAR SURFACE[a]

	Zone	Thumb (mm)	Index (mm)	Long (mm)	Ring (mm)	Little (mm)
Between tip and DIP joints	7	3–5	3–5	3–5	3–5	3–5
Between DIP and PIP joints	6		3–6	3–6	3–6	3–6
Between PIP and MP joints	5	4–7	4–7	4–7	4–7	4–7
Between web and distal palmar crease	4		5–8	5–8	5–8	5–8
Between distal palmar crease and center of palm	3		6–9	6–9	6–9	6–9
Rest of palm	1 and 2		7–10	7–10	7–10	7–10

[a]Reprinted with permission from G. E. Omer.[12]

research. Wolf *et al.*[13] describe application of pressure with a force transducer, measurement of sensory conduction velocity, and quantification of two-point discrimination measurements. Dyck *et al.*[15] describe a computerized system to evaluate touch-pressure, vibration, and temperature; a printout of results is immediately provided.

Interpreting the Results

Reliability of test results depends upon the skill and consistency of the tester to administer the tests and to record the results. Reliability also depends upon the ability of the patient to communicate accurate responses. As in any evaluation, reliability of retest results increases if the same person tests under conditions very similar to the previous test situation. Kent[11] tested 50 adult hemiplegic patients for sensory and motor deficits and retested the same persons 1 to 7 days later. She found the specific tests used to measure stereognosis and position sense highly reliable ($r = 0.97$ and $r = 0.90$, respectively). The test for two-point discrimination was not very reliable; the Pearson product moment coefficients ranged from 0.59 to 0.82, depending on the area of the body tested.

The location of absent and impaired responses must be compared to peripheral nerve and dermatomal distributions to determine the extent and specific nature of the sensory dysfunction. When peripheral nerves are involved, recovery of function proceeds proximally to distally. In the proximal area where the nerve is normal, you would expect intact functioning; where the nerve is recovering, you would expect impaired functioning; and where the nerve has not yet recovered, you would expect an absence of sensation. Reevaluation will indicate the recovery process.

In traumatic spinal cord injury, sensory loss will occur in the dermatomes below the level of the lesion. Dermatomal distribution is such that unless the spinal cord is anatomically or physiologically transected, or more than one dorsal root is involved in dorsal root damage, loss of sensation may be undetected because the areas served by dorsal roots overlap.

Sensory impairment as a result of cortical dysfunction does not follow the dermatomal distribution seen in dorsal root or spinal cord injury nor the peripheral nerve distribution as seen in injuries to specific peripheral nerves. Damage to the sensory cortex results in total or partial loss of discriminative sensations. Parts of the body are represented in the sensory cortex by a sensory homunculus located in an upside-down position similar to the homuncular distribution in the motor cortex. Because the sensory cortex covers a wide cortical area, a localized lesion usually affects a limited part of the contralateral side of the body. The loss is usually distal in either the upper or lower extremity, depending upon the site of the lesion,[16] because distal parts have a larger representation in the sensory cortex than do proximal parts, and there is therefore more likelihood that a lesion would affect these sites.

Lesions in the brain stem can involve all sensory modalities to a varying extent. If the thalamus is involved a "thalamic syndrome" results in which the threshold for touch, temperature, and pain sensations is decreased on the contralateral side, and there is an overreaction to stimuli. Even mild stimuli may produce exaggerated and painful sensations.[17]

TREATMENT

Hyposensitivity

As of this writing no consistently effective therapeutic regimen has been reported to restore or retrain sensory function. Treatment is primarily aimed at teaching the patient to compensate for lost or impaired sensation in order to avoid injury and to improve motor performance. Since sensation from the periphery is a major source of feedback necessary for coordinated limb movement, loss of this feedback must be compensated for visually. In order to protect himself from injury, as well as to move with some degree of coordination, the patient must watch the movements of his extremities. A patient with kinesthetic loss could not accurately use the involved limb in the dark. The patient must constantly attend to situations in order to anticipate potential dangers. Although vision is the primary means of compensation, auditory stimuli, such as a bell or bracelet attached to the distal part of the extremity, may be a worthwhile adjunct.

Sensory retraining is a potential method of treatment. Some attempts at sensory retraining have been made by therapists who used techniques of rubbing the limb vigorously with terry toweling before repetitively moving the limb. Another technique, used to improve stereognosis, involved having the patient feel the object first with the eyes occluded and then with the eyes open for immediate feedback and reinforcement. The therapist discusses the various qualities of the stimuli with the patient in an attempt to help the patient to note cognitively the characteristics of various stimuli in order to recognize them on subsequent presentations. The stimuli are graded in such a way to require only gross awareness or discrimination initially and more refined responses as the patient's accuracy improves. Vinograd *et al.*[18] used this method and reported limited success in increasing manual dexterity of patient with cortical sensory deficits in hemiplegia, but their patients failed to learn to use the arm spontaneously, as had been hoped. Ferreri[19] reports evidence that sensory retraining can alleviate astereognosis to some degree in spastic cerebral palsied adults. In both reports large objects were easier for patients to identify than small ones.

Wynn Parry[4] describes the use of different shapes, weights, and textures in sensory retraining of patients following peripheral nerve injury as soon as some appreciation of sensation has returned. Identification of items is first attempted when the patient is blindfolded. Then the blindfold is removed so that patient can see and feel the objects simultaneously for the purpose of reestablishing central nervous system temporal and spatial patterns and images. Four 10-minute sessions per day are recommended, and positive results have been noted. Retraining of localization of tactile stimuli was highly successful using a similar technique of attempting to localize a stimulus and then looking to see where the stimulus was applied.

Hypersensitivity

Hypersensitivity is a sensory problem which therapists have had success in modifying by treatment. Graded, repetitive tactile stimuli are used to desensitize. The material used and the force applied are graded in conjunction with each other. Materials are graded from soft to hard to rough; force is graded from touch to rub to tap. Due to the patient's anticipation of pain, a program of desensitization is best carried out by the patient himself under the direction of the therapist.[20] Use of activities which involve graded texture and force is a means of implementing this program. For an example of a touching sequence, a patient could finger-feed marshmallows, then raw carrots, and then progress to pretzels. For an example of a rubbing sequence, the patient could pet the family cat, then finger paint, and then build castles in the sand. For an example of a tapping sequence, the patient could juggle or toss cotton balls, then ping pong balls, and increasingly heavier or textured balls. One example of a combination sequence in which the patient touches, rubs, and taps graded textures would be as follows: by the time the patient can touch sandpaper, he may be able to rub wood and tap cotton. To compensate for hypersensitivity, objects may need to be padded or wrapped to soften the surface. Wynn Parry[4] reports success in the use of electrical stimulation to reduce hyperaesthesia from neuroma following suture of peripheral nerves.

Anesthesia

Absence of sensation, especially of a large area of the body as occurs in spinal cord injury, for example, is a particularly serious problem. The patient is neither aware of the discomfort of remaining in the same position for a long time, nor, due to accompanying paralysis, is he easily able to change his position to relieve pressure. Pressure over bony prominences causes redness of the skin which is treated by the use of a wheelchair cushion, an alternating air mattress or sheepskin in bed, and changing position to relieve the pressure. If unnoticed, however, continued pressure on these susceptible areas causes loss of blood supply and tissue breakdown, resulting in a decubitus ulcer. Therefore, skin which is anesthetic must be visually inspected with frequency and care to identify and begin treatment of minor problems before they intensify. Skin areas which are not easily seen may be inspected by use of mirrors. Burns and abrasions are other possible mishaps which should be detected and treated early.

Although it is usual to associate prolonged unchanged position with development of decubiti, any prolonged pressure, such as that produced by an ill-fitting hand splint, can cause decubiti. Patients can be trained to recognize potentially dangerous amounts of pressure concentrated in small areas and to take the responsibility for maintaining the integrity of their own skin.

Brand[21] offers practical suggestions for relief of localized pressure, temperature hazards, or mechanical stresses in insensitive extremities. For the lower extremity ideas include changing shoes several times a day, wearing insoles, reducing walking distances, and use of a carpet on the floor of the car where overheating is a frequent hazard. For the upper extremity it is suggested to replace small handles and knobs with larger and rounded ones, to vary the use of tools or wear gloves or change hands.

Adjuncts to sensory training are becoming available as biomedical engineering advances. Some that are currently in use include the following. Electronic pressure-sensitive transducers are useful to obtain information from circumscribed areas, but are inadequate for obtaining information about whole hand usage because the number of transducers required to cover all potential areas of pressure in the hand makes their use clinically impractical. Pressure-sensitive microcapsules, an idea developed by the staff at United States Public Health Service Hospital in Carville, Louisiana, are clinically useful. The microcapsules break down under pressure and produce a color change in the material in which they are imbedded in proportion to the pressure exerted.[22] The material in which the capsules are imbedded can be made into socks, gloves, or other garments. The patient learns to avoid excessive pressure by adjusting or adapting his methods of performing tasks according to the intensity of the dye released in a given area.[23]

References

1. Chusid, S. G. *Correlative Neuroanatomy & Functional Neurology*, 17th ed. Los Altos, Calif.: Lange Medical Publications, 1979.
2. Paine, R. S., and Oppé, T. E. *Neurological Examination of Children*. In *Clinics in Developmental Medicine*, Vol. 20–21. London: Spastics Society Medical Education and Information Unit in Association with William Heinemann Medical Books, 1966.
3. Ayres, A. J. *Sensory Integration and Learning Disorders*. Los Angeles: Western Psychological Services, 1972.
4. Wynn Parry, C. B. Management of peripheral nerve injuries and traction lesions of the brachial plexus. *Int. Rehabil. Med.*, *1*(1): 9–20, 1978.
5. Johansson, R. S. Tactile sensibility in the human hand: Receptive field characteristics of mechanoreceptive units in the glabrous skin area. *J. Physiol.*, 281: 101–123, 1978.
6. Johansson, R. S., and Vallbo, A. B. Tactile sensibility in the human hand: Relative and absolute densities of four types of mechanoreceptive units in glabrous skin. *J. Physiol.*, *286*: 283–300, 1979.
7. Alpers, B. J., and Mancall, E. L. *Essentials of the Neurological Examination*. Philadelphia: F. A. Davis, 1971.
8. Werner, J. L., and Omer, G. E., Jr. Evaluating cutaneous pressure sensation of the hand. *Am. J. Occup. Ther.*, 24(5): 347–356, 1970.
9. Von Prince, K., and Butler, B., Jr. Measuring sensory function of the hand in peripheral nerve injuries. *Am. J. Occup. Ther.*, 21(6): 385–395, 1967.
10. Bender, M. B. Modification of the sensory examination. *J. Mt. Sinai Hosp.*, 33(3): 221–224, 1966.
11. Kent, B. E. Sensory-motor testing: The upper limb of adult patients with hemiplegia. *J.A.P.T.A.*, 45(6): 550–561, 1965.

12. Omer, G. E. Evaluation and reconstruction of the forearm and hand after acute traumatic peripheral nerve injuries. *J. Bone Joint Surg.*, *50-A*(7): 1454–1478, 1968.
13. Wolf, S. L., Nahai, F., Brown, D., Jordan, N., and Kutner, M. Objective determinations of sensibility in the upper extremity. *Phys. Ther.*, *57*(10): 1132–1137, 1977.
14. Renfrew, S. Fingertip sensation. *Lancet*, February 22, 396–397, 1969.
15. Dyck, P. J., Zimmerman, I. R., O'Brien, P. C., Ness, A., Caskey, P. E., Karnes, J., and Bushek, W. Introduction of automated systems to evaluate touch-pressure, vibration, and thermal cutaneous sensation in man. *Ann. Neurol.*, *4*(6): 502–510, 1978.
16. Bannister, R. *Brain's Clinical Neurology*, 4th ed. London: Oxford University Press, 1973.
17. Noback, C. *The Human Nervous System.* New York: McGraw-Hill, 1967.
18. Vinograd, A., Taylor, E., and Grossman, S. Sensory re-training of the hemiplegic hand. *Am. J. Occup. Ther.*, *16*(5): 246–250, 1962.
19. Ferreri, J. Intensive stereognostic training: Effect on spastic cerebral palsied adults. *Am. J. Occup. Ther.*, *16*(3): 141–142, 1962.
20. Unpublished notes from course, "Hand Rehabilitation." Chapel Hill: University of North Carolina, 1968.
21. Brand, P. W. Management of the insensitive limb. *Phys. Ther.*, *59*(1): 8–12, 1979.
22. Brand, P., and James, E. A pain substitute pressure assessment in the insensitive limb. *Am. J. Occup. Ther.*, *23*(6): 479–486, 1969.
23. Wood, H. Prevention of deformity in the insensitive hand: The role of the therapist. *Am. J. Occup. Ther.*, *23*(6): 488–489, 1969.

Supplementary Reading

Dellon, A. L. *Evaluation of Sensibility and Re-education of Sensation in the Hand.* Baltimore: Williams & Wilkins, 1981.
Dellon, A. L. The moving two-point discrimination test: Clinical evaluation of the quickly adapting fiber/receptor system. *J. Hand Surg.*, *3*(5): 474–481, 1978.
Dellon, A. L., Curtis, R. M., and Edgerton, M. T. Evaluating recovery of sensation in the hand following nerve injury. *Johns Hopkins Med. J.*, *130* (April): 235–243, 1972.
Wynn Parry, C. B., and Salter, M. Sensory re-education after median nerve lesions. *Hand*, *8*(3): 250–257, 1976.

chapter

4

Evaluation of Motor Control

Anna Deane Scott, M.Ed., OTR

When evaluating a patient with central nervous system dysfunction, consideration must be given to all influences on coordinated voluntary control of movement. Perry[1] notes that motor control occurs at six levels, including the cerebral cortex, basal ganglia, midbrain, brain stem, spinal cord, and reflex arc. In normal motor performance the cerebral cortex discriminates sensory input and controls motor output with the assistance of the sensorimotor activity of lower centers moderating muscle tone and patterns of movement. Damage to the brain leaves the lower centers without cerebral control, and pathological motions and reactions appear. Although the problems are manifested and evaluated peripherally, the deficits are not actually of the peripheral structures but only observed in these structures due to their release from cortical control. Evaluation must consider sensation; range of motion; muscle tone; reflex integration, automatic reactions and control of postures; coordinated control of voluntary movement; strength; and endurance.

SENSATION

The evaluation of sensation has been described in Chapter 3. The importance of sensation in the regulation of motor control has been supported by many research studies in which deafferentation of an extremity resulted in incoordinated use of the extremity.[2]

RANGE OF MOTION

Passive range of motion is evaluated by moving the patient's joints slowly and carefully through as full a range of motion as possible at each joint and recording measurements taken. Chapter 7 describes the method of measuring and recording joint range of motion. In central nervous system dysfunction passive range of motion is influenced by muscle tone. If muscle tone is increased, resistance to movement will be felt. This resistance can be overcome by maintaining a steady force against the resistance until the muscles relax and permit movement to continue. In spasticity a faster speed of movement may increase the strength of resistance,[3] so range of motion should be done slowly to avoid eliciting the stretch reflex. If muscle tone is decreased, hypermobility of joints will be noted and hyperextension may be found in joints which do not normally hyperextend. The affected shoulder of hemiplegic patients is prone to subluxation as a result of weakness of the supraspinatus, stretching of ligaments supporting the superior capsule, and abduction of the humerus which prevents functioning of the locking mechanism of the glenoid fossa.[4] It would seem that range of motion of the shoulder of the hemiplegic patient should be done with approximation of the head of the humerus and care during rotation to avoid overstretching the muscles of the rotator cuff.

MUSCLE TONE

Muscle tone is defined as the resistance a muscle offers to passive stretch. When a muscle is elongated, or stretched, the muscle contracts to resist the stretch with the response proportionate to the magnitude of the stretch. There are both tonic and phasic components of the stretch reflex.

The primary afferent endings (Ia) respond to both static (tonic) and dynamic (phasic) stretch, have a low threshold for stretch,[2] and are the only afferents which respond to a single, brief stretch[5] and to vibration.[2, 5] Change in length of muscle and the rate or velocity of the change affect the response to stretch via the Ia fibers. A sudden length change produces a phasic or fast response due to the Ia endings around the nuclear bag fibers[2] and a tonic or more maintained response due to the Ia endings around the nuclear chain fibers which respond more slowly to a change in length but maintain the response longer.[6] The Ia afferents have a monosynaptic connection to the alpha motor neuron of the muscle stretched. The Ia facilitates the muscle stretched, inhibits the antagonist via an interneuron, and connects with polysynaptic spinal pathways which possibly alter the effect of stretch via other pathways. The knee jerk and other tendon tapping procedures which dynamically elongate a muscle or its tendon and cause a phasic response are examples of Ia activation.[2]

The secondary afferents (II) have a high threshold for stretch and respond to static stretch exclusively, *i.e.*, a tonic or maintained stretch.[2] As the muscle is lengthened the firing of II fibers is increased. The II afferents have polysynaptic connections in the spinal cord via interneurons. Facilitation or inhibition via interneurons is influenced by input from supraspinal centers to a great extent. The classical view on which some clinical procedures have been based holds that the II afferents facilitate flexors and inhibit extensors. According to this view, when an extensor muscle is lengthened the II fibers would inhibit this muscle and thus reduce its response to a Ia brief or dynamic stretch. However, if a flexor muscle is lengthened the II fibers would facilitate this muscle and increase its response to a quick stretch. Discrepancies and uncertainties remain with regard to the function of the II afferent fibers.[7]

Studies of patients with spinal cord injuries have supported this classical concept of the function of the II afferent fibers. In studies of patients with brain lesions, however, the lengthened position of muscles has produced varying responses with no consistency relative to the site of the lesion.[7]

The gamma motor neurons affect stretch sensitivity of the muscle spindle via dynamic and static fusimotor fibers. P. B. C. Matthews[2] proposes that the dynamic fibers bias or increase the tautness of the muscle spindle and thereby increase the sensitivity of the primary ending to small stimuli and increase the response to large stretches. The static fibers control intrafusal muscle shortening when the extrafusal muscle is shortening. When the gamma motor neuron fires, the ends of the intrafusal muscle fibers contract. Both ends shorten so that the centers of the fibers are stretched, stimulating the primary afferent fiber. This is called internal stretch to differentiate it from the stretch applied by direct lengthening of the entire muscles (Fig. 4.1).

The Golgi tendon organs are receptors for changes in muscle tension. Impulses from Golgi tendon organs are transmitted by the Ib fibers, which have polysynaptic connections in the spinal cord. The Golgi tendon organs have a high threshold for a stretch stimulus and are activated when a muscle is stretched beyond the maximal length it normally has in the body. The Golgi tendon organ, however, has a low threshold for tension created by muscle contraction and assists in regulating the strength of muscle contraction. When

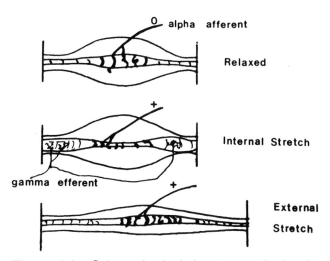

Figure 4.1 Schematic depicting two methods of causing stretch of muscle spindle, internal stretch and external stretch. (Modified from T. Twitchell.[36])

stimulated either by stretch or by contraction, the Golgi tendon organs inhibit development of tension in the same muscle and facilitate the antagonist.[2]

Evaluation of Muscle Tone

Since muscle tone is the resistance a muscle offers to passive stretch, passive movement of the extremities is used to evaluate tone. The range of motion (ROM) available in each joint should be determined before assessing muscle tone. A process often used in evaluation is to determine the available pain-free range for a joint by moving the part slowly; then the part is moved quickly within the available range to elicit a Ia response to stretch. If tone is increased there will be increased resistance to passive movement. The strength of the resistance increases with the velocity of movement[3]; therefore, the velocity must be similar at each testing in order for test-retest results to be reliable. In spasticity there will be a range of free movement, then a strong contraction of the muscle in response to stretch followed by free movement when the muscle relaxes with continued stretch. The sudden relaxation is termed the clasp-knife reaction and has been attributed to Golgi tendon organ inhibition. Matthews[2] suggests that such an abrupt cessation of contraction cannot be explained on that basis only and proposes that continued stretch exceeds the threshold of a central "all-or-none" mechanism which stops the stretch reflex. If present, spasticity of the muscle or muscle group being stretched is recorded as *mild* if a muscle can be lengthened quickly through most of its ROM with the stretch reflex occurring in the last one-fourth of the range, *moderate* if the stretch reflex occurs in midrange, and *severe* if it occurs in the initial one-fourth of the range in which the muscle is shortened. Questions occur concerning how to record spasticity when ROM is limited. Often the increased muscle tone has contributed significantly to the development of the range limitation. For example, if the elbow can be moved from full flexion to a position of 90° of flexion and a ROM limitation prevents further extension, a stretch reflex occurring just before 90° as the elbow is quickly extended would be recorded as moderate spasticity of the flexors and suspected of being contributory to the ROM limitation.

In rigidity there will be resistance to movement throughout the range of motion unless there is cogwheel rigidity, as in Parkinson's disease, in which the tremor superimposed on rigidity causes alternate contraction and relaxation throughout the range of the muscle being stretched.[8] Spasticity and rigidity may both be present in a muscle group; they are not mutually exclusive. In moving the part through a range of motion the resistance of rigidity will be felt initially, and a stretch reflex may be elicited later in the range.

In flaccidity, tone is decreased and there will be decreased resistance to passive movement. The extremity can be moved freely without the tension of stretch sensitivity present in normal muscles. Sometimes an entire extremity is flaccid, but in some patients there may be flaccidity in muscles of some joints of an extremity when muscles at other joints are spastic.

The distribution pattern of increased, decreased, and normal tone should be recorded as well as the severity of the dysfunction. The usual pattern of spasticity in brain-injured persons is increased tone in the flexor/adductor groups and decreased tone in the extensor/abductor groups.

The Bobaths assess tone by moving the person in normal postural patterns in order to evaluate the adaptation of different muscle groups to changes in body position involving both dynamic and static components of stretch. If reflex activity still dominates movement, tone will change in different body parts as body position changes. Therefore evaluation of tone in postural patterns is valuable in treatment planning. Resistance to movement into the different positions is noted. A quick, immediate adjustment of muscles to postural changes reflects normal tone. Undue resistance to changes in posture may be a result of rigidity or spasticity. Spasticity is described as severe, moderate, or slight. Undue lack of resistance and hypermobility of joints denotes flaccidity. In children with athetosis, tone may fluctuate from increased to absent resistance in response to change of position. The positions used by Bobath for evaluation of muscle tone in adult hemiplegia and cerebral palsy are described in Chapter 6.

THE INFLUENCES OF REFLEXES ON MOTOR FUNCTION

A reflex is an involuntary, stereotyped response to a particular stimulus. Reflex responses to stimuli develop in fetal life and continue to dominate motor behavior in early infancy.

Reflex motor behavior underlies many of the organized voluntary movements used in daily activities and sports[9]; these become increasingly apparent with increased stress and/or fatigue.[10] However, the reflexes demonstrated by the normal person differ in quality from those observed in persons with brain damage. The movement of the normal person is flexible; he can move in and out of reflex patterns while the stimulus remains in operation. However, the movement of the person with brain damage is often obligatory; he cannot change posture while controlled by the stimulus. Obligatory primitive reflexes occur as a result of CNS damage[10] and indicate the presence of severe motor disability.[11] When brain damage occurs in early development, as in cerebral palsy, the higher levels of control may be delayed in development, and the spinal cord and lower brain stem reflexes remain dominant beyond the age when they would normally diminish. Therapy is aimed at establishing maturationally based normal motor patterns. When cortical damage occurs in the adult, as in hemiplegia following a cerebrovascular accident, primitive reflexes may again be released from higher control and inhibition. However, in therapy the adult patients are working toward regaining motor patterns once established and now lost.

Voluntary movements are supported by automatic postural patterns—righting and equilibrium. Righting and equilibrium reactions enable the individual to move against gravity, align the body, and maintain balance.[10, 12] As these reactions develop, the more primitive reflexes diminish.[10] In normal development the integration of primitive reflexes is necessary for development of purposeful movements.[11]

Reflexes are a part of normal motor development, but if primitive reflexes persist beyond the appropriate age they interfere with development beyond that level. If brain damage occurs in persons who have already developed normally, it results in release of primitive reflexes from higher control; these stereotyped movement patterns reappear and interfere with regaining voluntary motor control.

Disturbances of reflex integration and tone produce stereotyped postures and movements in association with the person's voluntary attempts to move.

The influence of the positive supporting reaction is to increase extensor tone in standing, resulting in an inability to flex the lower extremities alternately in walking. The plantar flexion component of the positive supporting reaction places the weight on the balls of the feet and contributes to a lack of heel strike in the gait. When the lower extremities are flexed, when changing to or from sitting and standing positions, the individual is unable to support his weight on the flexed extremity. The crossed extension reflex may be combined with a positive supporting reaction in a standing position to reinforce extension of the affected extremity in spastic hemiplegia.[10] When the patient attempts to creep in a quadruped position the crossed extension reflex prevents reciprocal leg movement because the extended leg cannot be flexed.[13] Once the positive supporting reaction is inhibited and a negative supporting reaction develops the lower extremities can be flexed in walking, and extensor tone is modified to permit the slow relaxation required to raise or lower the body when rising from or assuming a sitting position, for ascending or descending stairs, and for reciprocal crawling.[10]

The asymmetrical tonic neck reflex prevents rolling from supine to prone because the scapula retracts on the skull side extremity, preventing bringing that arm across, and the arm extends on the face side extremity, the direction toward which rolling is attempted.[13] In sitting, flexion of the extremities on one side contributes to a loss of balance.[10] In a quadruped position the extremities on the skull side may collapse into flexion when the head is turned.[13] There may be an inability to maintain a standing position due to lack of stability resulting from flexion of the skull side lower extremity when the head turns. The asymmetrical tonic neck reflex may be so strong in patients with central nervous system damage that arm movement can be controlled only by turning the head. Contractures of the extremities, dislocated hip, and scoliosis may develop from a maintained position to one side due to a strong ATNR response.[10]

The symmetrical tonic neck reflex contributes to difficulty in maintaining a quadruped position. Flexion of the head causes the arms to flex and the patient collapses forward. Extension of the head causes the arms to extend and the legs to flex, and the patient sits back on the flexed legs.[10, 13] This sitting position is often observed in young children with spasticity and "bunny hopping" in this position can be the means of locomotion used.

The tonic labyrinthine reflex (TLR) prevents extension of the head in a prone position due to increased flexor tone. Strong extensor tone in a supine position prevents lifting the head in flexion and sitting up unassisted. If assisted to a sitting position the patient can remain sitting unless his head extends and increased extensor tone causes him to fall backwards.[10] The TLR also prevents rolling over from a supine position, and attempts to roll over increase extension to the extent that the back arches into hyperextension.[13] When the patient is supine, the TLR prevents flexion of the trunk and extremities, and bilateral hand activities requiring bringing the hands together in flexion cannot be accomplished.[14]

The tonic reflexes interact to reinforce or negate each other so that observed motor behavior is most often the interaction of several reflexes rather than the domination of any one.[10]

With the development of the labyrinthine righting reaction the tonic labyrinthine reflex is inhibited and the head can be lifted against gravity. The head can be extended in prone and the trunk then extends to a full prone extension position completely counteracting the influence of the tonic labyrinthine reflex in prone. Flexion of the head in supine is also possible when the labyrinthine righting reaction develops, and supine flexion counteracts the influence of the tonic labyrinthine reflex in supine[12, 14] and indicates integration of the tonic reflex. When the body righting reflex develops to replace neck righting, the trunk follows the head with trunk rotation. The influence of body righting is also seen in the labyrinthine righting and optic righting reactions when in upright position the body is moved laterally, forward, and backwards; the head rights itself to face vertical, and the trunk follows with a rotation component to align the trunk with the head. With a body righting reaction and inhibition of the tonic neck reflexes the individual can roll over to prone. A developmental sequence then follows in which the ability to roll over is combined with a labyrinthine righting reaction and inhibition of other tonic reflexes to a progression from rolling over to prone extension, on elbows, on hands and knees, to sitting and standing. Once a protective extension response develops the arms extend to protect the individual from falling over, and support on the extended arms helps to maintain a position. Cocontraction of proximal muscles in the supporting extremities develops from weight-bearing positions. Balance in each developmental position is achieved by equilibrium reactions in which the postural muscles contract to maintain or regain an upright position when equilibrium is challenged. Equilibrium reactions and protective extension are usually seen together as normal reactions to threatened loss of balance.

Reflex Testing of the Adult Patient

Reflex testing is done by applying the appropriate stimulus and observing the response. If the reflex response occurs, the reflex is *positive*; if the response does not occur, the reflex is *negative*. Neither positive nor negative can be equated with normal without considering whether a positive or negative response is normal for the age of the individual evaluated. When evaluating adults, no spinal or brain stem reflexes are normal.

Reflexes can be tested when the person is in various positions as long as the stimulus can be applied and the response is not prevented by the position or will not cause him harm.

Innate Primary Reactions

Innate primary reactions are reflexive primitive movements which involve total flexion and extension synergies of the proximal body parts. These reflexes may be present in the adult closed head injury patient. They are indicative of severe brain damage. Their absence on reevaluation is a sign of progress in recovery.

Automatic Walking[10] ***or Primitive Stepping.***[15] Birth to 1 month.[15]

Test Position. Hold the patient in an upright position allowing some weight bearing on his feet.[15]

Stimulus. Lean the patient forward.[10, 15]

Response. Automatic walking steps with regular rhythm and heel strike.[10, 15]

Placing Reaction of the Lower Limb. Birth to 1 month.[15]

Test Position. The adult patient can be supine or in a sitting position.

Stimulus. Brush the dorsum of the patient's foot against the edge of board or stiff cardboard.

Response. Flexion of the leg with placement of the foot as if to place the foot on top of the stimulating surface.[10, 15]

Placing Reaction of the Upper Limb. Birth to 6 months.[13]

Test Position. Place the adult patient in a sitting or supine position.

Stimulus. Brush the dorsum of one of the patient's hands against the under edge of a table[10, 13] or the edge of a stiff cardboard.

Response. Flexion of the arm with placement of the hand onto the table top.[13]

Moro Reflex. Birth to 6 months.[10, 15]

Stimulus. Several stimuli evoke the same response. A loud noise near the patient's head, sudden movement of the supporting surface, or dropping the patient backwards from a semisitting position may be used as the stimulus.[15] If the patient is in a wheelchair it can be tipped backward.

Response. Abduction, extension, and external rotation of the arms with abduction and extension of the fingers[16] followed by flexion to the midline.[13]

The Moro reflex as originally described was a response to the vestibular stimulation of being tipped off balance,[10] whereas the response to a noise was originally termed a startle reaction.[17] These are considered to be the same reaction in most neurology and developmental texts. By either name the response involves the total body and is differentiated from the jump or matured startle response to a loud noise seen in normal adults.

Grasp Reflex. Birth to 3 to 4 months.[13]

Stimulus. Apply pressure in the palm of the hand from the ulnar side.

Response. Finger flexion with a strong grip that persists and resists removal of the stimulus object.

Sucking Reflex. Birth to 3 to 4 months.[13]

Stimulus. Place a finger on the patient's lips.

Response. Sucking motion of the lips.

Rooting Reflex. Birth to 3 to 4 months.[13]

Stimulus. Stroke outward on the corner of the patient's mouth.

Response. The lower lip, tongue, and head move toward the stimulus.

Spinal Level Reflexes

These are phasic reflexes of total flexion or extension.[10, 16]

Flexor Withdrawal. Birth to 2 months.[15, 16]

Test Position. The patient is supine or sitting with head in midposition and legs extended.[16]

Stimulus. A quick tactile stimulus applied to the sole of one foot.[15, 16] A stimulus therapists often use is to scrape the thumbnail from the heel to the ball of the patient's foot.

Response. Uncontrolled flexion of the entire leg.[15, 16]

Extensor Thrust. Birth to 2 months.[16]

Test Position. The patient is supine or sitting with head in midposition. One leg is in extension and the other leg is fully flexed.[16]

Stimulus. Apply pressure to the ball of the foot of the flexed leg.[10, 15]

Response. Uncontrolled extension of the stimulated leg.[15, 16]

Crossed Extension. Birth to 2 months.[16]

Test Position. The patient is supine with head in midposition. One leg is in extension and the other leg is fully flexed.[15, 16]

Stimulus. Passively flex the extended leg.[15]

Response. Extension of the opposite leg with hip adduction and internal rotation.[15]

It is unsafe to test for this reflex while the patient is sitting. With a strong positive response, the patient could slide forward out of the chair. A patient with hemiplegia who can stand on both legs without exaggerated tone can be tested standing. The patient is asked to flex the noninvolved leg; a strong increase in extensor tone in the involved leg indicates a positive crossed extension reflex.[10] Guard the patient to prevent falling.

Brain Stem Reflexes

These are tonic or static reflexes which involve sustained changes in postural muscle tone affecting the whole body or more than one part of the body. By changing the position of the head relative to the body or the position of the head (and body) in space the proprioceptors located in the neck or in the vestibular apparatus are stimulated. The resultant changes in muscle tone are maintained as long as the stimulus is applied. These responses build up gradually, and the stimulus for each of the following reflexes should be held to allow time for the response in cases of less severe involvement when the response may occur more slowly after several seconds' delay.[10]

Asymmetrical Tonic Neck Reflex (ATNR). Birth to 4 months.[15]

Test Position. The patient is supine or sitting with arms and legs extended.[16]

Stimulus. Passively or actively turn the head 90° to one side.[15]

Response. Extension of limbs on the face side and flexion of limbs on the skull side. If the reflex response is weak there may be no motion of the extremities, but a change of tone can be noted in the extremities.[15, 16]

Repeat the stimulus to the other side.

Evaluation in quadruped position is more stressful and positive responses will be more readily elicited than in supine or sitting in patients with minimal reflex responses. Rotate the patient's head to the side; elbow flexion of the skull side arm indicates a positive response.

Sieg and Shuster[18] stress that the quality and intensity of the response should be observed. Speed of response and obvious attitudinal changes indicate the intensity of the response. Quality is observed in noting which components of the response are present under which conditions.

Symmetrical Tonic Neck Reflex (STNR). Birth to 4 to 5 months.[15, 16]

Test Position. The patient is prone over the therapist's knees, in a quadruped position,[16] or sitting.

Stimulus 1. Flex the patient's head, bringing his chin toward his chest.[15, 16]

Response. Flexion of the upper extremities and extension of the lower extremities.[15, 16]

Stimulus 2. Extend the patient's head.[15, 16]

Response. Extension of the upper extremities and flexion of the lower extremities.[15, 16]

If the reflex response is weak there may only be a change of tone noted rather than motion of the extremities.

Tonic Labyrinthine Reflex (TLR)—Prone. Birth to 4 months.[15, 16]

Test Position. The patient is prone with head in midposition.[16]

Stimulus. The test position is the stimulus.[16]

Response. Flexion of the extremities or increased flexor tone.[15]

If there is severe extensor spasticity there may still be extension in the prone position but with relatively weaker extensor tone than in a supine position.[10]

Tonic Labyrinthine Reflex—Supine. Birth to 4 months.[15, 16]

Test Position. The patient is supine with head in midposition.[16]

Stimulus. The test position is the stimulus.[16]

Response. Extension of the extremities or increased extensor tone.[15]

Positive Supporting Reaction. Birth to 6 months.[15]

Test Position. The patient is placed in an upright standing position,[15, 16] if possible, or supine or sitting.

Stimulus. Contact of the ball of the foot to the floor and stretch of the muscles of the foot.[10, 19]

Response. Extension of the lower extremity with cocontraction of flexors and extensors resulting in a stiff and rigid extension of the lower extremity.[10, 19]

Associated Reactions. These occur normally throughout life when attempting strenuous activities but are more widespread in central nervous system dysfunction when there is increased tone.[20] These are tonic reactions acting from one extremity to another.[10, 20]

Test Position. May be tested in any position.

Stimulus. Squeeze an object with one hand (the noninvolved hand if hemiplegic).[9, 16] Or resist any motion.

Response. Grasp[16] and flexion or an increase of flexor tone in the opposite upper extremity[10] will occur, or any motion used as stimulus will be mimicked.

In spastic hemiplegia associated reactions can also be elicited from one spastic extremity to the other spastic extremity on the same side of the body[10, 20] during stress.

Midbrain Reactions

These reactions permit a normal distribution of tone and active righting movements to bring the head and body into a normal relationship with each other in space.[16]

Neck Righting. Birth to 6 months.[16]

Test Position. The patient is supine with arms and legs extended.[16]

Stimulus. Passively turn the head to one side and hold it in this position.[15]

Response. The body rotates as a whole in the direction to which the head was turned.[16]

Body Righting Acting on the Body. Six months to 4 to 5 years.[10, 15]

Test Position. The patient is supine with arms and legs extended.[16]

Stimulus. Passively or actively turn the head to one side.[10]

Response. Segmental rotation around the body axis so that the body rotates at the shoulder, then the trunk, and then the pelvis.[15, 16]

The stimulus is the same for neck righting and body righting acting on the body. The therapist observes the patient's response in order to differentiate between the two reactions. The stimulus is also the same as that for the ATNR; therefore, the appearances of the neck righting reaction is heralded as a maturational step forward from brain stem level control to midbrain control.

Labyrinthine Righting Acting on the Head— Prone. From 2 months throughout life.[16, 20]

Test Position. Blindfold the patient and suspend him in a prone position.[10, 16]

Stimulus. The prone position in space.[10, 16]

Response. The head is brought to a face vertical position.[10, 16]

In normal development this reflex enables the baby to raise his head in a prone position.

Labyrinthine Righting Acting on the Head— Supine. From 6 months throughout life.[16, 20]

Test Position. Blindfold the patient and suspend him in supine position.[10, 16]

Stimulus. The supine position in space.[10, 16]

Response. The head is brought to a face vertical position.[10, 16]

In normal development this reflex enables the baby to raise his head when pulled to a sitting position.

When testing labyrinthine righting reactions in adults the original test position of suspension in space is modified to a prone or supine position on a mat. The ability to voluntarily raise the head in prone or supine is a positive response.[10] To do the test on larger children and adults in order to involve only the labyrinthine input, contact with the mat surface can be eliminated by positioning the person with the head extended over the edge of a raised mat.

Automatic Movement Reactions

Protective Extension (Parachute Reaction). From 6 months throughout life.[16]

Test Position. Suspend the patient upside down in the air by his pelvis.[15, 16]

Stimulus. Move the patient's head suddenly toward the floor.[15, 16]

Again, this test procedure used with babies must be modified for adults. Bobath lists detailed tests for evaluation of protective extension in the adult hemiplegic patient.[19] One example is the following.

Place a straight chair next to the patient's wheelchair on the patient's involved side. Remove the arm of the wheelchair, if detachable. Push the patient to the involved side and observe if the protective extension response occurs. Repeat to the other side if there is bilateral involvement. Guard to protect the patient from falling. The responses can be elicited in kneel-standing and also in standing positions in which the person is pushed toward a wall.

Response. Extension of the arms with finger extension and abduction in an effort to break a fall to protect the head.[15, 16]

Equilibrium Reactions.

These are all automatic, protective reactions to being tipped to one side so that the center of gravity is disturbed. They are tested in various developmental positions. In all positions the reaction typically involves an increase in tone and protective extension movement of the extremities on the lowered side with abduction and extension of the opposite extremities to help regain balance. Equilibrium reactions probably modify righting reactions and are necessary for progress beyond the quadruped position. The development of equilibrium reactions in each position can be seen when the next higher developmental position can be assumed by a child.[10]

Prone. From 6 months throughout life.[10, 16]
Test Position. The patient is prone on a board or a a mat.[15, 16]
Stimulus. Tilt the board or mat to one side.[15, 16]
Response. The patient's head and upper trunk turn toward the raised side with abduction and extension of the extremities on the raised side and protective extension of the extremities on the lowered side.[15, 16]

Supine. From 8 months throughout life.[10, 15]
Test Position. The patient is supine on a board or a mat.[15, 16]
Stimulus. Tilt the board or mat to one side.[15, 16]
Response. Same as for equilibrium reaction in the prone position.

Quadruped. From 8 months throughout life.[16]
Test Position. The patient is on his hands and knees on a flat surface.[16]
Stimulus. Tilt the patient to one side by pushing against one side of his trunk.[6]
Response. The patient will right his head and upper trunk. There will be abduction and extension of the extremities on the raised side with protective extension of the extremities on the side to which he was tipped.[16]

Sitting. From 10 to 12 months throughout life.[10, 16]
Test Position. The patient is sitting on a chair.[15, 16]
Stimulus. Tilt the chair[15] or tilt the patient to one side by pushing against one side of his trunk.[10]
Response. Righting of the head and upper trunk with abduction and extension of the extremities on the raised side and protective extension of the extremities on the lowered side.[15, 16]

Kneel-Standing. From 15 months throughout life.[16]
Test Position. The patient is on his knees with his body upright.
Stimulus. Tilt the patient to one side by pushing against one side of his trunk.

Response. Righting of the head and upper trunk with abduction and extension of the extremities on the raised side and protective extension of the extremities on the side to which the patient was tipped.[16]

Standing. From 15 to 18 months throughout life.[16]
Test Position. The patient is standing.
Stimulus. Tilt the patient to one side, holding him at the hips[10] or around the upper trunk.[20]
Response. Righting of the head and upper trunk with abduction and extension of the extremities on the raised side and protective extension of the extremities on the side to which the patient was tipped.[10]

Other Reactions in Standing. From 15 to 18 months throughout life.[16]
1. *Hopping.* Test Position. The patient is standing.
Stimulus. Hold the patient by his upper arms[16] or around the upper trunk[20] and move him forward, then backward and to each side.[16]
Response. Righting of the head and upper trunk with hopping steps in the direction of movement.[18]
2. *Dorsiflexion.* Test Position. The patient is standing.
Stimulus. Hold the patient around the upper trunk[10, 20] and tilt him backward unexpectedly.[10]
Response. Righting of the head and upper trunk with dorsiflexion of the ankles.[10, 16, 20]

Cortical Reactions

Optic Righting. From 6 months throughout life.[20]
Although these are righting reactions, they depend on the occipital cortex rather than the labyrinths.[10, 21]
Test Position. Suspend a child in prone or supine position in space without a blindfold.[10, 16]
Stimulus. The prone or supine position in space.
Response. The head is brought to a face vertical position.[10, 16]

When testing the optic righting reaction in adults use a prone or supine position on a mat. The ability to voluntarily raise the head in prone or supine is a positive response.

If the labyrinthine righting reactions are positive, the optic righting need not be tested because the response cannot be differentiated from the labyrinthine righting reaction. If labyrinthine righting is negative, however, the optic righting reaction may be used to compensate for the labyrinthine loss as a means of postural orientation.[10]

Each reflex response can be recorded on a record similar to the sample form presented in Table 4.1. Scoring is done by indicating whether the response was positive or negative, although some forms have another column to indicate whether a response was normal or abnormal as well. As mentioned before, the age of the person tested must be considered when determining whether positive or negative is the normal response. The comment section on the form may include such items as any change from standard test position, the strength of the response, or other descriptions of the response. After recording the results of testing, the highest level of reflex control achieved can be noted. If the level is age-appropriate then reflex development is normal, but if the level of control is lower than the normal expectancy for the age of the

Table 4.1
REFLEX TESTING[a]

Name: Date:

                                                         Therapist:

	Pos.	Neg.	Comments
Innate Primary Reactions			
a. automatic walking			
b. placing – upper extremity			
c. moro			
d. grasp			
e. sucking			
f. rooting			
Spinal Level Reflexes			
a. Flexor Withdrawal			
b. Extensor Thrust			
c. Crossed Extension			
Brain Stem Level Reflexes			
a. Asymmetrical Tonic Neck			
b. Symmetrical Tonic Neck			
c. Tonic Labyrinthine			
Supine			
Prone			
d. Positive Supporting Reaction			
e. Associated Reactions			
Midbrain Reactions			
a. Neck Righting			
b. Body Righting Acting on the Body			
c. Labyrinthine Righting Acting on the Head			
Prone			
Supine			
Automatic Movement Reactions			
a. Protective Extensor Thrust			
b. Equilibrium Reactions			
Prone			
Supine			
Quadruped			
Sitting			
Kneel-standing			
Standing			
Hopping			
Dorsiflexion			
Cortical Reflexes			
a. Optic Righting			

[a] Adapted from M. A. Fiorentino.[16]

person then the results must be interpreted in the light of other information to determine if treatment is appropriate. Factors to consider include the severity of the delay of reflex development and strength of the primitive reflexes, the age of the patient or the time elapsed since damage to the central nervous system occurred, and the extent of the damage.

The sooner after the insult to the central nervous system occurs and the less severe the damage, the greater are the chances of treatment being effective. For some patients with severe damage of long standing, the primitive reflexes may be used for locomotion and other activities and may be the person's only means of motor function. Treatment to inhibit these reflexes and to promote higher function may result in inhibition only and leave the person unable to function. If changes can be made, treatment is indicated and involves inhibition of the primary reactions of the spinal cord and brain stem by promoting the development of righting reactions and equilibrium responses.

CONTROL OF VOLUNTARY MOVEMENT

Motor development progresses from mass patterns of movement to more selective, specific movements as primitive reflex patterns are broken down into smaller units and reorganized into a wider choice of postures and movements.[22]

Development of conscious control progresses in a cephalocaudal direction from control of the head and eyes, to the trunk, then the upper extremities, and finally the lower extremities.[23] The sequence of development of sensory-motor control progresses from lifting the head in a prone position, to rolling over, to prone on elbows, to assuming a quadruped position, to sitting, to creeping on all fours, to kneel-standing, to standing and walking. This progression is reflected when watching a young child, approximately 1 year old, get up from a supine position. He rolls over, pushes up on his elbows and hands to all fours, and either pivots to sit and pulls up to stand from sitting or pulls from all fours to kneel-stand and stand. Visualization of this process of getting up may be helpful in recalling the general sequence of motor development.

Development proceeds from the mobility patterns of supine flexion, prone extension, and rolling to stability patterns in weight-bearing positions. Bilateral weight bearing distributes weight between the two extremities and is less demanding than unilateral weight bearing as seen when one hand is reaching.[24] In each weight-bearing position, mobility and stability are combined in a sequence from a bilateral position (stability) to rocking with bilateral support (mobility) to unilateral weight bearing (stability) while using the other extremity (proximal stability, distal mobility).

Adults have established patterns that become lost or interrupted with diffuse brain lesions. Evaluation and treatment are based on normal developmental sequences, and relearning may occur in some or all of these sequenced patterns. Some delimited lesions in adults, such as embolitic stroke, gun shot wounds, or tumors, may affect only specific functions For these, relearning focuses on reestablishing functional movements for which the patient has previously developed sensorimotor patterns.

Evaluation of motor control can be done using the evaluations of Rood, Bobath, or Brunnstrom described in Chapter 6. The evaluations are used to determine the highest level of consistent control that the patient evidences. Therapy then focuses on establishing the next level of control according to developmental sequences.

Coordination Tests

Control of acquired motor skills can be evaluated using coordination tests. Coordination is defined as the ability to control movements accurately and smoothly. Incoordination is a broad term for disabilities involving extraneous, uneven, and inaccurate movements. Deficits are related to the location of CNS damage, and planning effective treatment depends on understanding the cause and nature of the problems observed.

Cerebellum

Incoordination may be caused by dysfuntion of the unconscious cerebellar regulation of smooth voluntary movement and maintenance of upright posture.[8]

Cerebellar disturbances and methods of evaluation are as follows.

Tremor. An intention tremor occurring during voluntary movement and diminished or absent at rest.[8, 25] The tremor can be observed during the performance of activities or by asking the patient to alternately touch his own nose and then the examiner's finger, which is held in front of him and moved to various positions.[26] The tremor usually increases as the goal is approached.[27, 28] Observe the joints involved; this tremor usually occurs proximally due to lack of stability.[28] Other tests are the finger to finger test in which the patient reaches out to touch the examiner's finger[30] and the toe to finger test in the lower extremity.[27]

Dysdiadochokinesia. Impaired ability to accomplish repeated alternating movements rapidly and smoothly.[8] When asked to perform alternate movements, a patient with this symptom will perform the movements slowly with an incomplete range of motion or may be unable to perform alternate movements (adiadochokinesia). Tests include having the patient rapidly perform alternate supination-pronation or grasp-release.[8] Other tests include alternate rotation of the entire arm with arms fully extended in front of the patient,[29] tapping the table with extended fingers,[27] and tapping one wrist with the index and middle finger of the other hand.[29] In the lower extremity flexion-extension of the toes[8] and foot patting in which the heel remains on the floor and the foot rapidly pats the floor[30] are useful tests. Observe speed of performance and joints involved.[29] If tests are performed bilaterally differences between the two extremities can be determined by comparison. Speed of performance is recorded by noting the number of repetitions in a given time period.

Dysmetria. An inability to control muscle length[31] resulting in overshooting or pointing past an object toward the side of the lesion.[32] For example, if touching his face, a person might hit himself or if reaching for an object he might reach past the object. The finger to nose test is used for evaluation, and the ability to prevent past pointing is observed.[26, 27] In the lower extremity the toe to finger test is used; the patient touches the examiner's finger with his toe.[27]

Dyssynergia. A decomposition of movement with lack of smooth performance of movements because the synergistic action or reciprocation between agonists and antagonists is impaired or lacking (asynergia).[27, 28] In decomposition of movement each joint involved in a movement pattern functions independently so that the movement is broken up into its parts rather than being smooth and coordinated.[25, 32] Tests for other cerebellar functions also can provide an opportunity to observe dyssynergia.

In tests of alternate movements, note whether there is loss of rhythm and regularity in performance or whether the arms drift out to the sides.[28]

In the finger to nose test[26] or in reaching out to touch the examiner's finger in the finger to finger test[28] or toe to finger test, note whether movements are jerky and broken up into parts.[27] In the heel to shin or heel to knee test the patient is asked to place one heel on the opposite knee and slide the foot down the shin; dyssynergia may be observed.

Ataxic Gait. A wide-based, unsteady, staggering gait with a tendency to veer toward the side of the lesion.[25, 27] Observation of walking may suffice as an evaluation, or the patient may be asked to walk heel to toe along a straight line or to walk fast and turn quickly.[27, 28]

Rebound Phenomenon of Holmes. The lack of a check reflex to stop a strong active motion to avoid hitting something in the path of the motion. To test for this phenomenon the examiner resists the patient's elbow flexion and then releases the resistance; the patient may hit his own chest or shoulder if unable to check the motion.[27] The arm should be positioned to avoid having the patient hit his face.

Asthenia. Muscles are weak and tire easily.[32]

Hypotonia. Decreased muscle tone due to the loss of the cerebellum's facilitatory influence on the stretch reflex.[8] Granit[31] reports the results of many studies which lead to the conclusion that locomotor disturbances of cerebellar lesions suggest an absence of spindle control. After the removal of the cerebellum of a decerebrate cat there was reduction or loss of spindle stretch sensitivity which is controlled by gamma motor neurons. With no organized gamma activity muscle spindles cannot measure or send messages regarding muscle length which would then influence control of muscle length. Destruction of the cerebellar link to alpha and gamma motor neurons could

explain symptoms, such as dysmetria and adiodochokinesia.[31]

Posterior Columns

Posterior column damage with loss of proprioception also results in incoordination due to misjudgment of limb position and balance problems. Coordination deficits from a loss of proprioception and methods of evaluation are as follows.

Ataxia. A wide-based gait resulting from loss of position sense. The patient watches the floor and placement of feet to visually compensate for the loss.[28]

Romberg Sign. Inability to maintain balance in standing with the eyes closed. To test for this sign the patient stands with his feet together and then closes his eyes; loss of balance occurs.[27] Guard to prevent falling.

In posterior column deficits the finger to nose, heel to knee, and toe to finger tests may show dysmetria or overshooting, and the deficit is increased with the eyes closed.[28]

Basal Ganglia

The basal ganglia are thought to function in automatic patterned movements of locomotion[27] and to inhibit rhythmic movements.[27] Lesions of the basal ganglia result in a "release phenomenon" in which these rhythmic movements are released from inhibition and become apparent.[27] Basal ganglia lesions or diseases may result in one or more of the following abnormal involuntary movements.

Athetosis. Athetoid movements are characterized by slow, writhing, twisting, worm-like movements, particularly involving the neck, face, and extremities.[25] There is lack of postural stability in the neck, trunk, and proximal joints.[33] There is excessive mobility with increased speed,[27] but movements are involuntary and purposeless.[33] Muscle tone may be increased or decreased.[33, 34] Phelps[34] described 12 types of athetosis distinguished by type of motion, amount of tension, and other deficits of unique description. The site of the basal ganglia lesion that causes athetosis is not precisely localized.[8, 32] Observation should include notice of whether involvement is proximal or distal, which extremities are involved, whether motions are rotary or on a plane of flexion-extension, and whether tension is increased or decreased.[34]

Dystonia. A form of athetosis in which increased muscle tone causes distorted postures of the trunk and proximal extremities.[8] Involuntary contractions of trunk muscles result in torsion spasms,[25] and there is increased lumbar lordosis.[8] Athetosis is not present during sleep.[27]

Chorea. Choreiform movements are rapid, jerky, irregular movements primarily involving the face and distal extremities.[8, 25] The muscles are hypotonic. Chorea is related to degeneration of the putamen as in Huntington's chorea or may follow rheumatic fever, as in Sydenham's chorea.[8] Chorea may occur in sleep.[27]

Hemiballismus. Unilateral chorea in which there are violent, forceful, flinging movements of the extremities on one side of the body,[8, 25] particularly involving the proximal musculature.[25] It is caused by a lesion of the subthalamic nucleus.[8]

In summary, evaluation of coordination involves observation of the patient at rest and during activity to note the occurrence of any asynergic or involuntary movements as defined. Requests for the patient to perform particular movements, such as rapid, alternate supination and pronation, pointing to objects, or walking are made as necessary to observe the movements specified in the definition of a particular disturbance. Each problem of incoordination and its severity is noted. Involvement is often bilateral, but one side of the body may be more severely involved than the other. If damage is unilateral, the influence of the cerebellum is observed in the ipsilateral extremities, whereas the influence of the basal ganglia is on the contralateral extremities.

It is evident that problems of incoordination are associated with problems of muscle tone, muscle strength, proprioceptive sensations, speed of performance, and other areas of concern which must all be considered together when interpreting the results of evaluation in order to plan treatment.

Development of Hand Function

The ontogenetic development of sensory-motor control and hand function provides a basis for evaluation and treatment not only of children but also of adults who have suffered brain injury. The redevelopment of hand skill following a cerebrovascular accident, for example, closely parallels normal development.

The development of the motor patterns involved in hand function as described by A. Jean Ayres[23] progresses as follows: (a) control of neck and eye movements; (b) trunk stability and balance; (c) shoulder girdle and shoulder stability and movement; (d) elbow motion; (e) gross grasp; (f) wrist positioning and movement; (g) release of grasp; (h) forearm supination and pronation; and (i) individual finger manipulation. Each item in the progression overlaps the previous item(s) in time so that one component is still being completed as the next begins.

The ontogenetic development of reaching and prehensile behavior depends upon the coordination of visual and sensorimotor mechanisms and includes the entire development of head and eye control to digital release.[17, 35] Prehension includes reach, grasp, carry, and release.[35]

During the 18th prenatal week until the 16th to 24th postnatal week, the grasp reflex is evident.[35] The grasping reflex of the newborn reflects man's phylogenetic heritage, according to McGraw.[17] It is assumed to be under subcortical control because the human cortex is probably not functioning appreciably at birth.[17] If a rod is placed in the hand of a newborn, he grasps it with strength enough to support his body weight.[17] Twitchell[36] defines this as the traction response, the stimulus of which is stretch to the scapular adductors. Twitchell also identifies another reaction present at birth: the avoidance reaction. The hand shows a withdrawal or avoidance reaction to contact stimulation, the effect of which continues to contaminate voluntary hand function up to 5 or 6 years.[35, 36] During the newborn period (0 to 2 months), an object placed in the hand will be reflexly grasped, but there is no reaction to an object held in view.[17] A contact stimulation on the skin between the thumb and index finger also elicits automatic grasp.[36]

The 3- to 4-month-old infant displays motor responses, however disorganized, in response to objects within the visual field.[17, 35, 36] The true grasp reflex, flexion and adduction of the fingers, is evident and stimulated cutaneously by an object moving distally toward the medial palm.[36] When this reflex is fully developed, the traction response, with its attendant flexor synergy (flexion of all joints of the upper limb), can no longer be obtained.[36] Crude voluntary palmar grasp develops in the wake of the true grasp reflex. Palmar grasp does not include the thumb; it may be equated to hook grasp.[36]

At about 4 months, the sight of an object by the baby causes approaching movements of the digits and the entire upper extremity.[17] This response does not seem connected to a desire to have the object. The approach is primitive and may be done with fisted or open hand.[17] The instinctive grasp reaction is beginning to develop at this time also; in response to contact stimulation on the medial side of the hand, the forearm supinates to orient the hand toward the object.[36]

At 6 months, the child approaches an object with deliberateness once it is seen.[17] The child must give his undivided attention to securing the object, however, or the movement is interrupted.[17] There is excessive extension of digits during the approach and too forceful a grasp on contact at first.[17] The object is manipulated, once grasped.[17] The grasp is crude with the thumb used incidentally.[35]

At about 8 months, reach involves rotation at the shoulder, rather than at the forearm in order to orient the hand to objects. The elbow is more flexible[35] during reaching to secure close and far objects.

At about 9 to 10 months the child no longer must give full attention to approach and grasp of an object once he has seen it.[17] The wrist is more flexible.[35] The approach is still executed with excessive digit extension which moderates with maturation.[12] The instinctive grasp reflex is fully developed: in response to contact stimulation, the hand gropes for and adjusts to grasp the object.[36] Scissors grasp (thumb flexion and adduction) becomes a crude pinch. Opposition is achieved.[35, 36] The index finger pokes,[35] indicating that the grasp reflex is fully fractionated.[36] There is only advertent release of grasp, indicating a beginning cortical control of finger extension which takes place only after reaching and grasping have been perfected.[35]

At 11 months there is release of pincer grasp.[35] Refinement of release continues for the next several years.[17, 35] At 12 to 13 months supination comes under cortical control.[35] When the child reaches 12 to 14 years, all fine finger manipulation skills have developed.[35]

Dexterity Tests

Dexterity is defined as the ability to manipulate objects with the hands. Standardized dexterity tests such as the Crawford Small Parts Dexterity Test and the Minnesota Rate of Manipulation Test have been validated on populations of persons employed in jobs requiring a known degree of dexterity. The normative data are therefore very useful, especially in prevocational testing. Both these tests are commercially available. The Crawford test consists of pins, collars, and screws, and a board into which these fit. The pins and collars must be picked up and placed using tweezers. The screws are inserted to a certain depth using a screwdriver. Reliability data are: Tweezer $r = 0.80$ and screws $r = 0.82$.[37] The Minnesota test consists of a long frame (approximately 3 feet or 1 m long) having four horizontal rows of openings large enough to accommodate the round blocks (approximately 1½ inches or 3.8 cm in diameter). There are two subtests: Placing and Turning. Test-retest reliability ranges from $r = 0.84$ to $r = 0.91$.[37] The test has been adapted and standardized for the blind also. Information about purchase of these tests may be obtained from Buros' *Mental Measurement Yearbook*.[38]

Gross dexterity can be measured using the Box and Block Test (Figs. 4.2 and 4.3), which has norms established on 124 handicapped adults.[37] The score is the number of 1-inch (2.5-cm) cubes transferred from one well of the box to the other in 1 minute. One hundred cubes are used. The test can be used as a measure of endurance also; the number of blocks transferred before fatigue ensues is the score. This test can be used with patients who use prehension hand splints also. Norms for the Box and Block Test are in Table 4.2.

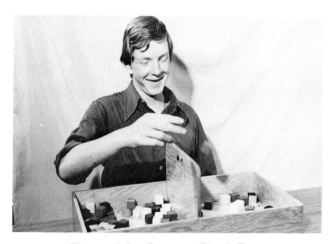

Figure 4.2 Box and Block Test.

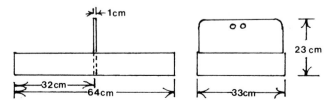

Figure 4.3 Dimensions of Box and Block Test.

Table 4.2
BOX AND BLOCK TEST: PERCENTILE NORMS OF NUMBER OF CUBES TRANSFERRED IN ONE MINUTE[a]

Best Hand	Centile	Worst Hand
89.0	99	78.5
83.3	95	73.3
79.1	90	69.1
73.8	80	59.5
68.3	70	52.0
62.0	60	44.4
57.1	50	38.0
52.1	40	32.3
44.9	30	26.1
33.7	20	18.0
25.7	10	12.7
17.5	5	9.3
3.5	1	2.5
N = 124		N = 113
Mean = 54.58		Mean = 39.44
Median = 57.1		Median = 38.0
Mode = 56.0		Mode = 20.0
SD = 20.11		SD = 21.99

[a] Based on adults with neuromuscular conditions.

An estimation of manual dexterity can be made from observing the patient do such tasks as thread a needle, button buttons, use scissors, pick up coins, write, transfer pegs or nails, or other similar tasks. If treatment is to be aimed at increasing hand function, however, more objective tests which will be sensitive to changes in the patient's performance are preferred.

STRENGTH AND ENDURANCE

When a patient lacks isolated control of voluntary movements he cannot accomplish one motion in isolation from the other motions in a movement pattern. Muscle testing requires isolated control and consequently cannot be done in its absence. When voluntary motor control of specific joint motions is lacking, strength is evaluated by describing the movement patterns which are present. Patterned movement of the extremities involve flexion or extension to a partial or full range of motion. The movement patterns of patients with hemiplegia have been carefully observed and described by Brunnstrom and are included in Chapter 6. When isolated control of voluntary movements develops or returns, muscle testing as described in Chapter 7 can then be used to evaluate strength.

Endurance for sustained activity may be limited in a patient with brain injury due to muscle weakness or increased cardiopulmonary demand of movements which have to overcome influences of increased muscle tone or primitive reflexes. In patients with hemiplegia cardiovascular problems may be a causal factor and a remaining influence on decreased endurance. Evaluation of heart rate is then used to monitor ability to perform or continue an activity. Endurance is evaluated in terms of rate of performance and length of time a repetitive effort is sustained. Holding of postures is evaluated by length of time only. Deficits of endurance were first recognized in association with lower motor neuron problems, and consequently the description of the evaluation of endurance is in Chapter 7 within the section concerning these problems.

References

1. Perry, J. Central control insufficiency: Pathomechanics. *Phys. Ther.* 58(3): 304–305, 1978.
2. Matthews, P. B. C. *Mammalian Muscle Receptors and Their Central Actions.* Baltimore: Williams & Wilkins, 1972.
3. Bishop, B. Spasticity: Its physiology and management. *Phys. Ther.*, 57(4): 385–395, 1977.
4. Basmajian, J. V. *Muscles Alive*, 4th ed. Baltimore: Williams & Wilkins, 1978.
5. Stuart, D. G., *et al.* Selective activation of Ia afferents by transient muscle stretch. *Exp. Brain Res.*, 10: 477–487, 1970.
6. Kottke, F. J. Reflex patterns initiated by the secondary sensory fiber endings of muscles spindles: A proposal. *Arch. Phys. Med. Rehabil.*, 56 (1): 1–7, 1975.
7. Urbscheit, N. L. Reflexes evoked by group II afferent fibers from muscle spindles. *Phys. Ther.* 59(9): 1083–1087, 1979.
8. Bannister, R. *Brain's Clinical Neurology*, 4th ed. London: Oxford University Press, 1973.
9. Hirt, S. The tonic neck reflex mechanism in the normal human adult. *Am. J. Phys. Med.* (NUSTEP Proceedings), 46(1): 362–369, 1967.
10. Bobath, B. *Abnormal Postural Reflex Activity Caused by Brain Lesions*, 2nd ed. London: Heinemann Medical Books, 1971.
11. Capute, A. J., Accardo, P. J., Vining, E. P. G., Rubenstein, J. E., Walcher, J. R., Harryman, S., and Ross, A. Primitive reflex profile: A pilot study. *Phys. Ther.*, 58(9): 1061–1065, 1978.
12. Ayres, A. J. *Sensory Integration and Learning Disorders.* Los Angeles: Western Psychological Services, 1972.
13. Fiorentino, M. A. *Normal and Abnormal Development.* Springfield, Ill.: Charles C Thomas, 1972.
14. Stockmeyer, S. Development from Prone to Upright Posture. A slide-tape lecture. Boston: Instructional Resource Center, Sargent College, Boston University, 1971.
15. Hoskins, T., and Squires, J. Development assessment: A test for gross motor and reflex development. *Phys. Ther.*, 53(2): 117–126, 1973.
16. Fiorentino, M. A. *Reflex Testing Methods for Evaluating C.N.S. Development*, 2nd ed. Springfield, Ill: Charles C Thomas, 1973.
17. McGraw, M. *The Neuromuscular Maturation of the Human Infant.* New York: Hafner Publishing Co., 1963.
18. Sieg, K. W., and Shuster, J. J. Comparison of three positions for evaluating the asymmetrical tonic neck reflex. *Am. J. Occup. Ther.*, 33(5): 311–316, 1979.
19. Bobath, B. *Adult Hemiplegia: Evaluation and Treatment*, 2nd ed. London: Heinemann Medical Books, 1978.
20. Bobath, K., and Bobath, B. Cerebral palsy. In *Physical Therapy Services in the Development Disabilities*, edited by P. H. Pearson and C. E. Williams. Springfield, Ill.: Charles C. Thomas, 1972.
21. Noback, C. *The Human Nervous System.* New York: McGraw-Hill, 1967, 214.
22. Milani-Comparetti, A., and Gidoni, E. A. Pattern analysis of motor development and its disorders. *Dev. Med. Child Neurol.*, 9: 625–630, 1967.
23. Ayres, A. J. Ontogenetic principles in the development of arm and hand functions. In *The Development of Sensory Integrative Theory and Practice*, edited by A. Henderson *et al.* Dubuque, Iowa: Kendall/Hunt Publishing Co., 1974.
24. Stockmeyer, S. A. A sensorimotor approach to treatment. In *Physical Therapy Services in the Developmental Disabilities*, edited by P. H. Pearson and C. E. Williams. Springfield, Ill. Charles C Thomas, 1972.
25. Carpenter, M. Cerebellum and basal ganglia. In *Physiological Basis of Rehabilitation Medicine*, edited by J. A. Downey and R. C. Darling. Philadelphia: W. B. Saunders, 1971.
26. DeJong, R. N., *et al. Essentials of the Neurological Examination.* Philadelphia: Smith Kline Corp., 1968.
27. Chusid, J. G. *Correlative Neuroanatomy and Functional Neurology*, 15th ed. Los Altos, Calif.: Lange Medical Publications, 1973.
28. Alpers, B. J., and Mancall, E. L. *Essentials of the Neurological Examination.* Philadelphia: F. A. Davis, 1971.
29. Klingon, G. H. Motor and reflex testing. *J. Mt. Sinai Hosp.*, 33(3): 225–235, 1966.
30. DeHaven, G. E., Mordock, J. B., and Loykovich, J. M. Evaluation of coordination deficits in children with minimal cerebral dysfunction. *Phys. Ther.*, 49(2): 153–157, 1969.
31. Granit, R. *The Basis of Motor Control.* London: Academic Press, 1970.
32. Noback, C., and Demarest, R. *The Nervous System: Introduction and Review.* New York: McGraw-Hill, 1972.
33. Guess, V. Central control insufficiency. II. Extraneous motion: A treatment approach. *Phys. Ther.*, 58(3): 306–312, 1978.
34. Phelps, W. M. Classification of athetosis with special reference to the motor classification. *Am. J. Phys. Med.*, 35(1): 24–31, 1956.
35. Ayres, A. J. Ontogenetic principles in the development of arm and hand functions. In *The Development of Sensory Integrative Theory and Practice: A Collection of Works of A. Jean Ayres*, edited by A. Henderson *et al.* Dubuque, Iowa: Kendall-Hunt Publishing Co., 1974.
36. Twitchell, T. Normal motor development. In *The Child with Central Nervous System Deficit.* Washington, D.C.: U.S. Government Printing Office, 1965.
37. Cromwell, F. S. *Occupational Therapist's Manual for Basic Skills Assessment: Primary Prevocational Evaluation.* Pasadena, Calif.: Fair Oaks Printing Co., 1965, pp. 25–31.
38. Buros, L. K. (ed.). *The Seventh Mental Measurement Yearbook*, Vol. II. Highland Park, N.J.: Gryphon Press, 1972, pp. 1043–1044.

Supplementary Reading

Bell, E., Jurek, K., and Wilson, T. Hand skill measurement: A gauge for treatment. *Am. J. Occup. Ther.*, 30 (2): 80–86, 1976.

Brennan, J. B. Clinical method of assessing tonus and voluntary movement in hemiplegia. *Br. Med. J.*, March 21, 1959, pp. 767–768.

Holt, K. S. The measurement of muscle tone and posture. In *Cerebellum, Posture and Cerebral Palsy*, edited by G. Walsh. London: The National Spastics Society Medical Education and Information Unit in association with Wm. Heinemann Books, 1963.

Jacobs, M. J. Development of normal motor behavior. *Am. J. Phys. Med.*, 46(1): 41–51, 1967.

Lagasse, P. P. Muscle strength: Ipsilateral and contralateral effects of superimposed stretch. *Arch. Phys. Med. Rehabil.*, 55(7): 305–310, 1974.

Sahrmann, S. A., Norton, B. J., Bomze, H. A., and Eliasson, S. G. Influence of the site of the lesion and muscle length on spasticity in man. *Phys. Ther.*, 54(12): 1290–1296, 1974.

chapter

5

Motor Control
Therapy

Catherine A. Trombly, M.A., OTR

The basic premise of current motor control therapy is that manipulation of the sensory input will effect a change in the resultant motor output of an individual. A second premise is that repetition of this sensory-motor-sensory sequence will bring this improved motor output within the person's repertoire of voluntary movement. A third premise is proposed: since recovery of motor control is relearning, therapeutic movement to be learned must be attended to and practiced as opposed to being elicited passively on a reflex basis. Research concerned with the acquisition of developmentally based motor skills and learning of acquired motor skills by normal persons would support these premises.

In the case of upper motor neuron lesions, planning and executing the more voluntary movements suffer most while the less voluntary movements are relatively spared. The patient is often unable to move a segment of a limb in isolation.[1]

Recovery usually follows a developmental sequence from reflex to voluntary control, from mass to discrete movements, and from proximal to distal control. Recovery can arrest at any level, and this is not wholly predictable. The speed of early spontaneous recovery offers a clue to the ultimate level of function to be gained.

Recovery will never be complete. Any cells in the brain that have been destroyed will not repair, and the function for which they were responsible will be diminished by the loss. Some believe that the amount of tissue damage is more disabling than the specific sites of destruction because remaining healthy tissue can, with relearning, assume lost functions.[2] There is developing evidence that neuronal plasticity, the tendency of new synaptic connections to be made among brain cells as a result of learning, may continue throughout life and could be expected to occur in the remaining, living cells.[3-5] It is safe to say, however, that if the pyramidal tract is destroyed, thereby preventing cortical motor control, discrete, skilled movement will not be regained.[6]

The question as to whether, and to what degree, therapist-manipulated input can improve the motor output of persons whose central mechanisms of motor control are abnormal is unanswered and awaits the data of occupational and physical therapy practitioners. There is evidence that in animals, training after brain damage resulted in improved function,[7] yet others have found recovery to be age-dependent.[8, 9]

Neurodevelopmental therapy began in the 1950s and 1960s when a few therapists began to modify their treatment approach to patients with central nervous system damage. These therapists based their treament on ideas generated from data available from neurophysiologists at that time. This data suggested that motor output was controlled by sensory (peripheral) input. The therapists attempted to bridge the gap between the data obtained from "pure", i.e., controlled, research on animals to clinical practice with humans. The treatment approaches of these therapists are described in the next chapter. When other therapists have applied techniques of these therapists, they have sometimes met with success and sometimes not. Having a conceptual framework about the control of movement allows the therapist versatility in choice of alternative therapy when "standard" procedures seem ineffective for a particular patient. For that reason it is helpful for the therapist to have a working model of movement control.

One model derived from information in the literature is proposed here. Perhaps the model you will propose would differ, depending on your experience in the literature. Unfortunately, there is not one known model of how movement is generated, learned, and controlled. Because of sophisticated technology and improved laboratory technique, much new information is being generated from experiments on awake monkeys and humans rather than anesthetized cats as before. This newer information suggest that peripheral control is subservient to central motor control.

The model presented here represents acquired motor skills and assumes prior maturation through the development of righting and equilibrium responses or at least the genetic organization that underlies these responses.[10, 11] Whether these maturationally based movement skills can be acquired through learning or manipulation of sensory inflow has not been addressed in the literature. Theories of motor learning presuppose their existence.[10]

ONE MODEL OF MOTOR CONTROL AND LEARNING

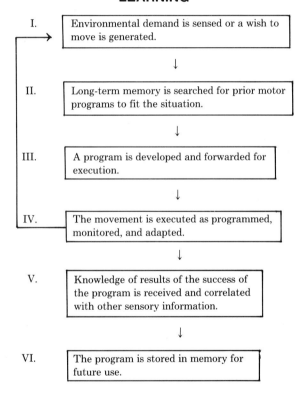

I. Environmental demand is sensed or a wish to move is generated.

↓

II. Long-term memory is searched for prior motor programs to fit the situation.

↓

III. A program is developed and forwarded for execution.

↓

IV. The movement is executed as programmed, monitored, and adapted.

↓

V. Knowledge of results of the success of the program is received and correlated with other sensory information.

↓

VI. The program is stored in memory for future use.

Obviously this simple model is not useful unless the elaborations assumed under each major step are familiar to the therapist. Each step will be discussed conceptually. The reader is referred to the references listed at the end of this chapter for greater detail. These concepts are hypotheses, for the most part, and are subject to modification through study and experience.

Environmental Demand is Sensed or a Wish to Move is Generated

Purposeful movement does not occur in the absence of a need to move.[11] This need is generated from within the person or as a response to sensory information from cutaneous, proprioceptive, auditory, or visual stimuli. Vision is a powerful stimulus for voluntary movement.[11, 12] A movement is organized and planned prior to initiation, that is, a program is developed.[13]

The somatosensory receptors provide the person, consciously and unconsciously, with knowledge of the whereabouts of the parts of his body before movement is programmed. The program must take into account the starting position.

Long-Term Memory is Searched

The idea to move, the "act of willing," simultaneously initiates search in long-term memory (LTM) for the memory trace and notifies the programming centers to begin strategy development.[15] The strategy consists of the details of which motor units are to contract or relax and when. Access to memory is achieved by concentrating on what it feels like to move for a particular purpose.[16]

Voluntary movement is based on previous movement.[10] Evidently, as part of the programming process, old programs, "perceptual traces,"[15] are activated, and the salient parts are salvaged and modified by new programming commands to fit the new situation. Movement memories that have been successful are stored in long-term memory (LTM) which seems impervious to forgetting. Successful means that the sensory inflow generated by the movement matched the sensory outflow at the time the program was generated and accomplished the goal.[17, 18] If attention is directed to the movement so that information concerning it remains in short-term memory (STM) for a time, then the memory becomes stored in the LTM for future use. However, if the information is lost from STM, then it does not become part of LTM.[19] Attention serves not only in the memory-building process, but also in increasing neuronal excitability, or the readiness of certain neurons to fire.[12, 20] These effects of attention, through the reticular activating system, are particularly important in readying motoneurons involved in associated or background contraction to fire.[20]

A Program is Developed and Forwarded for Execution

The program, or exact strategy, refers to a set of instructions of facilitation or inhibition to particular motoneurons and interneurons to fire at certain frequencies for certain periods of time.[21] Whether the movement is urged from external stimuli or by an act of willing, the same executive mechanisms are likely to be employed.[11] If agonist and antagonist are to contract simultaneously, the alpha motoneurons of both must be excited. If the agonist is to contract alone, the antagonist must be reciprocally inhibited; therefore, the circuits of inhibition involving the Renshaw cells and the Ia interneurons must be activated.[22, 23] To support the voluntary movement, postural muscles must also contract bilaterally to provide a stable base from which movement may occur; the neurons of these muscles are activated automatically as part of the program.[11] Also as part of the program the fusimotor neurons (also called gamma motoneurons) are programmed so that spindle sensitivity is exactly set, and accurate information concerning the length and speed of length change can be continually monitored.[23, 24] Thus, the alpha motoneurons and the gamma motoneurons are coactivated.[22, 25, 26] This coactivation, or forwarding of program for execution, is initiated by the motor cortex as well as by centers in the brain stem.[27, 28] Evarts[29] states that the motor cortex may participate in control of innate as well as learned movement. The brain stem, in response to its input from vestibular receptors, cerebellum, cortex, and basal ganglia, also contributes to control of the automatic postural aspect of the program.[23] The corticomotoneurons control both the voluntary aspect of the movement,[23] the part toward which attention is focused and the automatic, postural aspects.[29] Evarts[28, 29] further states that cells in the cerebellum and basal ganglia become active prior to movement. The basal ganglia are preferentially more active in slow movement, and the cerebellum seems to be more active in quick, ballistic movements. Both these areas have a critical role in controlling pyramidal output as they both feed the program through the motor cortex and the brain stem for execution.[29]

Alpha and gamma coactivation is not invariable, according to Matthews,[25] and he believes that either the alpha or the gamma motor neurons can be activated separately for maximal flexibility. Very fast movement, especially of distal muscles, may in fact be carried out by alpha motor neurons directly under cortical control. Evarts[29] would modify that to say, under cerebellar control mediated by the motor cortex.

The Movement is Executed, Monitored, and Adapted

The alpha motoneurons or ventral horn cells are the final common path from the central nervous system to extrafusal muscle fibers which effect movement. Each of these neurons and its muscle fibers is a motor unit. Depending on the number of motoneurons activated, a few or many motor units may be recruited to participate. Motor units are recruited to participate according to the *size principle*.[30, 31] Small motor units are recruited early. These are usually tonic, or holding, type units. If there is a demand for power or speed, the larger, phasic, units are recruited. The order of recruitment is the same whether volitionally or reflexly activated; one type of activation can enhance the recruitment of a unit subliminally activated by the other type of activation.[20] The frequency of firing of each recruited unit also increases with demand, so that some motor units fire at the same time as others and their effect summates to make a stronger contraction.[30] There is still enough asynchronous firing to result in a smooth contraction. When the muscle fa-

tigues, greater and greater synchrony occurs, which results in a noticeable tremor.[32]

During slow movement [approximately 650 msec[33] or more] or maintenance of a posture, ongoing sensory input from the muscle spindle, Golgi tendon organs, joint receptors, receptors in the skin, and vestibular receptors feed information back to the cerebellum, basal ganglia, and cortex.[22–25, 34–37] Visual monitoring of movement and auditory cues also provide powerful feedback. This is called a closed loop system.[14, 15] During fast movement [approximately 160 msec[33] or less] there isn't time to use feedback information for monitoring because the movement has ended before the feedback can be utilized. This type of control is termed open loop.[38] In this case, knowledge of results, compared with the sensory feedback received late, is very important in the shaping of future similar movements.[18]

If a slow ongoing movement is found to be wrong, an adjustment is made. You have experienced this if you have ever lifted a suitcase that you expected to be heavy (and so programmed your muscles for a mighty lift) but in fact it was light. You lifted much higher, faster, and with less precision than if your output matched the demand. In this case, your programming center was speedily informed, probably by tendon organs of your "lifter" muscles and the spindles of the stretched, noncontracting[39] antagonists, that too many motor units tensed and the antagonist was lengthening too fast. The spindles of the contracting muscles would go slack (unload) and stop firing because the extrafusal muscle fibers shortened faster than the intrafusal ones did, since the intrafusal ones were still following the program. Ordinarily there is greater Ia output from the spindles of the shortening agonist than from the lengthening antagonist due to the powerful gamma coactivation.[40] On the other hand, if you had expected, and so programmed for, a light suitcase, but in fact it was heavy then as the lift got underway, nothing happened at first because too few motor units were participating. Feedback would cause three adjustments to be made. Within 12 to 18 msec more alpha motoneurons would be recruited via the monosynaptic path of the segmental stretch reflex.[25, 39, 41, 42] Approximately 15 msec later more units would be recruited via transcortical loop stretch reflexes,[42, 43] which are the primary basis for load compensation.[6, 44–46] Thirdly, at about 120 msec a cerebellar assisted cortically controlled adjustment in the program would occur to meet the sensed demand.[42, 46]

What happened to bring about this flurry of activity is this: At the time of coactivation of the alpha and gamma motoneurons, the program is given to both. When movement is stopped by an outside (unplanned for) source, the extrafusal muscle fibers cannot contract as programmed. They remain lengthened, held by the outside force (extra heavy suitcase, therapist's hand, or whatever). Meanwhile, the intrafusal fibers keep contracting as programmed which keeps some stretch on their midsections. This contraction of the spindle is meant to keep the spindle at just the right length as the muscle shortens so it won't become slack or unloaded and become ineffective.[1, 47] However, the extrafusal muscle fibers aren't shortening, which puts enough added stretch on the spindle to fire the primary afferent endings which are sensitive to small additional increments of stretch. In so doing, the stretch reflexes are activated.

The secondary endings of the spindle, activated by prolonged, steady stretch,[23] may also be involved in activation of the tonic stretch reflex[46] which is facilitatory to the muscle in which it lies in contrast to the older belief that the secondary endings were facilitatory to the flexors and inhibitory to the extensors, regardless of origin.[22, 25, 48]

The Golgi tendon organs which lie in series with the muscle, in contrast to the spindles which lie in parallel, signal the tension of each motor unit.[26, 49] Joint receptors provide information concerning spatial location of the angle of the joint and the direction and speed of movement.[36, 37, 50] Location information is more primary than distance information in accurate reproduction of movement.[14]

Information from the spindles, tendon organs, and joint receptors has speedy access to the brain for use in reprogramming by way of the dorsal column-medial lemniscal system.[5, 23, 44] It is thought that the cerebellum may be the comparator, receiving the feedback and comparing it to the command for the program.

Cutaneous sensation has been found to be essential for adequate activation of the tonic stretch reflex,[44, 47, 51] and without it greater effort is required to move.[51] It has also been shown that cutaneous stimulation of a body part, especially the hand, activates corticomotor neurons that control that part.[11, 41] Cutaneous sensation seems to be direction-specific and proportional to speed of movement,[52] that is, impulses increase as the speed increases, and differences in impulses from receptors on the flexor and extensor surfaces give information concerning the direction.

Vestibular sense organs provide rapid information to the central nervous system concerning the stability of the center of gravity. Dynamic adjustments (equilibrium responses) are made to relocate the center of gravity over a stable base of support when the stability is threatened. Tonic adjustments (axial, antigravity muscle contraction) are made to keep the person upright and in balanced posture from which movement can take place. The adjustments are automatic and unlearned. The results are effected monosynaptically and polysynaptically by the vestibular nuclei in the brain stem primarily on the alpha and gamma motoneurons of the extensor (antigravity) muscles.[31, 53, 54]

If reprogramming must occur, the motor control process goes back to step I.

Knowledge of Results Is Received and Correlated with Other Sensory Information

A movement could be executed exactly as programmed and yet be inaccurate as far as accomplishing the goal.[38] Examples come readily to mind: a person throws a bowling ball to knock over 10 bowling pins and fails to hit any; a person is feeding himself candy while engrossed in reading and misses his mouth. In the first example knowledge of results is needed each time the person bowls; this is a motor task that uses voluntary control on an on-going basis to modify performance. The second example represents the type of voluntary motor task that, once learned by matching knowledge of results (KR) with kinesthetic feedback, requires direct control and attention only if something goes wrong. KR is crucial to motor learning. Deafferented monkeys were able to learn motor skills if they received clues that their performance was successful.[12, 23]

The early phase of motor learning can be termed the cognitive-motor stage. During this stage, the person actively plans the movement and cognitively correlates visual and auditory knowledge of results with somatosensory feedback.[14, 17, 19, 23] Vision usually guides the motor performance, either simultaneously with performance or later through the use of photographs (videotape replay, etc.). A conscious effort is made to match the "feel" of the performance with the visually perceived KR and/or ideal performance of an expert.[14, 19, 55] Adams[15] believes that this stage is guided by covert verbal behavior.

Athletes and people who train athletes or animals to do motor tasks emphasize practice, defined as correct repetition with knowledge of results and the goal to improve. Increased consistency of performance occurs with practice.[17]

With many repetitions, probably hundreds,[16] the cutaneous-kinesthetic-visual link is made, and knowledge of results and visual guidance are less needed to monitor the movement unless a target is involved.[11, 19, 55-57] This later phase of motor learning can be termed the kinesthetic stage. During this stage the learner concentrates on the feel of the movement and develops a knowledge of performance. Automatic motor performance is guided by knowledge of performance which is a synthesis of sensory inputs.[11, 52-55] However, well-learned movements run open-loop, that is, they do not rely on peripheral feedback.[33] Although it is known that practice is required, no one knows what central nervous system mechanism underlies the change from voluntary to automatic control.[14] It may be that synaptic transmission is facilitated for those circuits involved in the practiced movement, and others are inhibited or less facilitated.

The Program is Stored in Memory for Future Use

Short-term motor memory, located in frontal lobes of the cortex,[16] is immediately accessed by the sensory by-products of movement. Access to the memories is facilitated by familiar temporal/contextual situations.[58] If the sensations of movement are attended to so that they remain within the STM for a period of at least a few seconds, then they become committed to LTM. If not, no learning takes place.[19]

The most practiced movements are best imbedded in memory,[19] for example, walking, bicycling, writing a signature.

Merton[41] speaks of the tantalizing problem facing neurophysiologists and motor psychophysicists related to control of motor patterns: an individual's signature is the same, or at least so similar as to be detected if written by another, whether he writes it on paper using finger and wrist muscles or on the blackboard using shoulder muscles. In some way the pattern of the act is learned; the use of individual muscles is not.

By using this six-stage model of motor control, the therapist can evaluate where in the process the patient is having difficulty and can develop goals for treatment.

SOME GOALS OF MOTOR CONTROL THERAPY

Maintenance of Range of Motion

Maintenance of functional passive range of motion by slow, passive movement and positioning to discourage the effects of the tonic reflexes is important. The passive movement will probably not contribute to motor learning.[11, 59]

Therapeutic goals for persons with disturbed motor performance due to central nervous system damage include normalization of tone and normalization of movement.

Normalization of Tone so that Movement May be Executed

When there is excess tone (spasticity or rigidity) the goal is to decrease this background "noise" to allow freer movement. When there is too little tone, movement is weak or absent, and the muscle spindles have to be biased via the fusimotor neurons to accurately signal the state of the extrafusal muscle fibers so that both will be ready for executing the programs. Specific goals are: (1) If the flexor-adductors are hyperactive, inhibit them and facilitate the extensors; establish cocontraction, which is a balanced contraction of all the muscles around the joint. (2) If the extensor/abductors are hyperactive, inhibit them and facilitate the flexors; if the tonic muscles cocontract in a normal pattern, establish mobility patterns. (3) If the flexors are hypoactive, facilitate both the flexors and extensors to achieve balanced muscle contraction in stability and mobility functions. (4) If the extensors are hypoactive, facilitate them. Normalization of tone is achieved through use of controlled sensory stimulation.

Normalization of Movement

Depending on the patient, normalization of movement may involve integration of primitive reflexes by development of automatic postural adjustments; decrease of excess involuntary movement through re-learning (develop stability); learning to initiate voluntary movement where none exists (develop mobility); or evolvement of discrete movement from patterned responses through learning.

Integration of Primitive Reflexes

The primitive, usually tonic, reflexes need to be prevented from dominating the motor output of the patient. These reflexes underlie normal movement and posture and are evident in non-brain damaged persons when they are working under great stress (excess resistance or at the limits of endurance). Whether it is possible to integrate these reflexes through learning is unclear. However, procedures that therapists use to attempt to achieve this are: avoidance of situations in which these reflexes would manifest themselves even in normals (resistance or fatigue); positioning of the limbs opposite to the position they would assume in response to the stimulus; stimulating the righting, then later the equilibrium, responses while preventing a lower, more reflex-bound response. The correct response is assisted by guiding the patient passively. Some therapists believe the patient's attention should not be focused on the response, since righting and equilibrium reactions are considered automatic; others disagree and believe that since learning must take place, attention must be part of therapy. Much clinical research is needed here.

Relearning Functional Motor Patterns

There are essentially two motor patterns which interweave to accomplish the motor tasks of life. These are posture or stability and movement or mobility. Stability needs to be developed before accurate movement can occur. Axial and proximal limb stability precedes distal limb stability. For patients who exhibit too much mobility (athetosis, intention tremor) or the inability to control movement in midrange (athetosis), treatment is aimed at developing the needed stability. Persons who are unable to move (flaccidity) or who are bound by too much stability (spasticity or rigidity) need to develop mobility or phasic patterns in developmental sequence.

The development of these two patterns involves all the principles and methods of motor control therapy and will be specifically addressed after these methods are explained.

Developing Automaticity of Motor Performance

Once a correct response is elicited, it must be repeatedly practiced correctly to enable learning to occur. Learning will be evident by decreasing variability in performance which becomes increasingly more smoothly and accurately executed. Evolving more discrete movement from mass patterns is accomplished by introducing small variations from the mass pattern. The variations are introduced in developmental sequence. Variations in the movement must be developed by practice also. How much practice should be devoted to learning the movement before variations are introduced is not known.

Once the person has developed control of isolated movements, an indication of normal motor performance, then the goals become those of increasing strength, endurance, and the accuracy and speed of movement (coordination and dexterity). The use of principles described in the chapters on the biomechanical approach would then be appropriate.

THE PRINCIPLES AND METHODS OF MOTOR CONTROL THERAPY

Principle: Controlled Sensory Stimulation

Controlled sensory stimulation is used to provoke movement or to enhance weak ongoing muscle contraction. Movement is provoked as a reflex response to sensory stimuli. Increased motor output is the result of increasing the internal stretch sensitivity (spindle bias) through the effects of sensory stimulation that is amplified and directed to the gamma motoneurons through the reticular activating system. As a result of biasing, the spindles are set at a zero point which means they are taut and ready to react to external stretch or to supraspinal programming commands.

The use of controlled sensory stimulation presupposes that the firing of motor neurons can be affected by the number and nature (electrical charge) of impulses that impinge on them all at once (spatial summation) or in quick succession (temporal summation).

It is further hypothesized that the sign of the electrical charge can be manipulated by controlling the kind and amount of sensory input. Therefore, some sensory stimuli are termed facilitatory and some inhibitory. Facilitation, $\oplus$, refers to the state of readying the neuron to depolarize. Small subthreshold depolarizations occur as each facilitatory impulse arrives at a neuron, but these must summate to cause the impulse to be propagated by the neuron.[16, 23] Some of the impulses that arrive at the neuron are inhibitory, $\ominus$, that is, they hyperpolarize the cell membrane to decrease the likelihood of propagating the impulse.[22] The neuron becomes an algebraic adding machine; if there are more facilitatory than inhibitory impulses, then the neuron depolarizes and the impulse is propagated along to the next synapse. If the inhibitory influences are greater, however, no impulse is propagated. Facilitatory stimuli are generally of an arousing nature, while inhibitory stimuli are soothing and relaxing.

The intensity, duration, and frequency of sensory stimuli remain hypothetical. Margaret Rood has stated the values of these parameters based on her experience and study; however, no controlled study has supplied data confirming her recommendations. Nevertheless, Margaret Rood must be credited with emphasizing the importance of sensory input, and the specifics of her methods will be found in Chapter 6.

Although it seems a simple matter to apply stimuli and observe the results to discover which are therapeutically facilitating, in reality, with the possible exception of stretch, no stimulus seems to be universally facilitating or inhibiting.[60] The effect that any sensory

stimulus has on any individual may be different from its effect on any other individual. However, the response to a particular stimulus on repeated stimulation is usually the same for a particular individual.[60] The effect that any sensory stimulus has at the moment depends also upon the state of the central nervous system, or more specifically the interneurons or motor neurons in question, at the time of stimulation.[22, 31] All the cells of the central nervous system are firing all of the time at varying frequencies, which provides a dynamic background "noise" of excitation or inhibition.[31] If the stimulus from the periphery arrives at excited motor neurons, the effect of the stimulus will add to the background excitation, and the response may well be greater than anticipated; on the other hand, if the stimulus arrives at an inhibited central nervous system, the response will be less.

No one can exactly predict from known outward signs what the overall state of excitation of the central nervous system is. It is therefore important when using controlled sensory stimulation therapeutically to know what responses one seeks to achieve, to apply a chosen stimulus with care, and to observe carefully the reactions of the patient, however minute, in response to the stimulation. If the patient does not react as hoped, then the manner of application of the stimulus may need to be altered in regard to its intensity, the duration, or the location of its application. Before beginning to describe the effects of certain stimuli, as documented by research on animals or humans, the reader is reminded of a feature of neurophysiological organization called reciprocal inhibition. The antagonist muscle is automatically inhibited, due to the "wiring" of the nervous system which includes inhibitory interneurons, when the agonist and synergists are facilitated.[22] Therapeutically, the idea of reciprocal inhibition is used to inhibit spastic muscles by facilitating the antagonists.[61, 62] This effect will of course be subject to the limitations already mentioned for sensory stimulation.

Increase of Tone

To increase tone facilitatory sensory stimuli are used. Care is used to apply phasic stimuli to phasic muscles and tonic stimuli to tonic muscles. Most muscles are mixed but have a tendency to be more one type or the other.[31] Muscles considered phasic are pale, cross multiple joints, are superficial, used for mobility responses, e.g., extensor digitorum and biceps. Muscles considered tonic are red, cross a single joint, are deep, responsible for stability responses, e.g., interossei, small neck and back muscles, and the brachialis. Phasic stimulation is characterized by brevity and low intensity. Tonic stimulation is maintained, high intensity (many repetitions within a second) stimulation.

Tactile Stimulation. Stroking or brushing of the skin is applied over the muscles or muscle groups that are being treated.[63] The therapist can use her own fingertips, cotton, or a brush to deliver the tactile stimulus. A quick swipe is delivered for a phasic response and a sustained, rapid brushing for a tonic response. Hagbarth[63] discovered, by direct measurement on the alpha motor neurons, that tactile stimulation (light pinching) of the skin over flexor or extensor muscles of cats facilitated the alpha motor neuron firing of the muscle beneath and inhibited the motor neurons of its antagonist. Eldred and Hagbarth[64] found the same to be true for gamma motor neurons. They found that stimulation directly over the extensor muscle (cat's gastrocnemius) was facilitatory, but stimulation of any other skin area was inhibitory to the gamma motor neurons of the extensor muscles.

The importance of cutaneous stimulation to the enhancement of the tonic stretch reflex has been cited. Perturbation (movement) of a part has been found to initiate and enhance output of cortical motor neuron colonies related to the part moved.[42] Since the parts were handled and moved in the experiment, it can be assumed that skin, joint, and muscle receptor stimulation was involved.

Tactile stimulation should precede treatment because some of its effects are via the reticular activating system[5] (RAS), and the tonic response is bilateral and enduring.

Orthokinetics is a technique which may be considered tactile stimulation, although it is reported to stimulate the proprioceptors of muscles and tendon also.[65] A band of rubber-reinforced elastic bandage is made to fit around the limb at the area of the belly of the muscle to be stimulated. Several layers of bandage are used. The active part that is to be placed directly over the muscles to be stimulated is left free and stretchy; the remainder of the band, the inactive part, is sewn back and forth over and over to make it relatively inelastic. The cuff fits snugly but not tightly around the limb with the active field placed exactly over the muscles to be stimulated. As the patient exercises, especially by using reciprocal movements, or as he goes about his daily activities, the contraction and relaxation of muscles that lie under the cuff push the skin against the orthokinetic cuff, and the elastic part stimulates the skin by small pinches. The orthokinetic cuff has been found to decrease spasticity and increase range of motion in spastic patients when the active field is placed over the antagonist.[65, 66] This idea can be incorporated into splints for patients; the splint surface provides the inactive, inhibitory field and the elastic bandage, used as a strap, provides the active, facilitatory field.

Thermal Stimulation.

The brief application of ice to the skin over the muscles being treated or in the palm of the hand or on the soles of the feet is facilitating. A phasic response is obtained from a quick swipe on the palm or sole. A tonic response is obtained from a few seconds of maintained icing over the muscle. Swallowing can be initiated by swiping the skin over the sternal notch. Breathing (inspiration) can be activated by swiping along the borders of the rib cage. Icing is thought to work segmentally and through the RAS as does touch.[5]

Vestibular Stimulation.

These stimuli are used to challenge righting and equilibrium responses and to facilitate extensor (tonic) tone. The response is immediate and lasts only as long as the stimulus is applied.

Stimulation of the various vestibular receptors is attained by rotary movements; linear movements, especially those that include acceleration and deceleration; and by different positions of the head. Although knowledge is incomplete, it is believed that the semicircular canals are stimulated by changes in angular acceleration, while the otoliths are stimulated by position and linear acceleration.[31] Ayres[67] states that the most stimulating position is upside down, but that horizontal prone-lying is also very effective.

The tonic labyrinthine inverted (TLI) posture was found effective by Tokizane et al.[68] for facilitation of extensor tone. In the TLI, the head is upside down. They also found that the upright posture was least facilitatory to extensor tone; intermediate postures of the head produced intermediate amounts of extensor tonus. Flexor tone was evident in opposite directions according to the law of reciprocal innervation. Interestingly, the most pronounced effect of the TLI posture was observed in the distal muscles (extensor carpi radialis and ulnaris; flexor carpi radialis and ulnaris; soleus and tibialis anterior), while the least effect was evident in the proximal muscles (deltoid and gluteus maximus). The muscles were monitored electromyographically while the human subjects were lying on a flat surface which was rotated so that the muscular responses could be studied in all positions from upright to upside-down.

The TLI posture can be achieved through the use of a large inflatable pillow or ball, a cable spool, or a barrel. The person is positioned so that the head is down. Caution should be observed to detect unwanted changes in blood pressure. Of course the TLI should not be used for any patient for whom increased intracranial pressure is a precaution.

Acceleration and deceleration stimulates equilibrium responses as well as increased extensor tone. Acceleration and deceleration can be achieved by swinging the patient to and fro on a swing or in a net hammock suspended from one hook in the ceiling which encloses the person within the hammock and gives him a feeling of safety. By placing the person prone on a skooter board and letting him roll down an incline (Fig. 5.1), or by pulling on a rope attached to the skooter board, the therapist can also stimulate the various receptors. A skooter board is a flat board large enough to support the patient from midchest to hips and which has a free-wheeling universal caster at each corner.

Rotation can be achieved by having the person rotate his head; by twirling or "winding-up" a swing or the above-mentioned hammock and letting it go to spin around and unwind; or by twirling the person in a chair that rotates. Being rolled on a big ball, jumping up and down, rope jumping, pogo stick riding, and

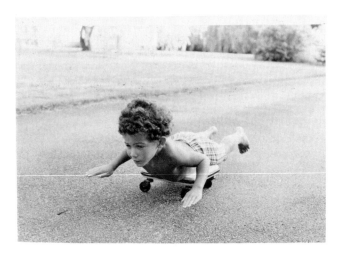

Figure 5.1 Skooter board on an incline eliciting the pivot prone position and providing vestibular stimulation.

tumblesaults are all methods to stimulate the vestibular receptors but are not useful with patients with brain damage, especially adults.

Fast rocking can be done in a rocking chair or by placing the person sidelying and, with the therapist's hands on the shoulder and hip, moving the person rapidly from side to prone and back repeatedly for several minutes.

The equilibrium board can be used to elicit equilibrium responses in supine-lying, prone-lying, sitting, quadruped, and kneeling. The board is tilted rapidly to the degree that it challenges the patient's balance but within recoverable limits. The equilibrium board is a flat board mounted on rockers at either end. The patient must be guarded.

The use of vestibular stimulation can result in an overfacilitation or an overinhibition. Ayres[67] states that if this should occur, the response can be normalized by asking the patient to make an adaptive response (planned movement) which balances the excitatory and inhibitory states in the brain.

Proprioceptive Stimulation. These stimuli are used to evoke reflex responses, to enhance ongoing movement or to increase awareness of movement. The effect is immediate and lasts as long as the stimulus is applied.

1. Vibration is a selective means of stretching in that it activates only the primary afferents of the muscle spindles and not the secondaries.[25] The tonic vibration reflex (TVR) is a polysynaptic stretch reflex which depends not only on spinal polysynaptic pathways, but also on supraspinal pathways. Vibration is facilitatory to tonic postural muscles.[69] When a muscle is vibrated at small amplitudes of a few millimeters at 50 to 500 Hz, a TVR is elicited and the muscle slowly contracts. Because the discharge of the primary afferent responds to each small stretch of the vibrator, the frequency of the vibrator is a most crucial parameter of this method of stimulation.

Application of the vibrator to the tendon is more

effective.[69, 70] But a similar response can be obtained if it is applied to the muscle belly and the amplitude is high.[69] There is a rise time of 20[70] to 30[71] seconds in normals, depending upon the amount of initial relaxation of the muscle, before the response reaches its maximum; this may take longer in patients with a damaged central nervous system.[70] The vibration of a muscle or tendon should last at least 30 seconds but not more than 1 or 2 minutes because the heat and friction produced by the vibrator may be uncomfortable.[62] The response lasts only as long as the vibration itself is applied.[62] Repeated short periods of vibration may lead to an increased response which approaches the maximum the muscle can exert.[25] A voluntary contraction of the muscle being stimulated enhances the vibratory effects, especially if the muscle is isometrically contracted in the shortened range[61, 69] (Fig. 5.2). The strength of the TVR varies with the length of the muscle at the time vibration is applied; it has been found to increase when the muscle is elongated.[61, 69] However, the TVR is more greatly enhanced by voluntary contraction, of less than maximal force, than by passive lengthening.[69] Vibration applied to a muscle that is voluntarily contracted maximally adds nothing more to the response.[69]

Vibration is an extremely effective method to increase the stretch sensitivity of tonic muscles and to inhibit antagonistic phasic muscles.[69, 71]

Hagbarth and Eklund[72] found that vibration of spastic muscles of hemiparetic patients caused an initial phasic response followed by a tonic response that lasted as long as the stimulus was applied. Synergistic muscles acting on neighboring joints, which were not

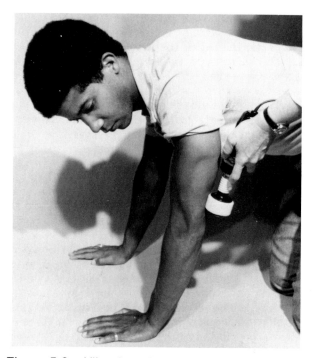

Figure 5.2 Vibration of triceps tendon contracted in a shortened range to assist achievement of full elbow extension in a weightbearing position.

vibrated, showed a sustained reflex contraction also. At times, even antagonists, usually reciprocally inhibited, were facilitated. Bishop[62] has reported the effects that other experimenters have found in the use of vibration on persons with motor disorders due to central nervous system disease or damage. In persons with spasticity, the usual result was relaxation of spastic antagonists and an increase in the response of the weak muscle which was vibrated. For patients with cerebellar disorders, vibration either aggravated their condition or had no effect. In patients with cerebral palsy some beneficial effects observed due to vibration in conjunction with "conventional therapy" were an increase in speed of movement, improved body image perception, and an improvement in memory for motor acts.

Bishop[62] has identified contraindications to the use of vibration on patients: as a general rule, vibration should not be applied if it accentuates a patient's motor disorder.

2. Stretch is used to elicit motion or to increase the contraction of a muscle. According to Granit,[22] the stretch reflex is a component of functionally organized movements, volitional or automatic. The fusimotor component is activated automatically in volitional movement due to the alpha-gamma linkage. Passive stretch of a muscle evokes unlinked spindle firing incapable of supporting stretch reflexes other than a monosynaptic burst—a tendon jerk.

Quick, light passive stretch is used to elicit a response from the primary afferent of the spindle to monosynaptically facilitate a dynamic response of the same muscle being stretched. Repeated brief, light, short stretches or tapping the tendons[25] results in brief unsustained outputs from the tapped muscle. It can augment the dynamic response of a contracting muscle or increase the likelihood of response from a hypotonic muscle. The movement must be resisted to cause an other-than-momentary effect. Due to the resistance more motor units will be programmed to fire, and learning will take place.

Although reciprocal inhibition of the antagonist is expected as a result of stretch, this is not always the case in normals.

Prolonged or firmer stretch, especially with the muscle in a lengthened position, is used to differentially elicit a response from the secondary afferents (IIs) of the muscle being stretched. Matthews[25] proposes that the IIs do not always inhibit extension and always facilitate flexion as once believed. He believes stimulation of these afferents results in autogenic excitation.[25, 73] Further, he believes that the higher levels of the central nervous system may switch the action of the secondaries ". . . so that they may produce sometimes excitation and sometimes inhibition of the motor neurons of their own muscle."[25]

Based on clinical observation, Kottke[74] postulates that stimulation of the secondary endings by stretching the proximal musculature to the end of range results in organized spinal reflexes termed the crossed extension reflex or the spinal reflex posture, described as flexion synergy of one upper extremity and the contralateral lower extremity and extension synergy of the other limbs. Flexion synergy includes flexion of most joints of the limb combined with external rotation and abduction of the proximal joint. Extension synergy includes extension of most joints of the limb combined with internal rotation and adduction of the proximal joint. Kottke further postulates that stretch to the distal musculature results in regional patterns of flexion or extension, depending on which muscles were stretched.

Although the newer ideas about the function of the II afferent await experimentation for validation, it appears that at the very least, therapists must be careful in their method of application of stretch stimulation and vigilant in their observation of the results.

Parameters of the method of using stretch to be noted include: (a) whether the muscles are elongated or in a shortened range at the start of stretch; (b) whether the muscle is relaxed or contracting; (c) the force of the stretch; (d) and the speed of the stretch. The flexors are started in a lengthened range and extensors in a shortened range. If the muscle is contracting, the effect of stretch will be increased because of the additive effects of external and internal stretch of the muscle spindle. The internal stretch occurs due to programming. It is believed that the force and speed of stretch differentially activate Ia's (light, quick) or IIs (firm prolonged). Any load added to a limb by adding weights to the limb or by having the person use tools may stretch muscles.

Kenny and Heaberlin[75] found in their electromyographic study of spastic children that when the limbs worked in eccentric or isometric contraction, which eliminated the stretch reflex, the EMG was similar to normals. However, during concentric contraction when gravity stretched the contracting muscles, the EMG showed that contraction occurred later and stopped later in relation to movement than it did in normals. In other words, voluntary control of concentric contraction was hindered by the stretch reflex in those for whom hyperactive stretch reflexes are a symptom.

The extensor (antigravity) muscles are responsible for posture. They are primarily tonic in nature.[71] Usually tonic muscle fibers contract readily to slight amounts of stretch. If the internal stretch sensitivity of the spindles is lacking then these muscles become less responsive; therefore, stability is poor. A technique first described by Rood, as interpreted by Stockmeyer,[76] to bias the spindles is shortened, held, resisted contraction (SHRC) in pivot prone. Pivot prone is a position by which a person lies prone and extends upper trunk and head; abducts, extends, and externally rotates shoulders; and extends hips and knees off the surface so that he rests on the pivot point at approximately T_{10}. The spindles of these muscles are programmed along with the extrafusal muscle fibers to shorten to hold this posture. The resistance of gravity exerts a constant force against the shortening, so that the central nervous system must reprogram more and more units to fire to complete and hold the posture. The use of the SHRC of extensor muscles while in prone position may more importantly serve to integrate the tonic labyrinthine reflex. A person whose TLR is incompletely integrated will have difficulty extending while prone, since the prone posture is the reflex stimulus for flexion. Such a person would need to be assisted to assume this posture by use of sensory stimulation to the extensor/abductor muscles.

3. Reflexes are used to evoke movement or postural responses when the patient is otherwise unable to initiate these responses. A reflex is defined as a more or less stereotyped response to a stimulus. Evoked reflexes are used with the expectation that by combining the motor response with a willed effort on the part of the patient, they will begin to form voluntary movement.

Voluntary motor control is encouraged by providing tasks for the patient to do which inherently demand the movement. In this way, the patient attempts to do the movement, which is based on the automatic reaction, purposefully; that is, he focuses attention on the intent to do something—reach for something, look at an interesting scene—rather than the actual step-by-step process of moving.

Reflexes are known to be the basis of voluntary motor patterns. Hirt[77] reviewed the literature of the first half of this century which establishes the now accepted premise that reflex motor behavior is present in normal children and adults and in fact underlies many of the organized voluntary movements used in daily activities and sports. However, the development of reflex movement, *per se*, would not be appropriate because it does not automatically become voluntary movement. Neither do therapists continue the stimulation of the reflex component of movement once the patient has begun to move with volition.

4. Resistance is used to increase the output of a muscle by adding it to an ongoing movement unexpectedly. This brings about the reaction described on page 61. Resistance also causes a cocontraction response of muscles around a joint. Too much resistance can increase the abnormality of movement by evoking primitive reflexes or by causing an overflow of excitation to synergistic muscles. This is a special consideration in patients with brain damage in whom these reactions would be unwanted.

The sensory stimuli can be combined to increase the effects. The least amount of stimulation that is needed to ensure movement is all that is used. When weaning the patient from stimulation applied externally, one stimulus is removed at a time so that the patient is still able to move successfully.

Decease of Tone

The difference between inhibiton and facilitation is in the mode of application rather than the kind of stimuli. Inhibitory stimuli are used or facilitation is applied to the antagonist muscle, and inhibition is brought about reciprocally. Care must be exercised that an inhibitory response is actually occurring because reciprocal inhibition seems to be faulty in persons with spasticity.[75]

Tactile Stimulation. Rood has identified a particular type of tactile stimulation for inhibition: slow stroking of the posterior primary rami. The effect is possibly through calming of the output of the sympathetic chain; the autonomic nervous system is known to affect gamma firing.[78] The person lies prone in a quiet environment. The therapist uses the palm of her hand or extended fingers to apply firm presure from occiput to coccyx in a slow, rhythmical manner. Relaxation can be seen to occur within minutes.

Thermal Stimulation. Prolonged icing over several minutes in duration inhibits muscle contraction,[5, 79] but after removal there is a rebound effect when the muscle warms; it exhibits greater tone.[76] Neutral warmth, in which the whole person or the hypertonic part is wrapped in a flannel blanket or similar material, results in relaxation of the hypertonic muscles without a rebound.[76] Therapists make form-fitting wraps from stockinette or sheepskin for the patient to wear to bed which results in decreased tone by morning. Also, therapists suggest that patients with spastic arms wear sweaters.

One group has had some success with the use of prolonged icing of the extensor muscles of patients with intention tremor; they did not report the rebound effect. The tremor was decreased as long as the ice was used. Warming the extensor muscles increased the tremor.[80]

Vestibular Stimulation. Slow, rhythmical movement is inhibiting, that is, relaxing. Slow rolling is done similarly to fast rocking except much more slowly. A decrease in hypertonicity should be seen within minutes.

Proprioceptive Stimulation. Vibration is inhibitory when it is applied to the antagonist.

Resistance can be used to inhibit or damp movement in persons with ataxia. It has been found that there is an optimal weight increment for each person and that to exceed that increment voids the effect of weighting.[81, 82] The optimal weight is determined by trial and error. Some ataxics are too weak to work against the amount of weight necessary to damp their involuntary movement.

Stretch, prolonged over several minutes during which the patient's limb is not moved, results in a "letting go" of the hypertonic muscle which the therapist can feel. Greater range of motion is gained by stretching in this manner increment by increment.

Principle: Willed Movement

Willed movement is defined as movement which the person pays attention to, makes an effort to accomplish, and which satisfies a goal. Without conscious attention to movement, learning will not take place.[10, 12]

Too much effort may disrupt the motor performance of a person learning a new skill whether his central nervous system is damaged or not. When first learning a new skill, more motor units are recruited in the agonist than are needed, and more synergists are also recruited.[32] As learning progresses, differentiation occurs, and only the most economical amount of muscle output is generated.[32] If the motor pattern is grossly distorted by excess effort, the person can be cued to relax, to exert less force, to move more slowly.

Using the principle of willed movement therapeutically is basic to occupational therapy. Occupational therapists have always used purposeful activity as their medium. The central control theory provides a good basis on which to continue.

Whereas up to this time, controlled sensory stimulation was the major tool used to attempt to improve motor control, we propose that the use of willed movement become the major emphasis. We, and others[83] hypothesize it to be *the most* effective tool when used in combination with awareness of result either through an intact sensory system or use of augmented sensory feedback (biofeedback). The therapist uses willed movement by making a demand, verbal or nonverbal, for movement to meet a demand. The response, or approximation of it, needs to be within the patient's capabilities. The patient needs to receive reliable feedback concerning the movement. Therefore, visual and auditory feedback may need to substitute for unreliable proprioceptive feedback (unreliable because spindle bias is under central control, which is disordered in patients with brain damage).[83]

The trainer can facilitate learning in the cognitive-motor stage through demonstration, provision of movies or videotapes of expert performance, provision of videotape feedback, and cueing the person to attend to specific somasthetic feedback, such as joint location, in relation to a visualized KR.[17, 19, 55] Also helpful is the mental rehearsal of the sequence of the motor task.[55] Prior instruction seems to preset the stretch mechanism, making it more responsive.[84]

Execution of a novel motor act requires that new minute neural changes occur until the pattern of movement is learned.[35] Miller et al.[13] proposes that adult humans learn by trial and error the tactical details of the strategy of a "communicated plan" which they have received from some source, such as another person, a movie, etc. The strategy is the sketchy directions, such as "saw this piece of wood in half." The tactical details include such facts as "hold the wood securely, grasp the saw tightly, extend and flex your elbow." Miller believes that it is unhelpful to instruct a person via the tactical details.

In the kinesthetic stage of learning, the trainer is most helpful by structuring the environment and the schedule of practice/rest. Cueing the person to attend to certain sensations helps him to develop knowledge of performance (KP).[16, 17, 19]

More specific therapeutic methods need to be developed for use with brain-damaged persons. The research of physical educators and motor learning specialists will be useful. Questions that need to be addressed are: which is better, verbal cueing or environmental set-up, to focus the patient's attention on the goal? What is the best way to help the patient to remember what it felt like to move to accomplish a certain goal? When and how should knowledge of results and of performance be provided? What patient characteristics are crucial to the success of these methods? What responses (maturational or acquired; stereotyped such as lower extremity function or adaptive such as upper extremity function) can and cannot be achieved using this principle?

Principle: Developmental Sequence

Each new skill is learned with the previous ones as its base. Therefore, therapeutic activities and exercises are chosen to match the person's level of development and to stimulate the next higher level of development. Development occurs spirally, that is, the next motor response can be introduced before the previous one is perfected.

Activities chosen for therapy must match the person's developmental level and must reflect these developmental sequences, all interwoven together for gradation. Reflexes must be integrated before voluntary movement can progress. Control must be achieved over the axial and proximal body parts before limb control is possible. Control develops cephalocaudally. Ulnar control (power) develops before radial (precision) in the develoment of hand usage. Gross, mass patterns of movement evolve into differentiated, discrete movement. Control of stability of the part is needed before control of mobility is possible.

Principle: Practice (Repetition)

Repetition is necessary for learning. It is believed that repetitious use of the same synaptic pathways enhances the likelihood of that pathway activating as a whole when the appropriate stimulus is encountered,[10] that is, the response becomes automatic. An automatic response is characterized by repeatability (decreased variability) and speed. Practice is repetition with an intention to improve.[19]

Practice sessions that distribute rest periods between bouts of practice have been found most effective in athletic training.[19] The fact that a patient is also weak from bedrest and from the recovery process necessitates rest periods.

Practice sessions can be continuous with brief rests up to fatigue, but should not extend beyond because performance deteriorates with fatigue. Alternately, practice can be distributed into periods of brief practice and extended rest.

Practice should occur using the implements and the environment that are natural for the response.[19] This idea, used in athletic training, is most appropriate for brain-damaged persons.

The whole response should be practiced using as close to normal timing as possible. Once the whole response is developing, perfection of each part can be stressed separately.[19]

METHODS TO DEVELOP STABILITY AND MOBILITY

Stability

Stability refers to the cocontraction of the agonist and antagonist muscles around a joint to maintain a posture against gravity. The antigravity extensor/abductor (tonic) muscles are usually in need of facilitation. Some neurophysiologists[85] think that in the upper extremity of man the flexors, which are the antigravity muscles in the upright posture, are the tonic muscles. This has not been tested out clinically, but certainly needs to be. We will continue to describe the extensors as the tonic muscles. Controlled sensory stimulation is used to prepare the tonic muscles for greater contraction. Brushing of the skin and application of ice for 3 to 5 seconds over the bellies of the extensor/abductor muscles have been suggested as appropriate stimuli to apply before any other treatment, since their effect is thought to be lasting. Other sensory stimulation is applied as the patient attempts to move or hold a posture. These include vibration, tapping of the muscle belly, and resistance. The use of shortened, held, resisted contraction (SHRC) to rebias the spindles of these muscles is used to prepare for assumption of a weight-bearing posture. Weight-bearing postures are thought to evoke cocontraction responses.[76] Through willed movement the persons responds to a developmentally appropriate demand for stability. This posture is held for some time (practiced).

The SHRC used is prone extension in which the person lies prone and extends the hips and knees off the surface so that he is resting on a pivot approximately opposite to T_{10}. The spindles of these muscles are programmed, along with the extrafusal muscle fibers, to shorten to hold this position. The resistance of gravity exerts a constant force against the shortening which causes the CNS to reprogram more and more units as well as causing the recruitment of more units through the stretch reflex servo-assist mechanism. It is reasoned that immediately following prone extension, the spindles are biased short and are very responsive to small increments of stretch. Therefore, if the person moved into prone on elbows or quadruped position, the shoulder and hip extensor/abductor muscles would be stretched relative to their new shortened range and thereby facilitated through the servo-assist mechanism. The flexor part of the cocontraction around the hips and scapulohumeral joints is probably brought about by central programming to maintain the position. Formerly, the IIs of the extensors were thought to be responsible before doubt was cast on the role of the IIs as exclusive facilitators of flexors. (See Urbscheit[48] for a discussion of the secondary ending.) It is now known that central control exerts much more input to the alpha motoneurons than peripheral sources of stimulation and that central control easily overrides peripheral control.[40]

If, however, the person were balanced in prone on elbows, little if any excitation of the shoulder/scapular muscles would occur because no demand existed. Preliminary electromyographic evidence has shown that if the parts are lined up, one on top of the other, no muscle output occurs in normals.[32] As soon as the person is off balance or must take a greater part of the weight distribution, however, the muscles do contract in response to the demand to maintain the posture. It would be interesting to see electromyographically the effect of use of unstable surfaces, e.g., soft mattress, water bed, etc. Cocontraction does occur and can be seen electromyographically in response to resistance or in preparation for hitting a target with the limb.[32, 62]

Once stability is beginning to develop in one posture, the person needs to learn to control movement in the midranges so that mobility responses can be developed with proper proximal stability. He learns this control by moving slightly away from the stable position in all directions. The distal part of the limb is still stabilized against a surface or by tightly grasping a heavy tool. The patient concentrates on controlled movement of the particular joint. Greater and greater range within limits of control are aimed for.

In summary, evocation of a stability response requires appropriate sensory stimulation to tonic muscles, a demand for the holding response in developmental sequence, and repetition to learn it. Stability is then integrated with control of mobility.

Mobility

For the person who is unable to move, movement is evoked by whatever means. Controlled sensory stimulation is used to provoke reflex responses. Reflexes that are useful are the withdrawal reflex (stimulus = brief light touch, thermal (ice), or pain on the distal part of the extremities); the stretch reflex (stimulus = quick, light stretch); associated reaction (stimulus = resistance to movement of the opposite side of the body), and the tonic neck and labyrinthine reflexes (stimulus = position of the head). Supporting the limb in a gravity-eliminated plane in either the therapist's hand, on a "skate" (Fig. 5.3), or in a mobile arm support allows the limb to move. The patient gets somatosensory and visual feedback because of the movement. Painful stimuli are used only as a last resort in the case of semicomatose patients on whom other stimuli are ineffective.

The reflex response is evoked in combination with a demand for voluntary effort to accomplish a movement goal. The response is reinforced by adding resistance to the evoked motion to recruit more motor units both through peripheral servo-assist and through central reprogramming of an ongoing motion. Other sensory stimuli may be added to enhance the movement as the pattern is learned through repetition.

The flexor/adductor (phasic) muscles are facilitated. The stimulation of the reflex component is deleted, and gradually all extra stimulation is withdrawn as the movement comes under voluntary control. Variations of the newly learned response are practiced and used functionally. Once gross, full limb movements are possible, more discrete control of each joint is attempted.

In summary, mobility is brought about by use of phasic reflexes preferentially, or tonic reflexes if necessary, by stimulation of the muscles responsible for the movement, by demanding a developmentally appropriate movement, and by practice.

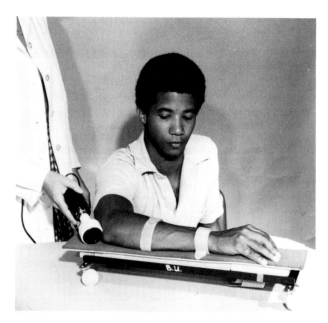

Figure 5.3 Arm is supported on therapeutic skate, and movement is elicited by use of vibration.

Obviously these treatment techniques need serious clinical research to validate their effectiveness. In any case, persons with central nervous system motor deficits rarely achieve full recovery, and some become progressively worse. We believe that teaching compensatory techniques to accomplish important daily tasks for which the person is responsible should be integrated into the therapy program to ensure success and feelings of competence. Function by whatever means is the goal.

References

1. Bannister, R. *Brain's Clinical Neurology*, 4th ed. New York: Oxford University Press, 1973.
2. Stein, D. G., Rosen, J. J., Graziadei, J. Mishkin, D., and Brink, J. Central nervous system: Recovery of function. *Science, 166:* 528-530, 1969.
3. Stenevi, U., Bjorklund, A., and Moore, R. Y. Morphological plasticity of central adrenergic neurons. *Brain Behav. Evol., 8:* 110-134, 1973.
4. Lynch, G. G., Smith, R. L. and Cotman, C. W. Recovery of function following brain damage: A consideration of some neural mechanisms. In *Neurophysiologic Aspects of Rehabilitation Medicine*, edited by A. A. Buerger and J. S. Tobis. Springfield, Ill.: Charles C Thomas, 1976.
5. Harris, F. A. Facilitation techniques in therapeutic exercise. In *Therapeutic Exercise*, 3rd ed, edited by J. V. Basmajian. Baltimore: Williams & Wilkins, 1978.
6. Phillips, C. G. Motor apparatus of the baboon's hand. *Proc. R. Soc. Lond. [Biol.], 173:* 141-174, 1969.
7. Yu, J. Functional recovery with and without training following brain damage in experimental animals: A review. *Arch. Phys. Med. Rehabil., 57:* 38-41, 1976.
8. Goldman, P. S. The role of experience in recovery of function following orbital prefrontal lesions in infant monkeys. *Neuropsychologia, 14:* 401-412, 1976.
9. Teuber, H-L., and Rudel, R. G. Behavior after cerebral lesions in children and adults. *Dev. Med. Child Neurol., 4:* 3-20, 1962.
10. Gardner, E. B. The neurophysiological basis of motor learning. *Phys. Ther. 47:* 115-122, 1967.
11. Granit, R. *The Purposive Brain*. Cambridge, Mass.: M.I.T. Press, 1977.
12. Klein, R. M. Attention and movement. In *Motor Control: Issues and Trends*, edited by G. E. Stelmach. New York: Academic Press, 1976.
13. Miller, G. A., Galanter, E., and Pribram, K. H. *Plans and the Structure of Behavior*. New York: Henry Holt & Co., 1960.
14. Kelso, J. A. S., and Stelmach, G. E. Central and peripheral mechanisms in motor control. In *Motor Control: Issues & Trends*, edited by G. E. Stelmach. New York: Academic Press, 1976.
15. Adams, J. A. Issues for a closed-loop theory of motor learning. In *Motor Control: Issues & Trends*, edited by G. E. Stelmach. New York: Academic Press, 1976.
16. Pribram, K. H. The neurophysiology of remembering. *Sci. Am., 220:* 73-86, 1969.
17. Gentile, A. M. A working model of skill acquisition with application to teaching. *Quest, 17:* 3-23, 1972.
18. Schmidt, R. A., and Wrisberg, C. A. Further tests of Adams' closed loop theory: Response produced feedback and the error detection mechanism. *J. Motor Behav., 5:* 155-164, 1973.
19. Sage, G. H. *Introduction to Motor Behavior: A Neuropsychological Approach*, 2nd ed. Reading, Mass.: Addison-Wesley, 1977.
20. Ashworth, B., Grimby, L., and Kugelberg, E. Comparison of voluntary & reflex activation of motor units. *J. Neurol. Neurosurg. Psychiatry, 30:* 91-98, 1967.
21. Gazzaniga, M. Sensory motor control mechanisms. In *The Bisected Brain*, edited by M. Gazzaniga. New York: Appleton-Century Crofts, 1970.
22. Granit, R. The functional role of the muscle spindles—facts and hypotheses. *Brain, 98:* 531-556, 1975.
23. Granit, R., and Burke, R. E. The control of movement and posture. *Brain Res., 53:* 1-28, 1973.
24. Vallbo, A. B. Discharge patterns in human muscle spindle afferents during isometric voluntary contractions. *Acta Psysiol. Scand., 80:* 552-566, 1970.
25. Matthews, P. B. C. *Mammalian Muscle Receptors and Their Central Actions*. Baltimore: Williams & Wilkins, 1972.
26. Moore, J. The Golgi tendon organ and the muscle spindle. *Am. J. Occup. Ther., 28:* 415-420, 1974.
27. Lawrence, D. G., and Hopkins, D. A. The development of motor control in the rhesus monkey: Evidence concerning the role of corticomotoneuronal connections. *Brain, 99:* 235-254, 1976.
28. Evarts, E. V. Brain mechanisms in movement. *Sci. Am., 224:* 96, 1973.
29. Evarts, E. V. The third Stevenson lecture: Changing concepts of central control of movement. *Can. J. Physiol. Pharmacol., 53:* 191-201, 1975.
30. Henneman, E. The Size Principle: How the Dimension of Motoneurons Influence their Properties and Those of the Muscle Fibers They Supply. Keynote Address. International Society of Electrophysiological Kinesiology, Boston, Aug., 1979.
31. Eyzaguirre, C., and Fidone, S. J. *Physiology of the Nervous System*, 2nd ed. Chicago: Yearbook Medical Publishers, 1975.
32. Basmajian, J. V. *Muscles Alive*, 4th ed. Baltimore: Williams & Wilkins, 1979.
33. Russell, D. G. Spatial location cues and movement production. In *Motor Control: Issues & Trends*, edited by G. E. Stelmach. New York: Academic Press, 1976.
34. Eldred, E., and Hagbarth, K.-E. Facilitation and inhibition of gamma efferents by stimulation of certain skin areas. *J. Neurophysiol., 17:* 59-65, 1954.
35. Eccles, J. C. *The Understanding of the Brain*. New York: McGraw-Hill, 1973.
36. Millar, J. Joint afferent fibers responding to muscle stretch, vibration, and contraction. *Brain Res., 63:* 382, 1973.
37. Freeman, M. A. R., and Wyke, B. Articular contributions to limb muscle reflexes. *Br. J. Surg., 53:* 66, 1966.
38. Schmidt, R. A. The schema as a solution to some persistent problems in motor learning theory. In *Motor Control: Issues & Trends*, edited by G. E. Stelmach. New York: Academic Press, 1976.
39. Gottlieb, G. L., and Agarwal, G. C. The role of the myotatic

reflex in the voluntary control of movements. *Brain Res.*, *40:* 139–143, 1972.

40. Bizzi, E., Dev, P., Morasso, P., and Polit, A. Effect of load disturbances during centrally initiated movements. *J. Neurophysiol.*, *41:* 542–556, 1978.

41. Merton, P. A. How we control the contraction of our muscles. *Sci. Am.*, *226*(5): 30–37, 1972.

42. Evarts, E. V. Motor cortex reflexes associated with learned movements. *Science, 179:* 501–503, 1973.

43. Vallbo, A. B. The significance of intramuscular receptors in load compensation during voluntary contractions in man. In *Advances in Behavioral Biology, Vol. 7: Control of Posture and Locomotion*, edited by R. B. Stein, K. G. Pearson, R. S. Smith, and J. B. Redford. New York: Plenum Press, 1973.

44. Marsden, C. D., Merton, P. A., and Morton, H. B. Is the human stretch reflex cortical rather than spinal? *Lancet*, April 7: 759–761, 1973.

45. Conrad, B., and Aschoff, J. C. Effects of voluntary isometric and isotonic activity on late transcortical reflex components in normal subjects and hemiparetic patients. *Electroencephalogr. Clin. Neurophysiol.*, *42:* 107–116, 1977.

46. Conrad, B., Matsunami, K., Meyer-Lohman, J., Wiesendanger, M., and Brooks, V. B. Cortical load compensation during voluntary elbow movements. *Brain Res.*, *71:* 507–514, 1974.

47. Marsden, C. D. Servo control, the stretch reflex and movement in man. In *New Developments in Electromyography & Clinical Neurophysiology* Vol III, edited by J. E. Desmedt. Basel: S. Karger, 1973.

48. Urbscheit, N. L. Reflexes evoked by group II afferent fibers from muscle spindles. *Phys. Ther.*, *59:* 1083–1087, 1979.

49. Vallbo, A. B. Slowly adapting muscle receptors in man. *Acta Physiol. Scand.*, *78:* 315–333, 1970.

50. Skoglund, S. Anatomical and physiological studies of knee joint innervation in the cat. *Acta Physiol. Scand.*, *36* (Suppl. 124): 3–101, 1956.

51. Marsden, D. C., Merton, P. A., and Morton, H. B. Servo action and stretch reflex in human muscle and its apparent dependence on peripheral sensation. *J. Physiol.*, *216:* 21P–22P, 1971.

52. Hulliger, M., Nordh, E., Thelin, A-E., and Vallbo, A. B. The responses of afferent fibers from the glabrous skin of the hand during voluntary finger movements in man. *J. Physiol.*, *291:* 233–249, 1979.

53. Greenwood, R., and Hopkins, A. Landing from an unexpected fall and a voluntary step. *Brain*, *99:* 375–386, 1976.

54. Wilson, V. J. The labyrinth, the brain and posture. *Am. Sci.*, *63:* 325–332, 1975.

55. Keele, S. W., and Summers, J. J. The structure of motor programs. In *Motor Control: Issues and Trends*, edited by G. E. Stelmach. New York: Academic Press, 1976.

56. Polit, A., and Bizzi, E. Characteristics of motor programs underlying arm movements in monkeys. *J. Neurophysiol.*, *42:* 183–194, 1979.

57. Smith, J. L., Roberts, E. M., and Atkins, E. Fusimotor neuron block and voluntary arm movement in man. *Am. J. Phys. Med.*, *51:* 225–237, 1972.

58. Atkinson, R. C., and Shiffrin, R. M. The control of short-term memory. *Sci. Am.*, *225:* 82–90, 1971.

59. Held, R. Plasticity in sensory-motor systems. *Sci. Am.*, *213:* 84–94, 1965.

60. Cohen, L. Manipulation of cortical motor responses by peripheral sensory stimulation. *Arch. Phys. Med. Rehabil.*, 495–506, 1969.

61. Hagbarth, K.-E., and Eklund, G. Motor effects of vibrating muscle stimuli in man. In *Muscular Afferents and Motor Control: Nobel Symposium I*, edited by R. Granit, New York: John Wiley & Sons, 1966.

62. Bishop, B. Vibratory stimulation. Part III. Possible applications of vibration in treatment of motor dysfunctions. *Phys. Ther.*, *55*(2): 139–143, 1975.

63. Hagbarth, K.-E. Excitatory and inhibitory skin areas for flexor and extensor motoneurones. *Acta Physiol. Scand.*, *27:* 129–160, 1952.

64. Eldred, E., and Hagbarth, K.-E. Facilitation and inhibition of gamma efferents by stimulation of certain skin areas. *J. Neu-*

rophysiol., *17:* 59–65, 1954.

65. Blashy, M., and Fuchs, R. Orthokinetics: A new receptor facilitation method. *Am. J. Occup. Ther.*, *13:* 226, 1959.

66. Whelan, J. Effect of orthokinetics on upper extremity function of the adult hemiplegic patient. *Am. J. Occup. Ther.*, *18*(4): 141–143, 1964.

67. Ayres, A. J. *Sensory Integration and Learning Disorders.* Los Angeles: Western Psychological Services, 1972.

68. Tokizane, T., Murao, M., Ogata, T., and Kondo, T. Electromyographic studies on tonic neck, lumbar, and labyrinthine reflexes in normal persons. *Jpn. J. Physiol.*, *2:* 130–146, 1951.

69. Eklund, G., and Hagbarth, K.-E. Normal variability in tonic vibration reflexes in man. *Exp. Neurol.*, *16:* 80–92, 1966.

70. Johnston, R., Bishop, B., and Coffey, G. Mechanical vibration of skeletal muscles. *Phys. Ther.*, *50:*(4): 499–505, 1970.

71. Lance, J. W., DeGail, P., and Neilson, P. D. Tonic and phasic spinal cord mechanisms in man. *J. Neurol. Neurosurg. Psychiatr.*, *29:* 141, 1966.

72. Hagbarth, K.-E., and Eklund, G. The effects of muscle vibration in spasticity, rigidity, and cerebellar disorders. *J. Neurol. Neurosurg. Psychiatry 31:* 207–213, 1968.

73. Matthews, P. B. C. A critique of the hypotheses that the spindle secondary endings contribute excitation to the stretch reflex. In *Advances in Behavioral Biology, Vol. 7: Control of Posture and Locomotion*, edited by R. B. Stein, K. G. Pearson, R. S. Smith, and J. B. Redford. New York: Plenum Press, 1973, pp. 227–243.

74. Kottke, F. Reflex patterns initiated by the secondary sensory fiber endings of muscle spindles: A proposal. *Arch. Phys. Med. Rehabil.*, *56:* 1–7, 1975.

75. Kenny, W. E., and Heaberlin, P. C. An electromyographic study of the locomotor patern of spastic children. *Clin. Orthop.*, *24:* 139–151, 1962.

76. Stockmeyer, S. An interpretation of the approach of Rood to the treatment of neuromuscular dysfunction. *Am. J. Phys. Med.* (NUSTEP Proceedings), *46*(1): 900–956, 1967.

77. Hirt, S. The tonic neck reflex mechanism in the normal human adult. *Am. J. Phys. Med.*, (NUSTEP Proceedings), *46:* 362–369, 1967.

78. Hunt, C. C. The effect of sympathetic stimulation on mammalian muscle spindles. *J. Physiol.*, *151:* 332–341, 1960.

79. Miglietta, O. Action of cold on spasticity. Am. J. Phys. Med., *52:* 198–205, 1973.

80. Chase, R. A., Cullen, J. K., and Sullivan, S. A. Modification of intention tremor in man. *Nature, 206:* 485–487, 1965.

81. Morgan, M. H. Ataxia and weights. *Physiotherapy, 61:* 332–334, 1975.

82. Hewer, R. L., Cooper, R., and Morgan, M. H. An investigation into the value of treating intention tremor by weighting the affected limb. *Brain, 95:* 579–590, 1972.

83. Harris, F. A. Exteroceptive feedback of position and movement in remediation for disorders of coordination. In *Behavioral Psychology in Rehabilitation Medicine: Clinical Applications*, edited by L. P. Ince. Baltimore: Williams & Wilkins, 1980, pp. 87–156.

84. Hammond, P. H. The influence of prior instruction to the subject on apparently involuntary neuromuscular responses. *J. Physiol.*, *132:* 17P–18P, 156.

85. Ashby, P., and Burke, D. Stretch reflexes in the upper limb of spastic man. *J. Neurol. Neurosurg. Psychiatry, 34:* 765–771, 1971.

Supplementary Reading

Kottke, F. J. From reflex to skill: The training of coordination. *Arch. Phys. Med. Rehabil.*, *61*(12): 551–561, 1980.

Newell, K. M. Knowledge of results and motor learning. *J. Motor Behav.*, *6*(4): 235–244, 1974.

Pedersen, E. Management of spasticity on neurophysiologic basis. *Scand. J. Rehabil. Med.*, *Suppl 7:* 68–79, 1980.

Rushworth, G. Some pathophysiological aspects of spasticity and the search for rational and successful therapy. *Int. Rehabil. Med.*, *2:* 10–16, 1980.

Tracey, D. J. Joint receptors and the control of movement. *Trends Neurosci.*, *29:* 253–255, 1980.

chapter

6

Neurophysiological and Developmental Treatment Approaches

Four neurophysiologically and developmentally based approaches for the treatment of patients with motor control problems are:

1. The Rood approach
2. The Bobath neurodevelopmental approach
3. The Brunnstrom approach: movement therapy
4. The Proprioceptive Neuromuscular Facilitation (PNF) approach

Each approach is described as it is presented in the most recently available literature. Additional information is available to those who attend training workshops. Primary sources of information have been supplemented by the writings of others to present as complete a description of each approach as possible. In only one case have we included any information from a conference that has not been reported in the literature.

The four approaches are more similar than divergent, which is not surprising, because each has the goal of improved motor control for patients with brain damage and because each is based on information about the same central nervous system. Similarities include the importance of sensation to movement, the importance of repetition for learning, and the need for the patient to develop or redevelop motor control sequentially. The differences have to do with the use of conscious attention to movement and the use of spinal and brain stem level reflexes to elicit movement. None of the approaches addresses methods of developing skilled movement; all emphasize the development of basic movement and postures that underlie skill.

There must be collaboration among members of the rehabilitation team when these approaches are used because all the stimulation offered the patient during each day will affect his motor control and because goals must be coordinated. For example, if the goal of one therapy is to inhibit associated reactions, treatment given by other therapies should not be directed toward facilitating them.

The reader is encouraged to develop his own theory of motor control or his own treatment approach based on a sound rationale of neurophysiology, motor learning, and motor development. The reader may decide to eclectically choose procedures from several of the approaches presented in this chapter as those procedures fit his own theoretical framework at his level of understanding. Every procedure, whether proposed by others or originally deduced by the reader, must be clinically tested for effectiveness.

The Rood Approach

CATHERINE A. TROMBLY, M.A., OTR

Margaret Rood is both an occupational and a physical therapist. She has made contributions to therapists' knowledge regarding the treatment of persons with brain damage. Her major contributions are the emphasis on controlled sensory stimulation, the use of ontogenetic sequence, and the need to demand a purposeful response by the use of activity. She interpreted the research data related to the development of movement and the neurophysiological basis of movement and attempted to bridge between facts learned from the animal research to clinical application. Rood spent many years studying and clinically testing treatment methods that she devised based upon her readings. Treatment was originally designed for cerebral palsy but she believes it is applicable to any patient with motor control problems.[1]

Rood shared her ideas with others through clinical and classroom teaching but has written very little. Because she so rarely writes, some of the ideas reported here are based on interpretations of her method by three other knowledgeable therapists: Joy Huss, A. Jean Ayres, and Shirley Stockmeyer, who have helped clarify for other therapists the procedures and their rationale. It is sometimes difficult to identify where Rood's thinking leaves off and the other therapists' begins.

Rood's basic premise was[2]:

Motor patterns are developed from fundamental reflex patterns present at birth which are utilized and gradually modified through sensory stimuli until the highest control is gained on the conscious cortical level. It seemed to me then, that if it were possible to apply the proper sensory stimuli to the appropriate sensory receptor as it is utilized in normal sequential development, it might be possible to elicit motor responses reflexly and by following neurophysiological principles, establish proper motor engrams.

There are four major components of Rood's theory[3,4]:

1. The normalization of tone and evocation of desired muscular responses is accomplished through the use of appropriate sensory stimuli. Correct sensory input is necessary for the development of correct motor responses. Controlled sensory input is used to evoke muscular responses reflexly[5] which Rood believes is the earliest developmental step in gaining motor control.

2. Sensorimotor control is developmentally based and therefore therapy must start at the patient's level of development and progress him sequentially to higher and higher levels of sensorimotor control according to sequences Rood has identified. Muscular responses reflexly obtained are used in developmental patterns[5] in an effort to develop supraspinal control of those responses.

3. Movement is purposeful. Rood uses activity to demand a purposeful response from the patient in order to subcortically elicit the desired movement pattern. The responses of agonists, antagonists, and synergists are reflexly programmed according to a purpose or plan.[5] When the cortex commands "pick up the glass," for example, all the subcortical centers involved in motor performance cause facilitation or inhibition of muscles as appropriate for that program to allow the accomplishment of the motion[4] in a coordinated manner. The cortex does not direct each muscle individually.[5] The patient's attention is drawn to the end-goal or purpose, not the movement. Sensation that occurs during movement is basic to motor learning. In this way, the patient is helped to gain control over movement elicited reflexly.[5]

Purposeful movement cannot be invariably used; it may not be possible for a severely involved patient to respond in this way. It is, however, important to use this method when possible.[4] It is especially applicable when the focus of treatment is the trunk, lower extremities, or the proximal segments of the upper extremities, all of which are more or less subcortically controlled.[4,5] If the focus of treatment is development of skill in the distal segments of the upper extremities, then the attention of the patient must be on the movement of these parts which are more directly cortically controlled.[4,5]

4. Repetition of sensorimotor responses is necessary for learning.[4,6] Activities are used to provide purpose and repetition.

SENSORY STIMULI TO EVOKE MUSCULAR RESPONSES

Rood has determined certain methods of influencing motor responses from trial and error in clinical practice, based on the results cited in studies of the effects of stimuli on animals. The following methods have been found to be facilitating or inhibiting as described. However, the reader is reminded that the actual response each patient will exhibit will be an algebraic summation of all internal and external stimuli he is experiencing. Therefore, as in any therapeutic procedure, the response of the patient is carefully monitored and the stimuli changed as necessary to elicit the desired response. The effects of the TLR and the TNR may assist or retard the effects of the applied stimulus, and therefore the positioning of the patient during stimulation is important.[6]

Facilitation Methods

Tactile stimulation is offered in two ways: fast brushing and light stroking. Fast brushing refers to brushing of the hairs[7] or the skin over a muscle[5] by the use of a soft camel hair paint brush that has been substituted for the stirrer of a hand-held battery-powered cocktail mixer[8,9] (Fig. 6.1) and is now commercially available as a battery-powered brush. The revolving brush is applied on each skin area over the muscles to be stimulated.[5,6] Brushing can be effectively done on the skin of the dermatome served by the same spinal segment as those muscles in which the therapist is attempting to sensitize the muscle spindles.[5] Brushing of the dermatone is done for 5 seconds for each area.[10] If there is no response to the brushing after 30 seconds, the brushing of each area should be repeated three to five times more.[5,6] Fast brushing is thought to be a high threshold stimulus to the C size sensory fibers that discharge into polysynaptic pathways that are involved in the maintenance of posture and background gamma efferent activity.[5] The spindle is biased by this gamma system activity. High threshold receptors, of which the C fiber is an example, are difficult to stimulate and require a high intensity stimulus.[5] Fast brushing is a high intensity stimulus because of the high rate of revolutions of the brush and the duration that it is used.[5] High threshold stimulation facilitates the gamma system to bias spindles to increase the response to added external or internal stretch.[5]

The effect of fast brushing is nonspecific and reaches its maximum 30 to 40 minutes after stimulation due to the enhancement of the reticular activating system into which the C fibers feed.[5,7,11] In controlled studies of normal and post-stroke persons, Spicer and Matyas demonstrated a significant immediate facilitatory effect of fast brushing but no long-lasting effect (45 seconds postapplication) could be demonstrated.[12,13] The first manifestation may be on the opposite side of the body, especially in the lower extremities.[6] Fast brushing of the skin over the distribution of the posterior primary rami adjacent to the vertebral column

facilitates the tonic, deep muscles of the back, not the superficial ones; whereas fast brushing of the skin over the rest of the body, supplied by the anterior primary rami, facilitates a tonic response of the superficial muscles if the dermatomes corresponding to the muscles are brushed.[5] As soon as the patient is able to voluntarily control movement, stroking (brushing) is no longer effective.[6]

There are some precautions to be observed in relation to fast brushing. Fast brushing of the pinna of the ear stimulates the vagus nerve which influences cardiorespiratory functions. The vagus nerve is part of the parasympathetic section of the autonomic nervous system. Activation of this nerve slows the heart, produces bronchial constriction, and bronchial secretion.[14] Fast brushing over the posterior primary rami of L_{1-2} will cause voiding; over S_{2-4} will cause bladder retention (improve incontinence).[5]

Light touch or stroking of the skin activates the low threshold A size sensory fibers to activate reciprocal action of the superficial phasic or mobilizing muscles.[5-8] Low threshold receptors are easily stimulated and effect a fast, short-lived response through facilitation of the extrafusal motor system. Light stroking of the dorsum of the webs of the fingers or toes, or of the palms of the hands or the soles of the feet, elicits a phasic withdrawal motion of the stimulated limb.[5] Repetitive use of this stimulus to these areas will result in a crossed extensor reflex pattern.[5]

Thermal facilitation is done by using ice.[5] Icing is thought to have the same effects as brushing and stroking through the same neural mechanisms.[5,7] A convenient way to administer icing is by the use of plastic popsicle molds, which gives the therapist a handle to hold while icing.[8] "C-icing" is a high threshold stimulus used to stimulate postural, tonic responses via the C size sensory fibers.[5] Icing to activate the C fibers is done by holding the ice cube pressed in place for 3 to 5 seconds,[5] then wiping away the water. The skin areas to be stimulated are the same as noted for fast brushing with the exception of the distribution of the posterior primary rami along the back, which is avoided because it may cause a sympathetic nervous system response.[5,10] The ice, a noxious stimulus, when applied over the sympathetic chain causes a protective response of that system (vasoconstriction).[14]

"A-icing" is the application of quick swipes of the ice cube to evoke a reflex withdrawal, similar to the response of light touch, when the stimulus is applied to the palms or soles or the dorsal webs of the hands or feet.[5] When a response occurs, resistance to the movement is usually given.[8]

Quick icing is for use with "flaccid-placid types only."[5] A-icing of the upper right quadrant of the abdomen in the dermatomal representation for T_{7-9} will result in stimulation of the diaphragm.[5] Touching the lips with ice opens the mouth (a withdrawal response), but ice applied to the tongue and inside the lips closes the mouth.[5]

There is a rebound effect to icing which occurs approximately 30 seconds after stimulation[5] in which

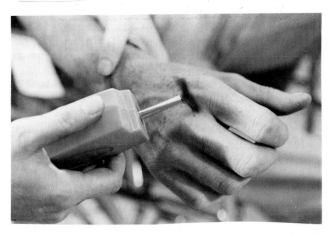

Figure 6.1 Battery-operated brush applied to facilitate finger extension.

the muscles so stimulated become temporarily inhibited. It is not clearly stated whether this rebound effect occurs with both types of icing.

Precautions about icing are similar to those for brushing. Icing of the pinna causes automatic vagal responses.[5] Ice to the trunk at the level of L_2 causes voiding and to S_{2-4}, urinary retention.[5]

Rider[15] found a statistically significant increase in strength of the triceps of normal children and children who had bilateral upper extremity flexor spasticity following a 2-week period of stimulation as compared to their strength scores before treatment. Stimuli used to facilitate the skin over the triceps were fast brushing, stroking, tapping, and C-icing. The level of significance was $p = 0.01$. There was also an increase in strength of triceps of both groups in the unfacilitated upper extremity, but this increase never exceeded the effect of direct stimulation. There was a significant mean decrease in strength of both elbow extensors of both groups following a 2-week period of no facilitation, with the exception that the strength of the extensor on the preferred side of the normal subjects leveled off at about the strength achieved postfacilitation and did not lose strength as all the others did.

In practice, high threshold stimulation precedes low threshold stimulation because of the longer lasting effects of the former.[5] It is suggested that since brushing and icing have a bilateral effect, stimulation of the unaffected side of a hemiplegic person prior to stimulation of his affected side would be beneficial.[6, 9]

The remainder of the stimuli to be discussed are proprioceptive stimuli; the effects of which last only for as long as the stimulus is applied.

Quick, light stretch of a muscle is a low threshold stimulus which activates a phasic response of the same muscles stretched through the primary (Ia) afferent endings of the spindles and the alpha motor neuron.[5] This is the phasic stretch reflex. The effect of quick, light stretch is immediate. Such stretch to a light work muscle, a physiological flexor or adductor, facilitates that muscle and inhibits its antagonist.[5]

Tapping of the tendon or the belly of the muscle to be facilitated is essentially the same phenomenon as quick stretch.[4] The therapist percusses the area using the fingertips.

Pressure on the muscle belly similarly elicits a stretch response by placing a stretch on the spindles.[4] It is done by manually pressing on the muscle or by the use of equipment which presses on the muscle.

Secondary stretch is a maintained stretch at the end of range used to facilitate the secondary (II) afferent fibers of the spindle. Secondary stretch of the heavy work muscles, the physiological extensors and abductors, facilitates their antagonists, the flexors and adductors, at the same time that these antagonists are in the shortened range.[4, 5] Research is needed here in light of newer hypotheses concerning the role of the secondary afferent.

Stretch to the intrinsic muscles of the hand or foot causes a facilitation of cocontraction of the proximal stabilizer muscles.[4, 8] Activities requiring forceful grasp stretch the intrinsics. If such activities can be combined in weight-bearing positions, the proximal stabilizers are further facilitated through the demand placed on them for cocontraction. In the prone-on-elbows position, a child can shoot water pistols to achieve this result. Grasping of handles of tools during their use also facilitates this response, especially if the handles have been modified to be cone shaped with the widest part of the cone at the ulnar border of the hand which further stretches the intrinsics. In one electromyographical study of the scapulohumeral muscles of normal adults, the weight-bearing position evoked little electrical activity ("extremely minimal"), unless used in combination with resisted grasp. Even then, the response was of low level.[16] Therefore, this question is opened for research.

Resistance is a form of stretch in which many or all of the spindles of a muscle are stimulated.[9] The spindle, of course, cannot know whether the discrepancy it senses is due to being stretched by a moving force or by resistance which is preventing the extrafusal muscle fibers from shortening as it shortens as programmed. The discrepancy causes the spindle to fire impulses in order to get more extrafusal muscle units firing. The electrical activity of the interneuronal pool is consequently high, and more and more motor units are more easily recruited to fire, a phenomenon called overflow. Resisting a phasic contraction prolongs the facilitation to bias the spindle and prevents immediate inhibition of the contracting muscles due to the effect of the GTO.[8] Resistance to contraction of muscles in a shortened range activates spindles and must be used to bias the spindles of the deeper, more tonic muscles used for posture which cannot be stimulated by C fiber stimulation which primarily activates peripheral muscles,[5] except in the back where C fiber stimulation is said to activate the deep muscles.[5]

A shortened, held, resisted contraction biases the spindles to a shorter length which makes them very sensitive to stretch.[5, 8]

Eccentric contraction against resistance provides a great amount of stretch, both external and internal, which maximally activates the primary afferents.

Heavy joint compression facilitates cocontraction of muscles around a joint. Heavy compression refers to resistance greater than body weight[5] which is applied so that the force is through the longitudinal axes of the bones whose articular surfaces approximate each other.[4] Resistance greater than body weight refers to that which is more than the weight of the body parts above the supporting joint. This type of stimulus activates high threshold receptors.[4] The stabilizing muscles need to go through a stage of holding against resistance in a shortened position before they are asked to cocontract as a response to heavy joint compression.[8] Weight-bearing positions of prone-on-elbows, prone-on-hands, quadruped, and standing are heavy joint compression positions if the patient lifts one or two extremities and bears weight on the other, weaker ones. Or, weights can be added: a hat or crown incorporating a ring of buckshot increases neck joint compression of a child, thereby improving head control.[11] Weighted bags, lead x-ray aprons, etc. can be placed on the shoulders, hips, or backs of patients, depending on their position, to increase the joint compression.

Pressure on bony prominences have both facilitatory and inhibitory results during normal purposeful movement.[4] For example, pressure over the lateral aspect of the calcaneous facilitates the medial dorsiflexors while inhibiting the calf muscles to allow dorsiflexion. Pressure on the medial aspect of the calcaneous facilitates the lateral dorsiflexors.[4]

Rood utilizes stimuli to special senses to facilitate or inhibit the skeletal musculature generally or that involved in vital functions more specifically. Olfactory and gustatory stimuli are facilitating or inhibiting through their influence on the autonomic nervous system. Unpleasant or potentially dangerous stimuli elicit a sympathetic ("fight or flight") reaction, and pleasant or nondangerous stimuli evoke a parasympathetic response and inhibit the sympathetic.[5] These stimuli will produce an emotional response as well as a physical response in the body.[5]

Auditory and visual stimuli can be used to generally facilitate or inhibit the central nervous system of the patient. Stimuli from all cranial nerves feed into the reticular formation,[5, 7] the alerting mechanism. Music with a definite beat would be facilitatory; soft, lullaby music would be inhibitory. A noisy, raucous clinic will be stimulating and may affect the performance of the patient with central nervous system dysfunction. The therapist's voice and manner of speech (fast and staccato vs. slow and calming, for example) may also affect the patient's performance. A drab, dull, colorless, and uninteresting environment will promote sleep and loss of tone.[7] A colorful, lighted, multistimuli environment will have a generalized facilitatory effect. Different colors may be more facilitating than others for each patient.

In summary, facilitation of phasic responses is done when no movement exists or following development of tonic responses. A-brushing and icing, quick, light stretch, and muscle or tendon tapping are used. Resistance to the movement may be added after it starts to reinforce it. Tonic responses are facilitated when there is too much movement or to develop postural stability. C-brushing and icing, secondary stretch, and heavy joint compression and resistance are used.

Inhibition Methods

Light joint compression, also called joint approximation, can be used to inhibit spastic muscles.[4] To use this method to relieve pain of spastic muscles of the shoulder, often seen in hemiplegic patients, hold the patient's elbow, abduct the arm to about 35 to 45°, and gently push the head of the humerus into the glenoid fossa and hold it there; the muscles will relax.[4, 11]

Slow stroking of the posterior primary rami with a firm but light pressure inhibits muscle tone in general and relaxes the patient.[4, 5] One of the therapist's hands starts at the back of the patient's head and strokes slowly and lightly but firmly along the vertebral musculature to the coccyx, at which time the therapist's other hand starts at the head and progresses likewise to the coccyx. This stroking using alternating hands is done for about 3 to 5 minutes[6, 9] or until the patient relaxes.[6]

Slow rolling of the patient from supine to side-lying is generally inhibitory.[10] The therapist holds the patient's shoulder and hip to slowly roll him. This continues until relaxation is seen. *Slow* rocking in a rocking chair, hollow barrel, etc. are variations. Self-administered rocking must be carefully monitored, because if it develops into fast rocking it will be facilitatory by way of vestibular stimulation.

Neutral warmth refers to maintaining the body heat by wrapping the specific area to be inhibited, or the area served by the posterior primary rami for a general effect, in a cotton blanket or down pillow or comforter for 10 to 20 minutes.[4, 10] Neutral heat is used because if heat greater than body temperature is used a rebound effect may occur in 2 to 3 hours which means the inhibited muscles become as facilitated as they were before this treatment or even superfacilitated.[5]

Pressure on the tendinous insertion of a muscle inhibits that muscle through the receptors located under the tendinous insertions, the Pacinian corpuscles.[4, 8, 10] The extrinsic flexors of the hand may be inhibited by applying constant pressure over the entire length of the long tendons.[8] Grasp of enlarged, firm or hard adapted handles of tools would provide this stimulation. Grasp also facilitates proximal cocontraction, as was stated previously.

A maintained stretch or maintenance of a lengthened position for a period of time ranging from several minutes to several weeks rebiases the spindle to the longer position. The lengthened muscle's spindles are rebiased longer and will not react to stretch as briskly at shorter ranges following this procedure. On the other hand, if a muscle is positioned in the shortened range, the muscle's spindles will be rebiased shorter and will react briskly to stretch beyond that shortened range. The balance of tone between agonists and antagonists will be disturbed if prolonged positioning is allowed. A contracture may ensue. Sometimes prolonged positioning is desired, e.g., when a spastic flexor muscle is held into a lengthened range by a cast or splint for several weeks, its spindles reset to the longer position and it is therefore less spastic. It has been demonstrated that a decrease of tone in the flexors of the hand and wrist, with a corresponding reciprocal increase of tone in the extensors, results.[17] A very weak muscle's spindles can also be biased shorter to increase tone in this passive way, although some of the more direct facilitatory methods that have been described that bias the spindle and increase internal stretch sensitivity are faster. Unresisted contraction can be used to inhibit the agonist by way of the low threshold GTOs; this would reciprocally facilitate the antagonists. To inhibit tight (spastic) muscles, Rood recommends that the patient be requested to contract maximally (brief, intense contraction[8]) before moving the limb into a lengthened position.[5] The brevity and intensity of the contraction is thought to activate a large number of GTOs at once which produces an overriding autoinhibition instead of the facilitation which is seen when resistance is added gradually during an on-going contraction.[8]

SEQUENCES OF MOTOR CONTROL

Rood has identified several sequences which she uses interrelatedly but which will be presented separately here for clarity. One sequence was already mentioned earlier, when the components of the Rood method were listed. To reiterate: a muscular response is first evoked reflexly, then responses so obtained are used in developmental patterns, and finally the patient uses the response purposefully to gain control over it.

Motor Patterns and Muscle Types

Two more sequences that Rood has identified have to do with differences in muscle responses due to their anatomical design. Light work muscles lie superficially, laterally, or distally and have a tendinous origin and insertion.[5] They are multiarthrodial; they are under more voluntary control and do phasic work.[5] They are activated by light stretch or low threshold exteroceptor stimulation and inhibited by unresisted contraction. Rood identifies the light work or mobilizing muscles as flexors and adductors, but this includes multiarthrodial extensors also. These muscles are termed physiologic flexors.[14] Heavy work muscles are deep, lie close to the joint, and are uniarthrodial. In the body, they are located proximally and medially. Heavy work muscles are tonic stability muscles. The tonic muscles are the antigravity extensor muscles capable of prolonged, sustained contraction.[14] They are under greater reflex control and are activated by heavy resistance or maintained stretch and high threshold receptor stimulation. These are the deep one-joint muscles, primarily extensors and abductors.[5]

Rood believes that neuromuscular integration is most normal if each muscle learns to contract first as it would normally be used phylogenetically and ontogenetically. Flexion precedes extension; adduction precedes abduction; ulnar patterns develop before radial ones; and rotation develops last.[11] She believes that if the normal first response of a muscle is a stabilizing contraction, it should be facilitated to contract in this manner and not in a mobilizing pattern. However, there is no convenient listing of what the original phylogenetic or ontogenetic function of each muscle was to guide this aspect of treatment. Therapists are guided by Rood's definitions of heavy work (tonic, stabilizing) muscles and light work (phasic, mobilizing) muscles in planning treatment. Therapeutic movement should be planned to be most advantageous to the particular muscle group being facilitated. Phasic flexors are facilitated if they are positioned so that their motion starts from the lengthened range, i.e., at the farthest point toward extension that can easily be

achieved, because flexors are facilitated by both their Ia and II afferents.[8, 9] Tonic extensors, on the other hand, should not be started in their lengthened range, due to the inhibitory effects of their own II afferents, but should rather start their contraction in the mid to shortened range.[8, 9] Because of the uncertainty of the effects of stimulation of the II afferents, as mentioned in the previous chapter, these suggestions need to be clinically tested. In the process of strengthening a muscle's responses, treatment must continue until the muscle is able to work strongly in all positions and the spindles exhibit a normal bias in all positions for voluntary motor control to be considered complete.

Another sequence that Rood identified has to do with the levels of developing motor control. There are four phases.

1. Muscles contract through their range with reciprocal inhibition of the antagonists.[4, 5] Stockmeyer[8] terms this the Mobility phase. Movement first appears as phasic, reciprocal shortening and lengthening contractions of muscles that cause movement which subserves a protective function.[4, 5] The stimulus for this type of response is quick, light stretch or stroking of the distal parts or other low threshold, A-fiber, types of stimulation. The movement of the neonate, waving his extremities back and forth in unresisted motion, typifies phasic movement.

2. Muscles around the joint contract simultaneously (cocontraction) to provide stability.[4, 8] This tonic, holding contraction is next to develop and is a basis for maintaining proximal posture to allow exploration of the environment and development of skill by the distal segments of the body.[4] Development of stability should precede work on developing phasic, skilled movement.[6] The stimuli for stability responses are high threshold stimulation: joint compression; stretch, especially of the intrinsic muscles of the hands and feet; fast brushing and other C-fiber stimulation; as well as resistance.[5] The reaction develops slowly over a period of 30 to 60 seconds, and maintained sensory input is necessary for a maintained response.[5, 8]

3. Proximal muscles contract to do heavy work superimposed on distal cocontraction.[4, 5] "Mobility superimposed on stability" is Stockmeyer's way of designating this level of motor control[8] in which the distal segment is fixed and the proximal segment moves. Sensory stimuli from high threshold spindle and joint receptors are involved in this response.[8] An example of this kind of motion occurs when an infant learns to assume the quadruped position but has not learned to move in that position yet: he rocks back and forth with his knees and hands planted firmly on the floor.

4. *Skill.* At this level of motor control, the proximal segment is stabilized and the distal segment moves.[4, 5] Examples of this level include walking, crawling, and use of the hands. Many occupational therapists are tempted to start therapy at this level; Ayres cautions against it.[4]

These levels of motor control are developed as the patient is paced through the skeletal developmental sequences which Rood refers to as ontogenetic motor

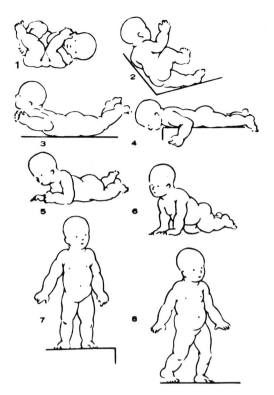

Figure 6.2 Ontogenetic motor patterns according to Rood. (*1*) Supine withdrawal; (*2*) Roll over; (*3*) Pivot prone; (*4*) Neck cocontraction; (*5*) On Elbows; (*6*) Quadruped; (*7*) Standing; (*8*) Walking. (Reproduced with permission from *Occupational Therapy*, 3rd ed, edited by H. S. Willard and C. S. Spackman. Philadelphia: J. B. Lippincott, 1963.)

patterns (Fig. 6.2). These eight patterns will be described, then the interrelationship may be studied using Table 6.1.

1. *Supine withdrawal,*[5] also called supine flexion, is a position of total flexion toward the vertebral level of T_{10}.[5, 8] The upper extremities cross the chest, and the dorsum of the extended hands touch the face. The lower extremities flex and abduct. The TLR is integrated through this posture by requiring a voluntary contraction of the flexors in spite of reflex facilitation of the antagonists. This pattern is used to obtain flexor responses when the patient has no movement or has predominant extensor responses. This pattern is used for patients who lack reciprocal phasic movement through normal range or who have not integrated the TLR.[5] This posture demands heavy work of the trunk and proximal parts of the extremities.[5] To elicit the withdrawal motor pattern, Rood[5] uses this method: fast brushing of the low back and the dermatomes of C_{1-4} posterior primary rami distribution. A small wedge is placed under the head and another under the pelvis to stretch the short extensors of the back which facilitates the flexors via the secondary endings. Putting the neck flexors and abdominals in a shortened position causes them to rebias their spindles to the shorter length, which puts them in a better condition

to maintain contraction. The extensors are facilitated through the influences of the TLR. If the extensor response is too strong to allow flexor movement, start treatment with the patient in a side-lying position.[5] A light work response of the limbs is then elicited by stroking or A-icing the sole or palm.

An activity is provided to demand the flexion/adduction pattern. A resistive activity is used to reinforce the ongoing movement; an unresisted contraction inhibits the muscle group responsible for the movement. Note that the force of the activity should be toward flexion/adduction. Suggestions are: tetherball using a lightweight ball, squeezing an accordian, and using a cylindrical cardboard balloon blower.

According to Rood,[5] this motor pattern also helps develop bowel and bladder function, eye convergence, and respiratory patterns.

2. *Roll over*—the arm and leg on the same side flex.[5] This pattern is appropriate for patients who are dominated by the primitive tonic reflexes, need mobilization of the extremities, or activation of lateral trunk musculature. Activity examples: roll over to reach an attractive object, roll down a hill, or provide something enticing for the patient to look at. Move it around to the side, thereby causing the patient's head to turn to maintain visual contact with it. The body will follow the head.

3. *Pivot prone,*[5] also called prone extension,[8] involves extension of the neck, trunk, shoulders, hips, and knees, abduction and external rotation of the shoulders, and elbow flexion. This is the first postural or stability pattern, on which all others depend. Assumption of the position is a phasic, reciprocal movement. Holding the position involves a shortened, held, resisted contraction of the extensor muscles which biases their spindles shorter so they are more sensitive. This facilitates extensor tone preparatory to weight bearing. When this position can be maintained, the STNR and the TLR are integrated. It is a chain response of the labyrinthine righting reaction. When working to achieve the whole pattern, the patient is prone on a firm, padded surface large enough to support the trunk only. If possible for the patient, the TLI posture is imposed while the patient's abdomen and pelvis are supported on a treatment ball (Fig. 6.3), barrel, small stool, etc. The area over the deep back extensors (distribution of the posterior primary rami) is C-brushed. The skin surfaces over the posterior deltoid, latissimus dorsi, trapezius, proximal hamstrings, and gluteus are C-brushed and iced if the skin is within the dermatomes. An activity is presented to demand and resist the response. Activity suggestions: pulling back on the string of a talking doll or toy, pulling back on an elastic-propelled plane in preparation for shooting it, using a sling shot (unilateral pattern),[8] riding prone on a skooter board (see Fig. 5.1), playing with a "button-on-string" toy, and rowing. Note that the force of the activity is in the direction of extension, although other movements are also involved in the activity. Simultaneously with the activity demand, vibration of the deep back and neck extensors

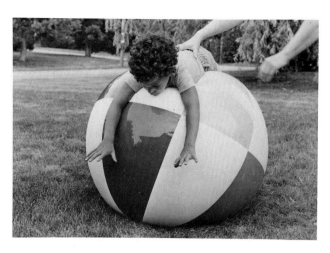

Figure 6.3 Large beach ball illustrating its use to elicit equilibrium reactions in prone and protective extensor thrust.

and other extensor muscles involved in the pattern is done, starting at the midline. The pivot prone position is held for a long period rather than relaxed and resumed repeatedly.

4. *Neck Cocontraction* is the pattern used to develop head control and is first activated in the prone position. Prior to putting the person prone, it is necessary to activate the flexors[6] if the flexors are not already active. The short neck flexors are activated first by C-brushing the flexor distribution of C_2. Next, the long neck flexors, the sternocleidomastoids, are activated. The person is then placed prone and is asked to raise his head against gravity. The labyrinth righting reaction stimulates the person to align his head so that his eyes are parallel and his nose is perpendicular to the surface on which he is lying. As the head bobs into flexion, the neck and trunk extensors are stretched and thereby facilitated to contract. The upper trapezius is activated to maintain the extension. Activation means the muscle is C-brushed 15 to 20 minutes before the demand for the pattern is made, and then during the attempt to complete the pattern, the muscles are squeezed (proprioceptive facilitation).[6] Sucking a resistive liquid through a straw or playing games in which a small object is picked up by sucking on a straw are activities that result in cocontraction of the neck muscles.[5, 8] Activities which require the person to look up while prone lying are used to demand the neck cocontraction pattern.

5. *On elbows*,[5] also called prone-on-elbows,[8] is a pattern of vertical extension. When the shoulders are brought into forward flexion so that the patient can bear weight on his elbows, the extensor muscles of the proximal upper extremity are stretched relative to the pivot prone position in which they are held shortened in extension and abduction. They are therefore facilitated to cocontract with the flexors and adductors at the shoulder in this position. A normal young child can be observed assuming the pivot prone position just prior to going into a prone-on-elbows position, as

if to "prime" his system. The child will progress to pushing backwards then forwards, like a marine belly crawling, and in time will progress to a prone position in which the arms are held straight with the hands bearing the weight. Unilateral weight bearing is more advanced than bilateral weight bearing. The prone-on-elbows pattern inhibits the STNR.[4] A procedure to achieve on elbows pattern is as follows: The back and neck extensors are C-brushed. The glenohumeral extensors and abductors are C-brushed and iced. The patient is asked to assume and hold the pivot prone position while resistance is added. Then the patient is placed in the prone on elbows position so that there is good joint compression at the shoulder. Pressure and vibration are applied to the extensor/abductor muscles of the glenohumeral joint as needed to gain cocontraction. An activity that demands resisted grasp is introduced to obtain reinforcement of shoulder cocontraction. One suggestion is for the child to shoot water pistols at a target placed in front of him. Another activity example: the person lies on the floor to watch TV which is placed so that the person must extend his neck and upper trunk to look at it. Other activities include playing board games or doing crafts while prone lying.[16] These activities begin to combine the static bilateral position with unilateral positioning and reaching. They could involve some crawling which is a higher level response (see Table 6.1).

6. *The all-fours* pattern,[5] also called quadruped,[8] occurs when the neck and upper extremities have developed stability; this position helps the trunk and lower extremities develop cocontraction. At first, the quadruped position is static; later the person is able to lift one or two of the points of support, *i.e.*, one arm and one leg. Later weight shifts backwards and forwards, from side to side, diagonally, and finally develops into crawling.[5, 8] A suggested procedure to develop the all-fours pattern is as follows: The back and neck extensors are C-brushed. The glenohumeral and hip extensors and abductors and the elbow extensors are C-brushed and iced. The patient assumes and holds the pivot prone position while resistance is added. Then the patient is placed into the all-fours position so that there is good joint compression at the elbows, shoulders, and hips. An activity that demands that the patient maintain the position is offered. Activity examples include holding a sling shot prepared to shoot (unilateral pattern while upright), weaving on a large loom adapted to resist elbow extension (while upright), holding wood in place while sawing it with the other hand, painting a large mural on the floor, and playing with a toy truck. While the activity is ongoing, stretch and vibration are applied to the muscles listed above as needed.

7. *Standing* is first done as a static bilateral posture, then progresses to a unilateral posture, and to shifting weight.[5] Activity suggestions include doing craft activities while standing at a high table and writing on a wall blackboard. Playing ball[18] or throwing bean bags help develop balance while standing.

8. *Walking* is the skill level of standing. It consists

Table 6.1
INTEGRATION OF ONTOGENETIC MOTOR PATTERNS WITH LEVELS OF MOTOR CONTROL[a]

Level I: Mobility[8]		Level II: Stability		Level III: Mobility on Stability[8]		Level IV: Skill	
Skeletal	Vital	Skeletal	Vital	Skeletal	Vital	Skeletal	Vital
1. Supine withdrawal	1. Inspiration	4. Pivot prone (held)	5. Phonation[b]	6. Neck cocontraction (orient head in space)	4. Swallow fluids	9. Prone-on-elbows, (head is doing skilled movement and one arm is free for skilled use. Belly crawling.)	5. Phonation
2. Roll over	2. Expiration	5. Neck cocontraction	3. Sucking	8. Prone-on-elbows, (shift from side to side, push backward and pull forward, unilateral weight bearing)	6. Chewing		8. Speech
3. Pivot prone (assume the position)		7. Prone-on-elbows		11. Quadruped (rocking, shifting, unilateral weight bearing)	7. Swallow solids	12. Quadruped (one arm free for skilled use. Creeping, trunk rotation and reciprocal movement, crossed diagonal.)	
		10. Quadruped		14. Standing (weight shift, unilateral weight bearing)		15. Standing and walking	
		13. Standing					

[a] The steps are numbered sequentially, but they blend together, i.e., one step is not completely mastered before the next begins at the most basic level.
[b] Although out of sequence, phonation is facilitated in the pivot prone position.[8]

of stance, push off, pick up (swing through), and heel strike.[5]

Rood's method undergoes continual evolution as current neurophysiological information becomes available. Although her newer ideas have not yet become part of the available literature, the author believes it important to report her latest ideas which she presented at a symposium cosponsored by the Massachusetts OT and PT Associations in Boston in July, 1976.[1] These ideas appear to amplify rather than negate the previous information.

Developmentally, total motor patterns are learned prior to differentiated patterns. Rood identified two total patterns: *Pattern I*, "toward pattern," is a phasic flexion pattern elicited by a light touch to the upper mouth at midline (cranial nerve V area). The patient's hands reach toward the mouth in response to this stimulus. The elbow and shoulder flex while the wrist and fingers extend. In a child, the legs also flex. In an adult, the legs flex only if the patient is touched on the abdomen near the umbilicus. Pattern I has a longer latency between stimulus and response than does pattern II. If no response is seen in supine, the patient should be positioned side-lying with the moving arm uppermost. This eliminates the contact stimulus to the extensor surface of the body and decreases the influence of the TLR which also facilitates extension. For young children and occasionally with adults, the light touch to the upper lip is followed by a maintained touch to the same area in order to balance the phasic response with a tonic response. A more discrete flexion pattern is elicited by applying the touch stimulus peripherally.[1] Pattern I seems to be equivalent to the first mobility response, the supine flexion or withdrawal pattern.

Pattern II, "away from pattern," is a tonic extensor pattern elicited by stimulation of the labyrinths, stretch receptors in muscle, and fast repetitive stimuli, such as fast brushing, which, Rood states,[1] has the effect of eliminating the stretch reflex in phasic muscles. Fast brushing precedes all other stimulation, since it requires 30 minutes to become maximally effective. The laybrinths are stimulated by use of the tonic labyrinth inverted (TLI) posture, although in adult hemiplegics, the patient is not inverted below horizontal due to the increase in cranial blood pressure that occurs when the head is dependent. The stretch receptors are stimulated by vibration; the midline deep back muscles are stimulated first before the more superficial, peripheral extensor muscles. A demand for extension against resistance is made on the patient through the use of activity.[1] Pattern II seems to be the first stability pattern, prone extension or pivot prone.

TREATMENT PROGRAMMING

Rood evaluates the patient to determine what the distribution of muscle tone is and to determine what level of motor control, according to her developmental sequences, the patient has achieved. Therapy starts by facilitating, using appropriate stimuli to facilitate the patient's muscles which will be needed to effect the pattern desired. If necessary, the patient is assisted into the desired pattern, and a purposeful activity that demands the movement and/or position and is within the capability of the patient, is immediately presented. The motor pattern chosen is the one which the patient can do. Then he is progressed through the sequences as he masters each skill. As he is perfecting a lower level skill, he may begin to learn a higher level skill. In Table 6.1 the steps are numbered sequentially for both the skeletal and vital function sequences, indicating the order used for evaluation and treatment planning.

In an attempt to illustrate the use of Rood's sequences, this example may be helpful. The evaluation of the hypothetical post-stroke patient indicated that he has some voluntary elbow flexion but his shoulder begins to abduct simultaneously with elbow flexion. He is able to grasp, but unable to release objects. He is able to roll over in bed and rotate his trunk while sitting. In sorting this data out, it is noted that the elbow flexors, probably primarily light work muscles, are contracting in that capacity, but the shoulder abductors, which are considered primarily heavy work muscles, should be contracting in a tonic pattern first. If they were doing so, the contraction would prevent the reflex abduction movement during elbow flexion. Flexion has developed at the elbow; extension is the next movement sought at that joint. Prone extension would be the next ontogenetic pattern to work for since roll over is already within his repertoire. Therefore, our treatment of this patient would involve controlled sensory stimulation of the tonic physiologic extensors of the shoulder and scapula and an activity which would demand a static prone extensor response at least unilaterally of the affected side. Stockmeyer[8] believes that it is unnecessary for the patient to actually be prone or that the activity be bilateral.

Rood suggests this plan for a post-CVA patient whose tonic muscles do not work well: 30 to 40 minutes before treatment, C-brush the tonic muscles of the unaffected side first, then those on the affected side. At treatment time, elicit pattern I (flexion) for feeding by touching the midline above the lip which will cause the hand to move to the mouth. The patient is back- or side-lying during this procedure.[1]

Joy Huss suggests some other treatment planning guidelines[9, 18]:

1. Hypotonia ("floppy baby syndrome," upper motor neuron flaccidity) is treated by overall general stimulation, especially swinging, rolling, spinning in all planes for labyrinth stimulation, and specific exteroceptive and proprioceptive stimulation for specific muscle stimulation. Activities are used to elicit specific motor patterns in sequence.

2. Hypertonia (spasticity which may be seen in spastic cerebral palsy, CVA, and multiple sclerosis patients, for example) is treated using neutral warmth for relaxation. Exteroceptive and proprioceptive stimulation of the antagonists of the spastic muscles is done. Activity is used in developmental sequence to reinforce normal movement.

3. Hypertonia (rigidity such as seen in Parkinson's disease) is treated using neutral warmth for relaxation. Reciprocal movement patterns are stimulated and reinforced using activity.

4. Hyperkinesis (uncontrolled movement such as seen in athetosis, chorea, ataxia) is treated by slow stroking for relaxation. Maintained holding patterns are stimulated at first and then patterns which involve keeping the distal segment stabilized while the proximal segment moves are used. When control is developed, the patient is progressed to movement patterns such as crawling, creeping. Activity is used to demand patterns of posture and movement.

Vital Function Developmental Sequence[11]

Functions involving food intake, respiration, and a combination of these two which are used for speech, compose this sequence, which is related to the skeletal sequence (See Table 6.1). Both sequences are handled concurrently in treatment, if appropriate. The vital function developmental sequence precedes speech. Therefore, the occupational therapist, who facilitates this sequence with the goal of decreasing dysphagia as part of a feeding program, collaborates with the speech therapist to achieve mutual goals. The sequence of development of speech mechanisms is:

1. Inspiration is effected at birth.[5]

2. Expiration is dependent on the depth of inspiration. The depth of inspiration is dependent on patterns set in the withdrawal pattern: cocontraction of the deep neck flexors and extensors and cocontraction of the low back musculature with the rectus abdominus.[5] The depth of inspiration can be further increased by icing the upper right quadrant of the abdomen to stimulate the diaphragm.[6] Crying, sneezing, and coughing are all expiration-type phenomenon.

3. Sucking. "Heavy work sucking is produced by the basic activation of cocontraction of the neck with the stabilizing influence of the infra- and suprahyoid muscles of the tongue, of cocontraction of facial muscles against the orbicularis oris above and below the mouth. Respiration and feeding depend on heavy work sucking."[5] If pressure is applied to the tip of the tongue, then sucking will ensue after five to seven repetitions of the pressure.[1] Resisted sucking facilitates neck cocontraction which in turns facilitates sucking.

4. Swallowing liquids may be activated by cutaneous stimulation of the mucous membranes of the palate, tongue, and uvula.[6] "The orbicularis oris is the key to swallowing as it activates, by direct stretch, the buccinators and superior constrictor of the pharynx."[5] Muscles of sucking and swallowing are activated, whereas voluntary muscles are relaxed, secondary to slow stroking of the cutaneous distribution of the posterior primary rami.[6] Stroking the chin will cause the patient to be unable to keep his mouth closed, resulting in drooling.

5. Phonation, defined as babbling, is controlled expiration.

6. Chewing

7. Swallowing solids

8. Speech, defined as production of recognizable words.

CONCLUSION

Rood's methods are in common usage by both occupational and physical therapists in the United States and other countries today. Nevertheless, controlled research on the effectiveness of this approach is extremely limited. As theses projects, some graduate students have conducted limited studies of isolated aspects of the approach on normal persons and patients with central nervous system deficits. However, the accessibility of their theses is limited. Other written case reports of successful results using this therapy are seemingly nonexistent. It becomes the need of present and future therapists to document the success of specific methods used to effect more mature motor responses in patients.

SECTION 2

The Bobath
Neurodevelopmental Approach
CATHERINE A. TROMBLY, M.A., OTR

Dr. and Mrs. Bobath, English neurologist and physiotherapist, respectively, have devised methods of evaluation and treatment for persons with cerebral palsy and hemiplegia. They believe the method would be effective for any patient having central nervous system deficit resulting in abnormal patterns of movement.[19]

The basic ideas from which the Bobaths devised their treatment approach are as follows. Sensations of movements are learned, not movements *per se*. Basic postural and movement patterns are learned which are later elaborated on to become functional skills. Every skilled activity takes place against a background of basic patterns of postural control, righting, equilibrium, and other protective reactions (such as the parachute reaction of the arms), reach, grasp, and release.[20]

When the brain is damaged, abnormal patterns of posture and movement develop which are incompatible with the performance of normal everyday activities. The abnormal patterns develop because sensation is shunted into these abnormal patterns. The law of shunting refers to a phenomenon the Bobaths describe as afferent inflow being

short circuited either temporarily (the athetoid patient) or more permanently (the spastic patient) into patterns of abnormal coordination released from higher inhibitory control . . . . A patient with abnormal motor output who moves abnormally in response to motivation and normal sensory input will still only experience and memorize the sensation of his abnormal movements, of excessive effort and lack of co-ordination. He will, therefore be unable to develop and lay down the memory of normal sensorimotor patterns.[20]

The abnormal patterns must be stopped, not so much by modifying the sensory input, but by giving back to the patient the lost or undeveloped control over his output in developmental sequence. The basic patterns of posture and movement, the righting and equilibrium responses, are elicited by providing the appropriate stimuli while the abnormal patterns are inhibited. In this way, the patient is given the opportunity to experience normal movement. The sensory information of correct movement is absolutely necessary for the development of improved motor control. Treatment, therefore, concentrates on handling the patient in such a way as to inhibit abnormal distribution of tone and abnormal postures while stimulating or encouraging the next level of motor control. The abnormal postures and tone are controlled at key points (proximal body parts, *i.e.,* head, neck, trunk, and sometimes distal parts, *i.e.,* thumb and finger) using reflex-inhibiting movements or patterns called RIPs. If the patient lacks tone, sensory stimulation or "tapping" is used while the RIP is applied so that the sensory inflow will not shunt into abnormal patterns. The Bobaths believe that once the patient can move easily in and out of normal basic patterns of posture and movement he will automatically be able to elaborate on these patterns to learn the more skilled activities required in daily living.[20-23]

Early treatment is considered ideal and necessary if true gains are to be made and fixed abnormal patterns, or contractures, avoided.[23, 24]

Evaluation is an integral part of treatment.[19] Within each treatment session the patient's progress is evaluated. Some measurable change should occur at every session and if it doesn't treatment must be modified.[23] The whole evaluation is not completed before treatment begins. The evaluations are designed in developmental sequence; once the patient's highest level of performance is ascertained, treatment begins and further evaluation is postponed until progress is noted.

The evaluations that the Bobaths do include the determination of the extent and distribution of hyper-

and hypotonus and the effect hypertonus in one part of the body has on other parts of the body. Tonus is estimated by placing the patient into developmentally sequenced postural patterns rather than testing at each joint.[19, 23] The therapist looks for the immediacy of adjustment of muscles to new positions (normal), for undue ease of placement and hyperextensibility (hypotonia), or for undue resistance to the test movement (hypertonia). The degree and pattern of spasticity are noted.

EVALUATION AND TREATMENT OF CEREBRAL PALSY

An overview of the procedures used in the evaluation and treatment of cerebral palsied children is included in this textbook because of the potential usefulness in the treatment of the severely brain-damaged or traumatic head-injured adult.

The Cerebral Palsy Assessment Chart and directions for administering the evaluation that was devised by Semans et al.[25] is included here (Table 6.2) because the book in which it was originally published is now out of print.

Throughout the testing, the therapist should ensure maximal freedom from emotional and physical tension through proper handling. In all tests, the therapist should first place the patient in the test position. Physical manipulation to reduce tension (a RIP) should be used if spasticity interferes with placement. If the therapist is unable to place the patient because of inability to relax tension or the presence of contractures or structural deviations, these are indicated on the form. Secondly, after being placed, the patient is asked to stay in the test position. As a third step, he is asked to move into the test position independently.

Grading Key for Cerebral Palsy Assessment Chart

A grading system with values from 0 to 5 is used as follows:

0—Cannot be placed in test posture.

1—Can be placed in test posture, but the position cannot be held.

2—Can hold test posture momentarily after being placed.

3—Can assume an approximate test posture unaided, in any manner.

4—Can assume and sustain test posture in a near normal manner (note any abnormal detail).

5—Normal.

Specific Instructions for Administering the Test Items

Each item in the test represents a necessary postural control for various functional activities. It is helpful to keep in mind the functional significance of each test while administering it in order to observe the most critical aspects contributing to the test score. The following groups are arranged in the approximate order of normal developmental sequence.

Supine

Test 1: Purpose—To test freedom from extensor hypertonus in the supine position. Emphasis in this test is on proximal joints.

Bring knees, one after the other, to chest with enough external rotation at hips to point knees toward axillae. This is needed to get complete flexion; if not attained, there is probably not full range of hip flexion. Steady knees in position with your body while placing child's arms as follows: Pull arms forward at shoulders, abducting the scapulae, and fold across chest so that his open palms cup his shoulders; arms should be up, away from chest wall; head should remain in a neutral position; feet should be relaxed in plantar flexion. If child assumes position except for dorsiflexed feet or incompletely relaxed hands, grade 4 should be given.

Test 2: Purpose—To test ability to flex or extend one leg at a time through full range.

Starting with hips and knees fully flexed and arms across chest or relaxed at side, bring right leg down to table into an extended position, avoiding internal rotation. Back should not arch. Return to starting position and repeat with left leg.

Test 3: Purpose—To test ability to raise head.

Place in a symmetrical supine position with legs extended and arms at sides. Raise head by flexing neck. The shoulders remain relaxed. If the child can raise the head but protracts the shoulder, a grade of 3 is given.

Prone

Test 4: Purpose—To test freedom from flexor hypertonus in prone position.

Place prone, lift under the shoulder to free the arms; place arms overhead one after the other, elbows and wrists extended, palms down, legs extended and relaxed. Head is raised in midposition. Replace arms below shoulder level before asking child to move into test position.

Test 5: Purpose—To test freedom of arms and shoulders from flexor hypertonus in prone position.

Place prone, arms externally rotated beside the body, palms down. Place the hands out a short distance from the body so that the arms are not pressed against the thorax. To assume position actively, start the child with his arms at shoulder level or above. Note any change of tension resulting from turning head from one side to the other.

Test 6: Purpose—To test selective control of hip and knee.

Place prone, arms relaxed beside head or at sides. Flex right knee to 90° without flexion at hip. The foot should not dorsiflex; other leg should remain relaxed. Repeat with left leg. For grade 4 or 5, there should be no appreciable motion in the hip.

In the next postures, righting reactions are required. Equilibrium and protective extension reactions are evaluated in each of the test postures. The righting reactions have to do with orienting the head relative to the body, or the body relative to the head and neck, or maintaining the head in a normal position in space.

Table 6.2
CEREBRAL PALSY ASSESSMENT CHART BASIC MOTOR CONTROL^a

Name:_____ Birthdate:_____ Diagnosis:_____

Test Postures and Movements	Examiner:	Name:		Name:		Name	
		Date	Remarks	Date	Remarks	Date	Remarks
Supine 1. Hips and knees fully flexed, arms crossed, palms on shoulders.							
2. Hips and knees fully flexed. (a) Extend right leg. (b) Extend left leg.		R. ___ L.		R. ___ L.		R. ___ L.	
3. Head raised.							
Prone 4. Arms extended beside head. Raise head in midposition.							
5. Arms extended beside body, palms down.							
6. (a) Flex right knee, hips extended. (b) Flex left knee, hips extended.		R. ___ L.		R. ___ L.		R. ___ L.	
7. Trunk supported on forearms, upper trunk extended, face vertical.							
8. Trunk supported on hands with elbows and hips extended.							
Sitting erect 9. Soles of feet together, hips flexed and externally rotated to at least 45°.							
10. Knees extended and legs abducted; hips 90°–100°.							

Table 6.2—*continued*

Name:_____ Diagnosis:_____ Birthdate:_____

Test Postures and Movements		Examiner: Name:		Name:		Name:	
		Date	Remarks	Date	Remarks	Date	Remarks
11. Legs hanging over edge of table. (a) Extend right knee. (b) Extend left knee.		R. L.		R. L.		R. L.	
Kneeling 12. Back and neck straight (not hyperextended). (a) Weight on knees. (b) Weight on hands.		a b		a b		a b	
13. Side sitting, upper trunk erect, arms relaxed: (a) On right hip. (b) On left hip.		R. L.		R. L.		R. L.	
14. Kneeling upright, hips extended, head in midposition, arms at sides.							
15. (a) Half kneeling: weight on right knee. (b) Half kneeling: weight on left knee.		R. L.		R. L.		R. L.	
Squatting 16. Heels down, toes not clawed, knees pointing in same direction as toes, hips fully flexed, head in line with trunk.							
Standing and components of walking 17. Standing, correct alignment.							
18. Pelvis and trunk aligned over forward leg. Both knees extended. (a) Right leg forward. (b) Left leg forward.		R. L.		R. L.		R. L.	
19. Bear weight on one leg in midstance. (a) Shift weight over right leg. (b) Shift weight over left leg.		R. L.		R. L.		R. L.	
20. Heel strike. Rear leg extended and externally rotated, heel down. Both knees straight: (a) Right heel strike. (b) Left heel strike.		R. L.		R. L.		R. L.	

a Reprinted with permission from S. Semans *et. al.*[25]

The equilibrium responses are automatic responses to a disturbance in balance by which the organism makes covert or overt motor adjustments to regain balance over his center of gravity. The protective extension patterns are automatic patterns of the upper extremities which cause the person to reach out in an attempt to break a fall and to protect the head from injury. The Bobaths attempt to elicit these responses at all developmental levels in their handling of the child.

Test 7: Purpose—To test postural control in spinal extension. This is important for beginning locomotion (crawling), erect sitting, and beginning use of hands.

Place prone, extend thoracic spine, and place arms one after the other in at least 90° shoulder flexion and slight abduction, supported on forearms. Head is raised with face vertical. Arms point straight ahead and hands are open.

Test 8: Purpose—To test ability to support weight on extended arms. This position is often difficult to attain, but it is necessary for creeping.

Start from test position 7. Lift child's head, giving gentle traction on cervical spine so that he supports himself on extended arms and the heel of his open hand; entire spine and hips are fully extended. Alternate method: Lift under shoulders or under chest.

Sitting Erect

Test 9: Purpose—To test control of hips in flexion, abduction, and external rotation.

Place in erect sitting position with hips abducted, flexed, and externally rotated to at least 45°, soles of feet together, arms relaxed. For grades 3 to 5, start in any sitting position on flat surface.

Test 10: Purpose—To test erect sitting with legs straight.

Place in erect sitting position with thighs abducted without internal rotation and with knees extended; flexion angle at hip should be 90 to 100°, arms relaxed.

Test 11: Purpose—To test selective control of hip and knee.

Place in erect sitting position, flexion angle at hip 90 to 100°, legs hanging vertically. Extend knee fully without further extension of hip. Other leg and arms should remain relaxed. (a) Right knee extended; (b) left knee extended.

Kneeling

Test 12: Purpose—To test weight-bearing and balance control on knees and heels of open hands.

Start in four-point kneeling (quadruped), back and neck straight (not hyperextended), legs parallel, elbows extended, hands pointing forward. (a) Weight predominantly on knees; (b) weight predominantly on hands.

Test 13: Purpose—To test ability of trunk to adapt to gravitational changes.

Place in side sitting from four-point or upright kneeling by lowering the hips to one side of feet. Head and upper trunk should be erect, arms free. (a) On right hip; (b) on left hip.

Test 14: Purpose—To test anterior-posterior control of pelvis and trunk on thighs.

Place in upright kneeling (kneel standing) position, hips extended, legs parallel, trunk and head erect, head in midposition, arms relaxed.

Test 15: Purpose—To test control of rotation at hip. Place in half-kneeling position from upright kneeling. The other foot is placed on floor in front and to the side for adequate supporting base. Hip, knee, and ankle of forward leg at 90°, toes not clawed. Pelvis and trunk face forward, knee slightly outward.

Squatting

Test 16: Purpose—To test control of extensor spasticity.

Place from squat sitting, *i.e.,* legs and hips fully flexed and outwardly rotated, feet flat on floor, toes not clawed, knees pointing in same direction as toes, arms forward for balance. Shift weight forward over feet into squatting position. Older child can be placed from a low stool. It is easier to assume this position if the legs are spread wide apart.

Standing and Components of Walking

Test 17: Purpose—To test normal distribution of tone in standing.

Place in standing position with body segments in normal alignment with relation to the line of gravity in midcoronal and midsaggittal planes, *i.e.,* weight evenly distributed over both feet, legs in midposition of rotation, and so on. Points of control might be the hip of one side and the knee of opposite side, or hip and opposite arm. A lift may be used to equalize leg length.

Test 18: Purpose—To test the ability to shift weight forward onto stance leg with rear leg extended for push off.

Place in forward step position. Shift weight over forward leg with trunk, pelvis, thigh, and leg correctly aligned over foot. Rear leg should be extended, outwardly rotated at hip, and resting on the normal, roll-off point (the head of the first metatarsal); arms should be relaxed. For grades 2 to 5, the therapist may steady child by holding one of his hands.

Test 19: Purpose—To test the ability to support the body over one leg (absence of Trendelenberg sign).

From a symmetrical standing position, shift weight laterally over one leg and lift the other free of the floor, as for the swing phase of walking. Trunk should remain erect. For grades 2 to 5, therapist may steady child by holding one hand.

Test 20: Purpose—To test heel strike.

One foot is advanced in dorsiflexion and heel placed on the floor. Weight is supported mainly on rear leg, hip extended, both knees straight. Ankles remain at approximately 90°. Arms should be relaxed. For grades 2 to 5, therapist may steady child by holding one of his hands.

Guiding questions that should be considered by the therapist during the evaluation include the following [22]:

1. Are the patient's motor abilities arrested at one level of development or are his abilities scattered in several different stages of development? The answer to this question will identify the gaps that must be filled in between the patient's lowest and highest levels of performance.

2. What abnormal postures does the patient exhibit and how do they interfere with his activities? The answer to this question indicates which patterns have to be inhibited in order to facilitate the normal patterns.

3. Does the patient have any abnormal postural patterns or persistent asymmetries that may in time develop into contractures and deformities? Treatment must be aimed at preventing deformities.

4. What is the distribution of abnormal tone? How

does tonus change with stimulation or effort? Is there abnormal tone only in certain positions and not others? Does movement affect tone? The answers to these questions will guide the design of reflex-inhibiting patterns and the selection of other treatment techniques.

Treatment planning for the spastic patient should include the inhibition of abnormal postures and tone while eliciting active motion in developmental sequence. After the patient develops the ability to maintain a posture, he is slowly moved to facilitate the righting and equilibrium reactions.

Reflex-Inhibiting Patterns

RIPs are used to inhibit patterns of abnormal muscle tone, such as those caused by the influence of predominating primitive tonic reflexes (tonic neck and tonic labyrinthine reflexes) so often seen in cerebral palsied children. Reflex-inhibiting patterns are partial patterns opposite to the typical abnormal patterns of postural tone that dominate the patient. The reflex-inhibiting patterns prevent shunting of the sensory inflow into abnormal patterns and redirect it into normal ones. As tone becomes more normal the child can learn to control the abating tonic reflex activity.[21] Inhibition of abnormal tone is always used concurrently with facilitation of the righting and equilibrium reactions. Severely involved patients, or older children, who have not been successfully treated previously, may need to be inhibited for a long time before a period of relative normalcy occurs during which they can actively move.[21, 22] Even these children are moved passively when postural tone decreases to begin stimulation of the righting reactions.[22] Reflex-inhibiting patterns are designed by examining the child in all patterns of posture (during the evaluation) to determine which distribution of abnormal tone is typical. By holding a key part of the child in an opposite pattern, the inhibiting pattern is tested to see if it tends to redistribute the tone of the whole child more normally as it should if it is to be used for treatment.[22] Key points of contacting the child are changed to allow the child to develop flexible control over his own movements and postures. Key points are usually proximal parts of the body (head, neck, shoulder girdle, pelvic girdle or trunk) from which abnormal reflexes seem to originate.[22] The key points are used to control tone distribution. Semans advises[25] that one should not yield to the temptation to start the reflex-inhibiting pattern where the spasticity is most obvious, but rather start more proximally, and then the distal parts will follow. If the therapist chooses the key point of control where hypertonus is greatest, the child will not be able to move that part and cannot develop control.[22] Full body reflex-inhibiting patterns are not used because the tone is liable to be shunted into a reverse pattern.[22] Rather, a key point is chosen which allows the full pattern of tone to be broken up during the handling.[22]

A few examples of reflex-inhibiting patterns will be listed here. However, the reflex-inhibiting patterns must be individualized for each person following a careful analysis of the patient's problems. These examples can be used as models. Raising the head into hyperextension facilitates extensor tone of the rest of the body and inhibits flexor tone.[22] Flexion of the head encourages flexion of the rest of the body and inhibits extensor hypertonicity.[19] Internal rotation of the limb inhibits extension, whereas external rotation inhibits flexion. Horizontal abduction or diagonal extension of the humerus inhibits flexion in the neck, arms, and hands. Lifting the arms overhead facilitates extension of the hips and trunk.[21] Flexion of the hip and knee combined with abduction of the hip inhibits extensor tone of the trunk and head and limbs. Symmetrical extension of the limbs, with the head in midline to rule out the influences of the asymmetrical tonic neck reflex, inhibits flexor spasticity of the arms. Rotation of the trunk between the shoulder and pelvic girdles inhibits both flexor and extensor hypertonus. Elevation of the arms inhibits flexor hypertonus.[22]

Handling

The Bobaths term their manner of control of the patient through reflex-inhibiting patterns and their movement of him to elicit righting and equilibrium responses, "handling."[21] This simulates handling of the normal infant by his mother. Handling is used to influence postural tone; to regulate coordination of agonists, antagonists, and synergists; to inhibit abnormal patterns; and to facilitate normal automatic responses. At first the therapist handles the patient to move him passively in correct patterns of posture or movement while the patient is encouraged to cooperate and help as he can. The therapist withdraws guidance and support as the patient is able to take over more and more initiative to move in correct patterns.

The handling is constantly changing to inhibit the undesired and to facilitate the desired responses in the dynamic treatment situation in which the patient's responses are changing due to the therapist's stimulation. It requires constant attention to the demands to be made of the patient, to the stimulation to be offered, and to the patient's responses to each. Abnormal tone or movement is prevented from happening at the first sign. The child is not allowed to exert effort because tone increases with effort and may become shunted into the abnormal patterns. Once the first normal reaction has occurred, it is repeated to establish new sensorimotor patterns and to make the reaction quicker and more reliable.[19]

Righting and Equilibrium Reactions

Reflex-inhibiting patterns are inhibitions imposed from the outside; true inhibition can be gained only through elicitation of the righting and equilibrium reactions. Righting reactions and equilibrium responses (including protective extension patterns) are elicited for each posture and movement that is being used in therapy. Many postures and movements are used during a treatment sequence to help the child develop dynamic control and to mimic normal development which occurs spirally: as one motor task is being elaborated on, others are beginning to enter the child's repertoire. "The movements (used in therapy) are the fundamental motor patterns which normal children develop during the first two years of life."[24]

The neck-righting reaction and the body-righting reaction on the body are evoked to assist the child to move from supine to prone, to on-elbows, to quadruped, to kneel-standing, and finally to standing. The child is moved in and out of the positions which are within his developmental capabilities using these reactions. He is moved to these postures in a variety of ways. For example, he does not always turn to the right when moving supine to prone but alternates moving toward the left. He is moved slowly at first, then with increasing speed as he is able to respond. When eliciting neck righting and body righting acting on the body the head is used as the key point. When eliciting labyrinthine righting reactions the key points used are scapulae or shoulders, and the head is left free to automatically adjust to the stimulus. When facilitating movements from the head and neck, the therapist places one hand lightly under the child's chin, the other against the back of his head. When facilitating movements from the shoulder girdle the therapist places the hands under the child's axillae, spreading the fingers in order to control the scapulae and upper arm. The child may be moved through a whole sequence of postures using these key points, or each segment of the whole process may be done separately for reinforcement. The child is not moved into postures he is not developmentally ready to assume.

Equilibrium reactions are elicited by displacing the person's center of gravity while he is in one of the developmental patterns. Elicitation of equilibrium reactions is not started until the person can maintain the position against gravity. He is, however, prepared for using these reactions by being moved passively to simulate these reactions while abnormal patterns are inhibited by a reflex-inhibiting pattern. Equilibrium reactions can be elicited by moving the person or the surface on which he is placed. For more advanced patients these responses may be elicited on mobile surfaces, such as an equilibrium board which is a flat surface on rockers; a very large beach ball; or inflatables which are large, rectangular, inflated plastic pillows that tip from side to side and back to front but less so than the ball. The therapist can exert more control moving the person rather than the surface. The person is moved in all directions within each posture: backward and forward, side to side, and obliquely. Elicitation of equilibrium responses is at first done slowly and gently; then the speed and range of displacement are increased as the patient is able to adjust. When moving the person, the therapist "taps" him off balance in one direction and then catches him with the other hand and taps him back to midline in the opposite direction.

The person is held by his hips or shoulders to leave his arms and head free to adjust the balance just as a tight rope walker does. He should not support himself with his hands. He should be held at the point in space where he is about to lose balance long enough for him to struggle a little to regain his balance. The therapist must withdraw support to the point that he feels the need to recover his own balance but not so much as to instill in him a fear of falling. Abnormal tone would increase due to a fear of falling.[23] When the person is able to do equilibrium reactions on a stable surface, he can be placed on a movable surface. The surface is tilted or moved to elicit the reaction.

Protective responses can be elicited at the same time as equilibrium reactions. The patient is held in a reflex-inhibiting pattern using the arm on the side opposite to the one on which the response will be elicited. He is pushed to the side, or forward slowly at first and later with more speed. He should respond by protecting himself by outstretching the free arm to meet the surface.

Sensory Stimulation

Sensory stimulation is used for hypotonic patients and others that appear to be "weak" when the abnormal tone is inhibited, or those who have a sensory disturbance. Sensory stimulation is never done unless the child is in a reflex-inhibiting pattern in order to shunt the inflow into desired channels. Sensory stimulation is done very carefully and stopped if the response becomes abnormal or hyperactive. It is aimed at local responses, and widespread associated reactions are avoided. The kinds of sensory stimulation advocated by the Bobaths include the following:

1. Weight bearing with pressure and resistance is used to elicit increased postural tone and a decrease of involuntary movements. This is especially good for ataxic and athetoid patients who need to develop static postures and slow movements within small ranges. Spastic patients need active movement; therefore, weight bearing is done in such a way that weight transfer is allowed.[22] Resistance and pressure may not be helpful in cases of spasticity because they would increase the likelihood of cocontraction.

2. Placing and Holding.[22, 23] Placing refers to the ability to arrest a movement at any stage automatically or voluntarily. The therapist moves the limb to various positions as the patient assists in this. Holding refers to the ability to hold a position without assistance once the limb is placed.

3. Tapping has several meanings. (a) Pressure (joint compression) tapping is used to increase tone for maintenance of an acceptable posture. (b) Inhibitory tapping is used to activate muscles that are weak due to reciprocal inhibition by spastic antagonists. The method used is to release the body part and to catch it as it falls a very small distance, thus stimulating the stretch reflexes. (c) Alternate tapping is used to stimulate balance reactions and is done by pushing the child by light "taps" back and forth from one position to midposition. (d) Sweep tapping is used to activate synergic patterns of muscle function and is done by

the therapist sharply sweeping his hand over the desired muscles in the direction of the desired movement.

"Only those techniques which bring about an immediate improvement of tone and active movement in any one treatment session should continue to be used."[26]

Treatment Program

Examples of combining a RIP with elicitation of a righting reaction and then equilibrium reactions are as follows: starting in supine, the neck is flexed to inhibit the extensor tone, then rotated to elicit the neck-righting reaction which is log roll to prone. The head is held in extension to inhibit flexor tone. If the patient is on an equilibrium board it is tipped to elicit a recovery response. (See Chapter 4 for descriptions of normal equilibrium responses.)

To progress, with the neck again extended to inhibit flexor tone, a gentle upward movement of the head prompts the patient to assume an on-elbows position. Again he is tipped or pushed off balance. Flexing the neck to encourage flexion of the hips combined with backward pressure against the top of the head can result in assumption of a quadruped position. Or, to alternately facilitate sitting up, the patient's head is lifted and rotated to one side. Then, before he reaches a side-lying position, pressure is exerted backward against the top of the head to flex the spine and hips while continuing with rotation of the spine. This results in sitting. Equilibrium responses would be elicited when the patient had control of each posture. Detailed directions concerning the use of righting reactions to attain each developmental posture are available in Bobaths' publications.

The occupational therapist will want to combine these suggestions for therapy with activity ideas to both motivate the patient and to encourage practice in functional situations. For example, handling the patient from supine to prone could be combined with the patient's interest in looking at something or need to reach to the side. Eventually, the therapist could use an enticing activity to stimulate the child to move in this pattern without the therapist handling him. If an object a person is looking at is raised higher after the person is prone, or if activities such as blowing bubbles are used, prone on elbow posture will be encouraged. Prone on hands can be encouraged by moving the stimulus object even higher. From an on-hands position, side sitting may be encouraged by having the person reach toward the back of himself to get an object such as game parts. Once achieved, the person can support himself on his affected extremity in order to develop postural supporting reactions in that limb.

From a side-sitting position, quadruped can be achieved by requiring that the person throw something using the limb that was supporting him, in order to build up momentum that is directed toward the quadruped position. To practice development of equilibrium reactions in quadruped, the patient could be presented with the need to reach for objects placed in front or to the side of him, or to move in the position. From quadruped, kneel standing can be achieved by making a demand for the person to reach up for an object. Of course activity demands must be within the capability of the patient. Excess effort produces tension which shunts into abnormal postures.

EVALUATION AND TREATMENT OF THE ADULT HEMIPLEGIC[23]

The Problem and Rationale

Instead of righting reactions, equilibrium responses and automatic adaptation of antigravity muscles to changes of posture seen in a normal person, a person with a lesion of the upper motor neuron exhibits static and stereotyped movement patterns (abnormal postural reflexes), spasticity, and exaggerated cocontraction that prevents free, coordinated movement. The abnormal postural reflexes that the hemiplegic patient most commonly exhibits are a symmetrical tonic neck reflex, the positive supporting reaction, and associated reactions. Associated reactions are not the normal, coordinated movement of the opposite side of the body often seen in children and new learners. They are tonic reflex movements of the affected side of the body which may outlast the duration of the stimulus. The stimulus is proprioceptive, *i.e.*, a forceful tonic contraction of the muscles of the sound side. Such a contraction occurs during excessive effort or in response to fear of falling; these are to be avoided.

Also contributing to the hemiplegic person's problem in initiating and performing movement is disturbed sensation and perception. Normally, movement is performed in response to perceived environmental stimuli. If the reception or perception of that stimuli is defective, then the motor response will also be defective.

Bobath treatment is "based on the view that spasticity is caused by the release of an abnormal postural mechanism which results in exaggerated static function at the expense of dynamic postural control. The aim of treatment is to help the patient gain control over the patterns of spasticity by inhibiting the abnormal reflex patterns." Spasticity underlies the abnormal reflex patterns and is reduced by counteracting their effect. Inhibition is combined with techniques of handling to elicit movement patterns of righting and equilibrium responses that underlie normal function. Emphasis is on changing motor output, thereby influencing sensory inflow necessary for learning of normal movement, as opposed to "putting in" sensory stimuli which are believed to be shunted by the lesion into the released abnormal patterns of spasticity.

Evaluation

The patient's postural and movement patterns are assessed to determine which functional patterns exist and whether abnormal patterns are present that may interfere with function. The strength and distribution of the spasticity is assessed simultaneously with the patterns. Due to spasticity, the postural patterns are usually restricted to one or two synergies, *i.e.,* the muscles are required to act only in stereotyped patterns.

Sensation is also evaluated. A persistent loss of sensation offers a poor prognosis for regaining motor control. Specifically, kinesthesia, proprioception, localization of pressure and light touch, and stereognosis are tested because of their predictive value.

The method of testing for tonus and postural reactions to being moved is called "placing." Placing is an important part of the treatment also. Evaluation and treatment are interwoven. The limb is moved by the therapist in exactly the movement patterns that the patient must eventually learn but which are at first interfered with by spasticity. As the therapist moves the limb, the patient's adaptation to the normal patterns of posture and movement imposed on him is assessed. Normal adaptation means that the person actively controls the weight of the limb; a holding response is immediately seen if the limb is left alone at any stage of the movement. Spasticity causes resistance if the movement is away from the pattern of spasticity or uncontrolled assistance to the passive or guided movement into the direction of the spasticity. Flaccidity causes the limb to feel heavy and abnormally relaxed; there is no active adjustment of the muscles to changes in posture and gravity and no holding of a position against gravity.

The patient's ability to perform specific movements is evaluated using two groups of tests: I. Tests for the Quality of Movement Patterns; and II. Tests for Balance and Other Automatic Protective Reactions. Test I has three grades of tasks, each more difficult than the previous one. The items within each grade are also arranged according to difficulty. Evaluation is stopped and treatment begins when the person is unable to do an item. Tests for balance and other automatic protective reactions are used for patients with slight disability only. The patient is tested only in those positions which he can maintain voluntarily.

Equilibrium (balance) reactions are tested by displacing the patient's center of gravity or by asking him to lift the unaffected limb while in a weight-bearing position, which automatically and naturally displaces the weight of his body onto the affected side and demands an automatic equilibrium adjustment. Note is made whether he can do this and how he responds when equilibrium reactions are elicited. These reactions are tested when the patient is prone, sitting, on all fours, kneel-standing, kneeling on one knee, standing with one foot in front of the other, and standing on one foot (first the unaffected, then the affected).

Protective extension of the affected arm is also tested in all these positions by pushing the patient off balance, while holding the patient by the unaffected hand with the arm held in extension and external rotation to facilitate extension of the affected arm and hand. Note is made whether he responds to each stimulus by reaching out to prevent a fall. The student

is referred to the original source for greater detail concerning the administration of these tests.

The test forms pertaining to the quality of movement of the upper extremity are reproduced here, with permission (Table 6.3).

In planning treatment, the therapist identifies from the evaluation (1) whether to increase, decrease, or stabilize tone; (2) which abnormal patterns need to be inhibited and which normal ones need to be facilitated; and (3) which functional skills the patient will need to relearn and the order of learning. The therapist then devises a "teaching plan" for these.

Treatment

Bobath believes that compensatory rehabilitation (ADL and gait training) results in increased spasticity and inactivity of the involved side and should be postponed until they naturally enter the treatment process that concentrates on restoration of motor control.

Spasticity must be prevented by use of the special techniques of handling that counteract the abnormal patterns of tonic reflex activity, called reflex-inhibiting patterns. The therapist changes the abnormal patterns by holding the limb so as to reverse the most important part of the pattern. The key points that are used are the neck, spine, pelvic and shoulder girdles. Spasticity distal to these points will be influenced. Other key points are distal ones (fingers and wrists, toes and ankles) which can influence proximal stability. Reflex-inhibiting patterns are designed for the individual patient and involve control of only the least number of points necessary to obtain relaxation of spasticity. In the hemiplegic, reflex-inhibiting patterns are used to counteract flexor spasticity in the upper extremity and trunk and extensor spasticity of the lower extremity.

The main reflex-inhibiting pattern used to counteract the flexor spasticity of the trunk and arm is extension of the neck and spine and external rotation of the shoulder with elbow extension. Extension of the wrist with supination of the forearm and abduction of the thumb may be added.

Rotation of the shoulder girdle in relation to the pelvis is another reflex-inhibiting pattern used to reduce flexor or extensor spasticity. To counteract flexor or extensor spasticity of the lower extremity, the pattern used is hip abduction and external rotation combined with extension of the hip and knee. Further reduction of extensor spasticity can be achieved by adding dorsiflexion of the ankle and toes and abduction of the great toe.

While spasticity is reduced by reflex-inhibiting patterns, the goal of therapy becomes one of providing the patient with the feeling of many different normal automatic and voluntary patterns of movement because it is the sensation of movement that is learned (stored in memory). Introduction of movement follows the developmental progressions of mass to isolated movement, proximal to distal control.

Sensory stimulation (tactile and proprioceptive) is

Table 6.3
TEST FORMS FOR THE QUALITY OF MOVEMENT OF THE UPPER EXTREMITY

I. Tests for the Quality of Movement Patterns

Tests for arm and shoulder girdle (to be tested separately in supine, sitting, and standing, as the result will be different in these positions.)

Grade 1	Supine		Sitting		Standing	
	Yes	No	Yes	No	Yes	No
a. Can he hold extended arm in elevation after having it placed there?						
With internal rotation?						
With external rotation?						
b. Can he lower the extended arm from the position of elevation to the horizontal plane and back again to elevation?						
Forward-downward?						
Sideways-downward?						
With internal rotation?						
With external rotation?						
c. Can he move the extended abducted arm from the horizontal plane to the side of his body and back again to the horizontal plane?						
With internal rotation?						
With external rotation?						
Grade 2						
a. Can he lift his arm to touch the opposite shoulder?						
With palm of hand?						
With back of hand?						
b. Can he bend his elbow with his arm in elevation to touch the top of his head?						
With pronation?						
With supination?						
c. Can he fold his hands behind his head with both elbows in horizontal abduction?						
With wrist flexed?						
With wrist extended?						
Grade 3						
a. Can he supinate his forearm and wrist?						
Without side-flexion of trunk on the affected side?						
With flexed elbow and flexed fingers?						
With extended elbow and extended fingers?						
b. Can he pronate his forearm without adduction of arm at shoulder						
c. Can he externally rotate his extended arm?						
(i) in horizontal abduction?						
(ii) by the side of his body?						
(iii) in elevation						
d. Can he bend and extend his elbow in supination to touch the shoulder of the same side? starting with:						
(i) arm by side of his body?						
(ii) horizontal abduction of the arm?						

Tests for wrist and fingers	Yes?	No?
Grade 1		
a. Can he place his flat hand forward down on table in front?		
Can he do this sideways when sitting on plinth?		
With fingers and thumb adducted?		
With fingers and thumb abducted?		
Grade 2		
a. Can he open his hand to grasp?		
With flexed wrist?		

Table 6.3—*continued*

	Yes?	No?
With extended wrist?		
With pronation?		
With supination?		
With adducted fingers and thumb?		
With abducted fingers and thumb?		

Grade 3
  a. Can he grasp and open his fingers again?
     With flexed elbow?
     With extended elbow?
     With pronation?
     With supination?
  b. Can he move individual fingers?
     Thumb?
     Index finger?
     Little finger?
     2nd and 3rd finger?
  c. Can he oppose fingers and thumb?
     Thumb and index finger?
     Thumb and 2nd finger?
     Thumb and little finger?

II. Tests for Balance and Other Automatic Protective Reactions[a]

	Yes?	No?

Balance reactions.
  Patient in prone lying, supporting himself on his forearms.
    a. His shoulder girdle is pushed toward affected side. Does he remain supported on affected forearm?
    b. His sound arm is lifted forward and up, as when reaching out with one hand. Does he immediately transfer his weight toward the affected arm?
    c. His sound arm is lifted and moved backward, and he is turned to his side, support on affected arm.
       Does he remain supported on affected arm?
  Patient sitting on the plinth, his feet unsupported.
    a. He is pushed toward the affected side. Does he stay upright?
       Does he laterally flex his head toward the sound side?
       Does he abduct his sound leg?
       Does he use the affected forearm for support?
       Does he use the affected hand for support?
    b. He is pushed forward.
       Does he bend affected hip and knee?
       Does he extend his spine?
       Does he lift his head?
    c. Both his legs are lifted up by the therapist, knees flexed.
       Does he stay upright?
       Does he move affected arm forward?
       Does he support himself backwards with affected arm?
  Patient in four-foot kneeling.
    a. His body is pushed toward the affected side.
       Does he abduct the sound leg?
       Does he remain on all fours?
    b. His sound arm is lifted and held up by the therapist.
       Does he keep affected arm extended?
    c. His sound leg is lifted.
       Does he keep affected leg flexed and transfer weight on to it?
    d. His sound arm and affected leg are lifted.
       Does he keep affected arm extended?

[a] In order to test these reactions the patient must be able to assume and hold the test position. He should react with specific movements in order to regain his balance or protect himself against falling when being moved or pushed unexpectedly.

Table 6.3—*continued*

	Yes?	No?
e. His affected arm and his sound leg are lifted. Does he remain on affected flexed leg?		
f. His sound arm and leg are lifted. Does he transfer his weight toward the affected side and maintain position?		

Patient in kneel-standing.

	Yes?	No?
a. He is pushed toward the affected side. Does he abduct the sound leg?		
Does he bend head laterally toward the sound side?		
Does he use his affected hand for support?		
b. He is pushed toward the sound side. Does he abduct the affected leg?		
Does he extend the affected arm sideways?		
c. He is pushed backward and asked not to sit down. Does he extend the affected arm forward?		
d. He is pushed gently forward, his sound arm held backward by the therapist. Does he use affected arm and hand for support on the ground?		
Does he lift affected foot off the ground?		

Patient half-kneeling, sound foot forward. (He should not use sound hand for support.)

	Yes?	No?
a. His sound foot is lifted up by the therapist. Does he remain upright?		
Does he keep affected hip extended?		
b. His sound foot is lifted by the therapist and placed sideways. Does he remain upright?		
Does he show balance movements with his affected arm?		
c. His sound foot is placed from the above position back to kneel-standing. Does he keep upright?		
Does he keep affected hip extended?		

Patient standing, feet parallel, standing base narrow.

	Yes?	No?
a. He is tipped backward and not allowed to make step backward with sound leg. (Therapist puts her foot on his sound one to prevent step.) Does he step backward with affected leg?		
b. He is tipped backward and not allowed to make steps with either leg. Does he dorsiflex toes of affected leg?		
Big toe only?		
Dorsiflex ankle and toes of affected leg?		
Does he move affected arm forward?		
c. He is tipped toward sound side. Does he abduct affected leg?		
Does he abduct and extend affected arm?		
Does he make steps to follow with affected leg across sound leg?		
d. He is tipped toward the affected side. Does he abduct the sound leg?		
Does he bend head laterally towards the sound side?		

Patient standing on affected leg only. (He is not allowed to use sound hand for support.)

	Yes?	No?
a. His sound foot is lifted by the therapist and moved forward as in making a step, extending his knee. Does he keep the heel of affected leg on the ground?		
Does he keep the knee of the affected leg extended?		
Does he assist weight transfer forward over affected leg with extended hip?		
b. His sound foot is lifted by the therapist and moved backward as in making a step backward. Does he keep the hip of affected leg extended?		
Does he assist weight transfer backward over affected leg?		
c. His sound foot is lifted by the therapist and held up while he is *pushed* gently sideways toward the affected side.		

Table 6.3—*continued*

	Yes?	No?

Does he follow and adjust his balance, moving the foot of the affected leg sideways by inverting and everting his foot alternately?
The same maneuver is done *pulling* him toward the affected side.
Does he follow and adjust his balance by moving his foot as above?

Tests for Protective Extension and Support of the Arm

When testing these reactions the patient's sound arm should be held by his hand, so that he cannot use it. It is advisable to hold the sound arm in extension and external rotation because this facilitates the extension of the affected arm and hand.

	Yes?	No?

a. The patient stands in front of a table or plinth. His sound arm is held backward and he is pushed forward toward the table.
   Does he extend his affected arm forward?
   Does he support himself on his fist?
   On the palm of his hand?
   His thumb adducted?
   His thumb abducted?
b. The patient stands facing a wall, at a distance which allows him to reach it with his hand. He is pushed forward against the wall, his sound arm held backward.
   Does he lift his affected arm and stretch it out against the wall?
   Does he place his hand against the wall, fingers flexed, thumb adducted?
   Fingers open, thumb abducted?
c. The patient is sitting on the plinth. His sound arm is held sideways by the therapist. He is pushed toward the affected side.
   Does he abduct the affected arm and support himself on his forearm?
   On his extended arm?
   Does he support himself on his fist?
   On his open palm?
   Thumb and fingers adducted?
   Thumb and fingers abducted?
d. The patient stands sideways to a wall, at a distance which allows him to reach it with his affected hand.
   Does he abduct and lift the affected arm?
   With flexed elbow?
   Does he reach out for the wall with extended elbow?
   Does he support himself with his fist against the wall?
   With his open hand?
   With adducted thumb and fingers?
   With abducted thumb and fingers?
e. The patient lies on the floor on his back. His sound hand is placed under his hip so that he cannot use it. The therapist takes a pillow and pretends to throw it towards his head.
   Does he move his affected arm to protect his face?
   With flexed elbow?
   With extended elbow?
   With internal rotation?
   With external rotation?
   With fisted hand?
   With open hand?
   Can he catch the pillow?

used for flaccid patients while the limb is held in a reflex-inhibiting pattern to prevent development of tone in the pattern of spasticity.

An introductory summary of treatment techniques used for the upper extremity will be presented here. The reader is referred to the original source, *Adult Hemiplegia: Evaluation and Treatment* (2nd edi-tion), and to the short courses offered by the Bobaths for detailed knowledge of the whole treatment program and to develop skill under supervision.

Treatment during the Initial Flaccid Stage

In this stage, tone is primarily absent, but there is intermittent spasticity in reaction to stretch. Treatment is a cooperative effort between therapists and nursing personnel. It focuses on positioning and movement in bed. The patient is encouraged and helped to use the affected arm for support as early as possible because weight bearing facilitates extensor tone. Frequent, passive turning by nurses to prevent deformity and decubiti ought to be done segmentally, as one normally would turn, so the patient will get the correct sensory input.[19]

Positioning. The patient should be encouraged to lie on either side for a time each day in order to be out of the supine position which encourages extensor tonus. The position of choice to inhibit the development of flexor tone in the upper extremity and extensor tone in the lower extremity, which is the usual picture in hemiplegia, is as follows: side-lying on the sound side with the head laterally flexed away from the affected side, the lateral trunk flexors lengthened and the affected arm propped on a pillow in front of the patient in order to bring the scapula forward from its retracted position. The elbow is extended. The affected leg should lie in a normal semiflexed position and not touch the foot of the bed which would elicit the positive supporting reaction.

While the patient is lying supine, the head should be laterally flexed away from the affected arm to counteract the tendency of the head to be drawn toward the affected side. There should be a pillow under the arm to pull the scapula forward and one under the knee to break up the lower extremity extension pattern. If the patient lacks extensor tone or has a tendency for flexor spasticity of the lower extremity, no pillow is used under the knee. Flexor contractures of the hip and knee and plantar flexor contractures must be avoided.

The patient must relearn segmental rolling over in bed to either side. The movement should be done actively if possible, or assisted or done passively at first if necessary. Typical postural patterns of hemiplegia must be avoided in every case, and movement is performed to reverse these patterns. The typical patterns in the upper extremity in detail are: the scapula is retracted and depressed, and the shoulder is adducted and inwardly rotated; the elbow, wrist, and fingers are flexed; the forearm is pronated; the wrist is ulnarly deviated; and the fingers are adducted. In the leg, simultaneous extension of the hip, knee, and ankle with inversion of the foot, inward rotation of the thigh, and backward rotation of the pelvic girdle are typical. The lateral flexors of trunk and head on the affected side shorten.

Movement in Bed. To turn over, the patient clasps his hands with fingers interlocked. He moves his clasped hands, with elbows extended, to a horizontal or overhead position. He can then move arms and trunk to either side and will then be able with some help to turn the pelvis and move the affected leg.

To sit on the edge of the bed, the person turns onto his side and rests on his forearm (hands still clasped if possible), lifts his head to vertical, then simultaneously pushes with the arm(s) to get his trunk upright, and brings the legs over the side of the bed. Early, he will need help with each step of this procedure and will find it easier to sit after rolling to his sound side, although it is more therapeutic for him to sit after rolling to the affected side.

While sitting, the affected arm should be used for weight bearing to gain balance that reduces the fear of falling, so he will learn to feel safe when bearing weight on the affected side. Also, by positioning the arm in extension, external rotation, and abduction of the shoulder, extension of the elbow, and supination of the forearm, flexor spasticity is inhibited and the extensor muscles are facilitated in a functional pattern. At first it may be necessary for the arm to be placed to the back of the person to get maximal external rotation and therefore greater inhibition of flexion. Later weight bearing on the arm can be done with the arm to the side, then in front of the person. At that point, the person should be able to use the non-weightbearing arm without reverting to excess flexion.

While still bed-bound the patient begins learning control of the arm at the shoulder. In order to allow full shoulder movement and prevent pain, the retracted, depressed scapula needs to be mobilized into protraction and upward rotation. To mobilize the scapula, the therapist supports the patient's arm with the elbow extended and the shoulder externally rotated. While holding along the lateral border and under the glenoid fossa of the scapula, the therapist moves the scapula upward, forward, and downward (but not backward into retraction). This movement can be done rhythmically and in a slow rotary fashion until mobilization is felt to occur. Then, holding and placing of the arm can begin. Keeping the scapula well forward, the extended arm is raised overhead. The patient tries to control it in positions in which it has been placed. Before he can move against gravity, he needs to be able to control his limbs against gravity. The arm is placed as described in the evaluation test I for arms and shoulder girdle Grade 1 (Table 6.3). Tapping as described previously is used to increase tone in flaccid muscles if necessary. *Associated reactions are steadfastly avoided.* As the patient is able to maintain the placed posture, he is asked to lower it slightly and hold at that position. He should then reverse the movement. When he can maintain the lowered position, he is asked to raise it actively from that position. If he cannot control it (move and reverse it), the arm is moved back to the last controlled position.

Treatment during the Spastic Stage

This stage is characterized by hypertonicity. The spasticity develops slowly with a predilection for the muscles involved in the typical hemiplegic posture described above. The patient moves in total patterns. Treatment in this stage is a continuation of that in the previous stage. Placing of the shoulder continues. "At whichever point the patient can arrest movement, he can also lift his arm from the point of placing." Distal reflex-inhibiting patterns are used as necessary. The total patterns are then further broken down and correspond to the movements described in the evaluation test I for arms and shoulder girdle Grades 2 and 3 (Table 6.3). These movements start while the patient is supine but progress to standing and then sitting as soon as possible.

Treatment during the Stage of Relative Recovery

Not all patients reach this level of recovery. During this stage, spasticity is slight. The patient is able to walk unaided and use the upper extremity for support and gross grasp. Treatment in this stage aims at improving the quality of gait and use of the affected hand. Treatment in the second stage overlaps with that of the third stage. Bobath sees the occupational therapist active in the patient's therapy to utilize the obtained movements in daily living, by use of bilateral and repetitive therapeutic tasks that reinforce the learned movements. Activities are illustrated in the original source.

Bobath cautions that the occupational therapist must also avoid letting the patient experience stress which reverts movement to spastic patterns. The therapist should provide opportunities for the patient to move automatically without having to think about the movement, *e.g.*, gestures, moving in rhythm with music, or movement while speaking or counting.

Simple movements of the hand, following developmental sequence, should be practiced before they are combined with the actual use of the hand in daily tasks. Bobath cites the hand skills of a 9- to 10-month-old child as examples of these simple movements: scratch, rake with fingers, poke with the index finger, pincer grasp, pull, push, wave, pat, throw, and release objects. He can transfer objects between hands, play games (such as "patty cake"). These same motions can be incorporated into adult games and activities.

The patient needs to learn to use whatever function is regained in the hand independent of the positions of the proximal segments of the limb.

Bobath suggests that the occupational therapist uniquely contributes to the treatment of the adult hemiplegic in the areas of hand function and sensory retraining.

In summary, the neurodevelopmental approach of Bobath involves (a) normalization of tone and (b) eliciting of righting and equilibrium responses first automatically and then gradually demanding more and more voluntary control.

SECTION 3

The Brunnstrom Approach: Movement Therapy

ANNA DEANE SCOTT, M.Ed., OTR

Signe Brunnstrom is a physical therapist who has been particularly concerned with the problems of patients with hemiplegia. Her approach to the evaluation and treatment of the adult hemiplegic patient is based on clinical observations, readings in neurophysiology, and trial of procedures to duplicate the conditions which produce spontaneous movements in hemiplegic patients. The principles of this approach and the evaluation and treatment procedures presented in this section are summarized and adapted from *Movement Therapy in Hemiplegia*[27] in which Brunnstrom describes her approach in detail.

In the spastic stage of hemiplegia, basic limb synergies, primitive postural reflexes, and associated reactions reappear, since the normally modifying influence of higher centers has been interfered with due to the cerebral vascular accident. The synergies and reflexes are those which are normal in early development, and Brunnstrom has concluded that they should be encouraged as a normal part of the sequence of the return of motor function in hemiplegia. Reflexes produce responses in muscles which then combine with voluntary effort to produce semivoluntary movements that can be strengthened. Proprioceptive and exteroceptive stimuli assist in eliciting the synergies. Resistance promotes a spread of impulses to other muscles of a pattern, whereas skin stimulation seems to be more applicable to reinforce particular muscles. Sensory and visual feedback, as well as success in achieving voluntary movement, serve as motivation to the patient. Relearning occurs in the sequence of anticipated recovery to ensure success. New motions are repeated to achieve smooth performance, and learned patterns of movement are reinforced by use in daily activities.

This rationale underlies the description and evaluation of the motor behavior of patients with hemiplegia and the treatment techniques of movement therapy.

EVALUATION

Evaluation is done to identify the primitive spinal or brain stem postural reflexes and associated reactions, the stage of recovery of voluntary control of movement, and sensory disturbances of the patient.

Tonic Reflexes

The primitive reflexes which may be present include the symmetrical and asymmetrical tonic neck reflexes, tonic labyrinthine reflexes, and tonic lumbar reflexes. With the exception of the tonic lumbar reflexes, the evaluation of these reflexes has been previously described in Chapter 4, Evaluation of Motor Control.

In the tonic lumbar reflexes, changes in the position of the upper trunk in relation to the pelvis influence tone of the muscles of the extremities. For example, rotation of the upper trunk to one side elicits increased flexor tone in the upper extremity and increased extensor tone in the lower extremity on the side to which the rotation occurred. Conversely, there is increased extensor tone in the upper extremity and increased flexor tone in the lower extremity on the side opposite to the direction of rotation.

Associated Reactions

Associated reactions are involuntary movements or reflexive increase of tone which are observed in the involved extremities of hemiplegic patients when other parts of the body are resisted during movement. These reactions are more easily elicited when spasticity is present. Some associated reactions are influenced by tonic neck reflexes, but resistance must be added in addition to the neck movements to gain the summation of sensorimotor influences which would elicit an associated reaction. Associated reactions in patients with hemiplegia include the following: Resistance to flexion of the noninvolved upper extremity can cause a flexor synergy of the involved upper extremity. Similarly, resistance to extension of the noninvolved upper extremity evokes an extension syngery of the involved upper extremity. Conversely, in the lower extremity, resistance to flexion of the noninvolved extremity causes extension of the involved extremity, and resistance to extension on the noninvolved side causes flexion of the involved extremity.

The interdependence of the upper and lower extremities on one side of the body is called homolateral synkinesis: a response in one extremity facilitates the same response in the other extremity. For example, flexion of the involved upper extremity facilitates flexion of the involved lower extremity.

Raimiste's phenomena are specific associated reactions of hip abduction or hip adduction, named for the French neurologist who described them. In the supine position resistance to hip abduction or adduction of the noninvolved extremity evokes the same motion of the involved extremity. There is a similar phenomenon in the upper extremities affecting horizontal adduction; however, it is not termed Raimiste's phenomenon.

Basic Limb Synergies

Limb synergies may be elicited as associated reactions or as voluntary movements in the early stages of

recovery when spasticity is present. When the patient initiates a movement of one joint, all muscles which are linked in a synergy with that movement automatically contract, causing a stereotyped movement pattern.

In the upper extremity, the flexor synergy is composed of scapular retraction and/or elevation, shoulder abduction and external rotation, elbow flexion, forearm supination, and wrist and finger flexion. Elbow flexion is the strongest component of the flexion synergy and the first motion to appear. Shoulder abduction and external rotation are weak components.

The extensor synergy of the upper extremity is composed of scapular protraction, shoulder adduction and internal rotation, elbow extension, forearm pronation, and variable wrist and finger motion, although wrist extension and finger flexion are usually seen. The pectoralis major is the strongest component of the extension synergy; consequently, shoulder adduction and internal rotation are the first motions to appear. Pronation is the next strongest component. Elbow extension is a weak component.

The upper extremity flexion synergy usually develops before the extensor synergy. When both synergies are developing and spasticity is marked, the strongest components of flexion and extension combine to produce the typical upper extremity posture in hemiplegia: The arm is adducted and internally rotated with the elbow flexed, forearm pronated, and the wrist and fingers flexed.

The lower extremity flexor synergy is composed of hip flexion, hip abduction and external rotation, knee flexion, dorsiflexion, and inversion of the ankle, and dorsiflexion of the toes. In this synergy hip flexion is the strongest component, whereas hip abduction and external rotation are weak components.

The lower extremity extensor synergy is composed of hip extension, hip adduction and internal rotation, knee extension, plantar flexion and inversion of the ankle, and plantar flexion of the toes. Hip adduction, knee extension, and plantar flexion of the ankle with inversion are all strong components. Weak components of this synergy are hip extension, hip internal rotation, and plantar flexion of the toes. Note that ankle inversion occurs in both lower extremity synergies.

The lower extremity extensor synergy is dominant in a standing position, due to the strength of this synergy combined with the influences of the positive supporting reaction and stretch forces against the sole of the foot which elicit plantar flexion.

Recovery Stages

Evaluation determines in which recovery stage a patient is functioning. Tables 6.4 and 6.5 list recovery stages in sequence.

Wrist stability and voluntary movements are also sequenced but do not have stage designations, although the sequence roughly parallels stages 4, 5, and 6. When the arm begins to develop movements deviating from synergy the wrist begins a sequence which

Table 6.4
RECOVERY STAGES OF THE UPPER EXTREMITY[a]

Stage: Arm	Stage: Hand
1. Flaccidity—no voluntary movement	1. Flaccidity
2. Synergies developing—flexion usually develops before extension (may be a weak associated reaction or voluntary contraction with or without joint motion); spasticity developing	2. Little or no active finger flexion
3. Synergies performed voluntarily Increased spasticity which may become marked	3. Mass grasp or hook grasp No voluntary finger extension or release

4. Some movements deviating from synergy:
  a. Hand behind body
  b. Arm to forward-horizontal position
  c. Pronation-supination with elbow flexed to 90°
    Spasticity decreasing
	4. Lateral prehension with release by thumb movement
	Semivoluntary finger extension (small range of motion)

5. Independence from the basic synergies:
  a. Arm to side-horizontal position
  b. Arm forward and overhead
  c. Pronation-supination with elbow full extended
    Spasticity waning
	5. Palmar prehension
	Possibly cylindrical and spherical grasp (awkward)
	Voluntary mass finger extension (variable range of motion)

6. Isolated joint movements freely performed with near normal coordination No spasticity	6. All types of prehension (improved skill) Voluntary finger extension (full range of motion) Individual finger movements

[a] Note: Perform upper extremity evaluation with the patient seated in a straight chair. If the evaluation in early stages must be done supine, note the position used.

Table 6.5
RECOVERY STAGES OF THE LOWER EXTREMITY

Stage:

1. Flaccidity
2. Minimal voluntary movements
3. Hip flexion, knee flexion, and ankle dorsiflexion performed as a combined motion in sitting and standing
4. In sitting:
   Knee flexion beyond 90°
   Ankle dorsiflexion with the heel on the floor
5. In standing:
   Isolated knee flexion with hip extended
   Isolated ankle dorsiflexion with knee extended
6. Hip abduction in standing
   Knee rotation with inversion and eversion of the ankle in sitting

progresses from wrist stability during active grasp, with the elbow flexed as well as with the elbow extended, wrist flexion and extension with the fist closed, and then wrist radial and ulnar deviation progressing to wrist circumduction.

The patient is asked to perform each motion of the stages. Instructions for the synergies should be goal-directed; for example, in the upper extremity, "Touch behind your ear" (flexor syngery) or "Reach out to touch my hand" (extensor synergy). The extensor motion is directed to the examiner's hand placed between the patient's knees. Demonstration of the desired motion is often helpful.

These stages represent the sequence of recovery which proceeds from one stage to the next, but may stop at any stage depending on the severity of the cortical damage. A patient is reported to be in the stage at which all motions can be completed. Since progress is gradual from stage to stage there may be instances when the patient is in transition between stages and a recording of stage 2 to 3, 3 to 4, etc. would more accurately describe the status of recovery.

Part of an evaluation form adapted from Brunnstrom[27] is included here (see Table 6.6). The lower extremity, ambulation, and gait analysis sections which are more pertinent to physical therapy evaluation and treatment planning have been omitted. Some forms include assessment of trunk balance, and a tendency to list to one side or an unstable sitting balance is noted.[28] Listing usually occurs to the involved side.[27] Another evaluation procedure describes scoring motor function and balance, sensation, and joint range of motion on an ordinal scale. Criteria are given as the basis for rating the patient's performance in each section and the totals can be used to give a maximum motor score for the upper extremity, lower extremity, or the involved side.[29]

When recording synergy patterns in stage 3, observe the motions present and the range of motion of each component of the synergy. The ranges are recorded in fractions or in percentages. For example, in the upper extremity flexor synergy the hand may be brought to

Table 6.6
HEMIPLEGIA—CLASSIFICATION AND PROGRESS RECORD:
UPPER LIMB—TEST SITTING

Name _____ Age _____ Date of Onset _____ Side Affected _____

Date   Stage
_____   1. No movement initiated or elicited. Flaccidity.

_____   2. Synergies or components developing. Spasticity developing. Note extent of response:
_____   Flexor synergy _____

              _____

_____   Extensor synergy _____

              _____

_____   3. Synergies or components initiated voluntarily. Spasticity marked.
                Flexor synergy   % Active Joint Range

_____   Shoulder girdle elevation   _____
_____   retraction   _____

_____   Shoulder joint abduction   _____
_____   external rotation   _____
_____   hyperextension   _____

_____   Elbow flexion   _____

_____   Forearm supination   _____

                Remarks: _____

                _____

                _____

                Extensor synergy   % Active Joint Range

_____   Shoulder girdle protraction   _____

_____   Shoulder joint adduction and internal rotation (pectoralis major)   _____

_____   Elbow extension   _____

_____   Forearm pronation   _____

                Remarks: _____

                _____

                _____

_____   4. Movements deviating from basic synergies.
                Spasticity decreasing

                                                                                    % ROM

_____   a. Hand behind back
                b. Raise arm to forward-horizontal   _____
_____   c. Pronation-supination, elbow at 90°   _____

                Remarks: _____

                _____

                _____

Table 6.6—*Continued*

Date   Stage

5. Relative independence of basic synergies.
Spasticity waning.

                                                            % ROM

   a. Raise arm to side-horizontal

   b. Raise arm forward overhead

   c. Pronation-supination, elbow extended

6. Movement coordinated and near normal. No spasticity.

Wrist   Describe Motion

4. Wrist stabilization for grasp
   a. Elbow extended
   b. Elbow flexed

5. Wrist flexion and extension, fist closed
   a. Elbow extended
   b. Elbow flexed
6. Wrist circumduction
   (stabilize forearm)

Digits

1. Flaccidity. No voluntary movement

2. Little or no active finger flexion

3. Mass grasp or hook grasp

4. a. Lateral prehension; release by thumb movement
   b. Semivoluntary mass extension-small ROM

5. a. Palmar prehension
   b. Voluntary mass extension-variable ROM
   c. Spherical grasp (awkward)
   d. Cylindrical grasp (awkward)

6. a. All types of grasp with improved skill
   b. Voluntary finger extension-full ROM
   c. Individual finger movements (do dexterity tests)

the mouth rather than the ear with complete elbow flexion, shoulder abduction approaching full range, supination to midrange, and external rotation only partially accomplished. These motions can be recorded as full, ¾, ½, and ¼ or 100%, 75%, 50%, and 25%. Occasionally in the flexor synergy the shoulder components may be so weak that shoulder extension is seen instead of abduction and external rotation,[27] although shoulder extension is a motion that is not considered to be part of the flexor synergy.[28] When recording motions in stages 4 and 5 the ranges obtained are also noted.

Careful recording of evaluation results enables the therapist to identify problems and establish treatment goals based on the needs of the individual and the various factors influencing performance ability.

Sensation

The results of a sensory evaluation provide necessary information for treatment planning. Evaluation of touch, pressure, kinesthesia, and proprioception are particularly important. The reader is referred to Chapter 3, Evaluation and Treatment of Sensation, for evaluation procedures.

TRAINING PROCEDURES

Trunk

Some patients with hemiplegia may have poor trunk balance and may require training to regain control of trunk movements. Brunnstrom's sequence of training would begin with activities to promote trunk balance and muscle contraction. First, balance is promoted by tipping the patient off balance in a sitting position to encourage righting reactions. The patient is gently pushed in forward, backward, and side-to-side directions to elicit balance responses. Emphasis is given to a push toward the involved side to promote contraction of trunk muscles on the noninvolved side to correct any listing tendency. Trunk training then progresses to activities to promote trunk flexion, extension, and then rotation. Practice in foward flexion of the trunk is assisted. The patient crosses his arms with the noninvolved hand under the involved elbow and the noninvolved forearm supporting the involved forearm. The therapist, sitting facing the patient, supports the patient under the elbows and assists in trunk flexion forward, avoiding any pull on the shoulders. Some pain-free shoulder flexion is accomplished during this forward movement. The patient is concentrating on trunk control, and shoulder movement occurs without conscious awareness. Return from trunk flexion is performed actively by the patient.

Forward flexion in oblique directions is then done to incorporate more scapular motion with the shoulder flexion already achieved. Brunnstrom recommends that the therapist stand to offer the best assistance to these oblique motions. Trunk rotation is then practiced with the patient supporting his involved arm and the therapist guiding trunk motion. Trunk rotation can be combined with head movements in the opposite direction of the trunk rotation, so that the tonic neck and tonic lumbar reflexes can be utilized to begin to elicit the shoulder components of the upper extremity synergies. The arms and trunk move in one direction while the head turns in the opposite direction. Head and trunk movements are combined with increasing ranges of movement of the shoulder, enabling pain-free shoulder and scapular abduction and adduction to be accomplished during trunk rotation. With increased shoulder abduction there is decreased tension in the pectoralis major and therefore a greater range of movement in abduction.

Upper Extremity: Stages 1 to 3

In stages 1 to 3 the goal of treatment is to promote voluntary control of the synergies and to encourage their use in purposeful activities. All movements occur in synergy patterns, but with increasing voluntary initiation and control of these patterns. Treatment principles involve the use of tonic reflexes, associated reactions, and proprioceptive and exteroceptive stimuli to develop muscle tension in preparation for voluntary movement. Associated reactions may evoke a muscle contraction which can then become semivoluntary so that "the patient experiences the sensation and statisfaction that accompanies a voluntary muscle contraction."[27] Facilitatory stimuli are used to evoke voluntary muscle contraction, and then graded resistance is applied. After voluntary effort is facilitated, the patient is asked to "hold" using an isometric contraction. Muscle contraction is graded from isometric to eccentric and then to concentric contraction with reversal from a lengthening to a shortening contraction. As voluntary effort becomes more effective, the facilitatory stimulation is reduced. The following techniques are summarized as examples of the use of these principles in the application of the Brunnstrom approach to treatment.

In the flexor synergy elbow flexion is the first motion that can be elicited.

Since many patients with hemiplegia have difficulty achieving shoulder movements and experience pain with passive range of motion, the shoulder and scapula are given special attention when initiating the flexor synergy. Efforts to achieve voluntary control of the synergy begin with scapular elevation which can then be combined with shoulder abduction so that increased shoulder range of motion can be painlessly achieved. Other components of the flexor synergy are then encouraged. Lateral flexion of the neck toward the involved side can be used to initiate scapular elevation. With the patient's arm supported on a table in shoulder abduction with elbow flexion, resistance to the head and shoulder are given while the patient is asked to "hold" the head and not let it move away from the shoulder to develop tension in the trapezius, which is both a lateral head flexor and a scapular elevator. Then both the patient's effort and the therapist's resistance emphasize shoulder elevation when lateral flexion of the neck is repeated. Active contraction may also be promoted by an associated reaction; as the patient attempts bilateral scapular elevation, resistance is given to the noninvolved scapula. If the involved scapula elevates as a result of an associated reaction, resistance is then added on the involved side as the patient is asked to "hold."

Unilateral scapular elevation of the involved arm is attempted next and may be achieved as a result of the previous procedures. If the patient is unable to accomplish the motion the therapist supports the patient's arm and assists the patient to elevate the scapula. Percussion or stroking over the upper trapezius will facilitate muscle contraction. The patient is then told to hold, "Don't let me push your shoulder down." After repeated holding with some resistance added, the patient does an eccentric contraction to let the shoulder down. Then a concentric or shortening contraction is attempted when he is told, "Now pull your shoulder up toward your ear." Active scapular elevation evokes other flexor components and tends to inhibit the pectoralis major. The patient repeats scapular elevation and relaxation as the therapist gently abducts the shoulder in increasing increments. Shoulder external rotation and forearm supination are then included in the movement. Activation of muscles around the shoulder also serves to prevent subluxation of the joint. Reversal of flexor motions to movements in the opposite direction begin to develop some components of the extensor synergy.

The extensor synergy tends to follow the flexor synergy and may need to be assisted in its initiation. Contraction of the pectoralis major, a strong component of the extensor synergy, can be elicited by an associated reaction similar to Raimiste's phenomenon in the lower extremities in which hip abduction or adduction is facilitated in the involved leg by resisting the movement in the noninvolved leg. To elicit this phenomenon in the upper extremities, the therapist supports the patient's arms in a position between horizontal abduction and adduction, instructs the patient to bring his arms together, and resists the noninvolved arm just proximal to the elbow. As contraction occurs bilaterally the patient is instructed, "Don't let me pull your arms apart." Then he attempts to bring his arms together voluntarily.

Because of the predominance of excess tone in the elbow flexors and relative weakness of elbow extensors in the extensor synergy elbow extension is usually more difficult to obtain but can be assisted by the following:

1. A supine position favors extension due to the influence of the TLR.

2. ATNR—head rotation toward the involved side promotes triceps tension.

3. Pronation of the forearm—the supinated position inhibits elbow extension.

4. Tonic lumbar reflex—rotation of the trunk to the noninvolved side facilitates extension of the involved arm. The patient attempts extension toward the non-involved knee.

5. Vigorous stroking of the skin over the triceps or tapping as the patient attempts extension.

6. Bilateral rowing with therapist and patient seated facing each other; the therapist's arms are crossed so that the therapist and patient grasp right hand to right hand and left hand to left hand. Rowing is done as in a boat with the therapist initially resisting the noninvolved arm and assisting the involved arm to get an associated reaction. Then resistance can be given bilaterally so that the movements toward extension combined with pronation are resisted, and the movements toward flexion combined with supination are guided. Quick stretch may be applied to the involved arm by lightly pushing back toward flexion as the patient is moving into extension to facilitate the extensors.

7. Unilateral resistance to the extension pattern may give direction to the patient's effort and facilitate a stronger contraction of the triceps.

8. "Hold-after-positioning" may also reinforce voluntary effort unilaterally. The patient's arm is positioned in the extensor synergy with the elbow in nearly full extension. The patient is asked to "hold" against resistance. Several quick stretches are used to facilitate contraction of the triceps.

9. Weight bearing on the extended arm by leaning forward with the involved arm on a sandbag placed on a low stool in front of the patient. The patient uses the noninvolved hand to position the involved hand with a clenched fist in an impression on the sandbag. Weight is then shifted onto the involved arm which supports the weight of the upper trunk.

10. Unilateral resistance to push the involved hand against the therapist's hand in full elbow extension. The therapist tries to guide the extremity toward shoulder abduction to break up the relationship of shoulder adduction to elbow extension, as a transition to stage 4.

As the synergies become established, they should be used in functional activities. The extensor synergy assists in holding objects for stabilization while the noninvolved hand functions, as in writing, and can be used to push the arm into the sleeve of garments. The flexor synergy assists in carrying items, such as a coat, handbag, or briefcase. Bilateral pushing and pulling activities reinforce both synergies. Sanding, weaving, and ironing are activities which use the flexor and extensor synergies alternately and repeatedly.

Upper Extremity: Stages 4 and 5

In stages 4 and 5 the goal of treatment is to promote voluntary movements which deviate from synergy so that willed movement overcomes the linkage between the various synergy components. Treatment principles involve the use of movement combinations which vary the direction of movements so that motions can be accomplished out of the synergy pattern. Movements begin with easier movements involving the strong components and progress to more difficult movements involving the weaker components. Proprioceptive and exteroceptive stimuli are still used in this phase of training, but tonic reflexes and associated reactions appropriate in the earlier stages when reflex behavior was desirable are no longer used now; willed movement with isolated control of muscle groups is the desired goal.

To promote deviation from synergies motions that begin to combine the synergies are encouraged as a transition from stage 3 to stage 4. Movement away from synergy is done in small increments. Patients are encouraged to do activities on their own for voluntary use of synergies and to attempt other motions. Functional activities are motivating, and activities such as eating, combing the hair, or washing the face require beginning motion out of synergy.

By resisting extension of the arm the therapist can guide the direction of motion and encourage a more lateral motion to break up the synergistic link of the pectoralis major with the triceps. When the triceps and pectoralis major are disassociated, the synergies no longer dominate.

Stage 4 Motions

To assist in getting the hand behind the body, a swinging motion of the arm with trunk rotation is helpful and, if balance is good, this can be more easily done when standing. Stroking the dorsum of the hand and arm is thought to give direction to the attempted voluntary movement. This technique is useful in achieving the hand behind back motion. With the patient sitting, the therapist can passively move the patient's arm to stroke it against the sacrum. Assisted motions into the pattern which are then reversed are used to introduce the desired pattern which gradually becomes voluntary. The patient can then use a stroking motion of the dorsum of the hand against the body to help complete the arm behind back movement. Finally the motion can be freely accomplished.

To achieve shoulder flexion to a forward-horizontal position active forward flexion can be attempted, with the therapist providing local facilitation and guidance of movement direction. If this is too difficult then another method may be used to assist in raising the arm forward to a horizontal position. The arm is positioned, and tapping over the anterior and middle deltoid is applied while the patient attempts to "hold" the position. If "hold after positioning" is accomplished active motion in a small range is begun, and the patient accomplishes lowering of the arm and active shoulder flexion in increasing increments until the full forward motion can be done. The range of active motion is increased from a small range near the full arm forward position to larger ranges of lowering and raising the arm until the full forward motion can be done actively. Stroking and rubbing of the triceps is used to assist in keeping full elbow extension as the arm is raised.

Pronation with the elbow flexed can be assisted by resisting pronation with the elbow extended and gradually increasing elbow flexion as the resistance to pronation is repeated. When resistance is no longer required and the patient can supinate and pronate the forearm with the elbow near the trunk, this motion has been achieved.

Stage 5 Motions

Disassociation of the pectoralis major and triceps as described above is most beneficial in achieving a side horizontal position. When these two motions are still under the influence of the extensor synergy the arm will drift toward horizontal adduction when the elbow is kept in extension. A strong triceps also helps prevent the elbow flexors from contracting with the synergistic influence of shoulder abduction.

In order to achieve an overhead arm position the serratus anterior must be strengthened. The scapula is passively mobilized by grasping the vertebral border to move the scapula as the arm is passively moved into an overhead position. Then the serratus anterior is strengthened in the forward horizontal position by asking the patient to push forward, applying quick stretches, and then asking the patient to "hold". Once resistance in a forward direction is achieved the forward motion is accomplished in increasing increments toward the arm overhead position.

Supination and pronation with the elbow extended is best achieved by using both hands in activities of interest to the patient that involve supination and pronation in various arm positions. The treatment progression is from supination-pronation accomplished close to the body with the elbow flexed to supination-pronation with the elbow extended. There are no special treatment procedures recommended to assist in developing disassociation of supination and elbow flexion.

All actions of stages 4 and 5 should be reinforced by use in meaningful and interesting activities. An example of an activity requiring placing the involved hand behind the back is dropping bean bags to hit into a container placed just behind the foot on the involved side. Another means of achieving this motion is to have pieces of an assembly project, such as mosaic tiles, placed on a table on the involved side and the project itself placed on the noninvolved side; the pa-

tient would pick up each tile on the involved side and pass it behind the back to the noninvolved hand. Raising the arm to forward-horizontal is involved in any vertically mounted game with velcro tabs, such as tic-tac-toe or checkers. Sponge painting is repetitive and essentially nonresistive and can be mounted on an easel. Activities using supination and pronation require turning objects, such as a knob or a screw driver. Resistance is to the direction in which the major force is exerted. Woodworking projects may involve sanding curved edges and are often assembled with screws. Some games are knob operated like Skittles, and other games can be vertically mounted and adapted to require supination and pronation. Checkers can be adapted by the use of threaded dowels that must be turned to remove and replace them for each move on the checkerboard. In stage 4 where resistance to pronation is suggested, first with the elbow extended and then with increasing amounts of elbow flexion, block printing could be positioned to resist pronation with gradual changes in the amount of elbow flexion. In order to achieve a side-horizontal position disassociation of the pectoralis major and triceps is necessary. Activities such as block printing or pressing clay into a flat piece for a large tile provide resistance to extension and can be gradually positioned from the extensor synergy to a more lateral position. The arm overhead position is achieved by strengthening the serratus anterior. Sanding on an inclined plane is an example of an activity requiring a forward push with an increasing range of movement in shoulder flexion.

Patients who recover comparatively rapidly after a stroke may spontaneously achieve stage 6; however, many hemiplegic patients do not achieve full recovery. Twitchell, as summarized by Brunnstrom,[27] states that patients who reached stages 3 and 4 within 10 days post-stroke recovered completely. Patients who failed to respond to proprioceptive facilitation did not recover willed movement at all. The longer the duration of the flaccid stage, the less likely was recovery.

Hand

Training techniques for return of function in the hand, although presented separately, parallel return of function in the arm in the various stages of recovery. Each hand stage may not, however, occur at the same time as the parallel stage of the arm. Hand motions require the greatest cortical control, and full recovery is rare.

If the patient is unable to initiate grasp, the traction response, with stretch of scapular adductors producing reflex finger flexion, may evoke grasp and assist voluntary effort. In hemiplegia, wrist flexion usually accompanies grasp initially, and stability in wrist extension must be developed. It is easier for the patient to stabilize the wrist in extension when the elbow is extended. With the elbow extended and wrist supported, percussion over the wrist extensor muscles together with the command, "Squeeze," promotes synergic contraction of the wrist extensors when the finger flexors contract. After repeated squeeze and relax alternation, wrist support is removed with the command, "Hold." Tapping on the wrist extensor muscles may facilitate holding. Once wrist extension and grasp are associated with the elbow extended, the process of positioning, percussion, and hold is repeated in increasing amounts of elbow flexion. Emphasis in training is on wrist stability, although wrist flexion and extension and circumduction may then be practiced.

Release of grasp and voluntary finger extension are then encouraged. Grasp is released by supinating the forearm and pulling the thumb away from the palm by moving the metacarpal into abduction and extension. Supination and pronation are repeated with emphasis on supination while the thumb is held out of the palm to achieve relaxation of the pronators. Cutaneous stimulation, stroking over the dorsum of the hand when the forearm is supinated, combined with repetition of thumb manipulation releases tension in the flexors. The patient can be taught to do this. With the forearm supinated, a rapid repeated stretch stimulus is applied to the dorsum of the fingers by rolling them toward the palm with a stroking motion to stretch finger extensors. When flexor tension is relaxed, the forearm is pronated and the arm elevated above horizontal (Souque's phenomenon), while stroking over the dorsum of the fingers and forearm continues and a tonic reflex extension can now be attempted, but effort exerted should be minimal to avoid a buildup of tension. Imitation synkinesis, in which the normal side performs a motion that is difficult to achieve on the involved side, may be observed when the patient attempts finger extension. After the fingers can be voluntarily extended with the arm raised, the arm is gradually lowered. If there is an increase of flexor tension reflected by decreasing range in extension, it is necessary to repeat the manipulations that inhibit flexion and facilitate extension.

Functional use of lateral prehension is encouraged. The patient must learn to move the thumb away from the index finger to gain release of lateral prehension. Percussion or friction over the abductor pollicis longus tendon can facilitate this motion. Activities are selected to encourage the use of other prehensile patterns as they develop. Palmar prehension is used to hold a pencil or paint brush. Spherical grasp is used to pick up round objects, and cylindrical grasp is used when holding the handles of tools.

Lower Extremity

Gait patterns, principles used in preparation for walking, and ambulation training are also described by Brunnstrom; these principles and procedures fall under the primary responsibility of the physical therapist.

CONCLUSION

Signe Brunnstrom has contributed significantly to our understanding of the motor behavior of the adult patient with hemiplegia. From her years of clinical observation and research of the literature she has devised a training program which follows neurodevelopmental principles and effective procedures in the professional literature for the benefit of others while continuing to acknowledge the need for further observations and the individuality of patient responses.

SECTION 4

The Proprioceptive Neuromuscular Facilitation (PNF) Approach

BEVERLY J. MYERS, B.S., OTR

INTRODUCTION

PNF embodies broad concepts of human motion derived from normal development. As such, PNF has value to occupational therapists in evaluating and enhancing motor performance. PNF has been defined as "a method of promoting or hastening the response of the neuromuscular mechanism through stimulation of the proprioceptors."[30] Various techniques are superimposed on patterns of movement and posture with attention to the sensory stimulation from manual contacts, visual cues, and verbal commands so as to bring as many favorable influences as possible to bear on the patient.

Applying PNF to the treatment of patients in occupational therapy requires that the therapist understands the concepts, learns the motor skills, and then incorporates the approach into activities that meet the individual patient's needs. This introduction presents the principles of PNF and some examples of application in OT. To learn the motor skills, the patterns and techniques must be performed under the supervision of a knowledgeable instructor. Learning by practicing with other students develops the feeling of how normal balanced antagonistic muscle groups respond in different developmental positions. Then learning may proceed to application and repeated use with patients.

HISTORY

Herman Kabat, Ph.D., M.D., neurophysiologist and physician, developed the method of proprioceptive neuromuscular facilitation at the Kabat-Kaiser Institute during the years 1946 to 1951. Sherrington's physiology and philosophy provided the foundation for many of the techniques. Some of the other experimenters who influenced the PNF approach were: Gellhorn, a neurophysiologist who studied proprioception and cortically induced movement; Gesell, who studied the development of motor behavior and patterned movement; McGraw, who studied the development of behavior as it relates to the maturation of neural structures; Hellebrandt, who studied combinations of movements and mass movements, finding that one can circumvent fatigue or speed recovery by changing the combination used; and Pavlov, who studied the mechanisms of learning and formation of habit patterns.

The diagonal patterns, PNFs unique feature, were the last aspect to be identified. Specific combinations of motion were carefully analyzed in 1951. Dr. Kabat found that when topographically aligned groups of muscles were stretched they produced a movement in a diagonal direction. Observation of functional movement and sport skills revealed the same spiral and diagonal characteristics.

Kabat began his work in the early 1940s in treating patients with cerebral palsy and multiple sclerosis. However, by the early 1950s PNF had been applied to the treatment of patients with all diagnoses, from those with central nervous system deficits to orthopedic conditions, arthritis, and peripheral nerve injuries.

In 1956 the first edition of the Knott and Voss book was published. Physical therapists who worked with Kabat wrote the PNF textbook,[30] the first book on the PNF approach to therapeutic exercise. The book was revised in 1968, and translations are available in six different languages. OTs used PNF as evidenced by the related articles published during the 1950s.[31-36] Ayres' series of three comprehensive articles[32] on PNF and application to OT were published in 1955. Voss also contributed a significant article on the same topic in 1959.[34]

No courses or workshops were offered for OTs until 1974 when Voss taught the first PNF course for OTs at Northwestern University. This course was cosponsored by the curriculum in OT, University of Illinois. Continuing education in the form of 1-week courses and 1-day workshops continues to be offered for occupational therapists.

PRINCIPLES

In developing the PNF method, Dr. Herman Kabat relied on authorities in the fields of neurophysiology,

motor learning, and motor behavior. The basic principles of PNF, as stated in 1966 by Voss, encompass the developmental concepts as drawn from these fields. The 11 principles follow.

1. *All human beings have potentials that are not fully developed.*[37] This first principle is a statement of philosophy. It provides the base for an attitude toward treating patients. The patient's abilities and potentials become the means to reduce his inabilities. When the patient's progress declines, the idea that the patient has reached a plateau is the last factor to be acknowledged. The cause may not be due to the patient's natural limitations, but rather due to the lack of experience and skills of the therapist, the lack of coordination with the rehabilitation team and the patient's family, the lack of time for appropriate treatment, or the lack of funds. PNF does not disregard the fact that some persons may reach a limit beyond which no further learning may occur. However, the emphasis is on bringing as many favorable influences to bear as possible on developing a patient's potential. Consider the common reaction of a person watching a tennis game for the first time. "Oh, I could never do that," he might exclaim. But after a few lessons, that same person may have channelled his potential and abilities to perform a skill which he previously thought was impossible. This philosophy, inherent in the PNF approach, is compatible with that of occupational therapy, where emphasis is placed on ability rather than disability.

Also, this philosophy underlies the approach of PNF in using the patient's stronger movement patterns to strengthen the weaker motions. Thus, an indirect approach results. In treatment, when the superior region is intact, as in a person with paraplegia, the movements of the head, neck, upper trunk, and upper limbs are used to facilitate and reinforce movements in the lower extremities. When the patient has one involved upper extremity, as in the person with a frozen shoulder, the motions of the intact upper extremity and inferior region are emphasized in bilateral combinations and total patterns to reduce the pain and increase movement in the affected arm.

2. *Normal motor development proceeds in a cervicocaudal and proximodistal direction.*[37] In treatment, this direction is heeded with attention given first to the development of motion in the head and neck, then in the trunk, and last in the extremities. For example, with the patient who is comatose, treatment would not begin by quietly performing range of motion on the hand but rather by first directing sensory stimuli to the head, as in greeting and talking to the patient, touching his face or head while talking, or providing other tactile input to the facial region. Positioning the patient in a total pattern, such as sidelying, would follow and would stimulate rotation of head, neck, and trunk. Then, if indicated, passive range of motion of the extremities could be administered.

As the head and neck lead the rest of the body in embryonic differentiation and reflex development,[41] so too the position of the head and neck influences the movement of the body's total pattern throughout life. For example, in standing when the head is quickly rotated to one side, the body weight shifts to that side. In treatment, this principle is applied when facilitating weight bearing. When a patient rises to stand from a wheelchair or bed, if weight is not equally distributed, asking the patient to look toward the inefficient side may promote a shift of weight toward that side. Likewise, when working on developing stability of the affected side of the patient who has hemiplegia, positioning the activity on the hemiplegic side will increase a weight shift toward the involved leg or arm, thus facilitating weight bearing on that side.

The development of movement and stability in the limbs proceeds in a proximodistal direction. In therapy, developing the function of the head, neck, and trunk precedes developing the function of the extremities, and that of the shoulder girdle before developing the fine motor skills of the hand. However, coordinated movement proceeds in a distal to proximal direction. When reaching for the telephone on a desk, the shoulder and elbow do not lead the movement; rather, the hand opens and reaches to grasp the phone. The rest of the arm supports and follows the movement of the hand.

3. *Early motor behavior is dominated by reflex activity. Mature motor behavior is reinforced or supported by postural reflex mechanisms.*[37] In other words, the reflexes present in the newborn do not disappear completely but become integrated into the child's nervous system as he matures. For example, the asymmetric tonic neck reflex (ATNR) supports rolling, the symmetric tonic neck reflex (STNR) supports the assumption of the hands-knees posture, and the body-on-body righting reflex supports the assumption of side-sitting from prone. In the adult, reflexes are available when needed to support movement. Evidence exists frequently in sports or when the body performs under stressful conditions.

Recognizing reflex responses in man requires good skills of observation, as the reflex response may not be complete. Tonus changes and partial movements are common. Hellebrandt *et al.*[42] studied the effect of the tonic neck reflex in the normal adult. An adaptation of one of her experiments can be easily performed with a partner. One person assumes a hands-knees position and the other person tests the triceps strength unilaterally four times. The first time, the person on hands and knees dorsiflexes her head and maintains this position. The tester waits 15 seconds, allowing for the latency of the tonus change, and then resists the triceps by attempting to passively flex the elbow. This procedure is repeated with the head ventroflexed, rotated away from the arm, and rotated towards the arm being tested. One would expect stronger responses when elbow extension is supported by the STNR, head dorsiflexed, and by the ATNR, head rotated towards the resisted arm. In treatment, application occurs when a patient with weakness on one side has difficulty assuming a hands-knees posture. Directing the patient to turn his head toward the weaker side will elicit the support of the ATNR to reinforce elbow extension. In PNF, a balance of reflex activity is sought.

4. *The growth of motor behavior has cyclic trends as evidenced by shifts between flexor and extensor dominance.*[37] For example, in the development of the sitting posture, the first cycle is flexion. The newborn child is positioned in sitting and with assistance, or with support of arms, remains sitting in a flexor-dominant posture. The next cycle is one of extension. Sitting is assumed independently, but usually with extension from prone to hands and knees and then with rotation to side-sitting and long-sitting. Finally, the cycle shifts to flexion again as the child learns to assume sitting symmetrically from supine.

Interaction between movements of flexion and extension is necessary for functional movement. In the action of rising to stand, one begins by flexing the superior region forward to shift weight onto the feet. Extension of the body follows as the upright position is attained. The normal child facilitates this interaction by rocking alternately from flexion to extension in various postures.[38] Gesell describes this process as reciprocal interweaving in which relationships of opposed functions are established.[43] These reciprocal relationships provide the basis for development of stability and balance of postures.

In treatment, the therapist applies this principle in observing the patient's movements. If flexor tone dominates, then extensor-dominant activities and methods of assumption will be selected. Like-wise, if extensor tone is dominant, activities stimulating flexor dominance will be chosen. Emphasis of treatment is rarely limited to one dominance, as an interaction between balanced antagonistic movements is sought.

5. *Goal-directed activity is made up of reversing movements.*[37] Early motor behavior occurs in random fashion through full range of motion. The spontaneous limb movements of the newborn usually fluctuate from extremes of flexion to extension. Yet the movements are rhythmic and reversing, qualities which continue throughout life. The act of eating is a reversing movement of the arm and jaw. Reversal of a total pattern is commonly found in removing a can of soda from the refrigerator. Initially the action includes walking forward to open the door and reaching forward to grasp the can. Reversal of direction follows to remove the can from the shelf and walk backward to close the door. If a patient cannot reverse directions, his functional ability will be limited. The rhythmic reversing of direction then becomes a goal of treatment, as reversing movements help to reestablish the balance and interaction between antagonists.

6. *Normal movement and posture are dependent upon "synergism" and a balanced interaction of antagonists.*[37] This principle encompasses the previous three and states the main goal in the PNF approach: to develop a balance of antagonists. A continual adjustment in reflex activity, dominance, and reversing or antagonistic movements is required for the constant changes of movement and posture that occur in func-

tional activity. For example, getting dressed demands interaction in all of these areas. Without a balance of antagonists, the quality of performance decreases, becoming more deliberate and losing its smooth and rhythmical characteristics. Thus, in treatment, prevention and correction of imbalances between antagonists is an objective.[37]

7. *Developing motor behavior is expressed in an orderly sequence of total patterns of movement and posture.*[38,40] The concept of recapitulating the developmental sequence is followed in treatment. The developmental sequence is considered a universal experience, common to all normal human beings. Thus, if a person, such as a child with cerebral palsy, has not experienced these total patterns, he has need to do so. With the patient who has developed normally and then becomes disabled, this sequence of developmental positions will have meaning to him.[37] In occupational therapy, the developmental sequence has direct application, as functional activities can be performed in a variety of postures. Thus, the patient not only experiences total patterns which facilitate the use of and integration of postural reflexes, but frustration is reduced. For example, his ability to dress is built through the total patterns of rolling, lower trunk rotation, bridging, and assumption to sitting, rather than through practice of inadequate or unstable sitting and standing positions.

The developmental sequence also includes the "combining movements" of the extremities as they interact with the head, neck, and trunk in total patterns (Table 6.7). The upper or lower extremity movements occur in an orderly sequence.[38,40] First to appear are bilateral symmetrical patterns, then bilateral asymmetrical, and bilateral reciprocal, and lastly unilateral patterns. When the upper and lower extremities move together, they begin in an ipsilateral pattern, then progress to alternating reciprocal, where contralateral extremities move in the same direction one at a time, while opposite contralateral extremities move in the opposite direction one at a time. For example, an infant beginning to creep uses an ipsilateral pattern. Later, the child uses an alternating reciprocal pattern, moving one extremity at a time. As coordination and rate of movement increase, the child progresses to the most advanced combination, diagonal reciprocal. This combination is similar to alternating reciprocal with only one difference: contralateral extremities move in the same direction at the same time, while the other contralateral extremities move in the opposite direction at the same time, as in normal creeping or walking. In occupational therapy, these combining movements may be used to assess a patient's level of performance or to design a treatment activity for stimulation of a response in the total pattern. For example, standing in a bilateral symmetrical combination will facilitate head, neck, and trunk flexion and extension. Swinging a bat or racquet in a bilateral asymmetrical combination will facilitate head, neck, and trunk rotation. Whereas, performing a reciprocal combination in

Table 6.7
COMBINED MOVEMENTS OF UPPER AND LOWER EXTREMITIES[a]

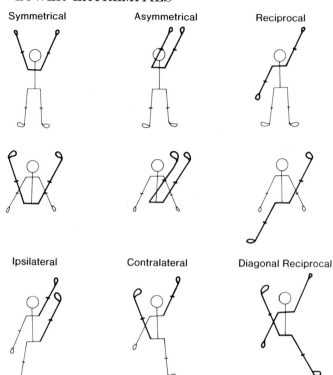

Symmetrical   Asymmetrical   Reciprocal

Ipsilateral   Contralateral   Diagonal Reciprocal

[a] Courtesy of D. E. Voss, Northwestern University Medical School, Chicago, Ill. Figures redrawn by Julie A. Livingston (Class of 1973).

throwing a ball or reaching for an item on a high shelf, will promote stability of head, neck, and trunk.

Direction of movement also develops in an orderly sequence. Gesell observed that the child follows a significant pattern in developing the ability to use a crayon. The strokes move from scrawl, to vertical, to horizontal, to circular, and oblique or diagonal. Comparable sequences of direction have been demonstrated in visual behavior eye-hand coordination, vocalization, percept-concept formation, and postural behavior.[44] Thus, the diagonal direction or pattern of movement is a combination of the previous three movements, and is the most advanced. Voss,[37] in citing Gesell, pointed out that in PNF, total patterns of movement are performed in a diagonal direction, as well as in forward, backward, sideward, and circular directions.

8. *Normal motor development has an orderly sequence but lacks a step by step quality. Overlapping occurs.*[37] In treatment, a patient does not remain in sitting until perfection of balance is achieved before attempting to stand. The order of the developmental sequence aids the therapist in finding a posture or a place to begin when treating the patient. A posture in which the patient is stable and can move successfully becomes a place to begin. The developmental se-

quence provides a direction in which to progress. However, the overlapping quality occurs as the patient may benefit from working on activities in postures above and below his level of ability.

Performing activities in developmental postures will enhance a person's adaptive response to the task or movement. However, the activity must be graded in keeping with the physical demands on the patient. If the physical demands are high, the activity must be simple. If the physical demands are low, the activity may be more complex. For example, a patient with brain damage may need to develop balance in kneeling and standing and improve his writing skills. In treatment, activities in kneeling may include simple gross motor activities, such as playing tic-tac-toe on the blackboard or sanding on an inclined board. However, when the patient practices writing, a fine motor activity, a more stable posture such as sitting is required. Besides kneeling and sitting the patient may engage in standing activities, walking to and from each activity, and gait training in physical therapy. Thus, overlapping of postures occurs in treatment during an individual therapy session or throughout the day.

9. *Improvement of motor ability is dependent upon motor learning.*[37] The concepts of motor learning that PNF applies to therapeutic exercise are similar to those used by occupational therapists in functional activity training. These concepts will be reviewed briefly with specific emphasis on the PNF approach.

Motor learning extends from the conditioning of responses to the learning of complex voluntary motor acts.[45] Harlow and Harlow[46] classified the conditioning of responses as the simplest form of learning. Proprioceptive feedback as received from receptors in the muscles, tendons, joints, and labyrinths plays a significant role in simple conditioned responses.[45] In addition, stress promotes maturation.[47] Levine[47] studied infant rats and their responses to the stresses of handling and electric shock. The rats who received either form of stress developed into normal active adults. Those rats who were not subjected to stress, defecated and urinated more frequently and did not explore their environment. Thus, motor learning is facilitated by stress coupled with sensory and environmental stimulation.

As maturation occurs, more complex acts may be learned. The sequence begins with conditioned responses progressing to an ability to discriminate between objects, to an ability to transfer learning from one problem to another, and then to the ability to solve complex problems requiring concept formation. Learning complex tasks can be facilitated by the use of "step-wise procedures," as demonstrated in Harlow's studies.[46] In PNF, the therapist helps the patient to learn many complex motor acts, such as transfers and other self-care skills. By selecting and providing appropriate sensory cues and through the use of techniques of facilitation, the demands of a task or parts of the task which the patient is unable to perform independently may be made more appropriate. PNF emphasizes the step-wise procedures of a task, yet allows the patient to complete the whole task. Thus, by training with repetition, the conditioning of responses occurs and leads to the achievement of the whole task.

Sensory cues include visual, auditory, and tactile stimuli. Vision and hearing give direction to movement.[48] Vision may lead movement or follow the movement. For example, in lifting an object up to a shelf, the person will look to the shelf first, then lift the object. Thus, if a patient is not engaging the movement with his eyes, he has a need to do so. Following the movement visually will enhance the motor performance. Verbal commands increase sensory stimulation and may facilitate movement. Tone of voice may influence the quality of the muscle response. A loud, sharp command will yield a quick response and recruit more motor units. A soft, low command will produce a slower response. In the presence of pain, soft commands are always used to avoid stimulating jerky movements and further increasing the pain.[37]

Tactile cues in PNF are mainly provided by the therapist's manual contacts which facilitate movement or promote relaxation. Also, stretch and resistance may be applied by opposing the patient effort and yet becoming part of his effort.[37] Additional tactile stimulation may be provided by adjuncts to treatment, such as vibration and cold.

Thus, motor learning is enhanced by tracking sensory cues. One may track a visual stimulus, the sound of a voice, or a touch. Tactual tracking is more efficient.[49] In cybernetics research, movement with visual tracking was discovered to be less accurate than movement with tactual feedback. In treatment, an application of tracking may occur when a patient reaches for an object and is unable to complete the range of movement. A light touch on the back of the patient's hand, guiding him toward the object may be the only cue he needs to achieve the goal. Another example may occur when a patient with unilateral weakness in the upper limb attempts to wipe the table with a sponge. The performance may quickly deteriorate with the patient complaining of fatigue. With a light touch on the back of the patient's hand from the therapist hand or with self-touch from the patient's uninvolved hand, the patient's movement becomes less deliberate, endurance improves, and the task is completed. In summary, the application of motor learning concepts in PNF becomes one of combining as many favorable influences as possible to achieve the desired response.

10. *Frequency of stimulation and repetition of activity are used to promote and for retention of motor learning and for the development of strength and endurance.*[37] Patients, as well as any child or adult learning a new skill, require frequent stimulation and opportunity to practice in order that the task being learned may be retained. Motor learning has occurred when the movement is repeated enough to become integrated into the body's repertoire of movements

and can be used automatically. In treatment, repetition cannot be overemphasized. Activity has an inherent advantage over exercise because during activity, repetition occurs naturally.

11. *Goal-directed activities, coupled with techniques of facilitation, are used to hasten learning of total patterns of walking and of self-care activities.*[37] Facilitation techniques or exercise alone are not as meaningful as when they are coupled with an activity. Activity which directs attention away from the motor aspects of the task and toward a purposeful goal enhances neurological integration.[50] Likewise, purposeful activity alone is not enough. It is necessary but not always sufficient to meet the patient's needs. Therapists need to relate the facilitation techniques to activity.[50]

EVALUATION

Assessment becomes an ongoing process in the PNF approach. Following the initial evaluation, a treatment plan is established with selected procedures and techniques. Modifications occur as the needs of the patient change or as the therapist observes a change in the patient's performance.

As PNF encompasses concepts that may be applied to many diagnoses, the evaluation is general in nature. Forms for evaluation, analysis, and planning treatment programs in physical therapy were developed by Voss[51] in 1967 and 1969. Descriptions of the evaluation process have been presented in detail in the literature.[30,48] The evaluation reflects the developmental sequence, proceeding from a proximal to distal direction. A brief summary of the evaluation process is presented here.

Vital and related functions of the body are considered first. Functions of respiration, swallowing, voice production, and facial and tongue motions are evaluated with impairments, weakness, or asymmetry noted. Also, movements in response to visual, auditory, and tactile stimuli are elicited to determine which sensory cues may be used to reinforce movement and posture.

Head and neck patterns, the key to upper trunk patterns, receive the next consideration. Observation of head and neck position is made during the performance of developmental and functional activities. The following are noted: dominance of tone (flexor or extensor), alignment (midline or asymmetrical), and stability *vs.* mobility (balanced or deficient in one or both areas).

Combinations of diagonal patterns of the extremities are next in the evaluation sequence. The patient is asked to perform bilateral symmetrical, bilateral asymmetrical, and bilateral reciprocal combinations. The following areas are assessed: influence of head, neck, and trunk; range of motion, remembering that rotation is not complete in any pattern; quality of movement, such as smooth and rhythmical; and normal timing, with the distal component leading in coordinated movement.

Developmental postures are observed by asking the patient to assume and maintain positions in the developmental sequence. These total patterns are assessed to determine how muscle groups function in relation to each other in a given pattern. Previous evaluation centered on individual segments and functions. During observations of total patterns a central problem or imbalance may be identified. For example, is more stability or mobility needed? Is there a dominance rather than a balance of flexor or extensor tone? And does the patient have difficulty shifting from one dominance to another?

Functional activities, as performed in self-care tasks and transfers, are observed finally to determine any discrepancies between the patient's ability to perform individual and total patterns and his ability to combine these movements in performance of a functional task.

TREATMENT PROCEDURES

Diagonal Patterns

For every major part of the body: the head, neck, trunk, and extremities, two pairs of diagonal patterns of movement exist. Each pair of antagonistic patterns consists of three motion components. Flexion or extension is always present as the major component. These flexion and extension components are combined with rotation, either external or internal, and with abduction or adduction. For example, in diagonal one (D1) flexion of the upper extremity, flexion combines with adduction and external rotation. In diagonal two (D2) flexion, flexion combines with abduction and external rotation. These diagonal patterns are described in the Knott and Voss book[30] according to shoulder motion components, the original designation by Kabat. The briefer designations of diagonal one and diagonal two were introduced by Voss.[37] In development, the diagonal patterns appear in the functional movements of rolling and prone locomotion. Diagonal one derives from rolling and diagonal two from crawling on the belly.

Five factors support the use of diagonal patterns in treatment. First, the patterns agree with the spiral and diagonal characteristics of normal functional movement. Most muscles, by virtue of their attachments and alignment of their fibers, support this movement. Second, scientists who have studied integrative function of the brain support the concept that voluntary movement consists of mass movement patterns rather than individual muscle action. Hughlings Jackson[52] was one of the first to stimulate specific areas of the motor cortex and discovered that mass movement patterns were produced. Third, Gesell noted that diagonal movement occurs last in the normal development of direction and is the most advanced motion.[44] Thus, diagonal movements are combinations of the three pairs of antagonistic motions of flexion or extension, abduction or adduction, and external or internal rotation. Fourth, all diagonal patterns cross the midline, thereby facilitating interaction between two sides of the body, which is important to perceptual motor and sensory integrative functioning. Fifth, the diagonal patterns always incorporate a rotation component. As rotation is one of the last movements to develop, it is usually the first to be lost following an injury or with aging.[37] Use of diagonal patterns in therapy reinforces the component of rotation, necessary to the performance of functional tasks.

Bilateral symmetrical patterns occur where paired extremities perform like movements at the same time. These combining movements are the first to develop, and therefore, they are often the easiest to learn. Also, as they influence head, neck, and trunk flexion and extension, they play an important role in facilitating a reciprocal relationship between flexor and extensor dominance. Bilateral symmetrical patterns of the upper extremities (Figs. 6.4 and 6.5, Figs. 6.10 and 6.11) are commonly observed in the daily activities of riding a bicycle, putting a roast in the oven, and removing a pullover shirt overhead. Bilateral symmetrical pat-

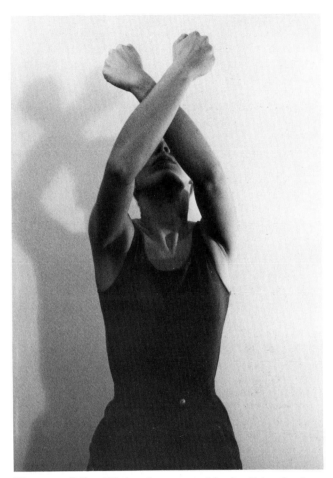

Figure 6.5 Bilateral symmetrical D1 flexion, shortened range; bilateral symmetrical D1 extension, lengthened range: *shoulders* flex, adduct, and externally rotate; *elbows* flex (intermediate joint, the elbow, may flex or extend), *forearms* supinate; *wrists* flex toward radial side; *fingers* flex and adduct; and *thumbs* flex and adduct.

terns of the lower extremities (Figs. 6.8 and 6.9, Figs. 6.14 and 6.15) are seen in the postures of standing and sitting.

Bilateral asymmetrical patterns occur when paired extremities perform movements toward one side at the same time. The limbs may move together free from contact as in bilateral asymmetrical flexion to the right, with the right arm in D2 flexion and the left in D1 flexion. The combining movement may also be performed with the arms in contact, as in the patterns of chopping (Figs. 6.6 and 6.7) and lifting (Figs. 6.12 and 6.13). Bilateral asymmetrical patterns influence the head, neck, and trunk movements in patterns of flexion with rotation or extension with rotation. When the arms perform in contact, the range of trunk flexion and extension with rotation increases. Swinging a baseball bat is an example of a bilateral asymmetric pattern in the upper extremities. The same combination in the lower extremities is found in the side-sitting position.

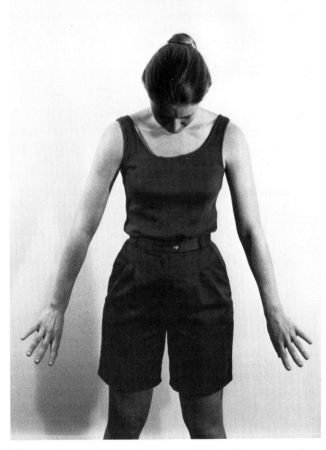

Figure 6.4 Bilateral symmetrical D1 extension, shortened range; bilateral symmetrical D1 flexion, lengthened range: *shoulders* extend, abduct, and internally rotate; *elbows* extend (intermediate joint, the elbow, may flex or extend), *forearms* pronate; *wrists* extend toward ulnar side; *fingers* extend and abduct; and *thumbs* extend and abduct.

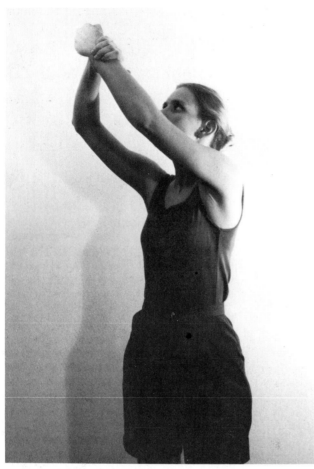

Figure 6.6 Bilateral asymmetric pattern with limbs in contact, as in "chopping." A chop to the left begins with the left arm in D1 flexion, and the right hand grasping the dorsum of the left wrist.

Bilateral reciprocal patterns occur when paired extremities perform movements in opposite directions at the same time. For example, in reciprocal movements of diagonal one, one arm begins in D1 extension, the other arm in D1 flexion. As one arm moves toward D1 flexion, the other arm moves toward D1 extension. Less flexion and extension of head, neck, and trunk are present in reciprocal motions as compared to other combined patterns. Rotation of head, neck, and trunk may occur, but the range is incomplete. When antagonistic patterns of both diagonals are performed at the same time, as in a reciprocal combination in combined diagonals with one arm in D1 extension and the other arm in D2 flexion, the movement of the head, neck, and trunk continue to decrease. The position of the head remains in midline. The reciprocal patterns have a stabilizing influence on head, neck, and trunk because one extremity flexes while the other extends, producing stability in the trunk. Examples of reciprocal movements are walking, running, and swimming the crawl stroke. They are also seen in activities which place an increased demand for equilibrium reactions on the body, such as in reaching for an item on a high

shelf, or performing a lay-up shot during a basketball game.

Unilateral patterns in developing motor behavior emerge from the bilateral patterns. The motions of the unilateral diagonal patterns are the same as those described in the bilateral symmetrical patterns (Figs. 6.4 and 6.5, 6.10 and 6.11). In skilled tasks the two diagonals may interact or one may dominate. Diagonal one in the upper extremities is observed in the basic activities of feeding and washing the face, right side with left hand. Diagonal two is seen in the self-care activities of zipping a front opening zipper and winding a watch. Diagonal one in the lower extremities is observed in pushing one foot through a pant leg and in crossing one leg to don a sock. Diagonal two is seen in hurdling and in swimming the breast stroke.

Examples of activities where the two diagonals interact are washing the face and waving. In washing the face (Table 6.8), when the right hand contacts the left side of the face, it is in D1 flexion. When the right hand washes the right side of the face, it is in D2 flexion with elbow flexed. Diagonals change and interact as the hand crosses the midline of the face and body. They also interact when the pattern crosses the

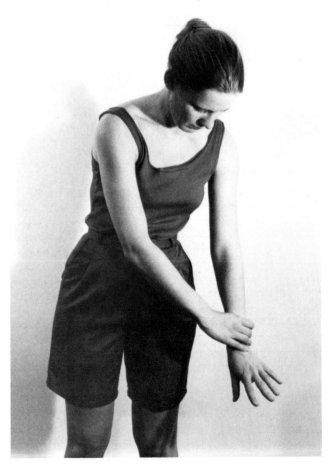

Figure 6.7 In chopping to the left, the left arm moves in D1 extension, with the right arm assisting in D2 extension.

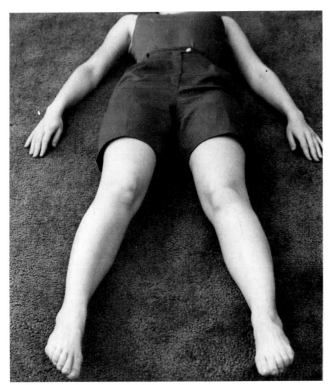

Figure 6.8 Bilateral symmetrical D1 extension, shortened range; bilateral symmetrical D1 flexion, lengthened range: *hips* extend, abduct, and internally rotate; *knees* extend (intermediate joint, the knee, may flex or extend), *ankles and feet* plantar flex and evert; and *toes* flex and adduct.

horizontal plane that transverses at the shoulders. An example occurs when waving goodbye. The right arm begins in extension on the same side of the body in D1 extension. When the arm raises above the shoulder to wave goodbye on the same side, it moves into D2 flexion with elbows flexed.

In all of the above bilateral and unilateral patterns, the intermediate joints, the elbow and the knee, may flex or extend. While the intermediate joints may change, the motions of the proximal and distal joints are consistent with each other. In the upper extremity, the consistency between the proximal and distal joints changes in a variation of the diagonal pattern called *thrusting* (Figs. 6.16 to 6.19).

The two pairs of upper extremity thrusting patterns are the ulnar thrust, D1, and the radial thrust, D2. In diagonal one flexion, external rotation is consistent with supination. In the D1 ulnar thrust, the shoulder remains the same, but the forearm is counterrotated in pronation, and the hand opens to the ulnar side. In diagonal two extension, internal rotation is consistent with pronation. In the D2 radial thrust, the shoulder remains the same, but the forearm is counterrotated in supination, and the hand opens to the radial side. All bilateral combinations can be performed with the thrusting patterns. In the lower extremities, mass extension of hip and knee is a powerful thrusting move-

ment. Thrusting patterns represent primitive patterns of protection, defense, reach, and grasp. The movement of thrusting occurs more forcefully than motions in other diagonal patterns. In treatment, thrusting is a good pattern in which to retrain elbow extension with wrist extension.

The diagonal patterns are used in OT to assess movement, as it occurs in specific combinations or in activities. Range of motion may also be performed in diagonal patterns. This method is more efficient than the traditional range of motion performed in anatomical planes. In addition, using diagonals constantly reinforces the rotation component. Lastly, the diagonal patterns provide a framework by which to train functional movements and to design goal-directed treatment activities.

Total Patterns

The sequence and procedures for assisting patients into the developmental postures were developed by Voss in 1971. A videotape was made in 1972 and

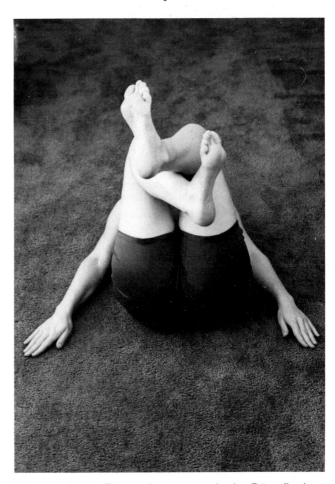

Figure 6.9 Bilateral symmetrical D1 flexion, shortened range; bilateral symmetrical D1 extension, lengthened range: *hips* flex, adduct, and externally rotate; *knees* flex (intermediate joint, the knee, may flex or extend), *ankles and feet* dorsiflex and invert; *toes*, extend and abduct.

Neurophysiological and Developmental Treatment Approaches **113**

with forearms pronated and wrist and fingers extended.

To assist a patient from prone to prone on elbows (Fig. 6.20), the *preparatory maneuvers* include placing the lower extremities in symmetrical extension and placing the head in a symmetrical position or turned to one side for comfort. Head, turned to one side, will be more difficult for the therapist to control as the shoulder toward which the head is turned will be elevated, with the other depressed against the mat. The upper extremities are placed in symmetrical D2 flexion with elbows flexed, fingers pointing to the nose. The *therapist positions* herself astride the patient if the patient is on the mat, or to one side if he is on a bed or cart. Therapist's hips and knees should be flexed.

Manual contacts, the hands in a mitt-like position, fingers and thumbs relaxed, apply stretch and assistance or resistance. The hands, placed over the pectoral

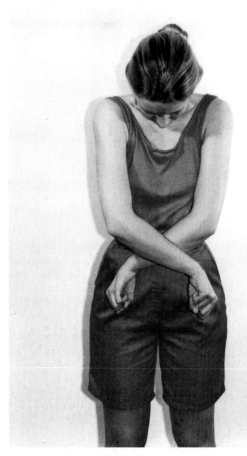

Figure 6.10 Bilateral symmetrical D2 extension, shortened range; bilateral symmetrical D2 flexion, lengthened range: *shoulders* extend, adduct, and internally rotate; *elbows* flex (intermediate joint, the elbow, may flex or extend); *forearms* pronate; wrists flex toward ulnar side; *fingers* flex and adduct; *thumbs* in opposition.

revised in 1973.[53] In 1981 the sequence and procedure for use in OT were produced by Myers.[54] In this sequence of total patterns, the therapist elicits reflex support in order to assist the more severely involved patient. With reflex support the assumption of postures may be achieved with minimal effort on the part of the therapist and patient. One procedure, assisting a patient from prone to prone on elbows, will be described in detail with application to activities.

Prone on Elbows

The prone on elbows posture may be used in daily living to watch TV or read on the floor. In *active assumption* prone on elbows is a symmetrical movement that is extensor-dominant. The tonic labyrinthine prone reflex must be overcome, while the optical and labyrinthine righting reflexes support the assumption. The pattern begins with head, neck, and upper trunk extension followed by adduction of shoulders

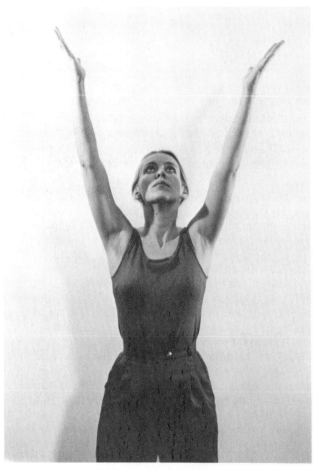

Figure 6.11 Bilateral symmetrical D2 flexion, shortened range; bilateral symmetrical D2 extension, lengthened range: *shoulders* flex, abduct, externally rotate; *elbows* extend (intermediate joint, the elbow, may flex or extend); *forearms* supinate; *wrists* extend toward radial side; *fingers* extend and abduct; *thumbs* extend and adduct.

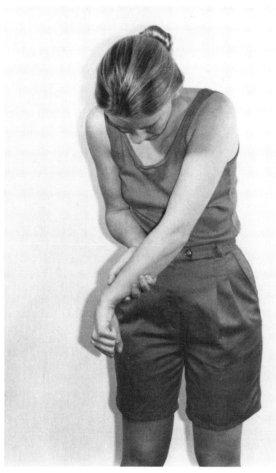

Figure 6.12 Bilateral asymmetric pattern with limbs in contact, as in "lifting." A lift to the left begins with the left arm in D2 extension and the right hand grasping the volar surface of the left wrist.

region with fingers pointing toward the umbilicus, stimulate a muscle response in the shoulder adductors which lends stability to the posture (Fig. 6.21). Hands should be placed medially to allow the patient's arms to assume a vertical position.

Auditory commands are "When I say three, look up. One, two, three, *look* up!" Simultaneously with the word, "up," the therapist leans backward, so that the patient's superior region is elevated with forearms falling into place.

In *application to activity* prone on elbows provides a good position in which to work for control of head and neck extension with weight bearing to facilitate stability in the scapulohumeral joint. Also any patients who need to spend time prone for healing or prevention of decubiti or to maintain muscle tone will need to be able to assume and maintain this posture to perform self-care activities. Various activities may be performed, depending on the patient's ability.

In level one, practicing assumption, rocking, raising and lowering the head, and depressing the scapula may be all that the patient can perform.

In level two, the patient is able to maintain an adequate posture for longer periods of time. Straw or mouth stick activities may be used. Margaret Rood has demonstrated that sucking and swallowing facilitate cocontraction of neck muscles and reinforce head and neck extension.[55] Control of the tongue may be enhanced in this primitive posture.

In level three, the patient will begin to perform manual activities with the elbows immobile and bearing weight. The activity will be confined to a small area as with a drawing or a title project. Eating finger foods is another facilitatory activity. The tongue receives a stretch stimulus in this position. With flaccidity or marked weakness, food may drop out of the mouth unless lip closure is maintained and the tongue is functional. The tongue and lips do not work as hard in the sitting posture. If a patient can perform for short periods in prone, his performance in sitting may improve faster.

In level four, the patient is able to decrease the support needed to maintain the posture and lift one extremity from the surface, as in playing a table game, typing one-handed, or combing one's hair. A brief outline of other sequences for assisting patients into developmental postures follows.

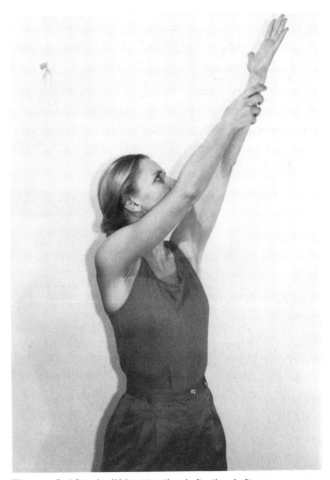

Figure 6.13 In lifting to the left, the left arm moves in D2 flexion, with the right arm assisting in D1 flexion.

Supine to Side-lying

Reflex support: ATNR
Preparatory maneuvers: Position uppermost leg and arms in D1 flexion.

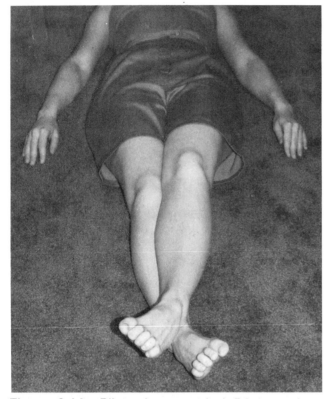

Figure 6.14 Bilateral symmetrical D2 extension, shortened range; bilateral symmetrical D2 flexion, lengthened range: *hips* extend, adduct, and externally rotate; *knees* extend (intermediate joint, the knee, may flex or extend); *ankles and feet* plantar flex and invert; *toes* flex and adduct.

Position of therapist: On side toward which patient will move
Manual contacts: Scapula and pelvis
Commands: "Look here!" Patient is assisted to side-lying.
Application to OT: Patients who must attend therapy on a cart may be positioned in side-lying. Also side-lying, a very stable posture, may be a "place to begin" treatment for the severely involved patient.
Examples of activities are: Use of a skateboard, stabilizing or rolling a ball, macramé, grasping and releasing objects in diagonal patterns, sliding the hand on the wall in various directions, and writing on the wall.

Side-lying to Side-sitting

Reflex support: Body on body righting
Preparatory maneuvers: Position legs in asymmetric flexion, and arms in asymmetric flexion at shoulder level.
Position of therapist: Behind patient's hips
Manual contacts: Shoulder girdle
Commands: "On the count of three, look back at me. One, two, three, *look* at me!" Patient is assisted to side-sitting.
Application to OT: Side-sitting is useful for increasing trunk rotation, facilitating equilibrium reactions, and movement of the free arm, while the supporting arm is stable with compression of joint surfaces and cocontraction of antagonistic muscle groups. Examples of activities are: table buffer exercises, stacking cones (reaching behind body to pick them up), turning pages of newspaper or magazine, playing chess, watching television, eating a snack, rug punching where the frame is stabilized in a vise. Response of supporting arm may be enhanced by vibration of elbow extensors.
Variation: The patient may move from side-lying to leaning on one elbow before progressing to side-sitting. Side-lying on elbow is often used by patients with paraplegia or quadriplegia during eating and hygiene activities performed on a cart or in a bed.

Supine to Long-sitting

Reflex support: Labyrinthine righting, optical righting
Preparatory maneuvers: Place legs in symmetrical extension and abduction.

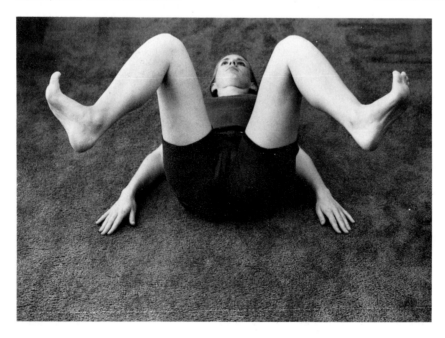

Figure 6.15 Bilateral symmetrical D2 flexion, shortened range; bilateral symmetrical D2 extension, lengthened range: *hips* flex, abduct and internally rotate; *knees* flex (intermediate joint, the knee, may flex or extend); *ankle and feet* dorsiflex and evert; *toes* extend and abduct.

Position of therapist: Astride patient at knees

Manual contacts: Dorsum of wrists

Commands: "On the count of three, look at your feet and sit up. One, two, three, *look* at your feet!" Patient is assisted to long-sitting.

Alternate sequence: Side-sitting to long-sitting

Preparatory maneuvers: Assist to side-sitting.

Position of therapist: Behind patient

Manual contacts: Shoulder girdle, one anteriorly, the other posteriorly

Commands: Tell patient to look in direction of turn and reach over for support with moving arm. Assist patient to rotate, distributing weight on both hips.

Application to OT: Long-sitting improves sitting balance and provides stability for dressing lower extremities in bed. It is easily applied to a variety of one-handed or two-handed activities. Some activities are: One-handed—Stack cones in a diagonal pattern, play checkers, throw bean bags, hit ball with stick, sanding project positioned on incline board, painting. Two-handed—Pull putty, throw and catch ball, roll ball around body, macramé, leather stamping, throw and mold clay, mix ingredients in a bowl, prepare vegetables.

Variation: Small lap board with legs placed over patient's legs provides a hard working surface and expands type of activities that can be done in this position.

Table 6.8
ACTIVITY FOR ANALYSIS: PRIMITIVE[a]
WASHING OF FACE AND NECK[b]

Hand(s)	Side(s) of Face	Diagonal and Sequence[c]	Combined Diagonals[d]
R	L, then R	D1, then D2	
L and R	Both sides	D1, then D2	BS
L contacts R wrist	L, then R	L, D2, then D1 R, D1, then D2	BA, chop and lift
R contacts L wrist	R, then L	L, D1, then D2 R, D2, then D1	BA, chop and life

[a] Primitive: Using hands and running water, without washcloth.

[b] Reprinted with permission from D. E. Voss, unpublished data.

[c] Diagonals change and interact as hand crosses midline of face, nose, or mouth.

[d] BS, both hands use *bilateral* symmetry, same diagonal; BA, one hand uses one diagonal as other hand uses the second, or other diagonal. Hands placed in contact as for "chopping and lifting" permits one hand to guide or "track" the other. This *bilateral asymmetrical* combination of diagonal patterns may be useful with hemiplegic patients among others.

Prone to Hands-Knees

Reflex support: STNR (head midline), or ATNR (head rotated)

Preparatory maneuvers: Position inferior region so that hips are flexed and thighs are vertical to floor.

Position of therapist: Astride patient holding hips securely between the therapist's knees

Manual contacts: Pectoral region

Commands: "On the count of three, look up. One, two, three, *look* up!" Patient is assisted to hands-knees.

Application to OT: Hands-knees posture promotes or enhances balance and stability in hips and shoulders.

Initially activity may include use of rhythmic stabilization following or preceding rocking in different directions—forward, backward, sideward, and diagonally to left and right. Simultaneous static/dynamic activity, *i.e.,* stacking cones, sanding, hammering, placing tiles in trivet, and figure eight board may follow as appropriate. Functional activities usually performed in this posture may be used, such as: washing and waxing floor, cleaning under bed, picking up item on floor, cleaning low shelves or oven, or working in garden.

Kneeling

Reflex support: Labyrinthine and optical righting, and equilibrium reactions

Procedure: Varies depending on method of assumption, *i.e.,* from heel-sitting, hands-knees, side-sitting.

Application to OT: Kneeling provides opportunity to develop upper extremity function for free standing, as well as hip extension, and hip extension with knee flexion necessary for gait. Activities will vary according to the patient's ability. Begin with both hands in contact with a supporting surface, as in rocking in various directions. Follow with a surface contact activity, such as sanding or dusting. Later, with both arms free, catch-

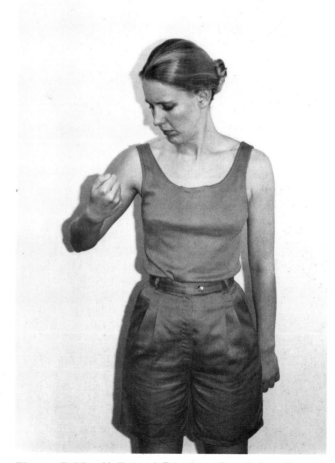

Figure 6.16 Unilateral D1 ulnar thrust, lengthened range; *shoulder* extends, abducts, and internally rotates; *elbow* flexes; *forearm* supinates; *wrist* flexes toward radial side; *fingers* flex and adduct; *thumb* flexes and adducts.

Assisting the patient into various postures helps him to experience functional movements with normal environmental and sensory stimulation to the total body. For example, the patient in the wheelchair, with lower limbs supported on footrests, is essentially suspended above the ground in a flexed posture. The sensory cues provided by gravity, body in contact with the ground, will be limited. If activities must be performed in a wheelchair, placing feet on the floor will facilitate a better response from the total pattern.

Selected Procedures and Techniques

Techniques for facilitation and inhibition include a battery of procedures that may be used singly or in combination, according to the abilities and needs of the patient. All techniques are superimposed on patterns of movement and posture.[37]

Sherrington described three principles of neurophysiology from which Kabat[56] developed many of the PNF techniques. *Irradiation*, the facilitation of one voluntary motion by another, is not haphazard but

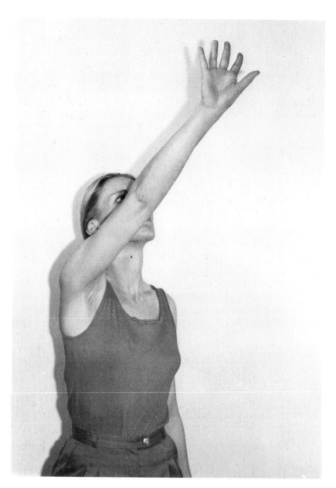

Figure 6.17 Unilateral D1 ulnar thrust, shortened range; *shoulder* flexes, adducts, and externally rotates; *elbow* extends; *forearm* pronates; *wrist* extends toward ulnar side; *fingers* extend and abduct; *thumb* extends and abducts.

ing and throwing a ball, writing on a blackboard, or cooking may be tried. Kneeling is the only position other than sitting and standing where both arms can be used free of the supporting surface.

Hands-Knees to Plantigrade

Reflex support: Labyrinthine and optical righting and equilibrium reactions
Preparatory maneuvers: Assist to hands-knees posture.
Position of therapist: Behind patient
Manual contacts: Pelvis
Commands: "Straighten your knees" or "Bring one foot forward and place it flat on the floor, then the other."
Application to OT: Plantigrade posture has minimal application to OT. However, a modified plantigrade posture with feet flat on the floor and hands or elbows resting on a supporting surface is easily used in many occupational therapy activities. A few are: washing dishes, wiping table, making bed, painting, grasping and releasing objects, playing cards with card holder, throwing bean bags in a game of "toss-a-cross," getting out of bathtub.

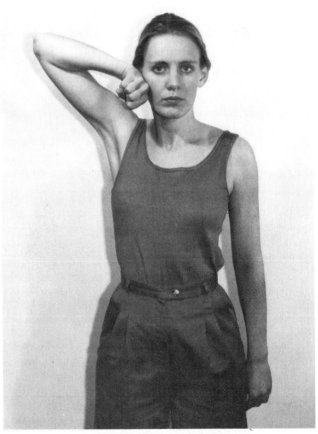

Figure 6.18 Unilateral D2 radial thrust, lengthened range: *shoulder* flexes, abducts, and externally rotates; *elbow* flexes; *forearm* pronates; *wrist* flexes toward ulnar side; *fingers* flex and adduct; *thumb* in opposition.

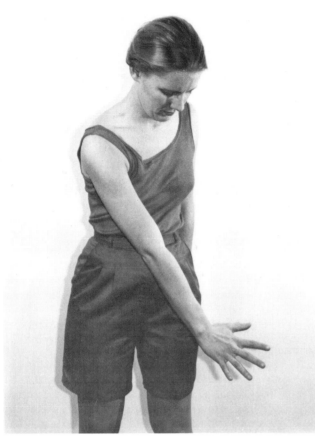

Figure 6.19 Unilateral D2 radial thrust, shortened range: *shoulder* extends, adducts, and internally rotates, *elbow* extends; *forearm* supinates; *wrist* extends toward radial side; *fingers* extend and abduct; *thumb* extends and abducts.

spreads in a specific pattern of muscle groups. The stimulus for irradiation is generated by tension in contracting muscles and related structures. In treatment, resistance coupled with stretch, as in repeated contractions, may elicit irradiation for the purpose of using the motions of the stronger muscle groups to facilitate the weaker motions of a pattern. *Successive induction* is also a process of facilitating one voluntary motion by another. However, the stronger antagonist facilitates the weaker agonist, as in resisted reversals of antagonists. In treatment when techniques of slow reversal and slow reversal-hold are used, a contraction of the stronger muscle groups is elicited first to more effectively facilitate the weaker muscle groups. If a muscle imbalance is present, this procedure carries the risk of increasing the imbalance. *Reciprocal innervation* is a process of inhibiting reflexes by voluntary motion. At the time that the agonist is facilitated or contracted against resistance the antagonist lengthens and provides control as the agonist contracts so that smooth movement is achieved. In treatment a slow reversal-hold-relax technique may be used to relax spastic or tight muscle groups. Relaxation of spastic antagonists can also be achieved by facilitation of the agonist through patterns of irradiation, stretch, and supporting reflexes.[56]

Techniques of *positioning, manual contacts,* and *verbal commands* may be used to promote a mobility or a stability response. Since these all have been discussed previously in this chapter, other techniques will be described. *Stretch* may be applied in two ways, as a stimulus for initiation of movement or as a quick stretch to initiate voluntary motion within the pattern and to increase strength and timing of a weak response. When applied as a stimulus, stretch must be given in the extreme lengthened range of the desired

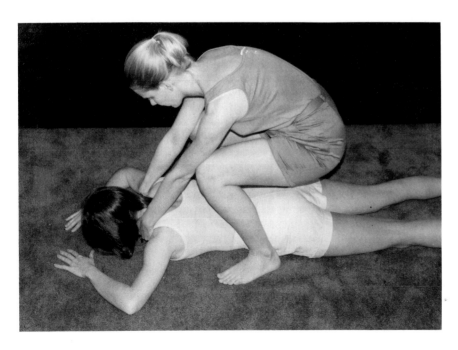

Figure 6.20 The position of the patient and the therapist for assisting a patient from prone to prone on elbows.

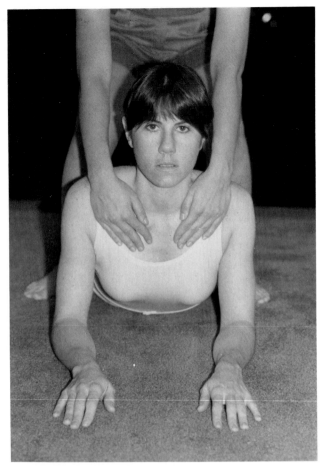

Figure 6.21 The manual contacts in assisting a patient from prone to prone on elbows. Hands are placed over the pectoral region with fingers pointing toward the umbilicus.

pressing joint surfaces. In treatment, approximation promotes stability and postural responses. Application in treatment occurs prior to demanding a voluntary contraction of muscle groups by the patient. In sitting, approximation or pressure may be applied in a downward direction over the shoulders. This technique may be applied as one sustained push or as repeated pushes. Approximation repeated quickly may be contraindicated for the patient with pain and with ataxia as seen in multiple sclerosis.[30]

Maximal resistance is probably the most misunderstood PNF technique. It does not refer to the maximal effort of the therapist, but rather to the maximal resistance that the patient can receive and still move smoothly through the full range of the pattern or maintain an isometric contraction. Manual contacts must be specifically applied over the agonists to facilitate a maximal response. For some patients, maximal resistance may only be a light touch, as resistance is graded to elicit the patient's maximal response. In treatment, maximal resistance is provided by the therapist on motions before and during activity or by equipment, such as pulleys and weighted tools.[30]

Two techniques directed to the agonist are repeated contractions and rhythmic initiation. *Repeated contractions* are used to increase range and endurance in weaker components of a pattern through a technique of emphasis. For example, if a patient is unable to reach his mouth for eating, he would be instructed to "hold," with an isometric contraction of all components at the point where the active motion decreases in power. Then the patient is asked repeatedly to "pull again" towards his mouth, shifting from isometric to isotonic contractions. *Rhythmic initiation* is used to improve the ability to initiate movement. This technique involves passive rhythmic motion, followed by active motion. Resistance may be gradually imposed as the patient's response increases. For example, a patient may lack the ability to initiate reaching for a glass on the table, due to rigidity from Parkinson's disease or severe spasticity. The therapist would ask the patient to relax and "let me move you." Then the therapist moves the part through the available range, until relaxation is felt. The patient is directed to begin moving actively with the command. "Now help me move you." As the patient's response increases, resistance may be added to reinforce the movement. The patient is then asked to move actively by himself and complete the task.[30]

The reversal of antagonists techniques, based on the principle of successive induction, include slow reversal, slow reversal-hold, and rhythmic stabilization. These reversal techniques are primarily used for strengthening or gaining range of motion. Either isotonic, isometric, or a combination of both types of contractions may be used. *Slow reversal* is an alternating isotonic contraction of antagonists. The procedure begins by asking the patient to perform the weaker agonistic pattern. In this example, D2 flexion will be the agonist. Manual contacts with maximal resistance are applied to determine the patient's response. The patient then

motion and coupled with the patient's voluntary effort. All motion components are stretched, especially rotation, as it is the rotary component which elongates the muscle fibers in a given pattern. A sudden or quick stretch is used primarily when there is no voluntary control of movement. For example, the hyperactive flexor reflex in a hand may be reduced by repeated quick stretch of the extensors. Quick stretch becomes an effective technique for the patient with quadriplegia in promoting a balance of reflexes below the level of lesion.

Use of the stretch stimulus and quick stretch aid the patient in learning to initiate and perform patterns with greater ease. Contraindications exist for the patient with pain, and with repaired tendons and other structures that should not be moved suddenly. Care should be exercised when stimulating flexion responses, as flexion reflexes may become dominant, creating an imbalance.

Traction, separating joint surfaces, stimulates joint receptors to promote movement. Traction is maintained throughout the active range of motion.[30] *Approximation* also stimulates joint receptors by com-

performs the antagonistic pattern D2 extension against maximal resistance. The agonistic pattern is now repeated, with an increase in power or range of motion expected due to the law of successive induction. Resistance must be graded to facilitate a strong contraction of the antagonist followed by maximal range of motion in the weaker agonist. Activities performed with the assist of a pulley automatically use the slow reversal technique. The pulley assists the gravity-resisted agonist and then resists the antagonistic movement. *Slow reversal-hold* proceeds in the same manner; however, an isometric contraction follows the completion of the isotonic contraction. Directions for a slow reversal-hold in the second diagonal would be: "Push your arm up and out toward me, and hold. Now, pull your arm down and across, and hold."[30]

Rhythmic stabilization is the simultaneous isometric contraction of antagonists, which results in cocontraction if the isometric contraction is not broken. This technique promotes stability by eliciting a more balanced response between antagonistic muscle groups. Relaxation is often achieved following the stabilization. As repeated isometric contractions are performed, circulation may increase. Also, the patient may hold his breath. Thus, only three or four repetitions are used.

This technique has numerous applications in therapy to provide increased stability and endurance for performance of a task. Rhythmic stabilization cannot be incorporated into an activity as it is an isometric exercise. However, it is used before an activity to enhance performance, during activity as the performance weakens, and after activity to prevent and correct imbalances built up during the activity.

This technique is contraindicated for patients with cardiac problems who are advised not to perform isometric contractions by their physician. Also rhythmic stabilization may be impossible for some patients, such as those with ataxia, who are unable to perform isometric contractions. These patients may be taught to stabilize by using the technique of slow reversal-hold through decrements of range until no motion occurs.[30]

Relaxation techniques include passive rotation, slow reversal-hold relax, contract-relax and hold-relax. *Passive rotation* coupled with range of motion is an effective technique used prior to dressing or splinting a limb in which the muscles are shortened or spastic. Place manual contacts on the intermediate and distal joints and perform range of motion. When restriction occurs, repeat rotation of all components of the pattern at the point of limitation, moving slowly and gently. As relaxation is felt, movement may continue through further range.

The procedures for the remaining three relaxation techniques follow the same sequence. Since only the stronger pattern of motion is resisted, a danger of creating further imbalances exists. These techniques rely upon the principle of reciprocal inhibition and can be effective when used appropriately. *Contract-relax* includes an isotonic contraction of the antagonist, relaxation, then passive movement of the agonistic pattern by the therapist. *Hold-relax* includes an isometric contraction of the antagonist, relaxation, then active movement of the agonist by the patient. *Slow reversal-hold-relax* includes as isotonic contraction followed by an isometric contraction of the antagonist, relaxation, then active movement of the agonist.[30]

CONCLUSION

Research to support the effectiveness of the PNF treatment approach is limited. The majority of the research reported in the last 10 years analyzed the response of able-bodied subjects to selected techniques by recording electromyographic (EMG) activity. Studies that support the principles and techniques are summarized briefly.

Holt et al.[57] tested the isometric strength of elbow flexion using EMG and dynamometer readings. Six subjects participated, three able-bodied and three with cerebral palsy. Four muscle contractions were measured with: (a) the head in anatomic position; (b) the head turned right; (c) the head turned left; and (d) a prior contraction of the antagonists. The results indicated that the reversal of antagonists was superior to the other independent variables in facilitating strength.

Tanigawa[58] compared the effects of the PNF hold-relax procedure and passive mobilization on tight hamstring muscles. He used a mathematical method to measure the angle of passive straight leg raising on 30 able-bodied male subjects. The results showed that subjects receiving the PNF hold-relax procedure increased their range of passive straight leg raising to a higher degree and at a faster rate than the subjects receiving passive mobilization.

Markos[59] compared the effects of the PNF procedures of contract-relax on active hip flexion in 30 able-bodied female subjects. The range of motion increased significantly more in subjects in the contract-relax group, both in the exercised and in the unexercised lower extremities. The author presented application of each technique to treatment, suggesting that contract-relax applied ipsilaterally may prevent disuse atrophy in specific muscles of the contralateral lower extremity.

Sullivan and Portney[60] monitored four shoulder muscles on 29 able-bodied subjects to confirm that each muscle tested would exhibit maximal EMG activity in an optimal diagonal pattern. The anterior deltoid demonstrated maximal activity in the D1 flexion pattern; the middle deltoid in the D2 flexion pattern; the posterior deltoid in the D1 extension pattern; and the sternal portion of the pectoralis major in the D2 extension pattern. The authors also reported that performing the patterns with elbows straight, flexing, and extending changed the amount of shoulder activity.

Pink[61] measured EMG activity in three muscles of the nonexercised upper extremity. The results from 10 able-bodied female subjects indicated that the following muscles do become active in the nonexercised limb. The sternal portion of the pectoralis major produced similar EMG activity during D1 flexion and extension of the contralateral limb. The infraspinatus was more active during D1 flexion, while the latissimus dorsi was more active during D1 extension. The author stated that these results could be used in treatment programs for patients who are unable to exercise one of their upper extremities.

In 1960 Mead[62] reported on a 6-year evaluation of PNF techniques. The author compared an experience using traditional therapeutic exercise to treat patients with poliomyelitis from 1948 to 1953 in a university physical medicine clinic to an experience using PNF to treat patients with varied diagnoses from 1954 to 1960 at the California Rehabilitation Center in Vallejo. Although a controlled study with statistical analysis was not done, the author found that the PNF approach was more effective than the traditional approach. Mead described the therapy program at Vallejo, and concluded that PNF techniques have application to all diagnoses.

Studies that question the principles and procedures are summarized as follows:

Arsenault[63] reviewed the literature and reported that success in using PNF techniques to treat neurological disorders was not universally true. Thus, he questioned the acceptance of using mass patterns of movement based on the lack of scientific support. Arsenault summarized Basmajian's studies on quadriceps function. Toe, ankle, and hip movements made no difference in the augmentation of quadriceps activity. Therefore, further research must be done to confirm the use of the PNF irradiation patterns.

Arsenault and Chapman[64] studied the effects of movement patterns used to promote quadriceps activity in seven able-bodied subjects over an 8-week period. No consistent response was found. In general, the D1 flexion pattern of the lower extremity increased the activity of the rectus femoris, but not the vastus medialis. The D2 flexion pattern produced a decrease of rectus femoris activity. The findings confirmed D1 flexion as the optimal pattern for the medial portion of the rectus femoris and disputed D2 flexion as the optimal pattern for the lateral portion of the rectus femoris. A proximal or distal resistance provided the ipsilateral overflow to the quadriceps. However, it is not clear whether precise PNF manual contacts and procedures were employed.

Synder and Forward[65] compared the sequential EMG activity in selected muscles of the lower limb during flexion and extension of the knee. Ten able-bodied female subjects performed active range of motion in the sagittal and diagonal planes of movement. An electrogoniometer was used to monitor the degree of knee flexion. The findings showed that selected muscles were more active in the sagittal plane than in the diagonal plane. Also, the authors observed the interaction of antagonists during fast and slow movements and following transiently induced pain in the semisquat position. They concluded that the assumption of increased activity in a diagonal plane of movement appears unjustified.

Surburg[66] studied the effects of maximal resistance with PNF patterns upon reaction, movement, and response time. Fifty able-bodied subjects participated for 6 weeks in one of three training programs: weight training, PNF patterning without resistance, and PNF patterning with maximal resistance. Analysis revealed no significant changes between the training groups.

In summary, scientific studies of the effectiveness of the PNF approach are limited to only one aspect of the approach. Research on the effect of total patterns and combining movements with functional application still needs to be done.

Acknowledgment. The author wishes to thank Dorothy E. Voss, Associate Professor Emeritus of Rehabilitation Medicine, Northwestern University Medical School, Chicago, Illinois, for her assistance and support in developing and reviewing this chapter. Also, the author is grateful to Mary Herbin, OTR, and Anne Overesch, OTR, for their time and technical skill in posing for the illustrations.

References

1. Rood, M. S. The Treatment of Neuromuscular Dysfunction: Rood Approach. Notes taken by C. Trombly at lecture delivered in Boston, Mass., July 9–11, 1976.
2. Rood, M. S. Neurophysiological reactions as a basis for physical therapy. *Phys. Ther. Rev., 34:* 444–449, 1954.
3. Curran, P. A study toward a theory of neuromuscular education through occupational therapy. *Am. J. Occup. Ther., 14:* 80–87, 1960.
4. Ayres, A. J. Integration of information. In *The Development of Sensory Integrative Theory and Practice,* edited by A. Henderson *et al.* Dubuque, Iowa: Kendall-Hunt Publishing Co., 1974.
5. Rood, M. S. The use of sensory receptors to activate, facilitate, and inhibit motor response, automatic and somatic, in developmental sequence. In *Approaches to the Treatment of Patients with Neuromuscular Dysfunction,* edited by C. Sattely. Dubuque, Iowa: Wm. C. Brown Book Co., 1962.
6. Rood, M. S. Neurophysiological mechanisms utilized in the treatment of neuromuscular dysfunction. *Am. J. Occup. Ther., 10:* 220–225, 1956.
7. Harris, F. Control of gamma efferents through the reticular activating system. *Am. J. Occup. Ther., 23:* 403–408, 1969.
8. Stockmeyer, S. An interpretation of the approach of Rood to the treatment of neuromuscular dysfunction. *Am. J. Phys. Med.* (NUSTEP Proceedings) *46* (1): 900–956, 1967.
9. Huss, J. An introduction to treatment techniques developed by Margaret Rood. In *Neuroanatomy and Neurophysiology Underlying Current Treatment Techniques for Sensorimotor Dysfunction.* edited by S. Perlmutter. University of Illinois, Division of Services for Crippled Children, undated, pp. 89–94.
10. Huss, J. Sensorimotor treatment approaches. In *Occupational Therapy,* 4th ed., edited by H. S. Willard and C. S. Spackman. Philadelphia: J. B. Lippincott, 1971.
11. Ayres, A. J. Occupational therapy directed toward neuromuscular integration. In *Occupational Therapy,* 3rd ed., edited by H. S. Willard and C. S. Spackman. Philadelphia: J. B. Lippincott, 1963.
12. Spicer, S. D., and Matyas, T. A. Facilitation of the tonic vibration reflex (TVR) by cutaneous stimulation. *Am. J. Phys. Med., 59*(5): 223–231, 1980.
13. Matyas, T. A., and Spicer, S. D. Facilitation of the tonic vibration reflex (TVR) by cutaneous stimulation in hemiplegics. *Am. J. Phys. Med., 59*(6): 280–287, 1980.

14. Eyzaguirre, C., and Fidone, S. J. *Physiology of the Nervous System*, 2nd ed. Chicago: Year Book Medical Publishers, 1975.

15. Rider, B. Effects of neuromuscular facilitation on cross transfer. *Am. J. Occup. Ther.*, 25: 84–89, 1971.

16. Zimny, N. *Effect of Position & Sensory Stimulation on Scapular Muscles*. Master's thesis, Sargent College of Allied Health Professions, Boston University, 1979.

17. Brennan, J. B. Response to stretch of hypertonic muscle groups in hemiplegia. *Br. Med. J.*, 1(5136): 1504–1507, 1959.

18. Huss, J. Application of the Rood techniques to treatment of the physically handicapped child. In *Occupational Therapy for The Multiply Handicapped Child*, edited by W. L. West. Proceedings of the 1965 Conference by the same name sponsored by the Childrens Bureau. Library of Congress Catalogue No. 65-64893.

19. Semans, S. The Bobath concept in treatment of neurological disorders. *Am. J. Phys. Med.* (NUSTEP Proceedings) 46: 732–985, 1967.

20. Bobath, K., and Bobath, B. The importance of memory traces of motor efferent discharges for learning skilled movement. *Dev. Med. Child Neurol.*, 16: 837–838, 1974.

21. Bobath, K., and Bobath, B. The facilitation of normal postural reactions and movements in the treatment of cerebral palsy. *Physiotherapy*, 50: 3–19, 1964.

22. Bobath, B. The neurodevelopmental approach to treatment. In *Physical Therapy Services in Developmental Disabilities*, edited by P. Pearson and C. Williams. Springfield, Ill.: Charles C Thomas, 1972.

23. Bobath, B. *Adult Hemiplegia: Evaluation and Treatment*, 2nd ed. London: Wm. Heinemann Medical Books, 1978.

24. Bobath, B. The very early treatment of cerebral palsy. *Dev. Med. Child Neurol.*, 9: 373–390, 1967.

25. Semans, S., *et al.* A cerebral palsy assessment chart. In *The Child with Central Nervous System Deficit*. Childrens Bureau Publication No. 432, U.S. Government Printing Office, 1965.

26. Bobath, B. Motor development, its effect on general development and application to the treatment of cerebral palsy. *Physiotherapy*, 57: 1–7, 1971.

27. Brunnstrom, S. *Movement Therapy in Hemiplegia*. New York: Harper & Row, 1970.

28. LaVigne, J. M. Hemiplegia sensorimotor assessment form. *Phys. Ther.*, 54(2): 128–134, 1974.

29. Fugl-Meyer, A. R., Jaasko, L., Leyman, I., Olsson, S., and Steglind, S. The post-stroke hemiplegic patient. *Scand. J. Rehabil. Med.*, 7: 13–31, 1975.

30. Knott, M., and Voss, D. E. *Proprioceptive Neuromuscular Facilitation: Patterns and Techniques*, 2nd ed. New York: Harper & Row, 1968.

31. Kabat, H., and Rosenberg, D. Concepts and techniques of occupational therapy neuromuscular disorders *Am. J. Occup. Ther.*, 4(1): 6–11, 79, 1950.

32. Ayres, A. J. Proprioceptive neuromuscular facilitation elicited through the upper extremities. Part I. Background 9 (1). Part II. Application 9 (2). Part III. Specific application 9 (3). *Am. J. Occup. Ther.*, 1955.

33. Cooke, D. M. The effects of resistance on multiple sclerosis patients with intention tremor. *Am. J. Occup. Ther.*, 12(2): 89–94, 1958.

34. Voss, D. E. PNF: Application of patterns and techniques in occupational therapy. *Am. J. Occup. Ther.*, 8(4): 191–194, 1959.

35. Whitaker, E. W. A suggested treatment in occupational therapy for patients with multiple sclerosis. *Am. J. Occup. Ther.*, 4(6): 247–251, 1950.

36. Carroll, J. The utilization of reinforcement techniques in the program for the hemiplegic. *Am. J. Occup. Ther.*, 4(5): 211–213, 239, 1950.

37. Voss, D. E. Proprioceptive neuromuscular facilitation. *Am. J. Phys. Med.*, 46(1): 838–898, 1967.

38. McGraw, M. B. *The neuromuscular maturation of the human infant*. New York: Columbia University Press, 1945. New York: Haftner Press, Reprinted edition, 1963.

39. Hooker, D. *The Prenatal Origin of Behavior*. Lawrence, Kansas: University of Kansas Press, 1952.

40. Gesell, A., and Amatruda, C. S. *Developmental Diagnosis*, 2nd ed. New York: Paul B. Hoeber, 1947.

41. Hooker, D. Evidence of prenatal function of the central nervous system in man. In *Scientific Bases for Neurophysiological Approaches to Therapeutic Exercise: An Anthology*, edited by O. Payton *et al.* Philadelphia: F. A. Davis, 1977.

42. Hellebrandt, F. A., Schade, M., and Carns, M. L. Methods of evoking the tonic neck reflexes in normal human subjects. *Am. J. Phys. Med.*, 41: 90–139, 1962.

43. Gesell, A. Reciprocal interweaving in neuromotor development. In *Scientific Bases for Neurophysiologic Approaches to Therapeutic Exercise: An Anthology*, edited by O. Payton *et al.* Philadelphia: F. A. Davis, 1977.

44. Gesell, A. Behavior patterns of fetal infant and child. *Genetics, (Proc. Assoc. Res. Nerv. Mental Dis.)*, 33: 114–123, 1954.

45. Buchwald, J. S. Basic mechanisms of motor learning. *J.A.P.T.A.*, 45: 314–331, 1965.

46. Harlow, H. F., and Harlow, M. K. Principles of primate learning lessons from animal behavior. In *Little Club Clinics in Developmental Medicine No. 7*, The Spastics Society, Ch. 5. London: Heinemann Medical Books, 1962.

47. Levine, S. Stimulation in infancy. *Sci. Am.*, 202(5): 80–86, 1960.

48. Voss, D. E. Proprioceptive neuromuscular facilitation: The PNF method. In *Physical Therapy Services in Developmental Disabilities*, edited by P. Pearson and C. Williams. Springfield, Ill.: Charles C Thomas, 1972.

49. Smith, K. U. Cybernetic foundations for rehabilitation. *Am. J. Phys. Med.*, 46(1): 379–467, 1967.

50. Ayres, A. J. Integration of information. In *Approaches to the Treatment of Patients with Neuromuscular Dysfunction*. Study Course VI, 3rd International Congress WFOT. Dubuque, Iowa: William C. Brown Book Co., 1962.

51. Voss, D. E. Teaching materials presented during short term courses and undergraduate curriculum at Northwestern University Medical School Programs in Physical Therapy. Evaluation Forms: Introduction and Sections 1–3, 1969.

52. Jackson, J. H. *Selected Writings*, Vol. 1., edited by J. Taylor. London: Hodder and Staughton, 1931.

53. Voss, D. E. Assistance in the Assumption of Total Patterns of Posture, PNF Approach (videotape). Chicago: Northwestern Medical School Program in Physical Therapy, 1973.

54. Myers, B. J. Assisting to Posture and Application in Occupational Therapy Activities (videotape). Chicago: Rehabilitation Institute of Chicago, 1981.

55. Stockmeyer, S. A. An interpretation of the approach of Rood to the treatment of neuromuscular dysfunction. *Am. J. Phys. Med.*, 46(1): 900–956, 1967.

56. Kabat, H. Proprioceptive facilitation in therapeutic exercise. In *Therapeutic Exercise*, 2nd ed. edited by S. Licht. New Haven: Elizabeth Licht, 1961, pp. 327–343.

57. Holt, L. E., Kaplan, H. M., Okita, T. Y., and Hoshiko, M. The influence of antagonistic contraction and head position on the responses of agonist muscles. *Arch. Phys. Med. Rehabil.*, 50(5): 279–291, 1968.

58. Tanigawa, M. C. Comparison of the hold-relax procedure and passive mobilization on increasing muscle length. *Phys. Ther.*, 52(7): 725–735, 1972.

59. Markos, P. D. Ipsilateral and contralateral effects of proprioceptive neuromuscular facilitation techniques on hip motion and electromyographic activity. *Phys. Ther.*, 59(11): 1366–1373, 1979.

60. Sullivan, P. E., and Portney, L. G. Electromyographic activity of shoulder muscles during unilateral upper extremity proprioceptive neuromuscular facilitation patterns. *Phys. Ther.*, 60(3): 283–288, 1980.

61. Pink, M. Contralateral effects of upper extremity proprioceptive neuromuscular facilitation patterns. *Phys. Ther.*, 61(8): 1158–1162, 1981.

62. Mead, S. A six-year evaluation of proprioceptive neuromuscular facilitation technics. *Phys. Med.*, 373–376, 1960.

63. Arsenault, A. B. Techniques of muscle re-education: Analysis of studies on the effect of techniques of patterning and neuromuscular facilitation. *Physiother. Can.*, 26(4): 190–194, 1974.

64. Arsenault, A. B., and Chapman, A. E. An electromyographic

investigation of the individual recruitment of the quadriceps muscles during isometric contraction of the knee extensors in different patterns of movement. *Physiother. Can.*, 26(50): 253–261, 1974.

65. Synder, J. L., and Forward, E. M. Comparison of knee flexion and extension in the diagonal and sagittal planes. *Phys. Ther.*, 52(12): 1255–1263, 1972.

66. Surburg, P. R. Interactive effects of resistance and facilitation patterning upon reaction and response times. *Phys. Ther.*, 59(13): 1513–1517, 1979.

Supplementary Reading

Bobath, B. The treatment of neuromuscular disorders by improving patterns of coordination. *Physiotherapy*, 55: 18–22, 1969.

Bobath, B. Treatment of adult hemiplegia. *Physiotherapy, 63:* 310–313, 1977.

Bobath, K., and Bobath, B. The neurodevelopmental treatment of cerebral palsy. *J.A.P.T.A.*, 47: 1039–1041, 1967.

Brunnstrom, S. Associated reactions of the upper extremity in adult patients with hemiplegia: An approach to training. *Phys. Ther. Rev.*, 36: 225–236, 1956.

Brunnstrom, S. Motor behavior of adult hemiplegic patients. *Am. J. Occup. Ther.*, 25(1): 6–12, 1961.

Brunnstrom, S. Motor testing procedures in hemiplegia. *J.A.P.T.A.*, 46(4): 357–375, 1966.

Brunnstrom, S. Training the adult hemiplegic patient: Orientation of techniques to patient's motor behavior. In *Approach to the Treatment of Patients with Neuromuscular Dysfunction*, edited by C. Sattely. Dubuque, Iowa: Wm. C. Brown Book Co., 1962, pp. 44–48.

Finnie, N. *Handling the Young Cerebral Palsied Child at Home*, 2nd ed. London: William Heinemann Medical Book, 1974.

Goff, B. The application of recent advances in neurophysiology to Miss M. Rood's concept of neuromuscular facilitation. *Physiotherapy, 58:* 409–415, 1972.

Hughes, E. Bobath and Brunnstrom: Comparison of two methods of treatment of a left hemiplegia. *Physiother. Can.*, 24(5): 262–266, 1972.

Kabat, H. Neuromuscular dysfunction and treatment of athetosis. *Physiotherapy*, 46(5): 125–129, 1960.

Knott, M. Bulbar involvement with good recovery. *J.A.P.T.A.*, 42(1): 38–39, 1962.

Knott, M. Neuromuscular facilitation in the treatment of rheumatoid arthritis. *J.A.P.T.A.*, 44(8): 737–739, 1964.

Knott, M. Report of a case of Parkinsonism treated with proprioceptive facilitation technics. *Phys. Ther. Rev.*, 37(4): 229, 1957.

Levy, J. *The Baby Exercise Book: For the First Fifteen Months*, translated by E. Gleasure. New York: Pantheon Books, a division of Random House, 1973.

Perry, C. E. Principles and techniques of the Brunnstrom approach to the treatment of hemiplegia. *Am. J. Phys. Med.*, NUSTEP Proceedings, 46(1): 789–812, 1967.

Voss, D. E., and Knott, M. The application of neuromuscular facilitation in the treatment of shoulder disabilities. *Phys. Ther. Rev.*, 33(10): 536–541, 1953.

PART THREE

Biomechanical Approach

The principles and methods that are presented in this section are appropriate for patients who have problems which directly affect their range of motion, strength, or endurance necessary to perform daily life tasks, but who have voluntary control of specific movements and/or motor patterns.

The biomechanical approach to treatment applies the mechanical principles of kinetics and kinematics to movement of the human body. Historically, the biomechanical approach preceded development of the neurodevelopmental approach. Physical activity for therapeutic exercise was used by occupational therapists in the 1940s and was then termed kinetic occupational therapy to signify its restorative rather than diversional goal. Exercise techniques were borrowed from other disciplines either directly or combined with activities. Restorative efforts focused on specific diseases or disability categories and emphasized the application of these techniques to particular problems without recognizing common or underlying principles.[1] At that time, activities were selected on the basis of their apparent value as determined by the therapist who first tried the activity to analyze it and then observed the patient performing it in the same manner. Since that time, studies have indicated what muscles are active during performance of different activities; that there is a specificity of training for whatever type of muscle contraction was used in training; and that indeed certain treatment regimes, administered under controlled conditions, are effective to restore function. Although the concept of biomechanical treatment has a long history, it is still developing with research studies of many disciplines helping to identify the effectiveness of techniques and the precautions to be observed.

Reference

1. Mosey, A. C. Occupational therapy— historical perspective. Involvement in the rehabilitation movement—1942–1960. *Am. J. Am. J. Occup. Ther.* 25(5): 234–236, 1971.

chapter

7

Evaluation

Anna Deane Scott, M.Ed., OTR and Catherine A. Trombly, M.A., OTR

Procedures for evaluation of range of motion, muscle strength, and endurance are described in this chapter. The clinical measures most commonly used by practicing therapists are presented in detail.

RANGE OF MOTION

Various physical problems can produce limited movement of joints. Each joint is potentially able to move in certain directions and to certain limits of motion due to its structure and the integrity of surrounding tissues. Trauma or disease which affect joints or surrounding tissues can alter the amount of motion at the joint. When there is alteration of joint motion, evaluation and treatment of this problem is indicated. Because it is the responsibility of the occupational therapist to document the effectiveness of treatment to increase range of motion, the therapist must be skilled in the measurement of joint range of motion. If you treat it, measure it!

The most widely used method of measuring joint motion is the system using the universal goniometer. Every goniometer has a protractor, an axis, and two arms. The stationary arm extends from the protractor on which degrees are marked. The other arm is termed the movable arm and has a center line or pointer to indicate the degrees of an angle measured. The axis is the point where these two arms are riveted together. Goniometers range in size from large goniometers which most accurately measure large joints to small goniometers which most accurately measure small joints. A full circle goniometer which measures degrees from 0° to 180° in each direction permits measurement of motion in both directions, i.e., flexion and extension, without repositioning the tool. Half-circle goniometers are also useful, and a small half-circle goniometer is preferred for measuring the forearm, wrist, and hand. When using a half-circle goniometer it is necessary to position the protractor opposite to the direction of

motion in order for the indicator to remain on the face of the protractor. A finger goniometer is of special design with a short movable arm and flat arm surfaces that fit comfortably over the finger joints (see Fig. 7.1).

In using the goniometer to measure joint motion care must be taken when placing the axis and the two arms in order to ensure accuracy and reliability. The axis of the goniometer is placed over the axis of joint motion which is the point around which the motion occurs. The axis of motion for some joints coincides with bony landmarks, whereas for other joints the axis of motion must be found by observing movement of the joint to determine the point around which motion occurs. Moore[1] describes the difficulty inherent in trying to place the axis of the goniometer over a specific landmark and stresses the importance of giving primary attention to alignment of the two arms. When the two arms of the goniometer are placed correctly they will intersect at the axis of motion. The stationary arm is positioned parallel to the longitudinal axis of the part proximal to the joint; the movable arm is positioned parallel to the longitudinal axis of the part distal to the joint. Which arm of the goniometer is used as the stationary arm and which is aligned with the moving part is not as important for accuracy of measurement as correct alignment of the arms parallel to the anatomical parts to measure the angle which intersects at the axis. In shoulder flexion, for example, the axis at the beginning of the motion is below the acromion process, but at the end of the motion the arm position has changed to the extent that the original axis position of the goniometer is no longer accurately placed over the joint. Because the anatomical landmark that corresponds to the axis of motion may shift during the movement, measurements are taken at the beginning and again at the end of the range of motion. These two measurements represent the limits of motion.

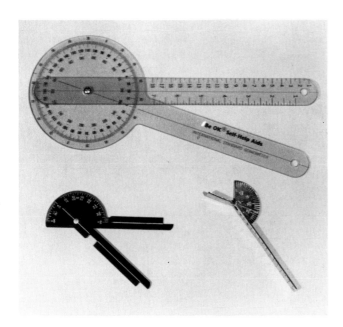

Figure 7.1 Full circle, half circle, and finger goniometers.

There are many factors of the test situation which influence accuracy and reliability. Care must be taken to reduce the effect of these factors. The tester supports both the body part and the goniometer in a way that does not interfere with movement of the joint, i.e., supports proximal and distal to the joint leaving the joint free to move. Because clothing may interfere with full movement of a joint and can obstruct the correct alignment of the goniometer, the patient's clothing is removed as necessary, but feelings of modesty are respected. In addition, accuracy and reliability can be influenced by environmental and patient-related factors. Environmental variables include the time of day, the temperature and atmosphere of the room, the kind of goniometer used, and the experience and rigor of the tester. Therefore, original and retest measurements must be taken at the same time of day by the same person using the same kind of goniometer and technique in the same or similar setting. Patient-related factors include reaction to pain and fatigue and feelings of fear, tension, or stress. Every effort is made to make the patient physically and emotionally comfortable. With careful adherence to technique in the use of the goniometer, measurements taken at different times by the same tester are accurate to within 3 to 5°.[2] Therefore, this is considered a highly reliable method of measuring joint motion.

RANGE OF MOTION MEASUREMENT TECHNIQUE

If there is no limitation in active range of motion (AROM) as determined by observation of the patient's ability to move or no limitation in passive range of motion (PROM) as determined by passively moving each joint to the limits of motion, a detailed measurement is not needed. Range of motion can be noted to

be within normal limits (WNL) as determined by observation. Detailed measurements of joints which have limitations are taken and recorded in order to objectively identify problems, to assist in treatment planning, and to document improvement following treatment.

Measurement of joint range may be done actively or passively. Passive range of motion indicates the amount of motion at a given joint when the joint is moved by the therapist. Measurement of active range of motion indicates the amount of motion at a given joint achieved by a patient using his own muscle strength. If active range of motion is less than passive range of motion this is a problem of muscle weakness. Active range of motion measurement is used as a supplement to muscle testing to indicate fine gradations of change in weak muscles. When joint limitation is the problem being evaluated, passive range of motion must be done. Measurements of the upper extremities are given in more detail here than those for the lower extremities because daily life tasks involve more refined upper extremity movement and necessitate more detailed consideration of hand function.

Some clinics still use a 180° starting position; anatomical position is 180° and motion occurs toward zero by this method. In the International SFTR (sagittal, frontal, transverse, rotation) Method the zero starting position is used, and ranges are recorded in terms of anatomical planes.[3]

A Neutral Zero Method for measuring and recording is recommended by the Committee on Joint Motion of the American Academy of Orthopaedic Surgeons[4] and is generally used. In this method anatomical position is considered to be zero, or a starting position different from anatomical position is defined as the zero starting position. Extension is the term used for the natural motion opposite to flexion, and hyperextension is used only when the motion is unnatural as occasionally seen, for example, in the elbow or knee joints. Ranges are compared to the noninvolved extremity or to average ranges expected for each motion. These average numbers are estimates, rather than exact standards, which have been stated by the Committee on Joint Motion and included here with the instructions for measurements and on the recording form.

Recording Range of Motion

Each measurement is accurately recorded on a range of motion form. The therapist must date and sign each evaluation and indicate whether measurements represent active range of motion (AROM) or passive range of motion (PROM). A sample form is provided here, although each treatment facility may have its own form (see Table 7.1). Some facilities use forms with graphic representation, in which case each range of motion is shaded on a diagram of the movement. Whether the recording is numerical or graphical, it represents the starting and ending positions (limits of motion) for each movement.

Table 7.1
RANGE OF MOTION

Patient's Name _____

AROM _____
PROM _____

Left			Right	
PROM	AROM	Date of Measurement	PROM	AROM
		Tester's Name		
		SHOULDER		
		Flexion 0-180		
		Extension 0-60		
		Abduction 0-180		
		Horizontal Abduction 0-90		
		Horizontal Adduction 0-45		
		Internal Rotation 0-70		
		External Rotation 0-90		
		Internal Rotation (Alternate) 0-80		
		External Rotation (Alternate) 0-60		
		ELBOW and FOREARM		
		Flexion-Extension 0-150		
		Supination 0-80		
		Pronation 0-80		
		WRIST		
		Flexion 0-80		
		Extension 0-70		
		Ulnar Deviation 0-30		
		Radial Deviation 0-20		
		THUMB		
		CM Flexion 0-15		
		CM Extension 0-20		
		MP Flexion-Extension 0-50		
		IP Flexion-Extension 0-80		
		Abduction 0-70		
		Opposition cm.		
		INDEX FINGER		
		MP Flexion 0-90		
		MP Hyperextension 0-45		
		PIP Flexion-Extension 0-100		
		DIP Flexion-Extension 0-90		
		Abduction No Norm		
		Adduction No Norm		

If starting position cannot be achieved due to a limitation, measurement is taken as close to starting position as possible and again at end position or as close to end position as possible. The limits thus obtained are recorded to indicate limitations in movement.

Examples using elbow flexion:

0 to 150°—No limitation
20 to 150°—A limitation in extension
0 to 120°—A limitation in flexion
20 to 120°—Limitations in both flexion and extension

Some therapists indicate a limitation in extension by recording the limitation negatively, for example, −20° of extension or lacks 20° of extension or −20 to 150. On the other hand, some therapists record −20 to 150 to indicate that there are 20 degrees of hyperextension in a joint where hyperextension is not normally present. If hyperextension as an unnatural motion is recorded as a separate measurement as recommended by the American Academy of Orthopaedic Surgeons then the elbow range would state 0 to 20° of hyperextension and 0 to 150° of flexion and would fully

Table 7.1—*continued*

		MIDDLE FINGER			
		MP Flexion	0-90		
		MP Hyperextension	0-45		
		PIP Flexion-Extension	0-100		
		DIP Flexion-Extension	0-90		
		Abduction (radially)	No Norm		
		Adduction (ulnarly)	No Norm		
		RING FINGER			
		MP Flexion	0-90		
		MP Hyperextension	0-45		
		PIP Flexion-Extension	0-100		
		DIP Flexion-Extension	0-90		
		Abduction	No Norm		
		Adduction	No Norm		
		LITTLE FINGER			
		MP Flexion	0-90		
		MP Hyperextension	0-45		
		PIP Flexion-Extension	0-100		
		DIP Flexion-Extension	0-90		
		Abduction	No Norm		
		Adduction	No Norm		
		HIP			
		Flexion	0-120		
		Extension	0-30		
		Abduction	0-45		
		Adduction	0-30		
		Internal Rotation	0-45		
		External Rotation	0-45		
		KNEE			
		Flexion-Extension	0-135		
		ANKLE			
		Dorsiflexion	0-20		
		Plantar Flexion	0-50		
		Inversion	0-35		
		Eversion	0-15		

Comments:

describe the available range of motion without confusion, while eliminating the use of unclear negative recordings. According to the American Academy of Orthopaedic Surgeons the following notations of range would be indicated to describe these elbow measurements:

0 to 150° of flexion
150 to 0° of extension
0 to 20° of hyperextension, if present

A recording of 20 to 150° of flexion would be termed a 20° flexion deformity.[4] Since these notations vary in their meaning it is important to clarify the intended meaning and to ensure consistency within the same treatment facility.

In a fused joint the starting and end positions will be the same with no range of motion. This is re-

corded as fused at x degrees. If a joint that normally moves in two directions is unable to be moved in one direction, this range of motion is recorded as None. For example, if wrist flexion is 15 to 80° with a 15° flexion deformity, the wrist cannot be positioned at zero or moved into extension. Wrist extension is therefore None.

If range of motion is limited by pain or other abnormalities, such as edema or adipose tissue, the reason for the limitation should be clearly indicated on the range of motion recording form.

Interpreting the Results

The recording of range of motion is reviewed to identify which joints are limited. A significant limitation is one which may lead to a deformity or decrease function. Some associated problems which may cause range of motion limitations are joint disease or injury, edema, pain, spasticity, skin tightness, muscle and tendon shortening, poor positioning, or muscle weakness. With the significant limitations and influencing factors in mind the short-term goals necessary to achieve the long-term goal of increasing range of motion can be identified. It is also necessary to check the muscle test results in relation to range of motion. When there is no limitation of range of motion but the muscle test indicates that the patient is too weak to complete the full range of any joint motion, treatment planning should include prevention of range of motion limitations in those joints.

MEASUREMENT OF THE UPPER EXTREMITY

For the measurements given here, the patient is seated with trunk erect against the back of an armless straight chair. The measurements may be taken with the patient standing or supine, if necessary, unless otherwise noted.

Shoulder Flexion

Movement of the humerus anteriorly in the sagittal plane (0 to 180° which represents both glenohumeral and axioscapular motion).

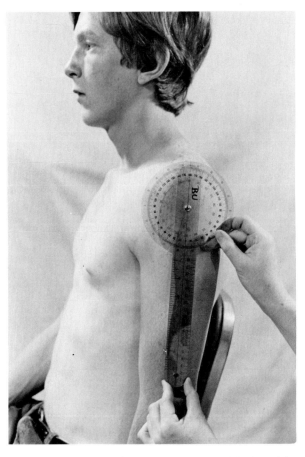

Figure 7.2 Starting position: Arm at side in midposition.

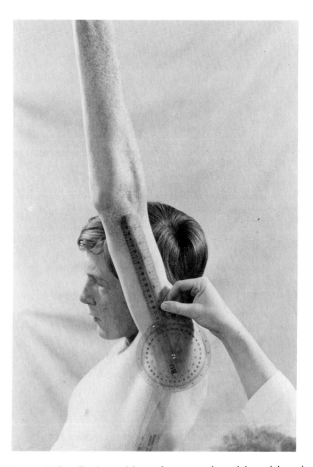

Figure 7.3 End position: Arm overhead in midposition.

Goniometer Placement

Axis. A point through the lateral aspect of the glenohumeral joint approximately 1 inch below the acromion process.

Stationary Arm. Parallel to the lateral midline of the trunk.

Movable Arm. Parallel to the longitudinal axis of the humerus on the lateral aspect.

Possible Substitutions. Trunk extension, shoulder abduction.

Shoulder Extension

Movement of the humerus posteriorly in a sagittal plane (0 to 60°).

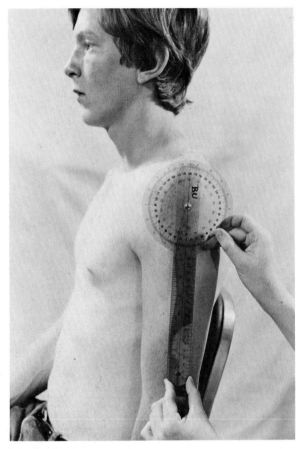 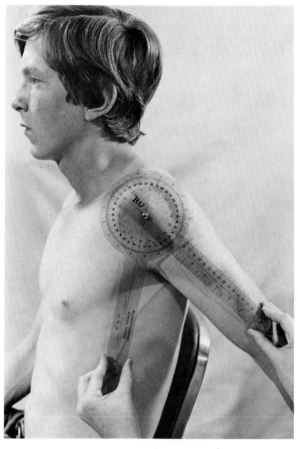

Figure 7.4 Starting position: Patient seated at the edge of the chair so there is no restriction behind humerus. Arm at side in internal rotation.

Figure 7.5 End position: Arm backwards at limit of motion.

Goniometer Placement

Axis. A point through the lateral aspect of the glenohumeral joint approximately 1 inch below the acromion process.

Stationary Arm. Parallel to the lateral midline of the trunk.

Movable Arm. Parallel to the longitudinal axis of the humerus on the lateral aspect.

Possible Substitutions. Trunk flexion, scapular elevation and downward rotation, shoulder abduction.

Shoulder Abduction

Movement of the humerus laterally in a frontal plane (0 to 180° which represents both glenohumeral and axioscapular motion).

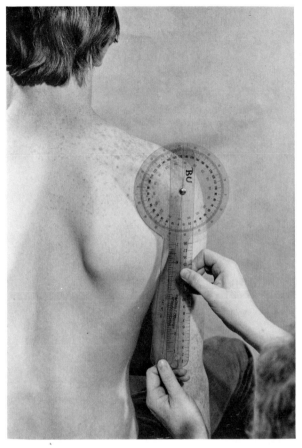

Figure 7.6 Starting position: Arm at side in external rotation which allows the humerus to clear the acromion process.

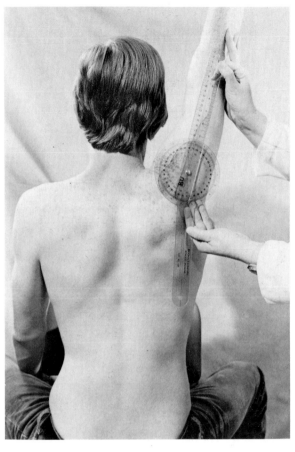

Figure 7.7 End position: Arm overhead with palm facing opposite side.

Goniometer Placement

Axis. A point through the anterior or posterior aspect of the glenohumeral joint. Some people consider measurement from the anterior aspect safer, since the patient's back can be supported against the chair, but it is preferable to measure adult female patients from the posterior aspect.

Stationary Arm. Laterally along the trunk, parallel to the spine.

Movable Arm. Parallel to the longitudinal axis of the humerus.

Possible Substitutions. Lateral flexion of trunk, scapular elevation, shoulder flexion or extension.

Horizontal Abduction

Movement of the humerus on a horizontal plane from a position of 90° of shoulder flexion to a position of 90° of shoulder abduction and to the limit of motion (0 to 90°).

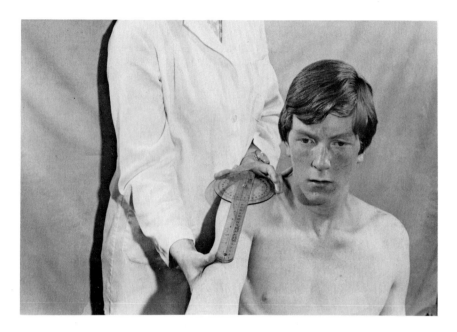

Figure 7.8 Starting position: Arm internally rotated and at 90° of shoulder flexion.

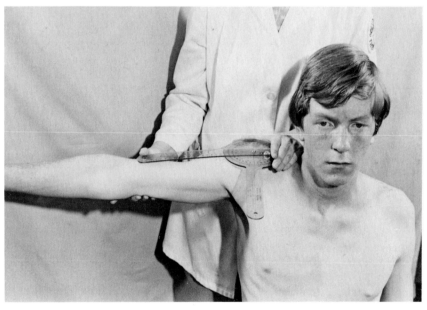

Figure 7.9 End position: Arm at 90° of shoulder abduction.

Goniometer Placement

Axis. On top of the acromion process.

Stationary Arm. To start, this arm is parallel to the longitudinal axis of the humerus on the superior aspect and remains in that position, perpendicular to the body, although the humerus moves away. (An alternative position of the stationary arm is across the shoulder, anterior to the neck, and in line with the opposite acromion process. In this alternate position the goniometer would read 90° at the start, and this must be considered when recording.)

Movable Arm. Parallel to the longitudinal axis of the humerus on the superior aspect.

Possible Substitution. Trunk rotation.

Horizontal Adduction

Movement of the humerus on a horizontal plane from a position of 90° of shoulder abduction through a position of 90° of shoulder flexion, across the trunk to the limit of motion. The 90° of return motion from horizontal abduction is not measured. The motion is measured from a position of 90° shoulder flexion across the trunk (0 to 45°).

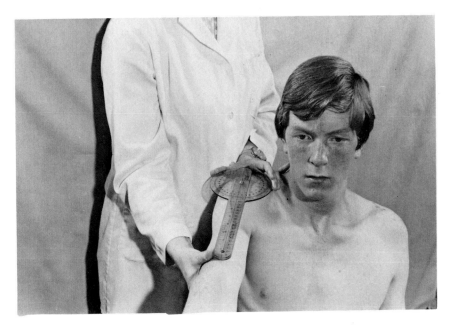

Figure 7.10 Starting position: Arm internally rotated and at 90° of shoulder flexion.

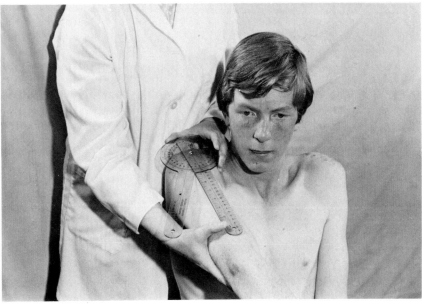

Fgure 7.11 End position: Arm across trunk at limit of motion.

Goniometer Placement

Axis. On top of the acromion process.

Stationary Arm. Parallel to the longitudinal axis on the superior aspect of the humerus in starting position and remains perpendicular to the body, although the humerus moves away. The alternative placement given for horizontal abduction also applies in this case.

Movable Arm. Parallel to the longitudinal axis of the humerus on the superior aspect.

Possible Substitution. Trunk rotation.

Internal Rotation

Movement of the humerus in a medial direction around the longitudinal axis of the humerus (0 to 70°).

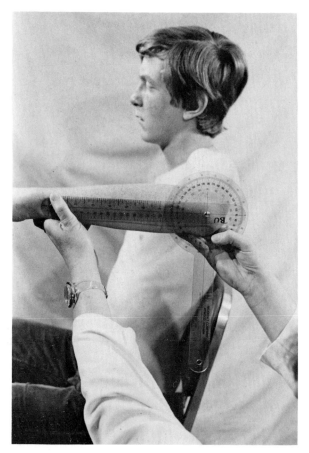

Figure 7.12 Starting position: The extremity is supported in a position of 90° of shoulder abduction and 90° of elbow flexion with the forearm pronated and parallel to the floor.

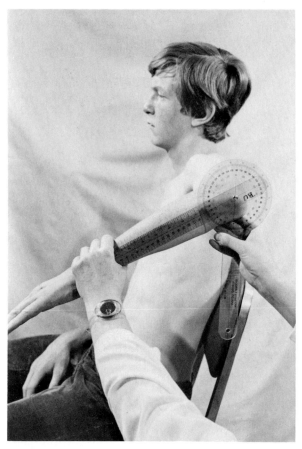

Figure 7.13 End position: The extremity is in a position of 90° of shoulder abduction and 90° of elbow flexion; forearm and hand have moved toward the floor to the limit of motion.

Goniometer Placement

Axis. Olecranon process of ulna.

Stationary Arm. Perpendicular to the floor and parallel to the lateral trunk. The goniometer will read 90° at the start, and this must be deducted when recording.

Movable Arm. Parallel to the longitudinal axis of the ulna.

Possible Substitutions. Scapular elevation and downward rotation, trunk flexion, elbow extension.

Note. In the supine position with the shoulder abducted to 90° and the elbow flexed to 90° the stationary arm is perpendicular to the floor with the movable arm along the ulna. The goniometer will read 0° at the start.[1]

External Rotation

Movement of the humerus in a lateral direction around the longitudinal axis of the humerus (0 to 90°).

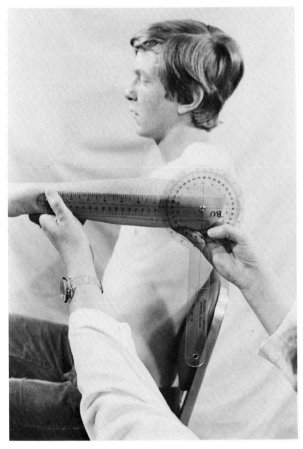

Figure 7.14 Starting position: The extremity is supported in a position of 90° of shoulder abduction and 90° of elbow flexion with the forearm pronated and parallel to the floor.

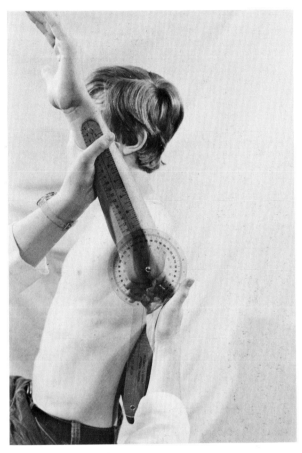

Figure 7.15 End position: The extremity is in a position of 90° of shoulder abduction and 90° of elbow flexion; forearm and hand have moved toward the ceiling to the limit of motion.

Goniometer Placement

Axis. Olecranon process of ulna.

Stationary Arm. Perpendicular to the floor and parallel to the lateral trunk. The goniometer will read 90° at the start, and this must be deducted when recording.

Movable Arm. Parallel to the longitudinal axis of the ulna.

Possible Substitutions. Scapular depression and upward rotation, trunk extension, elbow extension.

Note. In the supine position the humerus should be supported on a pad to place it in line with the acromion process. The measurement is the same as for internal rotation.[1]

Internal and External Rotation: Alternate Method

If shoulder limitation prevents positioning for the previously described method, the patient may be seated with humerus adducted to his side and elbow flexed to 90°. This method will be inaccurate in internal rotation if the patient has a large abdomen. (Internal rotation: 0 to 80°; external rotation: 0 to 60°).

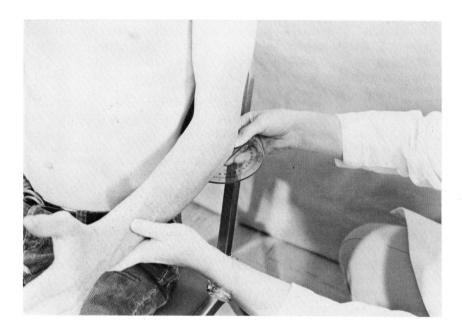

Figure 7.16 External rotation (alternate method): Start position.

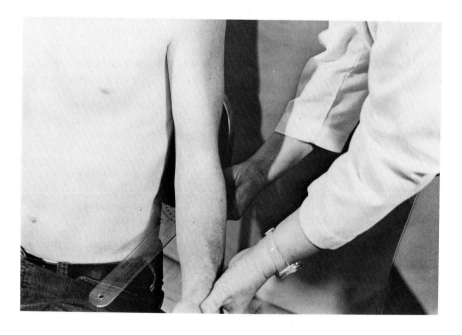

Figure 7.17 External rotation (alternate method): End position.

Elbow Flexion-Extension

Movement of the supinated forearm anteriorly in the sagittal plane (0 to 150°).

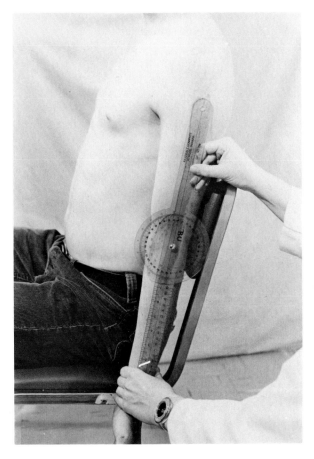

Figure 7.18 Starting position: Arm in anatomical position. This measurement is recorded as the limit of extension.

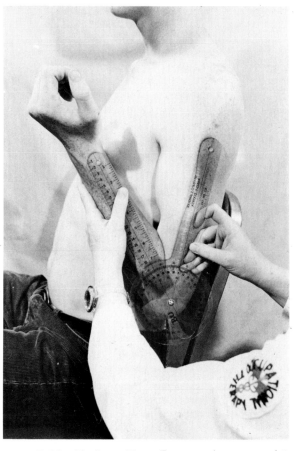

Figure 7.19 End position: Forearm has moved toward the humerus so that the hand approximates the shoulder to the limit of motion of elbow flexion.

Goniometer Placement

Axis. Lateral epicondyle of the humerus.
Stationary Arm. Parallel to the longitudinal axis of the humerus on the lateral aspect.

Movable Arm. Parallel to the longitudinal axis of the radius.

Forearm Supination

Rotation of the forearm laterally around its longitudinal axis from midposition (0 to 80°).

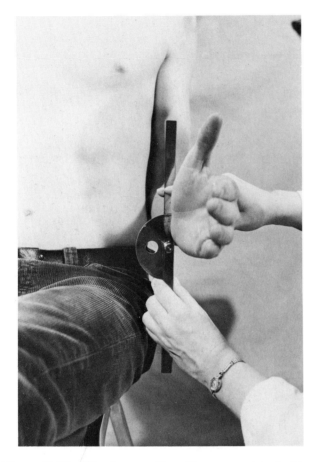

Figure 7.20 Starting position: Humerus adducted to the side and elbow flexed to 90° with the forearm in midposition.

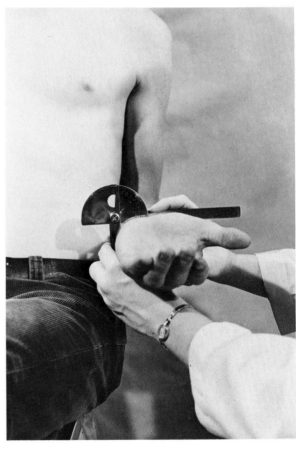

Figure 7.21 End position: Forearm rotated so that the palm faces up.

Goniometer Placement

Axis. Parallel to the longitudinal axis of the forearm displaced toward the ulna.
Stationary Arm. Perpendicular to the floor.
Movable Arm. Across the distal radius and ulna on the volar surface.

Possible Substitutions. Shoulder adduction and external rotation.

Forearm Supination: Alternate Method

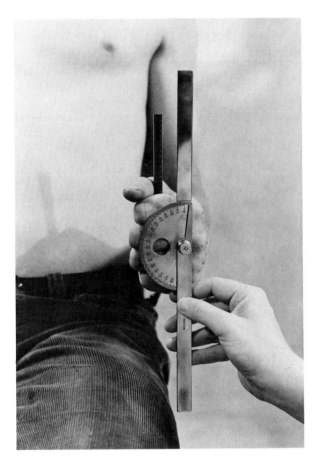

Figure 7.22 Starting position: Humerus adducted to the side and elbow flexed to 90° with the forearm in midposition. A pencil is held in the tightly closed fist with the pencil protruding from the radial side of the hand.

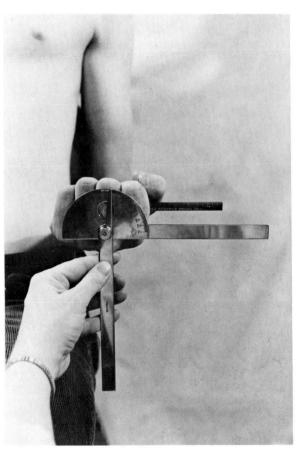

Figure 7.23 End position: The forearm is rotated so that the palm faces up. The pencil is still grasped tightly.

Goniometer Placement

Axis. Head of the third metacarpal which coincides with the longitudinal axis of the forearm.

Stationary Arm. Perpendicular to the floor.

Movable Arm. Parallel to the pencil.

Possible Substitutions. Movement of pencil by release of grasp or by wrist extension and deviation, shoulder adduction, and external rotation.

Forearm Pronation

Rotation of the forearm medially around its longitudinal axis from midposition (0 to 80°).

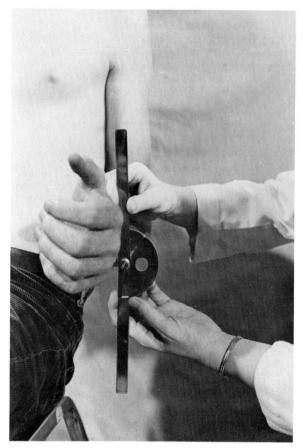

Figure 7.24 Starting position: Humerus adducted to the side and elbow flexed to 90° with the forearm in midposition.

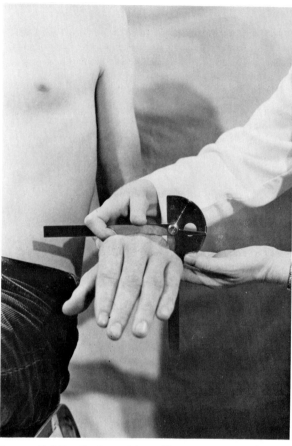

Figure 7.25 End position: Forearm rotated so that the palm faces down.

Goniometer Placement

Axis. Longitudinal axis of forearm displaced toward the ulnar side.

Stationary Arm. Perpendicular to the floor.

Movable Arm. Across the distal radius and ulna on the dorsal surface.

Possible Substitutions. Abduction and internal rotation of the shoulder.

Forearm Pronation: Alternate Method

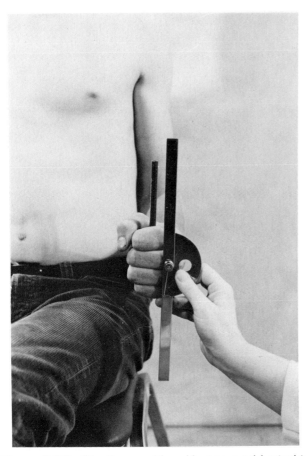

Figure 7.26 Starting position: Humerus adducted to the side and elbow flexed to 90° with the forearm in midposition. A pencil is held in the tightly closed fist, with the pencil protruding from the radial side of the hand.

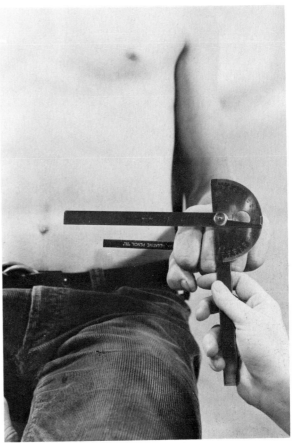

Figure 7.27 End position: The forearm is rotated so that the palm faces down. The pencil is still grasped tightly.

Goniometer Placement

Axis. Head of the third metacarpal which coincides with the longitudinal axis of the forearm.

Stationary Arm. Perpendicular to the floor.

Movable Arm. Parallel to the pencil.

Possible Substitutions. Movement of pencil by release of grasp or by wrist flexion and deviation, or abduction and internal rotation of the shoulder.

Wrist Flexion (Volar Flexion)

Movement of the hand volarly in the sagittal plane (0 to 80°).

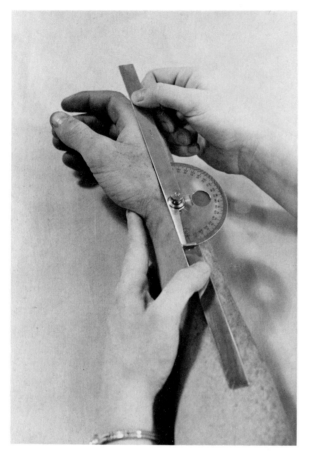

Figure 7.28 Starting position: Forearm rests on the table in midposition; wrist is in neutral position. The fingers are slightly extended or relaxed to eliminate the error that could occur dur to tenodesis effect: the finger extensor tendons are too short to allow full wrist flexion with full finger flexion.

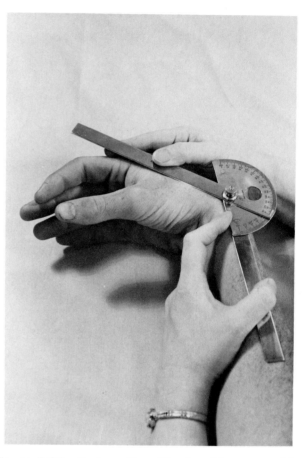

Figure 7.29 End position: The hand has moved toward the volar forearm to the limit of motion.

Goniometer Placement

Axis. Over the styloid process of the radius which is located on the lateral aspect of the wrist at the anatomical snuff box.

Stationary Arm. Parallel to the longitudinal axis of the radius.

Movable Arm. Parallel to the longitudinal axis of the second metacarpal.

Wrist Extension (Dorsiflexion)

Movement of the hand dorsally in the sagittal plane (0 to 70°).

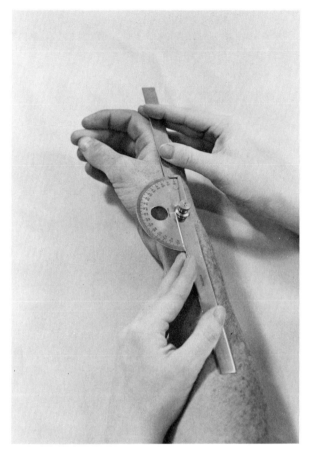

Figure 7.30 Starting position: The forearm rests on the table in midposition. The wrist is in neutral position. The fingers should be slightly flexed or relaxed to eliminate the error which could occur due to the finger flexor tendons being too short to allow full wrist hyperextension with full finger extension.

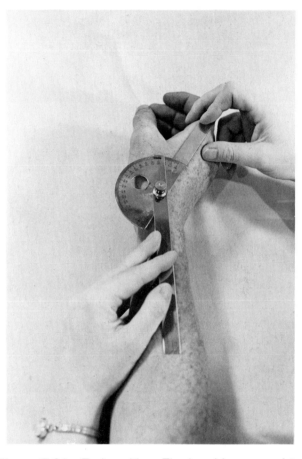

Figure 7.31 End position: The hand has moved toward the dorsal forearm to the limit of motion.

Goniometer Placement

Axis. Over the styloid process of the radius.
Stationary Arm. Parallel to the longitudinal axis of the radius.

Movable Arm. Parallel to the longitudinal axis of the second metacarpal.

Wrist Ulnar Deviation

Movement of the hand toward the ulnar side in a frontal plane (0 to 30°).

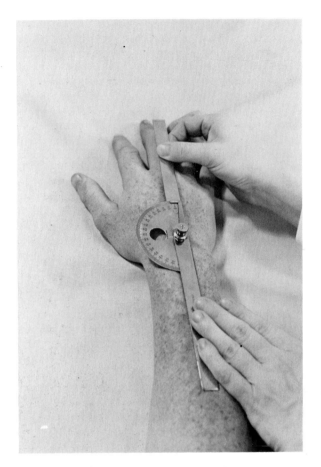

Figure 7.32 Starting position: The forearm is pronated with the volar surface of the forearm and palm resting lightly on the table. The wrist is in neutral position, with fingers relaxed.

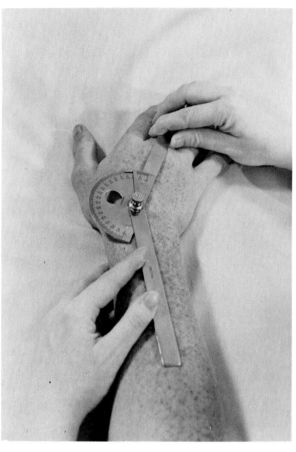

Figure 7.33 End position: The hand has moved so that the little finger approximates the ulna to the limit of motion.

Goniometer Placement

Axis. On the dorsal aspect of the wrist joint in line with the base of the third metacarpal.

Stationary Arm. Along the midline of the forearm on the dorsal surface.

Movable Arm. Along the midline of the third metacarpal.

Possible Substitutions. Wrist extension, wrist flexion.

Wrist Radial Deviation

Movement of the hand toward the radial side in a frontal plane (0 to 20°).

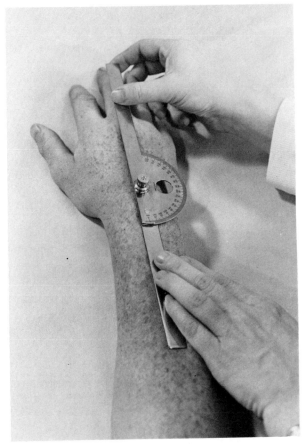

Figure 7.34 Starting position: The forearm is pronated, with the volar surface of the forearm and the palm resting lightly on the table. The wrist is in neutral position, fingers relaxed.

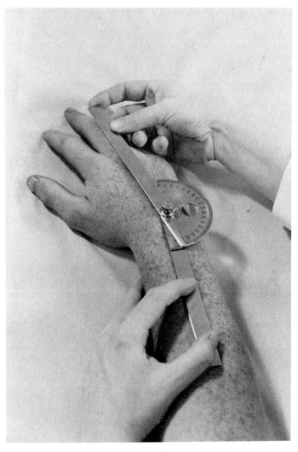

Figure 7.35 End position: The hand has moved so that the thumb approximates the radius to the limit of motion.

Goniometer Placement

Axis. On the dorsal aspect of the wrist joint in line with the base of the third metacarpal.

Stationary arm. Along the midline of the forearm on the dorsal surface.

Movable Arm. Along the midline of the third metacarpal.

Possible Substitution. Wrist extension.

Thumb Carpometacarpal Flexion

Movement of the thumb across the palm in the frontal plane (0 to 15°).

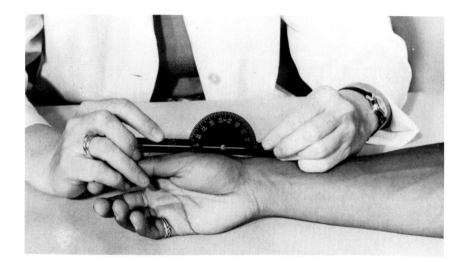

Figure 7.36 Starting position: The wrist is in neutral or slight ulnar deviation to align the second metacarpal and the radius. The CM joint is in neutral, with the thumb next to the volar surface of the index finger.

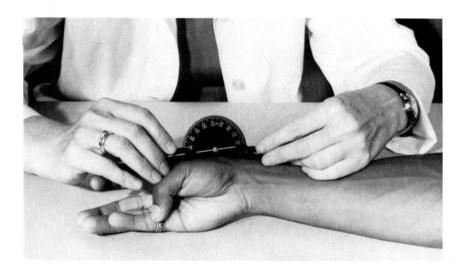

Figure 7.37 End position: The thumb has moved across the plane of the palm toward the ulnar side to the limit of motion in flexion.

Goniometer Placement

Axis. On the radial side of the wrist at the junction of the base of the first metacarpal and the radius.

Stationary Arm. Parallel to the longitudinal axis of the radius.

Movable Arm. Parallel to the longitudinal axis of the first metacarpal.

Thumb Carpometacarpal Extension

Movement of the thumb away from the palm in the frontal plane (0 to 20°).

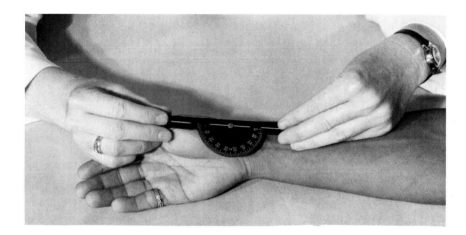

Figure 7.38 Starting position: The wrist is in neutral or slight ulnar deviation to align the second metacarpal and the radius. The CM joint is in neutral with the thumb next to the volar surface of the index finger.

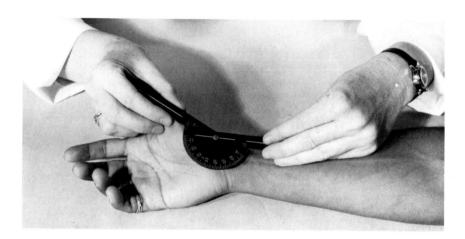

Figure 7.39 End position: The thumb has moved into full extension away from the palm toward the radial side to the limit of motion in extension.

Goniometer Placement

Axis. On the volar side of the wrist at the junction of the base of the first metacarpal and the radius.

Stationary Arm. Parallel to the longitudinal axis of the radius.

Movable Arm. Parallel to the longitudinal axis of the first metacarpal.

Thumb Metacarpophalangeal (MP) Flexion-Extension

Movement of the thumb across the palm in the frontal plane (0 to 50°).

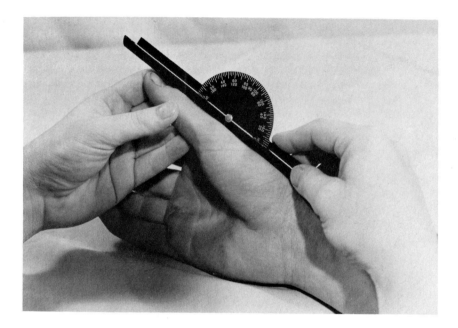

Figure 7.40 Starting position: The wrist is in neutral position or slight extension. The MP joint is in extension.

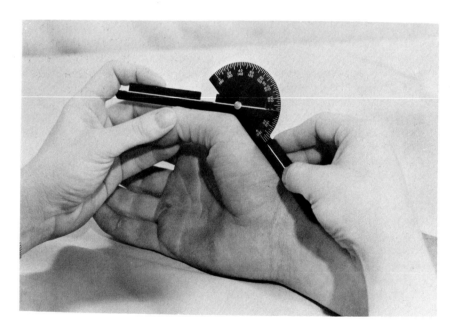

Figure 7.41 End position: The thumb has moved across the plane of the palm toward the ulnar side of the hand to the limit of motion in flexion.

Goniometer Placement

Axis. On the dorsal aspect of the MP joint.

Stationary Arm. On the dorsal surface, along the midline of the first metacarpal.

Movable Arm. On the dorsal surface, along the midline of the proximal phalanx of the thumb.

Note. The arms of the goniometer must remain in full contact with skin surfaces over the bones for accuracy. Do not apply excessive pressure with the edge of a half-circle goniometer. These statements apply to all flexion-extension measurements of the fingers and thumb.

Thumb Interphalangeal (IP) Flexion-Extension

Movement of the distal phalanx of the thumb toward the volar surface of the proximal phalanx of the thumb (0 to 80°).

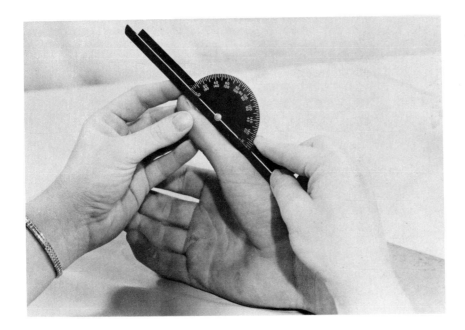

Figure 7.42 Starting position: The wrist is in neutral position or slight extension. The IP joint is in extension.

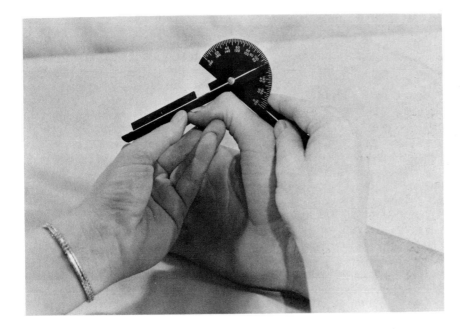

Figure 7.43 End position: The volar surface of the distal phalanx approximates the volar surface of the proximal phalanx to the limit of motion in flexion.

Goniometer Placement

Axis. On the dorsal aspect of the IP joint.

Stationary Arm. On the dorsal surface, along the proximal phalanx.

Movable Arm. On the dorsal surface, along the distal phalanx.

Note. If the thumbnail prevents full goniometer contact, shift the movable arm laterally to increase accuracy.

Alternate Goniometer Placement

Thumb MP and IP flexion-extension can be measured on the lateral aspect of the thumb using lateral aspects of the same landmarks.

Thumb Abduction

Movement of the thumb anteriorly in the sagittal plane, up away from the palm of the hand in line with the index finger (0 to 70°).

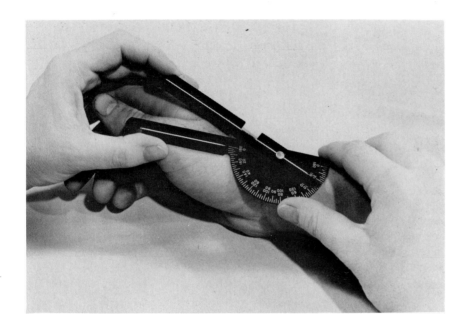

Figure 7.44 Starting position: The wrist is in neutral position and the thumb is touching the volar surface of the palm and index finger. *Note.* This is the zero starting position; although the goniometer may indicate 20 to 30° it is recorded as zero.

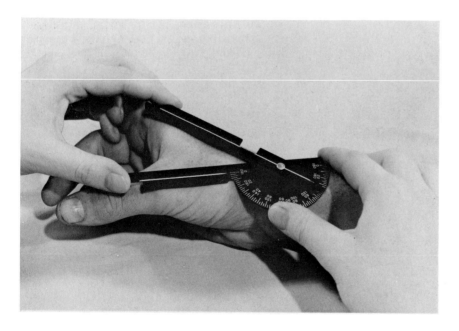

Figure 7.45 End position: The thumb has moved away from the palm in line with the index finger to the limit of motion.

Goniometer Placement

Axis. On the radial side of the wrist at the junction of the bases of the first and second metacarpals.

Stationary Arm. Along the second metacarpal on its lateral aspect.

Movable Arm. Along the first metacarpal on its dorsal surface.

Thumb Abduction and Opposition: Ruler Measurements

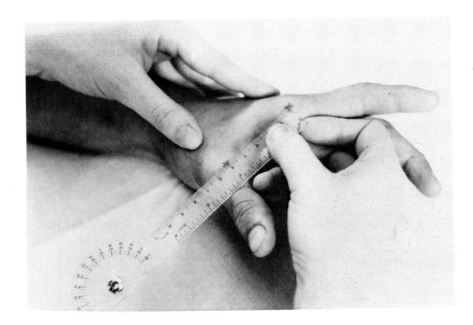

Figure 7.46 Thumb abduction: Ruler measurement of web space.

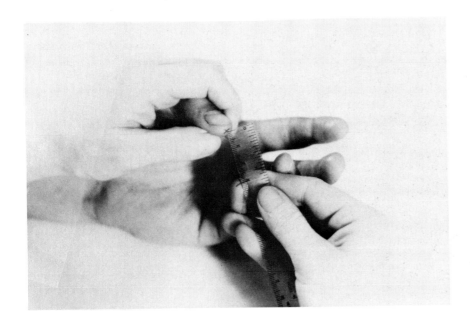

Figure 7.47 Thumb opposition: Ruler measurement.

Abduction. Take the measurement from the midpoint of the head of the first metacarpal to the midpoint of the head of the second metacarpal while the thumb is in full abduction.

Opposition. Rotary movement of the thumb to approximate the pad of the thumb to pads of the fingers. Normally, a person can oppose to each of the fingers.

Measure the distance from the tip of the thumb (not the thumbnail) to the tip end of the little finger to record any deficit of opposition.

Finger Metacarpophalangeal (MP) Flexion

Movement of the finger at the MP joint in a sagittal plane (0 to 90°).

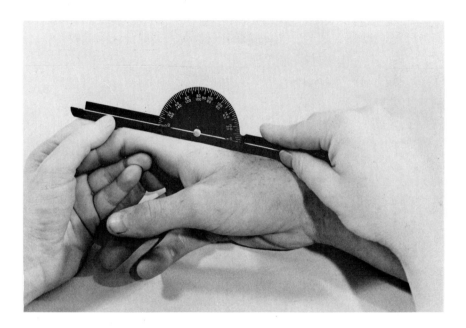

Figure 7.48 Starting position: The wrist is in neutral position or slight hyperextension. The MP joint is in extension.

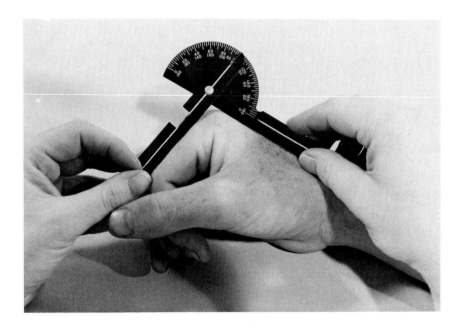

Figure 7.49 End position: The volar surface of the proximal phalanx approximates the palm to the limit of motion of flexion.

Goniometer Placement

Axis. On the dorsal aspect of the MP joint of the finger being measured.

Stationary Arm. On the dorsal surface along the midline of the metacarpal of the finger being measured.

Movable Arm. On the dorsal surface along the midline of the proximal phalanx of the finger being measured.

Finger Metacarpophalangeal (MP) Hyperextension

Movement of the finger at the MP joint dorsally in a sagittal plane (0 to 45°).

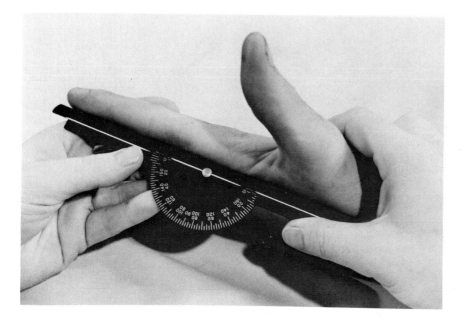

Figure 7.50 Starting position: The wrist is in neutral position or in slight flexion. The MP joint is in zero degrees (neutral position). The IP joints are relaxed.

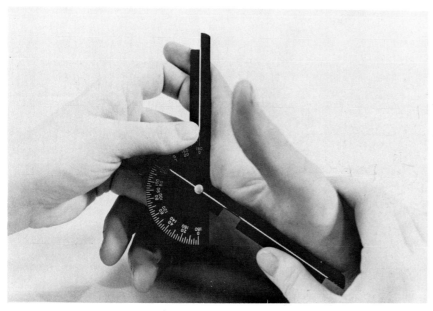

Figure 7.51 End position: The dorsal surface of the proximal phalanx moves toward the dorsum of the hand to the limit of motion.

Goniometer Placement

Axis. On the volar aspect of the MP joint of the finger being measured.

Stationary Arm. Along the volar aspect of the midline of the metacarpal of the finger being measured.

Movable Arm. Along the volar aspect of the midline of the proximal phalanx of the finger being measured. Allow the PIP and DIP joints to flex.

Alternate Goniometer Placement

MP flexion and hyperextension can be measured from the lateral aspect of the index and little fingers by using the lateral aspects of the same landmarks noted here. The long finger and ring finger measurements are estimated by sighting in from the adjoining fingers. This alternate method may be more accurate in cases where there are enlarged joints or excess tissue on the patient's palm.

Finger Proximal Interphalangeal (PIP) Flexion-Extension

Movement of the middle phalanx toward the volar surface of the proximal phalanx in the sagittal plane (0 to 100°).

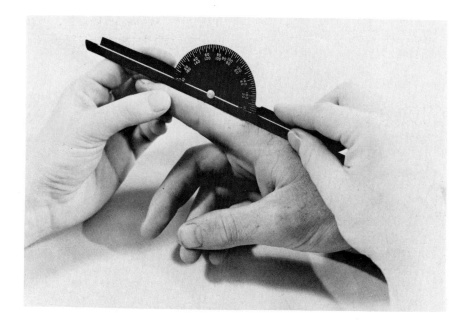

Figure 7.52 Starting position: The wrist is in neutral position or slight hyperextension. The PIP joint is in extension.

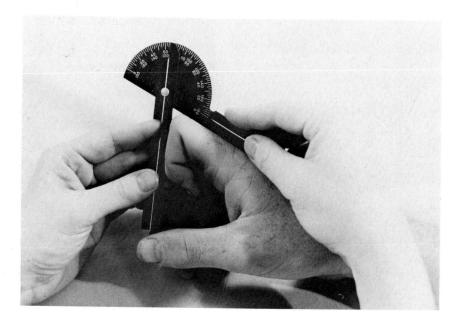

Figure 7.53 End position: the volar surface of the middle phalanx approximates the volar surface of the proximal phalanx to the limit of motion in flexion.

Goniometer Placement

Axis. On the dorsal aspect of the PIP joint of the finger being measured.

Stationary Arm. On the dorsal surface along the midline of the proximal phalanx of the finger being measured.

Movable Arm. On dorsal surface along the midline of the middle phalanx of the finger being measured.

Finger Distal Interphalangeal (DIP) Flexion-Extension

Movement of the distal phalanx toward the volar surface of the middle phalanx in a sagittal plane (0 to 90°).

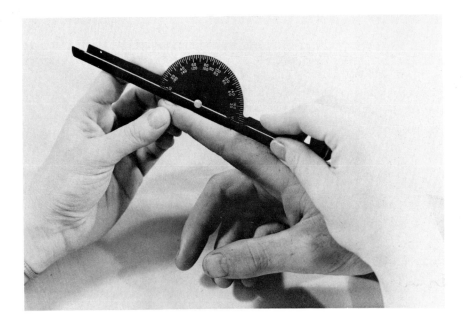

Figure 7.54 Starting position: The wrist is in neutral position or slight hyperextension. The DIP joint is in extension.

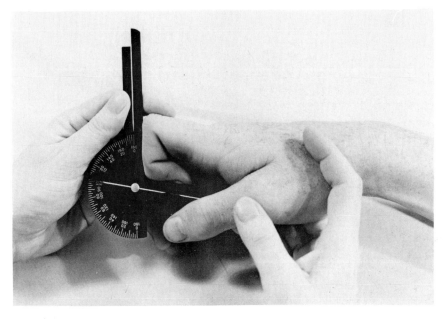

Figure 7.55 End position: The volar surface of the distal phalanx approximates the volar surface of the middle phalanx to the limit of motion in flexion. The PIP joint should flex to permit full DIP flexion.

Goniometer Placement

Axis. On the dorsal aspect of the DIP joint of the finger being measured.

Stationary Arm. On the dorsal surface along the midline of the middle phalanx of the finger being measured.

Movable Arm. On the dorsal surface along the midline of the distal phalanx of the finger being measured.

Note. If the fingernail prevents full goniometer contact, shift the movable arm laterally to increase accuracy.

Alternate Goniometer Placement

Finger PIP and DIP flexion-extension can be measured from the lateral aspect of each finger using the lateral aspect of the same landmarks. This method may be more accurate when joints are enlarged.

Finger Flexion: Ruler Measurements

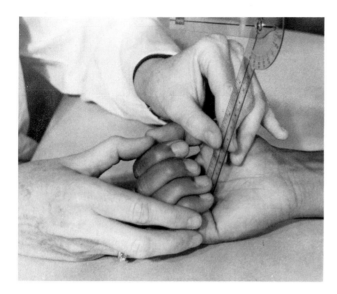

Figure 7.56 PIP and DIP flexion: Ruler measurement.

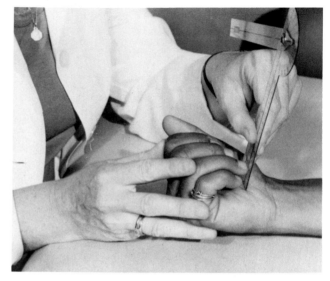

Figure 7.57 MP, PIP, and DIP flexion: Ruler measurement.

PIP and DIP Flexion

Measure from the tip of the finger to the distal palmar crease.

MP, PIP, and DIP Flexion

Measure from the tip of the finger to the base of the palm.[1]

Finger Abduction

Movement of the index, ring, and little fingers away from the midline of the hand in a frontal plane. The middle finger, which is the midline of the hand, abducts in both radial and ulnar directions.

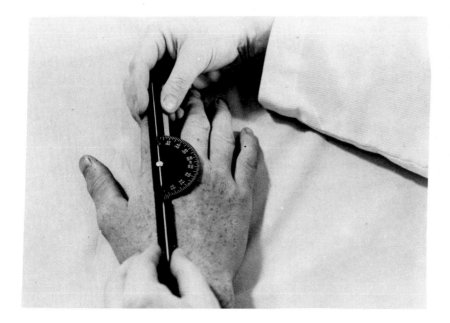

Figure 7.58 Starting position: The volar surface of the forearm and palm are resting lightly on a table. The metacarpal and the proximal phalanx of the finger being measured should be in a straight line.

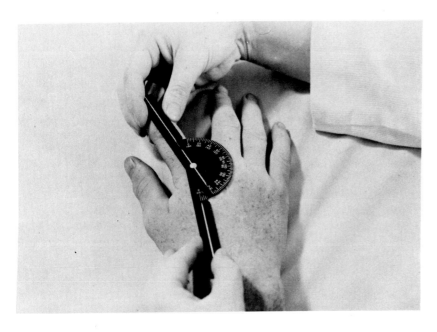

Figure 7.59 End position: The finger has moved away from the midposition to the limit of motion.

Goniometer Placement

Axis. On the dorsal aspect of the MP joint of the finger being measured.

Stationary Arm. Along the dorsal surface of the metacarpal of the finger being measured.

Movable Arm. Along the dorsal surface of the proximal phalanx of the finger being measured.

Alternate Measurement. Ruler measurements may be taken from the midpoint of the tip of each finger to the midpoint of the tip of the adjacent finger.

Finger Adduction

Movement of the index, ring, and little fingers toward the midline of the hand in a frontal plane.

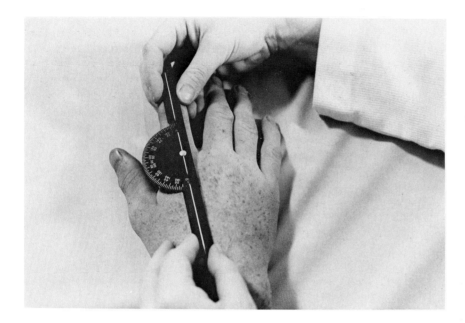

Figure 7.60 Starting position: The volar surface of the forearm and palm are resting lightly on a table. The metacarpal and the proximal phalanx of the finger being measured should be in a straight line.

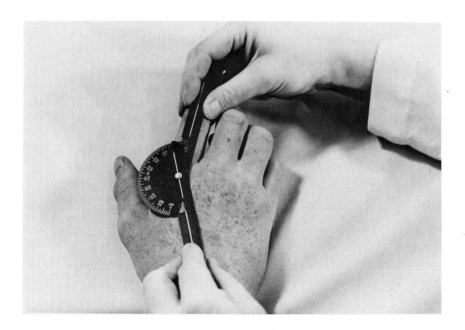

Figure 7.61 End position: The finger has moved toward the middle finger to the limit of motion. Move adjacent fingers out of the way if necessary to allow full excursion of movement.

Goniometer Placement

Axis. On the dorsal aspect of the MP joint of the finger being measured.

Stationary Arm. Along the dorsal surface of the metacarpal of the finger being measured. The middle finger is not measured.

Movable Arm. Along the dorsal surface of the proximal phalanx of the finger being measured.

MP Deviation Correction Measurement

In the case of ulnar deviation deformity of the metacarpophalangeal joints often seen in rheumatoid arthritis, this additional measurement is taken.

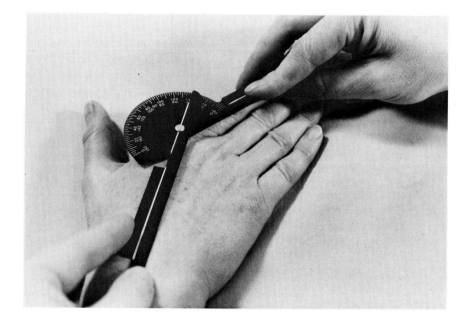

Figure 7.62 Starting position: The hand and forearm rest pronated on a flat surface. The finger is in the position of ulnar deviation in which the finger normally lies.

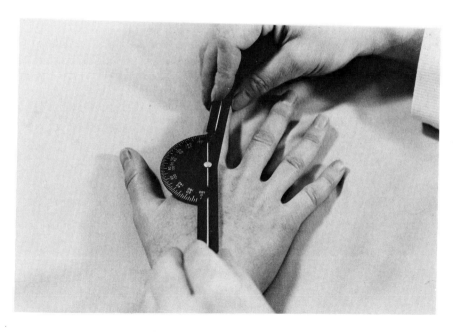

Figure 7.63 End position: Radial deviation of the finger.

Goniometer Placement

Axis. Over the MP joint of the finger being measured.

Stationary Arm. Placed along the dorsal midline of the metacarpal.

Movable Arm. Placed along the dorsal midline of the proximal phalanx.

The active range is compared to the passive range to determine if muscle weakness is present. Passive range of motion is compared to the norm of 0° deviation to determine if a fixed deformity exists.

MEASUREMENT OF THE LOWER EXTREMITY

Hip Flexion

Movement of the thigh anteriorly in a sagittal plane (0 to 120° with the knee flexed).

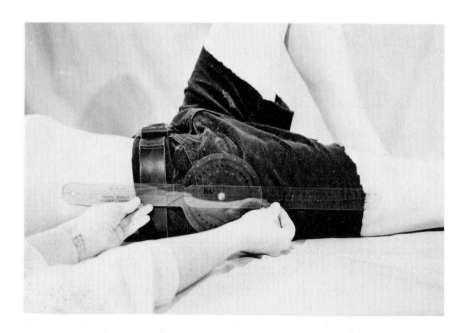

Figure 7.64 Starting position: Patient is supine. The leg being measured is fully extended. The opposite leg may be flexed or extended at the hip and knee.

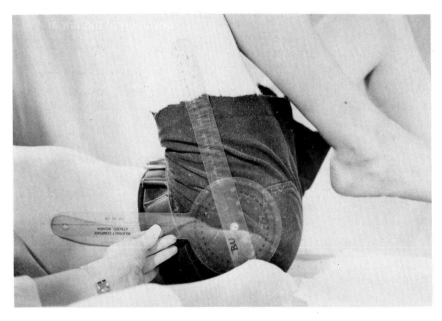

Figure 7.65 End position: As the hip is flexed, the knee is allowed to flex. The anterior thigh approximates the anterior trunk to the limit of motion.

Goniometer Placement

Axis. On a point on the lateral aspect of the hip opposite the greater trochanter.

Stationary Arm. Perpendicular to a line drawn from the anterior superior iliac spine to the posterior superior iliac spine of the pelvis.

Movable Arm. Along the midline of the femur on the lateral aspect of the thigh, pointing toward the lateral epicondyle of the femur.

Hip Extension

Movement of the thigh posteriorly in a sagittal plane (0 to 30° with the knee extended).

This average range was determined by using the lateral trunk as a reference for placement of the stationary arm. Mundale et al.[5] measured hip extension in 36 normal subjects using the relationship of the femur to the pelvis as described below; they found only one subject with hip extension beyond zero. Kottke and Kubicek[6] described the relationship of pelvic tilt to stable posture and supported Mundale's method of measurement for hip extension.

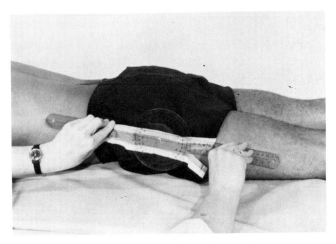

Figure 7.66 Starting position: The patient is prone with both legs fully extended.

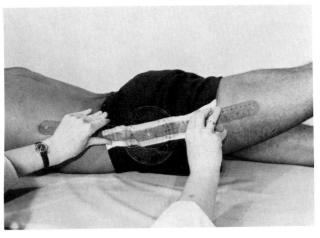

Figure 7.67 End position: The thigh is moved up off the table to the limit of motion. The knee remains extended.

Goniometer Placement

Axis. On a point on the lateral aspect of the hip opposite the greater trochanter.

Stationary Arm. Perpendicular to a line drawn from the anterior superior iliac spine to the posterior superior iliac spine of the pelvis.

Movable Arm. Along the midline of the femur on the lateral aspect of the thigh in line with the lateral epicondyle of the femur.

Note. Clayson et al.[7] described an adapted goniometer for measuring hip extension; one arm of the goniometer has a flexible metal band which can be secured to the anterior and posterior superior iliac spines.

Hip Abduction

Movement of the thigh laterally away from the midline of the body in a frontal plane (0 to 45°).

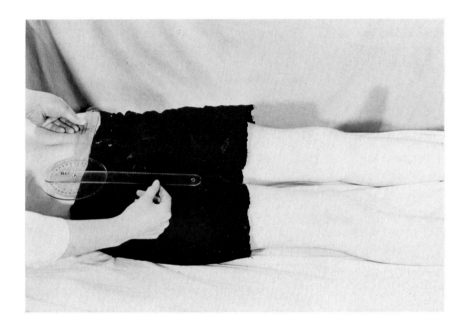

Figure 7.68 Starting position: Patient is supine with legs extended.

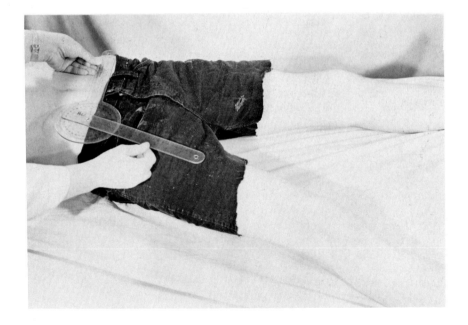

Figure 7.69 End position: The leg being measured is moved laterally to the limit of motion. Knee remains extended.

Goniometer Placement

Axis. The anterior superior iliac spine of the side being measured.

Stationary Arm. On a line between the two anterior superior iliac spines.

Movable Arm. Parallel to the midline of the femur on the anterior surface of the thigh; it points toward the patella.

Possible Substitution. Hip external rotation.

Hip Adduction

Movement of the thigh medially across the midline of the body in a frontal plane (0 to 30°).

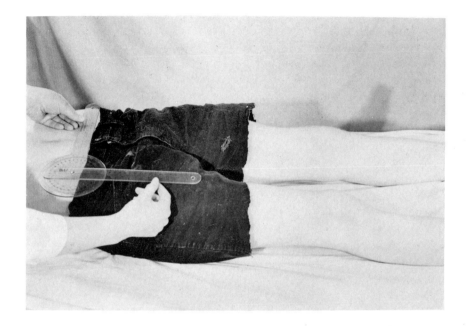

Figure 7.70 Starting position: The patient is supine with the legs extended.

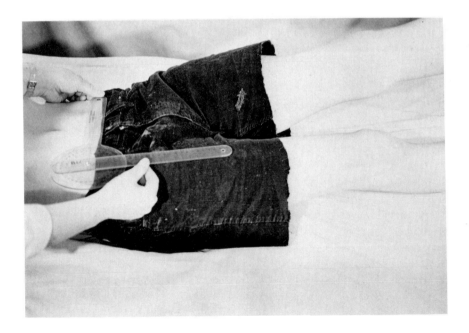

Figure 7.71 End position: The leg not being measured is flexed at the hip to move it out of the way. The leg being measured is moved medially across the midline of the body to the limit of motion.

Goniometer Placement

Axis. Anterior superior iliac spine of the side being measured.

Stationary Arm. On a line between the two anterior superior iliac spines.

Movable Arm. Parallel to the midline of the femur on the anterior surface of the thigh and pointing toward the patella.

Possible Substitution. Hip internal rotation.

Hip Internal Rotation

Movement of the femur medially around its longitudinal axis (0 to 45°).

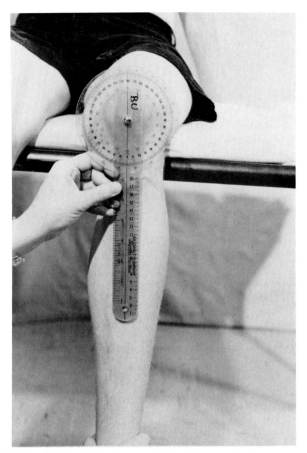

Figure 7.72 Starting position: The patient is seated with the hip flexed to 90°. The lower leg hangs over the edge of the plinth.

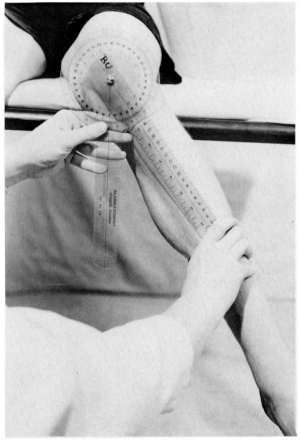

Figure 7.73 End position: The foot and lower leg are moved laterally while the thigh rotates medially but is not permitted to adduct or flex.

Goniometer Placement

Axis. Centered on the knee joint over the patella.
Stationary Arm. Perpendicular to the floor.

Movable Arm. Along the midline of the tibial shaft.

Hip External Rotation

Movement of the femur laterally around its longitudinal axis (0 to 45°).

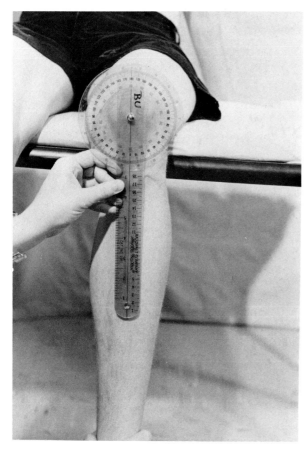

Figure 7.74 Starting position: The patient is seated with the hip and knee flexed to 90°. The lower leg hangs over the edge of the plinth.

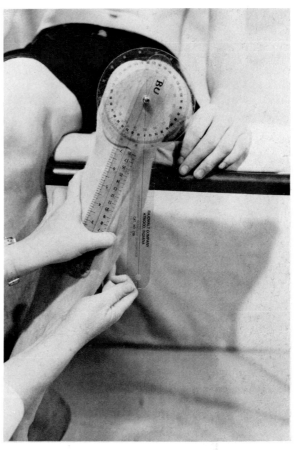

Figure 7.75 End position: The foot and lower leg are moved medially while the thigh rotates laterally but is not permitted to flex or abduct.

Goniometer Placement

Axis. Centered on the knee joint over the patella.
Stationary Arm. Perpendicular to the floor.

Movable Arm. Along the midline of the tibial shaft.

Hip Internal and External Rotation: Alternate Method

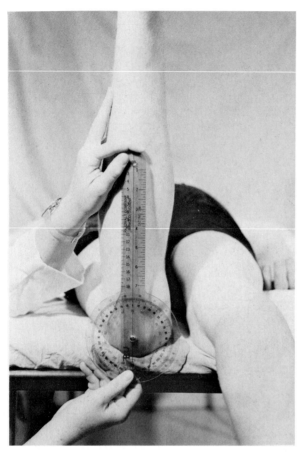

Figure 7.76 Starting position: Patient is prone with knee flexed to 90° and lower leg perpendicular to the plinth.

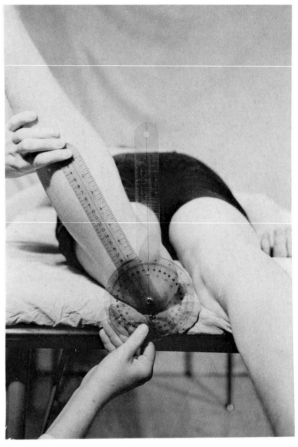

Figure 7.77 End position for internal rotation: The foot and lower leg are moved laterally to the limit of motion while the thigh rotates medially. No thigh adduction is permitted. For external rotation the foot and lower leg are moved medially while the thigh rotates laterally. No thigh abduction is permitted.

Goniometer Placement

Axis. Centered on the knee joint over the patella.
Stationary Arm. Perpendicular to the floor.

Movable Arm. Along the midline of the tibial shaft.

Knee Flexion-Extension

Movement of the lower leg posteriorly in a sagittal plane (0 to 135°).

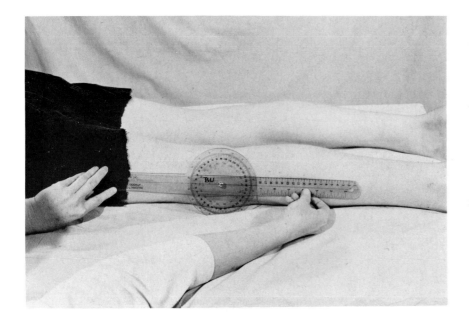

Figure 7.78 Starting position: Patient is prone with both legs fully extended and feet over the table edge. Alternate position: Patient sits with knees flexed and lower legs over the table edge.

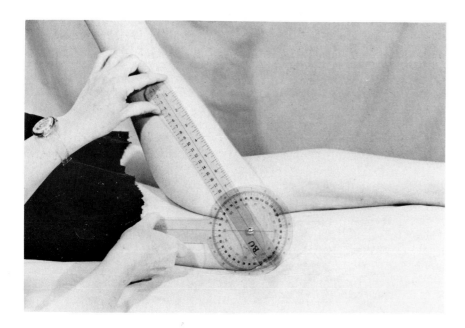

Figure 7.79 End position: The lower leg is moved so that the calf approximates the posterior thigh to the limit of flexion.

Goniometer Placement

Axis. The knee joint at the lateral tibial condyle.
Stationary Arm. Along the midline of the femur on the lateral aspect of the thigh.

Movable Arm. Along the lateral midline of the lower leg in line with the lateral malleolus.

Ankle Dorsiflexion-Plantar Flexion

Dorsiflexion is movement of the foot anteriorly in the sagittal plane (0 to 20°). Plantar flexion is movement of the foot posteriorly in a sagittal plane (0 to 50°).

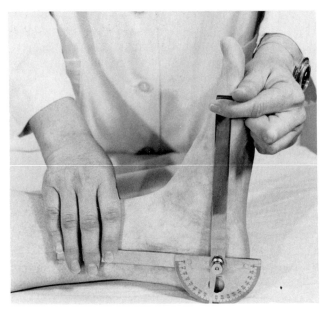

Figure 7.80 Starting position: The patient is sitting or supine with knee flexed. The foot is in neutral position (90°).

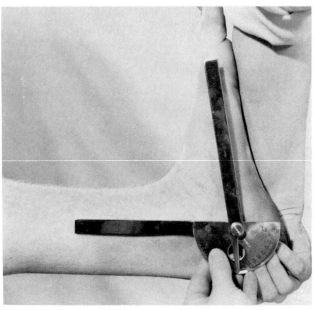

Figure 7.81 End position for dorsiflexion: The foot is moved so that the toes point up.

Goniometer Placement

Axis. On the medial aspect of the ankle joint approximately 1 inch below the medial malleolus.

Stationary Arm. Along the midline of the medial aspect of the lower leg.

Movable Arm. In line with the first metatarsal. The goniometer will read 90° at the start of the measurement, and this must be deducted when recording.

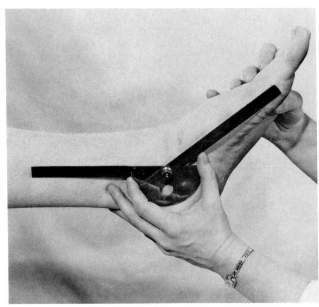

Figure 7.82 End position for plantar flexion: The foot is moved so that the toes point down.

Ankle Inversion

Inversion is movement of the forefoot to bring the sole of the foot to face medially (0 to 35°).

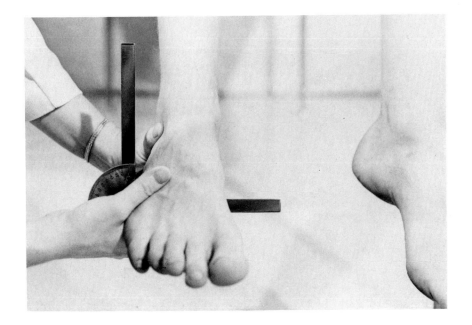

Figure 7.83 Starting position: The patient is supine or sitting with the knee flexed. The foot is in neutral position.

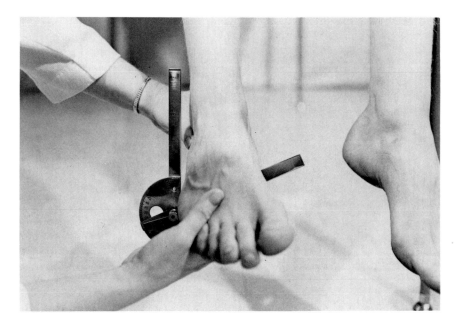

Figure 7.84 End position: The sole of the foot faces medially to the limit of motion. External rotation of the hip is prohibited.

Goniometer Placement

Axis. A point parallel to the longitudinal axis of the foot, displaced laterally.

Stationary Arm. Along the midline of the lateral aspect of the lower leg.

Movable Arm. Across the sole of the forefoot.

Note. The goniometer will read 90° at the start of the measurement and this must be deducted when recording.

Ankle Eversion

Eversion is movement of the forefoot to bring the sole of the foot to face laterally (0 to 15°).

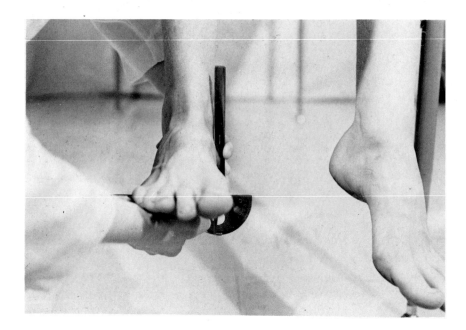

Figure 7.85 Starting position: The patient is supine or sitting with the knee flexed. The foot is in neutral position.

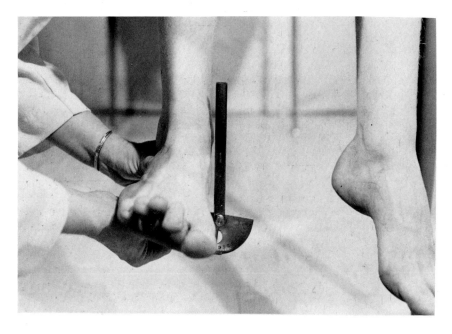

Figure 7.86 End position: The sole of the foot faces laterally to the limit of motion. Internal rotation of the hip is prohibited.

Goniometer Placement

Axis. A point parallel to the longitudinal axis of the foot displaced medially.

Stationary Arm. Along the midline of the lower leg on the medial aspect.

Movable Arm. Across the sole of the forefoot.

Note. The goniometer will read 90° at the start of motion, and this must be deducted when recording.

Other Methods Used to Record Range of Motion

Palm Prints[8, 9]

Imprints of the palm of the patient's whole hand are made on paper using either finger paint or a water-based ink stamp pad. This presents a graphic record of deformities. Sequential palm prints indicate changes in these deformities over time. This method is frequently used to record the changes in deformities of the hands of rheumatoid arthritic patients.

Xerography[10]

Xerox photographs of the patient's whole hand are made for the same reasons that palm prints are made. Xerography, however, gives a clearer representation.

Outline

The hand is placed on a paper and a tracing is made around the entire hand with the fingers in both an abducted and an adducted position. This is an alternative graphic representation of abduction and adduction of the fingers often used instead of, or as an adjunct to, goniometric measurement or ruler measurement.

Bubble Goniometer

This is a measuring tool that uses the principle of a carpenter's level in which a bubble of air within a column of liquid moves when the angle of the carpenter's level is changed. The bubble goniometer is designed like a watch in which the bubble rests at the highest point (equivalent to 12 o'clock), and the face is marked off in degrees rather than in minutes. It is currently most often used to measure the cervical spine.

Gravity Goniometer

This is a tool which resembles a round lollipop and is used to measure supination and pronation of the forearm. The round face of the instrument is marked off in degrees and has an indicator like a compass point which always points up due to the force of gravity. Its accuracy depends upon careful positioning as described for the alternate method of measuring supination and pronation using a pencil.

Electrogoniometer[11]

This is a device which records electrically the position of the joint or joints to which it is applied. A potentiometer whose resistance changes with changes in position is mounted at the joint to be measured. The electrical signal is electronically recorded on paper as a graphic representation of the position of the joint. The degrees of change can be mathematically determined, or the electronic signal can be run through an on-line computer and a computer readout obtained. It is currently a research tool. Figure 7.87 shows a finger electrogoniometer which measures movement of the MP and PIP joints of the middle finger.

Functional

Range of motion is observed during the performance of activities to see if there are any limitations which interfere with function. This type of observation assists in determining if the patient's ROM limitations are significant.

MUSCLE STRENGTH

When weakness limits function it is necessary to determine the degree and extent of the weakness. In

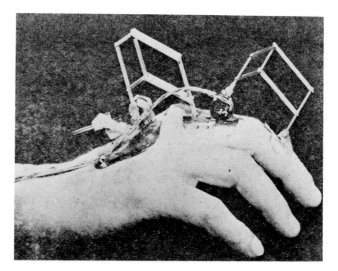

Figure 7.87 Electrogoniometer placed to measure MP and PIP flexion and extension of the long finger. (Reproduced with permission from C. Long and M. E. Brown: *Journal of Bone and Joint Surgery* 46-A(8), 1964.)

some cases, such as Landry-Guillain-Barré syndrome, weakness will be generalized, and therefore testing will be extensive. In other cases, such as a peripheral nerve injury, weakness will be limited to muscles innervated by the damaged nerve, and muscle testing will usually involve only these muscles. In other words the therapist tests those muscles which are involved and toward which treatment will be directed. If you treat it, measure it!

Strength of muscle contraction can be measured by means of spring scales, tensiometers, dynamometers, weights, or manual resistance.[12] Although the measurement of strength taken using apparatus is more exact, it is difficult and time-consuming to set up the apparatus as precisely as it must be in order to get accurate measurements of each muscle group. Therefore, clinicians use manual muscle testing which they have found to be adequate for most clinical purposes. Manual muscle testing is the application of resistance by the therapist to the voluntary maximal contraction of the patient's muscles.

There are several different methods of manual muscle testing currently used. Force applied after the motion is completed to assess the isometric holding strength has been traditionally used rather than resistance to the ongoing movement of an isotonic contraction. Carlson[13] tested elbow flexion strength of 36 normal subjects comparing tests of isometric and isotonic strength and found that isometric strength was significantly greater than isotonic strength in these subjects, but there was a high positive relationship between the two types of contraction. Caldwell *et al.*[14] noted that the differences in existing tests of muscle strength have led to difficulty in comparison of results obtained by various sources due to lack of agreement on terminology and methods. They state that results of strength testing or of any investigation are only useful if test procedures are reported to the extent of being reproducible. Isometric testing is currently used for clinical testing of muscle strength; an outside force (*i.e.*, manual resistance) is applied to test the muscle's ability to hold after the motion is completed. Kendall *et al.*[15] describe procedures for testing individual muscles and use a grading scale based on percentage of performance. Daniels and Worthingham[16] also describe tests of individual muscles with force applied at the end of the motion to test isometric strength; grades are reported from zero or trace to poor, fair, good, and normal. Both of these sources use movement against the resistance of gravity for evaluation of weaker muscles. Kendall *et al.*[15] do not consider the influence of gravity important for testing supination and pronation or the fingers and toes. Daniels and Worthingham[16] sometimes consider a partial range against gravity as a poor grade when it is not practical to eliminate gravity or for tests of fingers and toes where gravity is not considered to be an important influence.

The evaluation of muscle strength presented here uses force applied to isometric holding after the completion of the movement of the part. Gravity as resistance is considered an important variable and is used for all motions where practical and possible, including supination and pronation, as well as motions of the fingers and toes. In the authors' experience elimination of gravity has been observed to alter the performance ability of muscles of the fingers and is considered to be an important variable, even though the weight of a small lever arm is, of course, less than the weight of a large lever. When standard procedures for evaluation against gravity and gravity eliminated are given in the literature or are in general use these are described. When a gravity eliminated position is not described in the literature the authors applied the concepts to these muscles to describe a gravity eliminated position. Tests of the upper and lower extremities described here are motion tests for the purpose of evaluating strength in terms of ability to perform functionally. Tests of individual muscles in the wrist and hand are given because of the clinical need for specific assessment to determine correct treatment procedures for hand rehabilitation and splinting.

Other factors also influence the outcome of a manual muscle test. Caldwell *et al.*[14] mentioned that it was important to avoid factors that influenced motivation or performance, including spectators, fear, noise, rewards, and competition. Neutral conditions and factual instruction were preferred. It was recommended that test procedures be clearly described, the smooth motion requested with a build up of effort and a hold of 4 seconds against resistance required. A rest of 2 minutes between similar efforts was suggested. Nicholas *et al.*[17] found that the testers' perception of strength correlated with the two variables of force and time; strength was determined by the combined perception of the amount of force exerted by the tester and the time before the limb was unable to hold the position as a result of the applied force.

Manual Muscle Testing Grading System

The muscle or muscle group is assigned a grade according to the amount of resistance it can take. Two of the many grading systems that have evolved are presented here. Therapists customarily use the letter grading system, although numerical scales are sometimes used. Table 7.2 equates one numerical scale with the letter grading system.

Manual Muscle Testing Procedures

The therapist moves each of the patient's joints through passive range of motion to estimate what range of motion is available at each joint. The available range is considered to be "full range of motion" for the purposes of muscle testing. However, notation is made that a limitation exists if it does.

There are established procedures for muscle testing in order to make this evaluation as valid and reliable as possible. The patient is *positioned* so that the direction of movement will be against gravity, or with gravity eliminated as appropriate to the strength of the muscle. As a consideration for the patient's com-

Table 7.2
MUSCLE TESTING GRADING SYSTEMS: NUMERICAL SCALE EQUATED WITH LETTER GRADING SYSTEM

Against Gravity	5	Normal	N	= The part moves through full range of motion against maximum resistance and gravity. "Normal" differs for each muscle group and in persons of different ages, sex, and occupations.
	4	Good	G	= The part moves through full range of motion against gravity and moderate resistance.
		Good minus	G−	= The part moves through full range of motion against gravity and less than moderate resistance.
		Fair plus	F+	= The part moves through full range of motion against gravity, takes minimal resistance, and then "breaks," i.e., relaxes suddenly.
	3	Fair	F	= The part moves through full range of motion against gravity with no added resistance.
		Fair minus	F−	= The part moves less than full range of motion against gravity.
Gravity Eliminated		Poor plus	P+	= The part moves through full range of motion on a gravity eliminated plane, takes minimal resistance, and then "breaks."
	2	Poor	P	= The part moves through full range of motion on a gravity eliminated plane with no added resistance.
		Poor minus	P−	= The part moves less than full range of motion on a gravity eliminated plane.
	1	Trace	T	= Tension is palpated in the muscle or the tendon but no motion occurs at the joint.
	0	Zero	0	= No tension is palpated in the muscle or tendon

fort, all testing is done in one position before changing to another position. For efficient movement of the part distal to the joint, the proximal attachment must be *stabilized*. For weak patients, the therapist must provide this stability but must avoid placing hands over the muscles that are contracting. The prime movers are *palpated* to ascertain that they are functioning during the motion. Palpation is, in fact, the basis for assigning a trace grade. The technique of palpation involves the therapist placing the finger pads firmly but lightly over the belly or tendon of the patient's muscle. It is sometimes necessary to have the patient try to do the motion, then relax, which causes the muscle to alternately contract and relax and allows verification that the correct muscle is being palpated. *Resistance* is applied on the distal end of the moving bone *i.e.*, the bone into which the muscle insert. If resistance is applied at any other point, the lever arm is lengthened or shortened and therefore the resistance is changed. Resistance is applied in a direction opposite to the motion after the patient has completed the motion, a procedure which is called the *break test*.[16] Gravity and/or muscles other than those being tested may *substitute* to cause the motion. Careful positioning, palpation, and observation can identify these substitutions.

The photograph of each against-gravity position shows the completed test motion and the application of resistance. The photograph of each gravity-eliminated position shows the support of the part during motion.

Scapular Elevation

Prime Movers
   Upper trapezius
   Levator scapulae

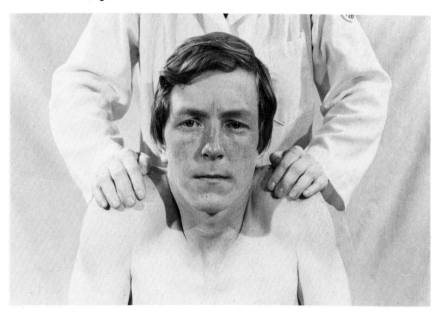

Figure 7.88 Resistance in the against-gravity position. Movement starts with patient sitting erect with arms at the side. Patient raises his shoulders toward his ears.

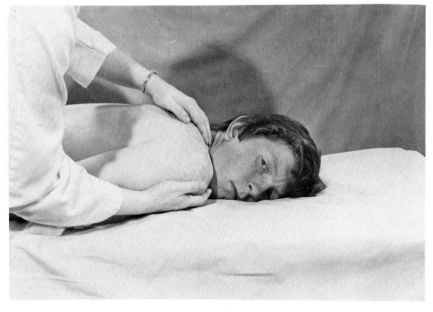

Figure 7.89 Gravity-eliminated position. With the patient prone, arms at the side, the therapist supports the shoulder as the patient attempts to move his shoulder toward his ear. The shoulder is lifted so the scapular motion will be on a gravity-eliminated plane.

Stabilize. Trunk.

Palpation. Upper trapezius is palpated on the shoulder at the curve of the neck. The levator is palpated posteriorly to the sternocleidomastoid on the lateral side of the neck.

Resistance. The therapist's hand is placed over the acromion and pushes down toward scapular depression. A normal trapezius of an adult cannot be "broken" using the break test.

Substitution. Pushing on knees with hands.

Scapular Depression

Prime Movers
  Lower trapezius
  Latissimus dorsi

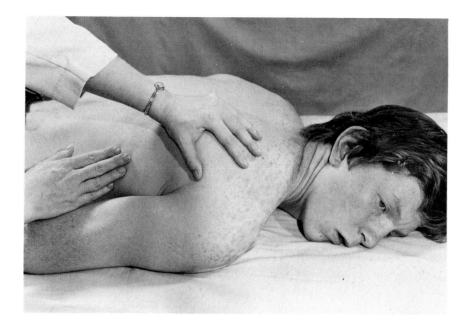

Figure 7.90 Resistance in the gravity-eliminated position. The patient is prone with the arm internally rotated and at the side. From resting position, patient moves the scapula caudally.

Against gravity position. This is tested in the gravity-eliminated position, since the patient cannot be positioned to move against gravity.

Stabilize. Trunk.

Palpation. The lower trapezius is palpated laterally to the vertebral column as it passes diagonally from the lower thoracic vertebrae to the spine of the scapula. The latissimus dorsi is palpated along the posteriolateral rib cage or at its point of distal attachment in the posterior axilla.

Resistance. The therapist's hand is cupped over the inferior angle of the scapula and pushes upward to-ward scapular elevation. When the inferior angle is not easily accessible due to tissue bulk, resistance can be applied at the distal humerus *if* the shoulder joint is stable and pain-free.

Grading. Because of the positioning, it is not possible to accurately grade shoulder depressors for against gravity grades. Experienced therapists estimate these grades and place a question mark (?) beside the grade.

Substitutions. In an upright position, gravity can substitute. In a prone position, the arm can be inched downward using the finger flexors.

Scapular Adduction

Prime Movers—
  Middle trapezius
  Rhomboids

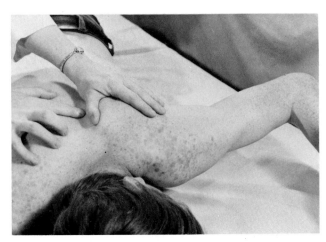

Figure 7.91 Test for middle trapezius against-gravity and resistance. The shoulder is externally rotated. The patient lifts his arm up off of the plinth to move the scapula toward the vertebral column.

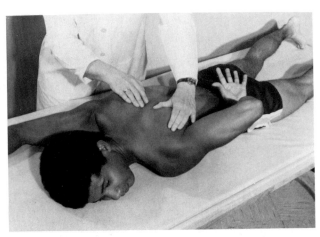

Figure 7.92 Test for rhomboids against-gravity and resistance. The shoulder is internally rotated with the hand held over the lumbar region. The patient lifts his hand up off of the buttocks to move the scapula toward the vertebral column.

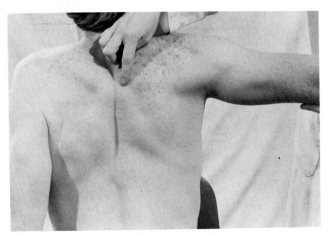

Figure 7.93 Gravity-eliminated position. The patient sits erect with the humerus abducted to 90° and supported. He attempts to move the scapula toward the vertebral column.

Stabilize. Trunk.

Palpation. Middle trapezius is palpated between the vertebral column and vertebral border of the scapula at the level of the spine of the scapula. With the arm in internal rotation and held over the back, the rhomboids are palpated along the vertebral border of the scapula, near the inferior angle.

Resistance. The whole length of the therapist's thumb is placed along the vertebral border of the scapula and the rest of the hand is placed on the dorsal surface of the scapula. The therapist pushes laterally.

Substitutions. None.

Scapular Abduction

Prime Mover
  Serratus anterior ✓

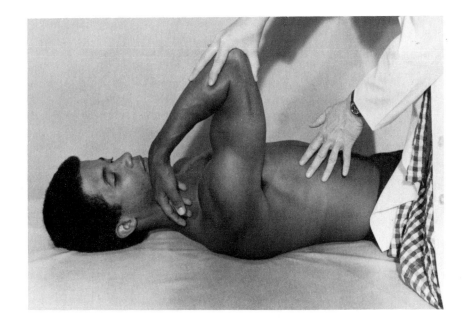

Figure 7.94 Resistance in the against-gravity position. The patient is supine with the humerus flexed to 90°; the elbow may be flexed or extended. The patient abducts the scapula so that the arm moves upward.

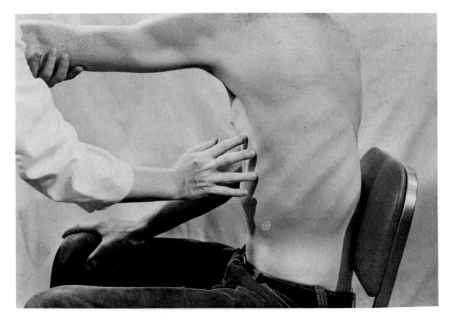

Figure 7.95 Gravity-eliminated position. The patient sits erect with the humerus flexed to 90° and supported; the elbow may be flexed or extended. He abducts the scapula so that the arm moves forward.

Stabilize. Trunk.

Palpation. Serratus anterior is palpated on the lateral ribs just lateral to the inferior angle of the scapula.

Resistance. Therapists have traditionally resisted this motion either by grasping the distal humerus or by cupping the hand over the patient's elbow and pushing down or backward toward adduction. *Note:*

This cannot be done safely if the shoulder is unstable. Application of resistance in this manner varies from the stated rules because it is difficult to apply resistance along the axillary border of the scapula.

Substitutions. This motion can be achieved by inching the arm forward on the supportive surface using the finger flexors.

Shoulder Flexion

Prime Movers
  Anterior deltoid
  Coracobrachialis
  Pectoralis major—clavicular
  Biceps—both heads

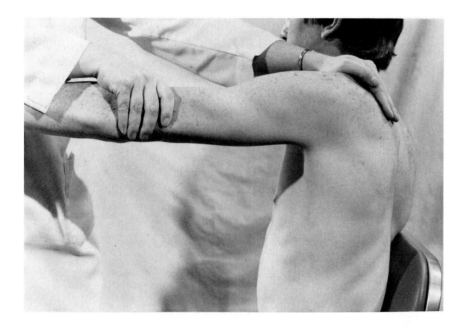

Figure 7.96 Resistance in the against-gravity position. The patient sits erect with the arm at the side in midposition. He flexes the humerus to 90° with the elbow extended.

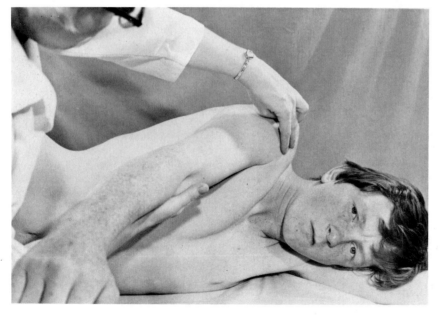

Figure 7.97 Gravity-eliminated position. The patient is side-lying with arm in midposition along the side of the body. The arm is supported by the therapist or by a smooth testing board while the patient attempts to flex the humerus to 90° with the elbow extended.

Stabilize. Scapula.

Palpation. Anterior deltoid is palpated immediately anterior to the glenohumeral joint. Coracobrachialis may be palpated medially to the biceps, which are palpated on the anterior aspect of the humerus. The clavicular head of the pectoralis major may be palpated below the clavicle on its way to insert on the humerus below the anterior deltoid.

Resistance. The therapist's hand is placed over the distal end of the humerus and pushes down toward extension. Movement above 90° involves scapular upward rotation; these motions are separated for muscle testing, although they are not separated for range of motion measurement.

Substitutions. Shoulder abductors; trunk extension.

Shoulder Extension

Prime Movers
  Latissimus dorsi
  Teres major
  Posterior deltoid
  Triceps—long head

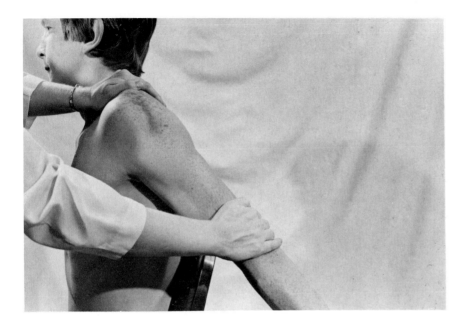

Figure 7.98 Resistance in the against-gravity position. Patient is sitting with the humerus internally rotated and the arm by the side. He extends the humerus. An alternate starting position is with the patient prone. *Note.* The therapist stands in front of the patient for safety to prevent the trunk from bending forward when resistance is applied.

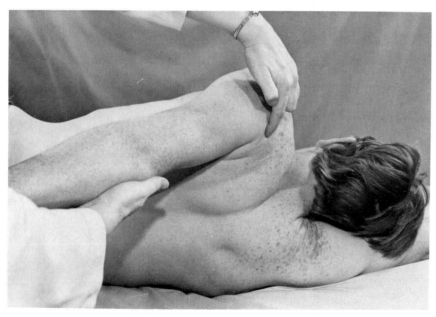

Figure 7.99 Gravity-eliminated position. The patient is side-lying with the humerus internally rotated and the arm supported with the elbow extended. Patient attempts to hyperextend the humerus.

Stabilize. Scapula.

Palpation. The latissimus dorsi and the teres major form the posterior border of the axilla. The latissimus dorsi is located inferiorly to the teres major. The posterior deltoid is located immediately posterior to the glenohumeral joint. The triceps is palpated on the posterior aspect of the humerus.

Resistance. The therapist's hand is placed over the distal end of the humerus and pushes forward toward flexion.

Substitutions. Shoulder abductors; tipping the shoulder forward.

Shoulder Abduction

Prime Movers
  Supraspinatus
  Middle deltoid

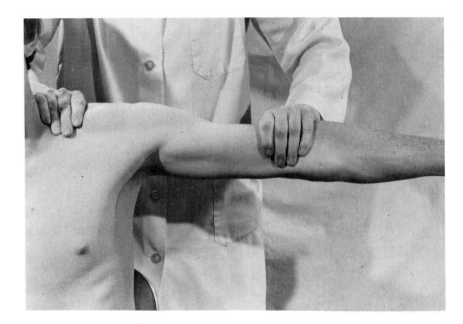

Figure 7.100 Resistance in the against-gravity position. The patient sits erect with the arm at the side in midposition. He abducts the humerus to 90° with the elbow extended.

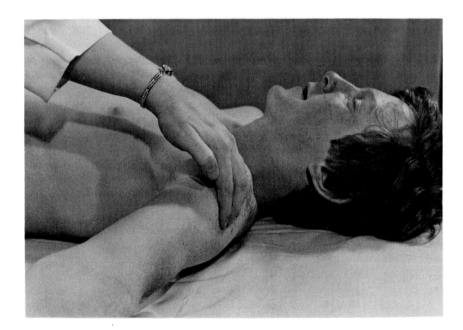

Figure 7.101 Gravity-eliminated position. The patient lies supine with the arm supported at the side in midposition. He attempts to abduct the arm to 90° with the elbow extended.

Stabilize. Scapula.

Palpation. The supraspinatus lies too deep for easy palpation. The middle deltoid is palpated below the acromion and laterally to the glenohumeral joint.

Resistance. The therapist's hand is placed over the distal end of the humerus and pushes the humerus down toward the body. Movement above 90° involves scapular upward rotation and is not measured.

Substitutions. The long head of the biceps can substitute if the humerus is allowed to be moved into external rotation; trunk lateral flexion.

Shoulder Adduction

Prime Movers
Pectoralis major
Teres major
Latissimus dorsi

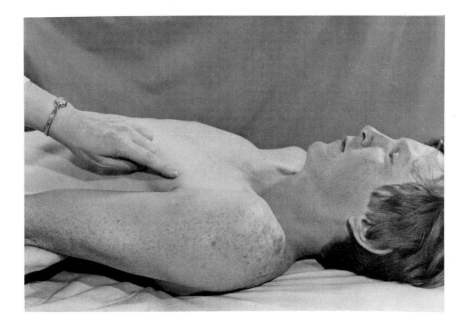

Figure 7.102 Resistance in the gravity-eliminated position. The patient is supine with the humerus abducted to 90° and in midposition. He adducts the humerus.

Against gravity position. Test in the gravity-eliminated position since the patient cannot be positioned for this motion against gravity.

Stabilize. Trunk.

Palpation. The pectoralis major forms the anterior border of the axilla where it may be easily palpated. The teres major and the latissimus dorsi have been previously described.

Resistance. The therapist's hand is placed on the medial side of the distal end of the humerus and pulls the humerus away from the patient's body.

Grading for antigravity grades again can only be estimated and a question mark entered beside the grade on the form. With experience, the therapist develops the skill to estimate reliably.

Substitutions. In an upright position gravity can substitute. On a supporting surface, the arm can be inched down using the finger flexors.

Shoulder Horizontal Abduction

Prime Mover
 Posterior deltoid

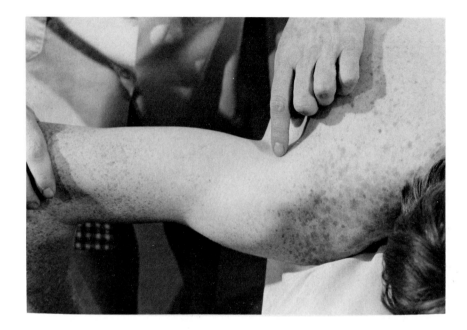

Figure 7.103 Resistance in the against-gravity position. The patient is positioned prone with the arm hanging in internal rotation over the edge of the table. He horizontally abducts the humerus, allowing the elbow to flex.

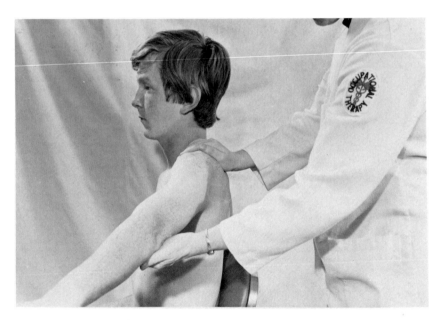

Figure 7.104 Gravity-eliminated position. The patient sits with the humerus flexed to 90° and the arm supported. He attempts to horizontally abduct the humerus.

Stabilize. Scapula. In the sitting position stabilize the trunk against the back of the chair.

Palpation. Posterior deltoid is palpated immediately posterior to the glenohumeral joint.

Resistance. Therapist's hand is placed on the posterior surface of the distal end of the humerus and pushes the arm downward or forward toward horizontal adduction.

Substitution. Trunk rotation in a sitting position.

Shoulder Horizontal Adduction

Prime Movers
  Pectoralis major
  Anterior deltoid

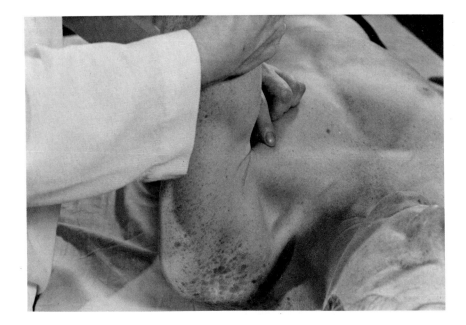

Figure 7.105 Resistance in the against-gravity position. The patient lies with the humerus abducted to 90°. The patient horizontally adducts the humerus to 90° of shoulder flexion. *Note.* In the supine position, if the triceps is weak, prevent the patient's hand from hitting his face.

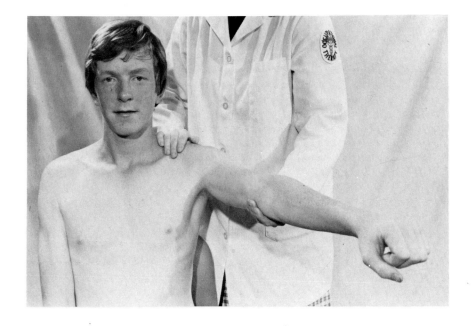

Figure 7.106 Gravity-eliminated position. The patient sits with the humerus abducted to 90° and attempts to horizontally adduct the humerus.

Stabilize. Scapula. In the sitting position stabilize the trunk against the back of the chair.

Palpation. The pectoralis major can be palpated along the anterior border of the axilla. The anterior deltoid is located immediately anterior to the glenohumeral joint below the acromion process.

Resistance. The therapist's hand is placed on the anterior surface of the distal end of the humerus and pushes the arm backward toward horizontal abduction.

Substitutions. In a sitting position, trunk rotation can substitute. The arm can be inched across the supporting surface using the finger flexors.

Shoulder External Rotation

Prime Movers
  Infraspinatus
  Teres minor
  Posterior deltoid

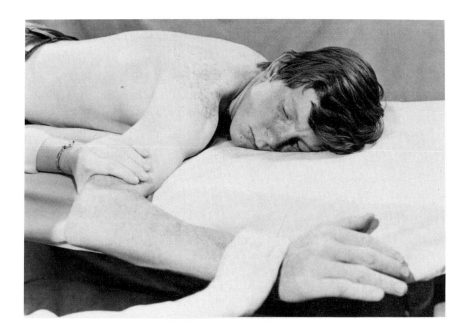

Figure 7.107 Resistance in the against-gravity position. The patient lies prone with the humerus abducted to 90° and supported on the table and the elbow flexed to 90° with the forearm dangling over the edge of the table. The patient externally rotates the humerus, bringing the dorsal surface of the hand toward the ceiling.

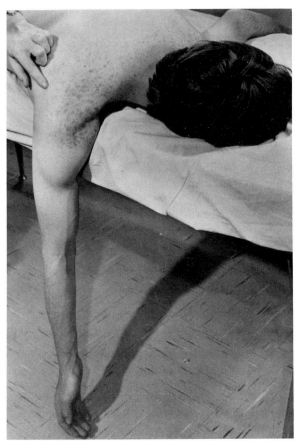

Figure 7.108 Gravity-eliminated position. The patient lies prone with the entire arm dangling over the edge of the table. He attempts to externally rotate the humerus.

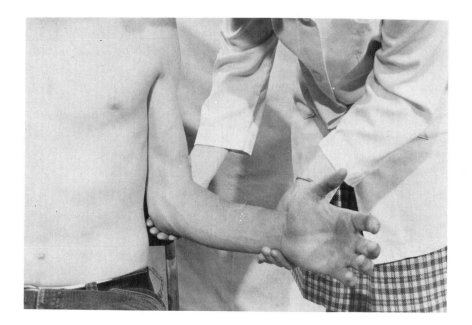

Figure 7.109 Alternate gravity-eliminated position. The patient sits with the humerus adducted and the elbow flexed to 90°. The hand moves laterally as the patient externally rotates the humerus.

Stabilize. Humerus above the elbow to allow only rotation.

Palpation. The infraspinatus is palpated inferiorly to the spine of the scapula. The teres minor is palpated between the posterior deltoid and the axillary border of the scapula; it is located superiorly to the teres major. Palpation of the posterior deltoid has been described.

Resistance. (1) Against gravity—the therapist's hand is placed on the dorsal surface of the distal end of the forearm and pushed toward the floor, keeping the patient's elbow supported and flexed to 90° to prevent supination. (2) Gravity-eliminated—the ther-

apist's hand encircles the distal end of the humerus and turns the humerus toward internal rotation.

Alternate gravity-eliminated position: the therapist's hand is placed on the dorsal surface of the distal end of the forearm and pushes forward, keeping the elbow flexed to 90°.

Substitutions. Scapula adduction combined with downward rotation can substitute. The triceps may substitute when resistance is applied in an against gravity position or in the alternate gravity-eliminated position. Supination may be mistaken for external rotation in a gravity-eliminated position.

Shoulder Internal Rotation

Prime Movers
  Subscapularis
  Teres major
  Latissimus dorsi
  Pectoralis major
  Anterior deltoid

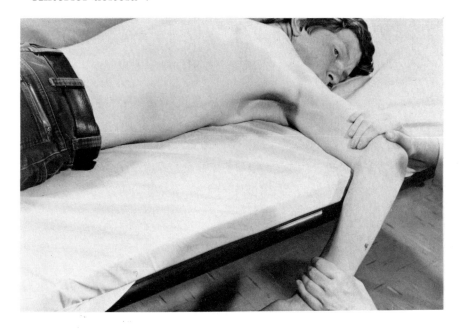

Figure 7.110 Resistance in the against-gravity position. The patient lies with the humerus abducted to 90° and supported on the table and the elbow flexed to 90° with the forearm dangling over the edge of the table. The patient internally rotates the humerus, bringing the palmar surface of the hand toward the ceiling.

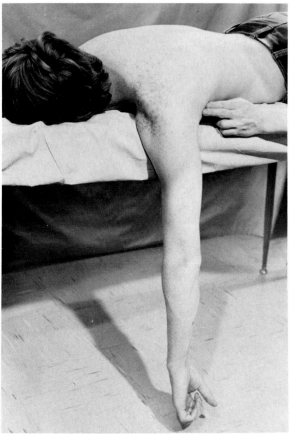

Figure 7.111 Gravity-eliminated position. The patient lies prone with the entire arm dangling over the edge of the table. He attempts to internally rotate the humerus.

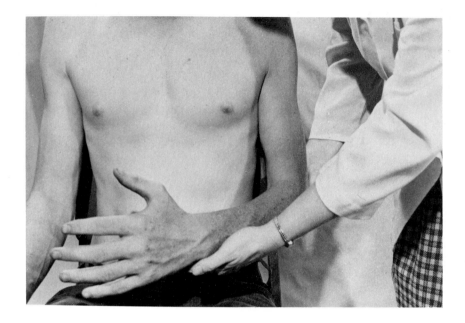

Figure 7.112 Alternate gravity-eliminated position. The patient sits with the humerus adducted and the elbow flexed to 90°. Patient's hand moves toward the abdomen as he internally rotates the humerus.

Stabilize. Humerus above the elbow to allow only rotation.

Palpation. The subscapularis is not easily palpated but may be palpated in the posterior axilla. The teres major, latissimus dorsi, pectoralis major, and anterior deltoid are palpated as previously described.

Resistance. (1) Against gravity—the therapist's hand is placed on the volar surface of the distal end of the forearm and pushes toward the floor, keeping the elbow supported and flexed to 90°. (2) Gravity-eliminated—the therapist's hand encircles the distal end of

the humerus and turns the humerus toward external rotation.

For alternate gravity-eliminated position: the therapist's hand is placed on the volar surface of the distal end of the forearm and pulls away from the abdomen, keeping the elbow flexed to 90°.

Substitutions. Scapula abduction combined with upward rotation can substitute. The triceps can substitute, as it did in external rotation. Pronation may be mistaken for internal rotation in a gravity-eliminated position.

Elbow Flexion

Prime Movers
Biceps
Brachialis
Brachioradialis

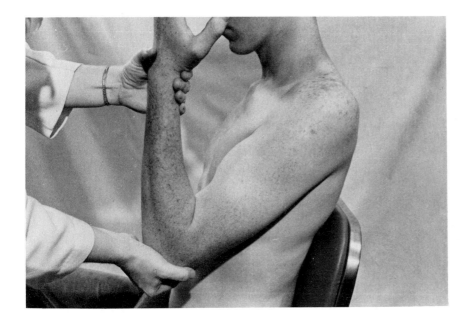

Figure 7.113 Resistance in the against-gravity position. The patient sits with his arm at the side in anatomical position. He raises his forearm so that the hand approximates the ipsilateral shoulder.

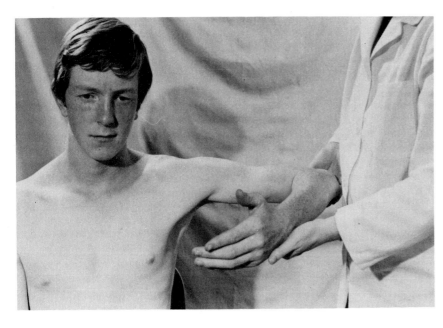

Figure 7.114 Gravity-eliminated position. The patient sits with the humerus abducted to 90° and the elbow extended, supported if necessary. The hand is relaxed. The patient attempts to flex the elbow.

Stabilize. Humerus.

Palpation. The biceps is easily palpated on the anterior surface of the humerus. With the biceps relaxed and the forearm pronated, the brachialis is palpated just medial to the distal biceps tendon. With the forearm in midposition the brachioradialis is palpated along the top of the proximal forearm.

Resistance. The therapist's hand is placed on the volar surface of the distal end of the forearm and pulls out toward extension.

Substitution. In a gravity-eliminated plane, the wrist extensors may substitute.

Elbow Extension

Prime Mover
  Triceps

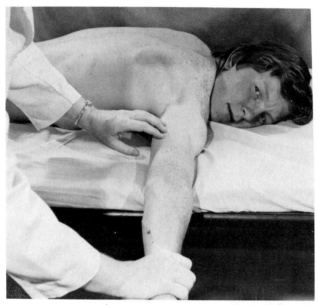

Figure 7.115 Resistance in the against-gravity position. The patient lies prone with the humerus abducted to 90° and supported on the table; the elbow is flexed and the forearm is hanging over the edge of the table. The patient extends the elbow.

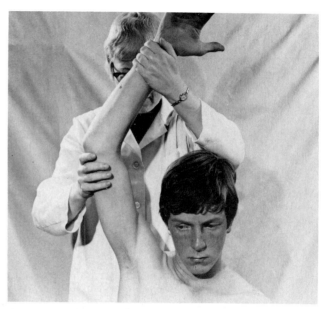

Figure 7.116 Alternate against-gravity position. The patient sits with the humerus flexed to 180° and the elbow fully flexed. He extends the elbow.

Note. If the shoulder is flaccid, avoid shoulder abduction and external rotation when moving the arm into a position of full shoulder flexion. Without the protection of its cuff musculature, abduction and rotation may place stress on the joint capsule and may dislocate the head of the humerus.

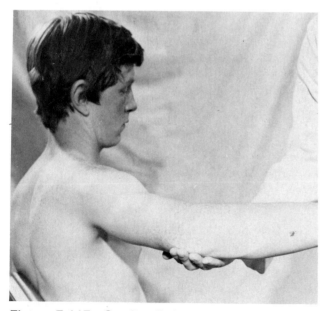

Figure 7.117 Gravity-eliminated position. The patient sits with the humerus abducted to 90° and supported if necessary; the elbow is fully flexed. The patient attempts to extend the elbow.

Stabilize. Humerus.

Palpation. The triceps is easily palpated on the posterior surface of the humerus.

Resistance. The therapist's hand is placed on the dorsal surface of the patient's forearm and pushes it toward flexion. Resistance is applied with the elbow in a position 10 to 15° less than full extension so that the elbow does not lock into position which could unreliably indicate strength where none existed.

Substitutions. Gravity may substitute in a sitting position. In the gravity-eliminated position, no external rotation of the shoulder is permitted in order to avoid letting extension occur due to the assistance of gravity. On a supporting surface, finger flexion may be used to inch the forearm across the surface.

Pronation

Prime Movers
    Pronator teres
    Pronator quadratus

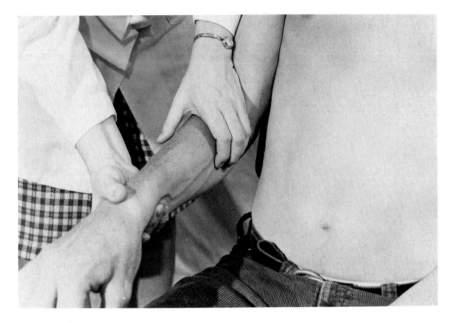

Figure 7.118 Resistance in the against-gravity position. The patient sits with the humerus adducted, the elbow flexed to 90°, the forearm supinated, and the wrist and fingers relaxed. The patient pronates to turn the palm down. *Note.* Gravity assists the motion beyond midposition.

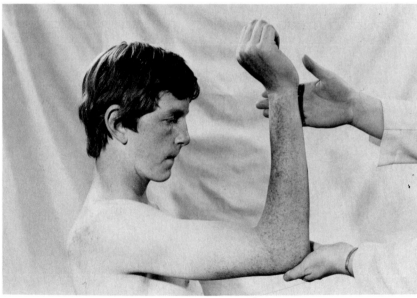

Figure 7.119 Gravity-eliminated position. The patient sits with the humerus flexed to 90° and supported, the elbow flexed to 90°, the forearm supinated, and the wrist and fingers relaxed. The patient pronates to turn the palm away from the face.

Stabilize. Humerus

Palpation. The pronator teres is palpated medially to the distal attachment of the biceps tendon on the volar surface of the proximal forearm. Pronator quadratus is too deep to palpate.

Resistance. The therapist's hand encircles the patient's volar wrist with the therapist's index finger extended along the forearm. The forearm is turned in the direction of supination.

Alternate methods of applying resistance are: (1) The therapist encircles the distal forearm by cupping the forearm between his thenar eminence and four fingers to avoid hurting the patient by applying force through the tips of the fingers and thumb. (2) The therapist interlaces the fingers of both his hands, and the patient's distal forearm is cupped between the therapist's opposing palms.

Substitutions. The wrist and finger flexors may substitute.

Supination

Prime Movers
Supinator
Biceps

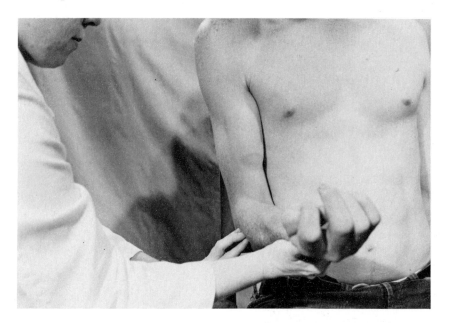

Figure 7.120 Resistance in the against-gravity position. The patients sits with the humerus adducted, the elbow flexed to 90°, the forearm pronated, and the wrist and fingers relaxed. The patients supinates to turn the palm up. *Note.* Gravity assists the motion beyond midposition.

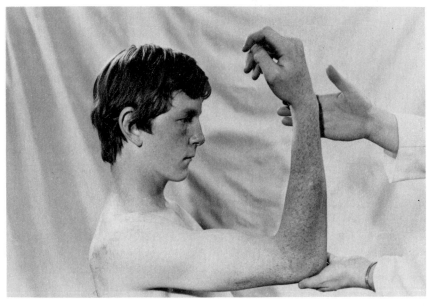

Figure 7.121 Gravity-eliminated position. The patient is positioned the same as for pronation, but with the forearm pronated. He attempts to turn the palm toward his face.

Note. To differentiate the supinator from the supination function of the biceps, test the supinator with elbow extended. The biceps does not supinate the extended arm unless resisted.[19]

Stabilize. Humerus.

Palpation. The supinator is palpated on the dorsal surface of the proximal forearm just distally to the head of the radius. Palpation of the biceps has been described.

Resistance. Same as for pronation except that the forearm is turned in the direction of pronation.

Substitutions. The wrist and finger extensors may substitute.

MUSCLES OF THE WRIST AND HAND

Many tendons of wrist and hand muscles cross more than one joint. For this reason test positions for individual muscles must include ways to minimize the effect of other muscles crossing the joint. As a general rule, to minimize the effect of a muscle, place the part to minimize or prevent its prime action. For example, to minimize the effect of the extensor pollicis longus on extension of the proximal joint of the thumb, the distal joint is flexed.

Wrist Extension

1. Extensor carpi radialis longus (ECRL)

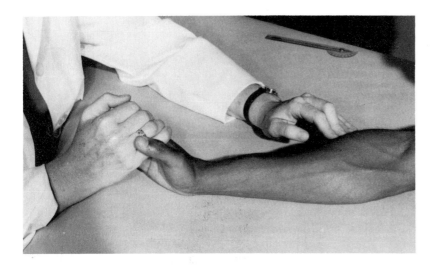

Figure 7.122 Resistance and palpation in the against-gravity position.

Position. (1) Against gravity—Forearm pronated to 45°, wrist flexed and ulnarly deviated, and the fingers and thumb relaxed. (2) Gravity-eliminated—Forearm in midposition, wrist flexed, fingers and thumb relaxed.

Stabilize. Forearm.

Test Motion. The patient extends the wrist toward the radial side.

Palpation. The tendon of the ECRL is palpated on the dorsal surface of the wrist at the base of the second metacarpal. The muscle belly is found on the dorsal proximal forearm adjacent to the brachioradialis.

Resistance. The therapist's palm is placed across the dorsum of the patient's hand on the radial side and pushes toward combined wrist flexion and ulnar deviation.

Substitutions. Extensor pollicis longus, extensor digitorum.

2. Extensor carpi radialis brevis (ECRB)

3. Extensor carpi ulnaris (ECU)

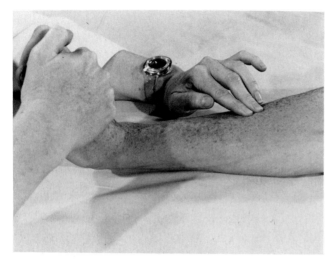

Figure 7.123 Resistance and palpation in the against-gravity position.

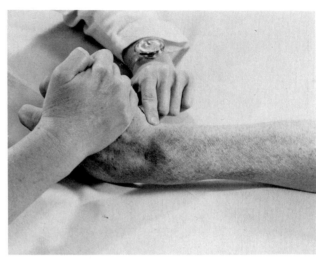

Figure 7.124 Resistance and palpation in the against-gravity position.

Position. (1) Against gravity—Forearm is fully pronated, the wrist is flexed and undeviated, the fingers and thumb are relaxed. (2) Gravity-eliminated—Same as for ECRL.

Stabilize. Forearm.

Test Motion. The patient extends the wrist without deviation.

Palpation. The tendon of the ECRB is palpated on the dorsal surface of the wrist at the base of the third metacarpal adjacent to the ECRL. The muscle belly of ECRB is found distal to the belly of ECRL on the dorsal surface of the proximal forearm.

Resistance. The therapist's palm is placed across the dorsum of the patient's hand and pushes directly toward flexion.

Substitutions. Extenxor pollicis longus; extensor digitorum.

Position. (1) Against gravity—Shoulder internally rotated, forearm fully pronated, wrist flexed and radially deviated, and fingers relaxed. (2) Gravity-eliminated—Forearm pronated to 45°, wrist flexed and radially deviated, fingers relaxed.

Stabilize. Forearm.

Test Motion. Patient extends the wrist toward the ulnar side.

Palpation. The ECU tendon is palpated on the dorsal surface of the wrist between the head of the ulna and the base of the fifth metacarpal. The muscle belly is found approximately 2 inches distal to the lateral epicondyle of the humerus.[18]

Resistance. The therapist's palm is placed across the dorsum of the patient's hand on the ulnar side and pushes toward combined wrist flexion and radial deviation.

Substitutions. Extensor digitorum.

Wrist Flexion

1. Flexor carpi radialis (FCR)

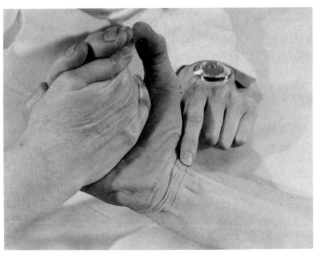

Figure 7.125 Resistance and palpation in the against-gravity position.

2. Palmaris longus

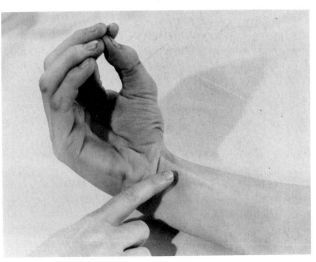

Figure 7.126

Position. (1) Against gravity—Forearm supinated, wrist extended, and fingers and thumb relaxed. (2) Gravity-eliminated—Forearm in midposition, wrist extended, and fingers and thumb relaxed.

Stabilize. Forearm.

Test Motion. Patient flexes the wrist.

Palpation. The FCR tendon is palpated on the volar surface of the wrist in line with the second metacarpal and radial to the palmaris longus (if present).

Resistance. The therapist's fingers are placed across the patient's palm and pull toward wrist extension.

Substitutions. Abductor pollicus longus; flexor pollicis longus; flexor digitorum superficialis; and flexor digitorum profundus.

The palmaris longus is a weak wrist flexor which has a small muscle belly and long tendon. The tendon crosses the center of the volar surface of the wrist. It is not tested for strength and may not even be present. However, if it is present, it will stand out prominently in the middle of the wrist when wrist flexion is resisted or the palm cupped.

3. Flexor carpi ulnaris (FCU)

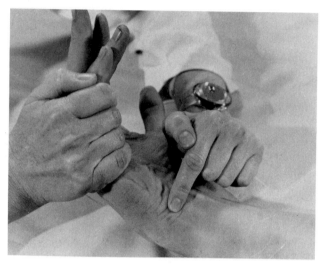

Figure 7.127 Resistance in the against-gravity position. The therapist's finger points to the tendon.

Position. (1) Against gravity—Shoulder adducted and externally rotated, forearm fully supinated, wrist extended, and fingers relaxed. (2) Gravity-eliminated—Forearm supinated to 45°, wrist extended, and fingers relaxed.

Stabilize. Forearm.

Test Motion. Patient flexes the wrist toward ulnar deviation.

Palpation. The FCU tendon is palpated on the volar surface of the wrist just proximally to the pisiform bone.

Resistance. The therapist's fingers are placed across the patient's palm and pull toward wrist extension and radial deviation.

Substitutions. Flexor digitorum superficialis; flexor digitorum profundus.

Finger DIP Flexion

Flexor digitorum profundus (FDP)

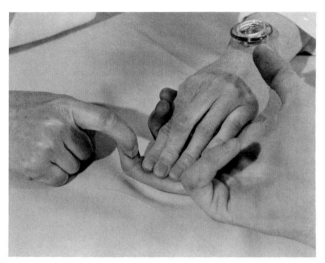

Figure 7.128 Resistance in the against-gravity position.

Position. (1) Against gravity—Forearm supinated and supported on a table; wrist and interphalangeal joints relaxed. (2) Gravity-eliminated—Forearm in midposition, resting on ulnar border on a table; wrist and interphalangeal joints relaxed in neutral position.

Stabilize. Middle phalanx of each finger as it is tested to prevent flexion of the proximal interphalangeal joint; wrist should remain in neutral.

Test Motion. Flexion of the distal phalanx toward the middle phalanx.

Palpation. The belly of the FDP is palpated just volarly to the ulna in the proximal third of the forearm. The tendons are sometimes palpable on the volar surface of the middle phalanges.

Resistance. The therapist places one finger on the pad of the patient's finger and pulls toward extension.

Substitutions. Rebound effect of apparent flexion following contraction of extensors. Wrist extension causes tenodesis action.

Finger PIP Flexion

Flexor digitorum superficialis (FDS)
Flexor digitorum profundus

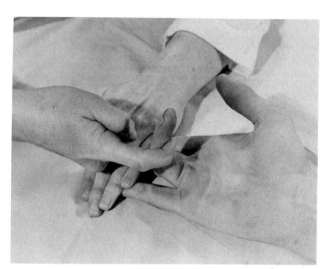

Figure 7.129 Resistance in the against-gravity position for flexor digitorum superficialis.

Position (for flexor digitorum superficialis). (1) Against gravity—Forearm supinated and supported on the table; wrist and metacarpophalangeal (MP) joints relaxed. To rule out the influence of the profoundus when testing the superificialis, hold all interphalangeal joints of the fingers not being tested into full extension. Because the profundus is essentially one muscle with four tendons, by preventing its action in three of the four fingers, it cannot work in the tested finger. In fact, the patient is unable to flex the distal joint of the tested finger at all! In some people the profundus slip to the index finger is such that this method cannot rule out its influence on the PIP joint of the index finger. This should be noted on the test form. (2) Gravity-eliminated—Forearm supported in midposition, with the wrist and MP joints relaxed in neutral position. Again rule out the influence of the FDP by holding all the joints of the nontested fingers in extension.

Stabilize. Proximal phalanx of the finger being tested and hold all joints of the other fingers into extension; the wrist should remain in neutral.

Test Motion. Patient flexes PIP joint.

Palpation. The superficialis is palpated on the volar surface of the proximal forearm toward the ulnar side. The tendons may be palpated at the wrist between the palmaris longus and the flexor carpi ulnaris.

Resistance. Using one finger, the therapist pulls the head of the middle phalanx toward extension.

Substitutions. Flexor digitorum profundus. Wrist extension caused tenodesis action.

Finger MP Flexion

Flexor digitorum profundus
Flexor digitorum superficialis
Dorsal interossei
Volar (Palmar) interossei
Flexor digiti minimi

The tests for the first four muscles have been or will be discussed under their alternate actions. The flexor of the little finger has no other action and is described here.

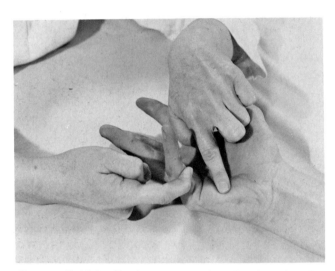

Figure 7.130 Resistance and palpation in the against-gravity position for flexor digiti minimi.

Position (for flexor digiti minimi). (1) Against gravity—Forearm supported in supination. (2) Gravity-eliminated—Forearm supported in midposition.

Stabilize. Other fingers in extension.

Test Motion. Patient flexes fifth finger at MP joint without flexing the interphalangeal joints.

Palpation. On the volar surface of the hypothenar eminence.

Resistance. Using one finger, the therapist pushes the head of the proximal phalanx toward extension. The therapist must be sure the interphalangeal joints remain extended.

Substitutions. Flexor digitorum profundus; flexor digitorum superficialis; third volar interosseus.

Finger Adduction

Volar (Palmar) interossei (3)

[handwritten: difficult to palpate middle finger doesn't have palmar interossei]

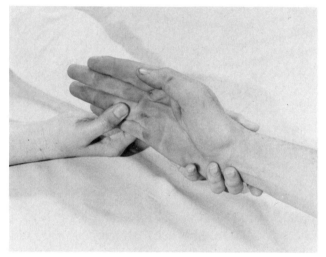

Figure 7.131 Resistance in the against-gravity position for palmar interossei 2 and 3.

Position. (1) Against gravity—For palmar interossei 2 and 3, support the forearm on the ulnar border of the wrist with the fingers extended and abducted. For palmar interosseus 1, the arm is internally rotated, the forearm fully pronated so that the hand can be supported on the radial border, with the hand free and the fingers extended and abducted. (2) Gravity-eliminated—Forearm is supinated and supported.

Stabilize. Support the hand lightly.

Test Motion. As each is tested, the patient moves the index, ring, or little finger toward the middle finger.

Palpation. The palmar interossei are usually too deep to palpate with certainty. When these muscles are atrophied the areas between the metacarpals on the volar surface appear sunken.

Resistance. One by one, the therapist pulls the head of the proximal phalanx of each finger being tested away from the middle finger.

Substitutions. Extrinsic finger flexors; gravity, depending upon the position of the hand, most usually substitutes for the first palmar interosseus.

Finger Abduction

Dorsal interossei (4)
Abductor digiti minimi

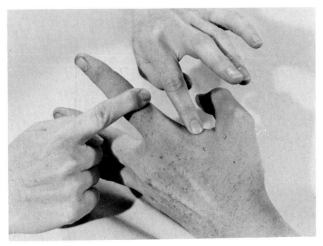

Figure 7.132 Resistance and palpation in the against-gravity position for dorsal interosseus 1.

Position. (1) Against gravity—For dorsal interossei 1 and 2, the forearm rests on the ulnar border on a supporting surface with the hand free and MPs adducted and slightly flexed. For dorsal interossei 3 and 4 and abductor digiti minimi, the arm is internally rotated, with the forearm fully pronated so that it can be supported on the radial border. The MPs are adducted and slightly flexed. Flexion of the MPs minimizes the abduction caused by the angle of pull of the extensor digitorum. (2) Gravity-eliminated—Forearm is pronated and supported with the hand free and MPs adducted and slightly flexed.

Stabilize. Support the hand lightly.

Test Motion. One by one, the patient moves the index finger away from the middle finger, the middle finger toward the index, the middle toward the ring finger, the ring finger toward the little finger, and the little finger away from the ring finger.

Palpation. The first dorsal interosseus fills the dorsal web space and can be easily palpated there. The abductor digiti minimi is palpated on the ulnar border of the fifth metacarpal. The other interossei lie between the metacarpals on the dorsal aspect of the hand where they may be palpated and on some people the tendons can be palpated as they enter the dorsal expansion near the heads of the metacarpals. When the dorsal interossei are atrophied, the spaces between the metacarpals appear sunken.

Resistance. The therapist pushes the head of the proximal phalanx of each finger, in turn, toward the direction opposite to its test motion.

Substitutions. Extensor digitorum; gravity, especially for dorsal interossei 3 and 4 and the abductor digiti minimi.

Finger MP Extension

Extensor digitorum (ED)
Extensor indicis proprius
Extensor digiti minimi

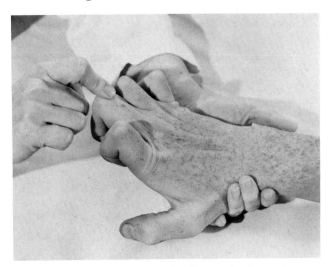

Figure 7.133 Resistance in the against-gravity position for extensor digitorum.

Position. (1) Against gravity—Forearm pronated and supported, wrist supported in neutral position, and fingers flexed at all joints. (2) Gravity-eliminated—Forearm supported in midposition, wrist in neutral, and fingers flexed.

Stabilize. Wrist and metacarpals.

Test Motion. Patient extends MP joints keeping the PIP and DIP joints flexed.

Palpation. The muscle belly of the ED is palpated on the dorsal-ulnar surface of the proximal forearm. Often the separate muscle bellies can be discerned. The tendons of this muscle are readily seen and palpated on the dorsum of the hand.

The extensor indicis tendon is located ulnarly to the extensor digitorum tendon. The belly of this muscle is palpated on the mid- to distal dorsal forearm between the radius and ulna.

The extensor digiti minimi tendon is palpated ulnarly to the ED. Actually, it is the tendon that looks as if it were the ED tendon to the little finger because the ED to the little finger is only a slip from the ED tendon to the ring finger.

Resistance. Using one finger, the therapist pushes the head of each proximal phalanx toward flexion, one at a time.

Substitution. Apparent extension of the fingers can occur due to the rebound effect of relaxation following finger flexion. Flexion of the wrist can cause finger extension through tenodesis action.

Finger Interphalangeal Extension

Lumbricales
Interossei
Extensor digitorum
Extensor indicis proprius
Extensor digiti minimi

According to electromyographical evidence, the intrinsics, especially the lumbricales, are the primary extensors of the interphalangeal joints.[20, 21] Except for the lumbricales, the other muscles have been discussed. The lumbricales, arising as they do from the flexor profundus and inserting on the extensor digitorum, have a unique duty in regard to finger extension. Contracting against the noncontracting flexor profundus, the lumbricales pull the tendons of that muscle forward toward the fingertips. This slackens the profundus tendons distal to the insertion of the lumbricales, allowing the extensor digitorum to fully extend the interphalangeal joints, regardless of the position of the MP joints.[21, 22] It has been electromyographically demonstrated that the profundus and the lumbricales operate out of phase with each other except during flexion of the metacarpophalageal joints while the interphalangeal joints are extended or extending.[21] Electromyographic evidence exists which shows that the interossei flex the MP joints while extending the interphalangeal joints and, in fact, operate to extend only when the MP joint is flexed or flexing.[21]

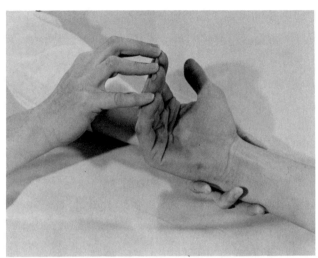

Figure 7.134 Resistance in the against-gravity position for testing lumbricales.

Position (lumbricales). There is no reliably good test for lumbrical function. Test 1 is the traditional test used. Test 2 is an hypothesized test. (1) Against gravity—Test 1: forearm supinated and supported. Wrist in neutral position, MPs extended, IPs flexed. Test 2: (alternate) MPs flexed and IPs extended. (2) Gravity-eliminated—same as above except that the forearm is supported in midposition.

Stabilize. Metacarpals.

Test Motion. Test 1—From the starting position, the patient simultaneously flexes his MP joints while extending his IP joints. The concept of this motion is difficult for patients to understand and will need practice.

Test 2—A perfectly adequate test, based on the electromyographical evidence, could be to have the patient maintain full IP extension while moving from a position of MP flexion to MP extension.

Palpation. Lumbricales lie too deeply to be palpated.

Resistance. Test 1—The therapist holds the tip of the finger being tested and pushes it toward starting position.

Test 2—The therapist places one finger on the patient's fingernail and pushes toward flexion.

Substitution. Nothing substitutes for DIP extension in the event of the loss of lumbrical function when the MP joint is extended. Other muscles of the dorsal expansion can substitute for DIP extension when the MP joint is flexed.

Thumb IP Extension

Extensor pollicis longus (EPL)

Thumb MP Extension

Extensor pollicis brevis (EPB)
Extensor pollicis longus

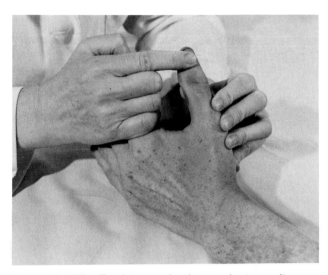

Figure 7.135 Resistance in the against-gravity position.

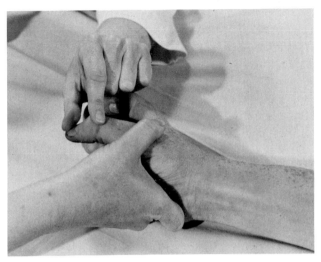

Figure 7.136 Resistance in the against-gravity position for extensor pollicis brevis.

Position. (1) Against gravity—Forearm supported in midposition, thumb flexed. (2) Gravity-eliminated—Forearm pronated, thumb flexed.

Stabilize. Proximal phalanx.

Test Motion. Patient extends the IP joint of the thumb.

Palpation. The tendon of the EPL may be palpated on the ulnar border of the anatomical snuff box and also on the dorsal surface of the proximal phalanx of the thumb.

Resistance. The therapist places one finger over the dorsum of the distal phalanx (thumbnail) and pushes toward flexion.

Substitutions. Relaxation of the flexor pollicis longus will result in apparent extensor movement due to rebound effect.

Position (test for extensor pollicis brevis). (1) Against gravity—Forearm supported in midposition, MP joint flexed, IP joint flexed. (2) Gravity-eliminated—Forearm pronated, MP joint flexed, IP joint flexed.

Stabilize. First metacarpal in abduction.

Test Motion. The patient extends the MP joint, keeping the IP joint flexed to minimize the effect of the extensor pollicis longus. The EPB may not be present.

Palpation. The tendon of the EPB is palpated on the radial border of the anatomical snuff box medial to the tendon of the abductor pollicis longus.

Resistance. The therapist's finger is placed on the dorsal surface of the head of the proximal phalanx and pushes toward flexion.

Substitution. Extensor pollicis longus.

Thumb Abduction

Abductor pollicis longus (APL)
Abductor pollicis brevis (APB)

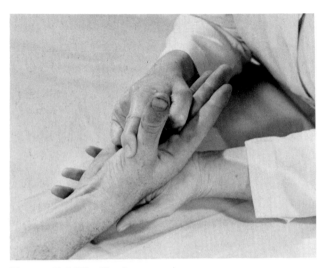

Figure 7.137 Resistance in the against-gravity position for abductor pollicis longus.

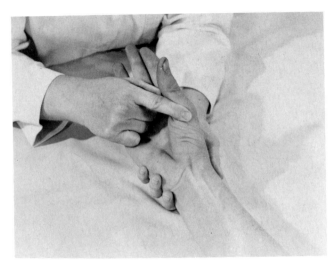

Figure 7.138 Resistance in the against-gravity position for abductor pollicis brevis.

Position (for abductor pollicis longus). (1) Against-gravity—Forearm supinated to 45°, wrist in neutral, thumb adducted. (2) Gravity-eliminated—Forearm pronated to 45°, wrist in neutral, thumb adducted.

Stabilize. Support the wrist on the ulnar side and hold it in neutral position.

Test Motion. Patient abducts the thumb in a radial direction on a diagonal plane between extension and true abduction.

Palpation. The tendon of the APL is palpated at the wrist joint just distally to the radial styloid and laterally to the EPB.

Resistance. The therapist's finger presses the head of the first metacarpal toward adduction.

Substitutions. Abductor pollicis brevis; extensor pollicis brevis.

Position (for abductor pollicis brevis). (1) Against-gravity—Forearm is supported in supination, wrist in neutral, thumb adducted. (2) Gravity-eliminated—Forearm is supported in midposition, wrist in neutral, thumb adducted.

Stabilize. Support the wrist in neutral position by holding it on the dorsal and ulnar side.

Test Motion. The patient abducts the thumb, bringing it straight up from the palm.

Palpation. APB is palpated over the center of the thenar eminence

Resistance. The therapist's finger presses the head of the first metacarpal toward adduction.

Substitution. Abductor pollicis longus.

Thumb MP Flexion

Flexor pollicis brevis (FPB)
Flexor pollicis longus (FPL)

Thumb IP Flexion

Flexor pollicis longus

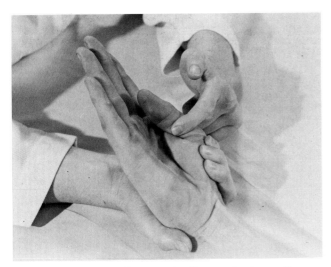

Figure 7.139 Resistance in the against-gravity position for flexor pollicis brevis.

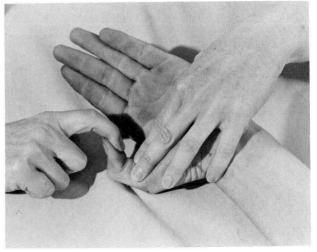

Figure 7.140 Resistance and palpation in the against-gravity position for flexor pollicis longus.

Position (for flexor pollicis brevis). (1) Against-gravity—Elbow flexed and forearm supinated so that the palmar surface of the thumb faces the ceiling; thumb is extended at both the MP and IP joints. (2) Gravity-eliminated—Forearm supinated to 90° so that thumb can flex across the plane of the palm.

Stabilize. First metacarpal.

Test Motion. Patient flexes the MP joint but keeps the IP joint extended to minimize the influence of the flexor pollicus longus.

Palpation. The FPB is palpated on the thenar eminence just proximal to the MP joint, and medial to the abductor pollicis brevis.

Resistance. The therapist's finger pushes the head of the proximal phalanx toward extension.

Substitution. Flexor pollicis longus.

Position (for flexor pollicis longus). (1) Against-gravity—Elbow flexed and forearm supinated so that the palmar surface of the thumb faces the ceiling; thumb extended at the MP and IP joints. (2) Gravity-eliminated—Forearm supinated to 90° so that the thumb can flex across the palm.

Stabilize. Proximal phalanx, holding MP joint in extension.

Test Motion. Patient flexes IP joint.

Palpation. The FPL tendon is palpated on the palmar surface of the proximal phalanx.

Resistance. The therapist's finger pushes the head of the distal phalanx toward extension.

Substitution. Relaxation of the extensor pollicis longus causes rebound movement.

Thumb Adduction

Adductor pollicis

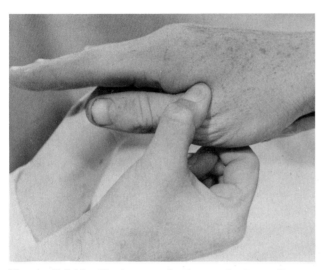

Figure 7.141 Resistance in the against-gravity position.

Position. (1) Against gravity—Forearm pronated, wrist and fingers in neutral, thumb abducted and MP and IP joints of the thumb in extension. (2) Gravity-eliminated—Same, except forearm in midposition.

Stabilize. Metacarpals of fingers, keeping the MP joints in neutral.

Test Motion. Patient brings the thumb toward the palm, without hyperextending the MP joint or flexing the MP or IP joints.

Palpation. Adductor pollicis is palpated on the palmar surface of the thumb web space.

Resistance. The therapist grasps the head of the proximal phalanx and pulls it away from the palm toward abduction.

Substitutions. Extensor pollicis longus; flexor pollicis longus; flexor pollicis brevis.

Opposition

Opponens pollicis
Opponens digiti minimi

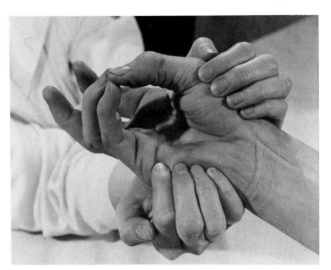

Figure 7.142 Resistance in the against-gravity position.

Position. (1) Against-gravity—Forearm supinated and supported, wrist in neutral, thumb adducted and extended. (2) Gravity-eliminated—Elbow resting on the table with forearm perpendicular to the table, wrist in neutral, thumb adducted and extended.

Stabilize. Hold the wrist in a neutral position.

Test Motion. The patient brings the thumb away from and across the palm rotating it so that the pad of the thumb approximates the pad of the little finger. The little finger rotates around to meet the thumb.

Palpation. Place fingertips along the lateral side of the shaft of the first metacarpal where opponens pollicis may be palpated before it becomes deep to the abductor pollicis brevis. The opponens digiti minimi can be palpated volarly along the shaft of the fifth metacarpal.

Resistance. The therapist holds along the first metacarpal and "derotates" the thumb or holds along the fifth metacarpal and "derotates" the little finger. These can be resisted simultaneously using both hands (see Fig. 7.142).

Substitutions. Abductor pollicis brevis; flexor pollicis brevis; flexor pollicis longus.

MEASUREMENT OF THE LOWER EXTREMITY

Hip Flexion

Prime Movers
  Iliopsoas
    Iliacus
    Psoas major

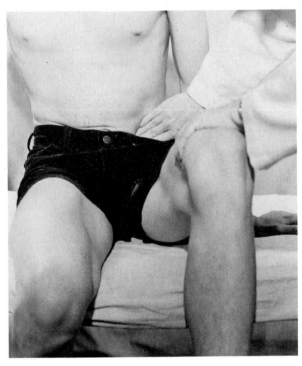

Figure 7.143 Resistance in the against-gravity position. The patient sits with his lower leg hanging over the edge of the sitting surface. He raises the thigh up from the surface; the knee remains flexed.

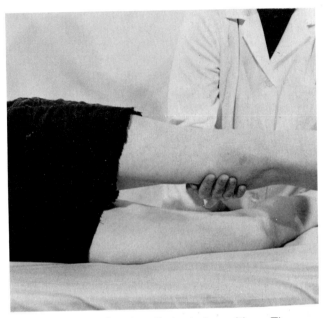

Figure 7.144 Gravity-eliminated position. The patient is side-lying on the side opposite the leg being tested. The leg to be tested is supported in extension at the hip and knee and in a position of 0° of abduction to align the leg and trunk. The patient flexes the hip as the therapist supports the leg in abduction; the knee may flex.

Stabilize. Pelvis.
Palpation. The iliacus is too deep to be palpated. In a sitting position the psoas major can be palpated with the patient bending forward to relax the abdominal muscles. The therapist's fingers are placed at the waist between the ribs and the iliac crest and pressure is applied posteriorly to feel the contraction of the psoas major as the hip flexes.[18]

Resistance. The therapist's hand is placed on the distal anterior thigh and presses downward toward extension.
Substitution. The abdominals can tilt the pelvis posteriorly to substitute for hip flexion in a gravity-eliminated position.

Hip Extension

Prime Movers
    Gluteus maximus
    Biceps femoris[19]

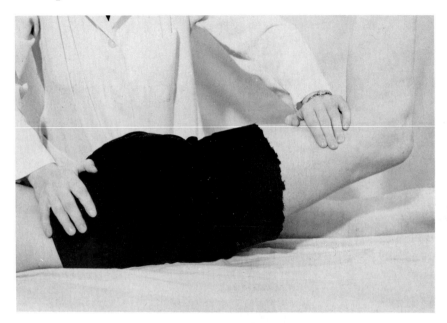

Figure 7.145 Resistance in the against-gravity position. The patient lies prone with knee flexed to shorten and weaken the hamstrings.[15, 16, 23]* (Hamstrings will be tested as knee flexors.) The patient extends the hip keeping the knee flexed.

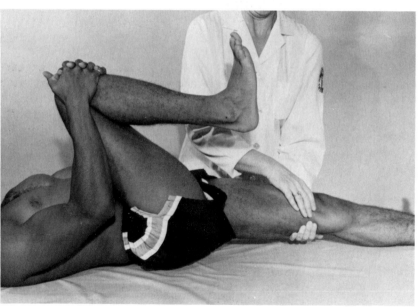

Figure 7.146 Alternate against-gravity position. The patient lies supine and holds the opposite leg in flexion at the hip and knee. The therapist holds the leg to be tested just above the knee and instructs the patient, "Do not let me raise your leg."[24] Grading: normal if trunk comes up from table; fair if the hip "gives" as the trunk begins to come up from the table.

---

* This idea needs to be supported by electromyographic kinesiological study, since it is contrary to the principle of minimizing the effect of a two-joint muscle which was stated earlier. Concepts based on anatomical analysis only have begun to be proven inadequate now that better technology exists for studying complex patterns of muscle action.

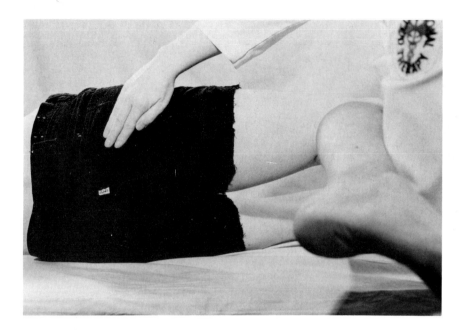

Figure 7.147 Gravity-eliminated position. The patient is side-lying with hip in neutral and knee flexed. The leg to be tested is on top. The patient extends the thigh.

Stabilize. Pelvis and lumbar spine.

Palpation. The gluteus maximus is the larger muscle of the buttock and can be easily palpated. The biceps femoris can be palpated on the posterior aspect of the thigh; its tendon bounds the popliteal fossa laterally.

Resistance. The therapist's hand is placed over the distal posterior thigh and presses downward or forward toward flexion.

Substitutions. Extension of the lumbar spine. The semimembranosus and semitendinosus assist resisted hip extension if the hip is abducted.[19]

Note. Gluteus maximus and hamstrings may be tested together as hip extensors with the knee extended.

Hip Abduction

Prime Movers
   Gluteus medius
   Gluteus minimus

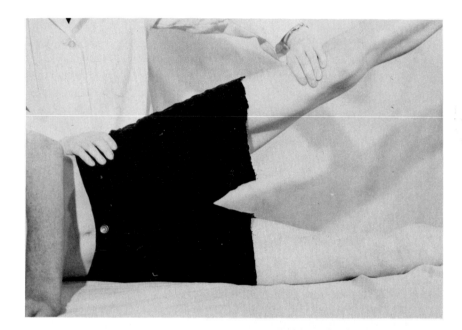

Figure 7.148 Resistance in the against-gravity position. The patient is side-lying on the side opposite the leg to be tested with that leg flexed at the hip and knee for balance. The leg to be tested is extended at the hip and knee and in alignment with the trunk. The patient moves the leg away from the midline of the body.

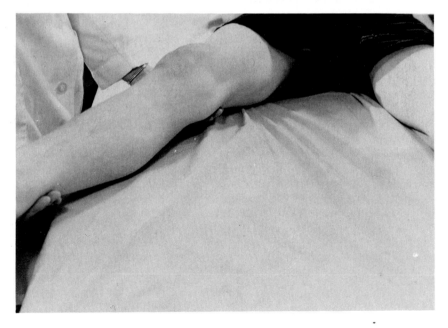

Figure 7.149 Gravity-eliminated position. The patient lies supine with hip and knee extended. He moves the leg away from midline.

Stabilize. Pelvis.
Palpation. The gluteus medius and minimus are palpated together laterally to the hip joint below the iliac crest.

Resistance. The therapist's hand is placed on the distal lateral thigh and pushes the leg toward the midline of the body.
Substitutions. Lateral flexion of the trunk; hip external rotation and flexion.

Hip Adduction

Prime Movers
   Adductor magnus
   Adductor longus
   Adductor brevis

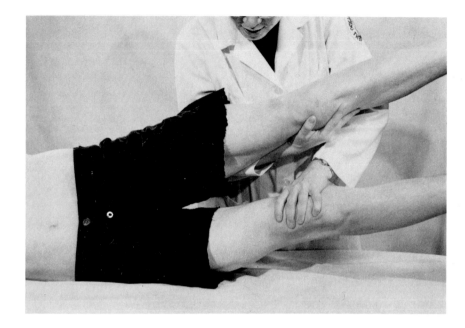

Figure 7.150 Resistance in the against-gravity position. The patient is side-lying on the leg to be tested with the other leg supported in abduction. Both legs are in extension at the hip and knee. The patient adducts the leg being tested, without rotating, to bring it toward the other leg and across the midline.

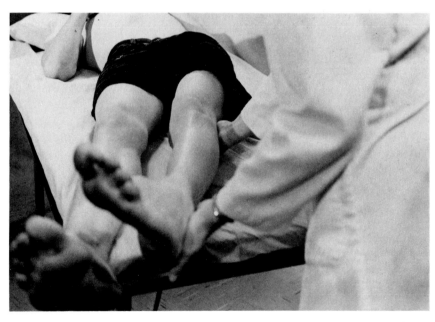

Figure 7.151 Gravity-eliminated position. The patient lies supine with both legs in abduction and extended at the hips and knees. The therapist supports the leg as the patient attempts to adduct across midline.

Stabilize. Pelvis.

Palpation. The adductors are palpated on the medial thigh.

Resistance. The therapist's hand is placed on the distal medial thigh and pushes the leg downward or outward toward abduction.

Substitutions. In the sidelying position hip internal rotation and flexion may substitute. In the supine position hip external rotation may substitute.

Hip Internal Rotation

Prime Movers
  Gluteus medius
  Gluteus minimus
  Tensor fasciae latae

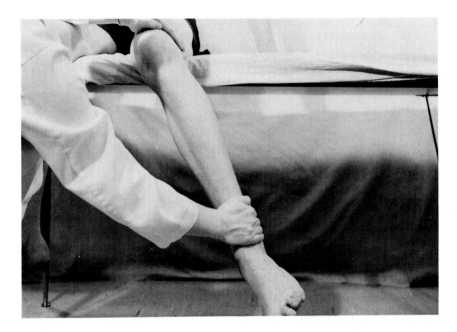

Figure 7.152 Resistance in the against-gravity position. The patient sits with the lower leg hanging over the edge of the sitting surface. The patient internally rotates the thigh, moving his foot laterally.

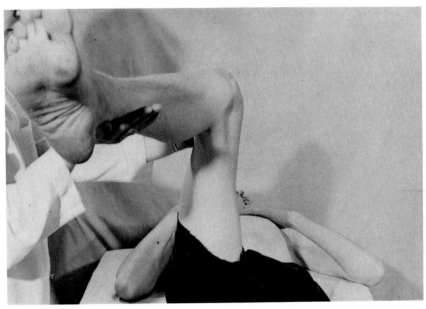

Figure 7.153 Gravity-eliminated position. The patient lies supine with hip flexed to 90°. The leg which is not being tested remains in extension. The patient internally rotates the thigh moving his foot laterally.

Stabilize. Femur above the knee to allow only rotation.

Palpation. Palpate the gluteus medius and minimus laterally to the hip joint. The tensor fasciae latae is located just anteriorly to the gluteus medius and below the anterior superior iliac spine.

Resistance. The therapist's hand is placed on the distal lateral part of the lower leg and pushes the foot medially, applying force toward external rotation.

Substitutions. Hip adduction and flexion.

A Knee Extension

Prime Movers
 Quadriceps
  Rectus femoris
  Vastus medialis
  Vastus intermedius
  Vastus lateralis

Hip External Rotation

Prime Movers
 Gluteus maximus
 Obturator internus and externus
 Gemellus superior and inferior
 Piriformis
 Quadratus femoris

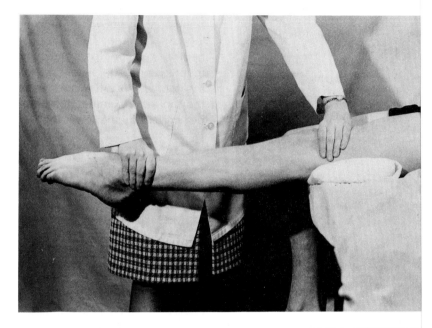

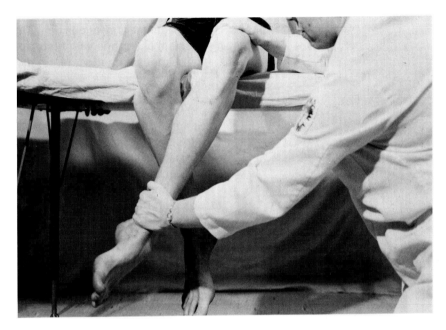

Figure 7.154 Resistance in the against-gravity position. The patient sits with the lower leg hanging over the edge of the sitting surface. The patient externally rotates the thigh, moving his foot medially.

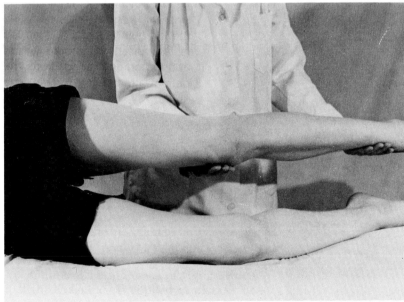

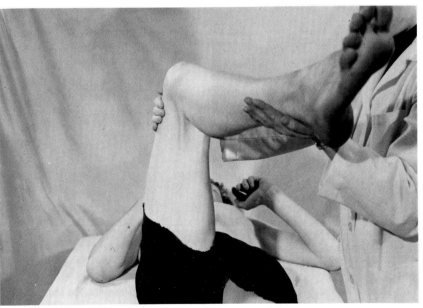

Figure 7.155 Gravity-eliminated position. The patient lies supine with the hip flexed to 90°. The leg not being tested remains in extension. The patient externally rotates the thigh, moving his foot medially.

Stabilize. Thigh.

Palpation. The tendon of the quadriceps may be palpated as it approaches the patella. Except for the vastus intermedius the muscle bellies can be palpated on the anterior surface of the thigh; the rectus is in the center and lies over the intermedius; the other vasti are palpated medially and laterally to the rectus.

Resistance
distal end of
ance is app
maximum in
can result fi
ance. It is
quadriceps.[2]
Substitution

Stabilize. Femur above the knee to allow only rotation.

Palpation. Palpation of the gluteus maximus has been described. The six small rotators are palpated as a group posteriorly to the greater trochanter.

Resistance. The therapist's hand is placed on the distal medial part of the lower leg and pulls the foot laterally toward internal rotation.

Substitutions. Hip abduction and flexion.

Evaluation **213**

Knee Flexion

Prime Movers
  Hamstrings
    Semimembranosus
    Semitendinosus
    Biceps femoris

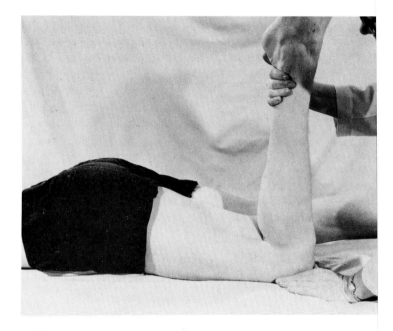

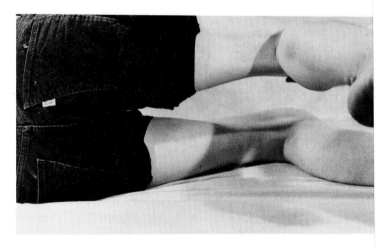

Stabilize. Thigh.

Palpation. These three muscles can be palpated on the posterior surface of the thigh. The tendon of the biceps femoris can be palpated on the lateral side of the popliteal space, and the tendon of the semitendinosus may be palpated on the medial side of the popliteal space. Both tendons become prominent when resistance is applied.[18] The biceps femoris can be isolated from the other muscles by rotating the ankle laterally while the lower leg is flexed. The semimembranosus and semitendinosus will contract more strongly if the ankle is rotated medially.

Re
dista
push
to on
medi
Su
beyo

Ankle Inversion

Prime Movers
  Tibialis posterior
  Tibialis anterior

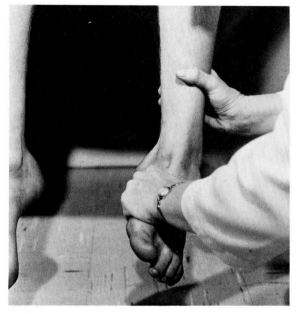

Figure 7.165 Resistance in the against-gravity position. The patient sits erect with the lower leg hanging free. Foot is in neutral position. The patient moves the foot so that the sole of the foot faces medially.

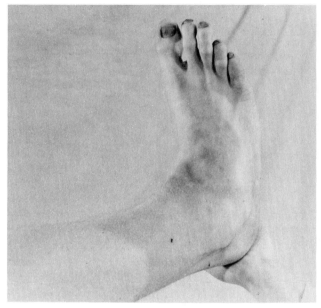

Figure 7.166 Gravity-eliminated position. The patient lies supine with the hip and knee flexed to 90°. Foot is in neutral position. The patient moves the foot so that the sole of the foot faces medially.

Stabilize. Distal part of the lower leg.

Palpation. The tendon of the tibialis posterior may be palpated on and above the medial malleolus. Palpation of the tibialis anterior has been described.

Resistance. The therapist places his hand on the medial surface of the forefoot and holds the first metatarsal between the heel of his hand and his fingers. He pulls the forefoot toward eversion.

Substitutions. Extrinsic toe flexors; external rotation of the hip when the patient is lying down with hips and knees extended.

Ankle Eversion

Prime Movers
    Peroneus longus
    Peroneus brevis
    Peroneus tertius

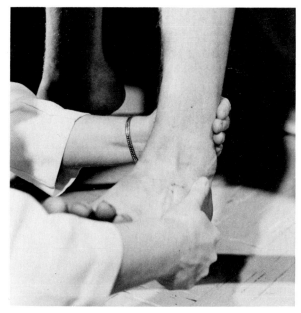

Figure 7.167 Resistance in the against-gravity position. The starting position is the same as for inversion; however, the patient moves the foot so that the sole of the foot faces laterally.

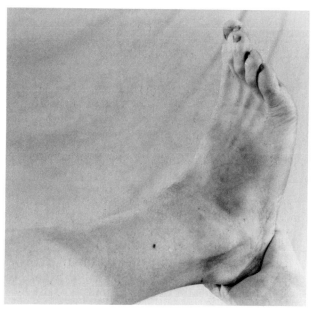

Figure 7.168 Gravity-eliminated position. The starting position is the same as for inversion; the patient moves the foot so that the sole of the foot faces laterally.

Stabilize. Distal lower leg.

Palpation. Peroneus longus is palpated just below the head of the fibula. The tendons of peroneus longus and brevis pass behind the lateral malleolus. The tendon of the peroneus brevis can be seen as it passes to its insertion on the fifth metatarsal. In some persons, the tendon of the longus may be distinguished from the brevis above the malleolus: the longus is adjacent but more posterior. Peroneus tertius is anterior to the lateral malleolus and is palpated lateral to the tendon to the fifth toe.[18]

Resistance. The therapist's hand is placed on the lateral surface of the forefoot and holds the fifth metatarsal between the heel of his hand and his fingers. He pulls the forefoot toward inversion.

Substitutions. Internal rotation of the hip when the patient is lying down with hips and knees extended; extensor digitorum longus.

Tests of Additional Muscles

The movements of head, neck, trunk, and toes have not been included here. However, if the treatment program is to include strengthening of any of this musculature, then the therapist is responsible for the measurement and is referred to texts listed in the references for guidance in doing so.

Recording Muscle Strength

The grade for each motion or muscle, in the case of wrists and hands, is accurately recorded in the appropriate column on the form. The form has columns to record the grades for the right and left sides of the body. The therapist must sign and date each test; if a test continues over several days, the dates should reflect that. A sample form is presented here (Table 7.3). The peripheral nerve and segmental levels are listed beside each muscle to assist the therapist in interpreting the results of the muscle test.

Normal strength of each muscle varies according to a person's age, sex, size, body type, and occupation. In manual muscle testing it is necessary for the therapist to develop a kinesthetic sense of what "normal" strength for each different muscle feels like. For example, the "normal" strength of the biceps far exceeds the "normal" strength of the adductor pollicis in a given individual. The "normal" strength of the biceps of a 6-year-old boy, however, might equal the "normal" strength of the adductor pollicis of a professional wrestler. The number and size of fibers in a muscle determines its strength: the larger and more numerous the fibers, the stronger the muscle. In order to develop a kinesthetic sense of "normal" a therapist must test many people who are able-bodied. When first beginning to test persons with muscle weakness, it is helpful to compare results with an experienced therapist.

Reliability, that is, the reproducibility of scores when no change has occurred, is essential for meaningful evaluation. Reliability of muscle testing data is affected by the interest and cooperation of the patient, by the tester, by the temperature of the day and the limb, by distractions to the patient and the tester, and by other environmental conditions.[25] To increase reliability, the variables should be controlled as much as possible from test to test. Of greatest importance to the reliability of the score of repeated tests is the strict adherence to the exact procedures of muscle testing.

If the muscle test is a reevaluation, the scores are compared to the previous test to note changes. The frequency of reevaluation depends upon the nature of the diagnosis. Where recovery is expected to be rapid, reevaluation is done frequently. In any case, reevaluation is done at least once a month as long as the patient is receiving therapy. If the repeated muscle tests show that the patient is making gains, the therapeutic program is considered beneficial. When repeated muscle tests show no gains despite programming adaptations, the patient is considered to have reached a plateau and may be considered to be no longer benefiting from restorative therapy. Each institution defines for itself the amount of time a patient is allowed to remain on a plateau before being considered for discharge. However, remember that the occupational therapist will be concerned with helping the patient compensate for his remaining disability by means of rehabilitative therapy before discharge.

Patients with degenerative diseases are expected to get weaker, and therefore therapy is aimed at maintaining their strength and function as long as possible. Repeated muscle tests are done to confirm that effect of therapy. A plateau for these patients is desirable, and therapy for maintaining strength should be continued.

Interpretation

After the muscle test scores have all been recorded, the therapist reviews the scores and looks for the muscles that are weak as well as the distribution and significance of the weakness. Any muscle which grades good minus (G−) or below is considered to be weak. Good plus (G+) muscles are functional, and usually no therapy is indicated for these. Good (G) muscles may or may not be functionally adequate for the patient, depending on his occupation. The pattern of muscle weakness is important to notice; the pattern may reflect the spinal cord level of segmental innervation, a peripheral nerve distribution, or an imbalance of forces which is potentially deforming. Noticing the pattern of muscle weakness may locate not only indications of significant weaknesses, but also indications of significant strengths. For example, a muscle test of a spinal cord-injured patient which indicates some strength in a muscle innervated by a segment below the level of his other functional muscles is a hopeful sign for more potential recovery. As another example, muscles recover proximally to distally following peripheral nerve injury, and records indicating return of function in muscles help to trace the progress of regeneration.

Granger[26] supports the use of a muscle test as a measure of muscle tension but emphasizes the need to interpret muscle performance with consideration of pathology and other clinical signs that influence motor output. These variables include muscle size, rhythm and efficiency of contraction, and mechanical factors such as joint disease, pain, or inflammation. Muscle performance must be interpreted in terms of all the direct and indirect influences on muscle strength characteristic of pathology of different components of the motor system that form a chain of pathways and mechanisms from the brain to myoneural junctions affecting the eventual motor output. Understanding the causes of muscle weakness influences treatment planning in terms of precautions and treatment principles used.

Other Methods Used to Record Muscle Strength

Frequently therapists supplement manual strength testing with dynamometer measurements of grasp and pinch for which norms have been established.[27, 28]

The grasp dynamometer measures the strength of

Patient's Name: _____

Diagnosis: _____

Patient's Case Number: _____ Date of Onset: _____

LEFT   RIGHT

			Examiner		
			Date		

		S C A P U L A	**ELEVATION**
			    Upper Trapezius (accessory) CR XI, C_{3-4}
			    Levator Scapulae (dorsal scapular)C_5, C_{3-4}		

			DEPRESSION
			    Lower Trapezius (accessory) CR XI, C_{3-4}
			    Latissimus Dorsi (thoraco-dorsal) C_{6-8}		

			ADDUCTION
			    Middle Trapezius (accessory) CR XI, C_{3-4}
			    Rhomboids (dorsal scapular) C_5		

			ABDUCTION Serratus Anterior (long thoracic) C_{5-7}		

		S H O U L D E R	**FLEXION**
			    Anterior Deltoid (axillary) C_{5-6}
			    Coracobrachialis (musculocutaneous) C_{5-6}
			    Pectoralis Major-clavicular (pectoral) C_5-T_1
			    Biceps (musculocutaneous) C_{5-6}		

			EXTENSION
			    Latissimus Dorsi (thoraco-dorsal) C_{6-8}
			    Teres Major (lower subscapular) C_{5-6}
			    Posterior Deltoid (axillary) C_{5-6}
			    Triceps-long head (radial) C_{7-8}		

			ABDUCTION
			    Supraspinatus (suprascapular) C_5
			    Middle Deltoid (axillary) C_{5-6}		

			ADDUCTION
			    Latissimus Dorsi (thoraco-dorsal) C_{6-8}
			    Teres Major (lower subscapular) C_{5-6}
			    Pectoralis Major (pectoral) C_5-T_1		

grasp in pounds (Fig. 7.169). Norms based on a sample of 250 normal adults have been established for males and females from 20 years through 80 years using the Jamar Dynamometer.[27] Norms extrapolated from Kellor's article are included here (Table 7.4). The standard method of measurement upon which the norms are based is as follows. The handle of the dynamometer is set to fit the patient's hand size, adjusted to allow metacarpophalangeal flexion. During the test, the patient may rest his forearm on the table top if he wishes but may not rest the dynamometer on anything. The patient squeezes the dynamometer with as

Table 7.3—*continued*

LEFT				RIGHT	
			Examiner		
			Date		
	SHOULDER Cont'd.		**INTERNAL ROTATION** Subscapularis (upper & lower subscapular)C_{5-6} Teres Major (lower subscapular) C_{5-6} Latissimus Dorsi (thoraco-dorsal) C_{6-8} Pectoralis Major (pectoral) C_5-T_1 Anterior Deltoid (axillary) C_{5-6}		
			EXTERNAL ROTATION Infraspinatus (suprascapular) C_{5-6} Teres Minor (axillary) C_{5-6} Posterior Deltoid (axillary) C_{5-6}		
			HORIZONTAL ABDUCTION Posterior Deltoid (axillary) C_{5-6}		
			HORIZONTAL ADDUCTION Pectoralis Major (pectoral) C_5-T_1 Anterior Deltoid (axillary) C_{5-6}		
	ELBOW		**FLEXION** Biceps (musculocutaneous) C_{5-6} Brachioradialis (radial) C_{5-6} Brachialis (musculocutaneous) C_{5-6}		
			EXTENSION Triceps (radial) C_{7-8}		
	FOREARM		**SUPINATION** Supinator (radial) C_6 Biceps (musculocutaneous) C_{5-6}		
			PRONATION Pronator Teres (median) C_{6-7} Pronator Quadratus (median) C_8-T_1		
	WRIST		**EXTENSION**		
			Ext. Carpi Radialis Longus (radial) C_{6-7}		
			Ext. Carpi Radialis Brevis (radial) C_{6-7}		
			Ext. Carpi Ulnaris (radial) C_{7-8}		
			FLEXION		
			Flexor Carpi Radialix (median) C_{6-7}		
			Palmaris Longus (median) C_8		
			Flexor Carpi Ulnaris (ulnar) C_{7-8}		
	FINGERS	P.I.P.	**FLEXION**		
			Flexor Superficialis 1st (median) C_7-T_1		
			Flexor Superficialis 2nd (median) C_7-T_1		
			Flexor Superficialis 3rd (median) C_7-T_1		
			Flexor Superficialis 4th (median) C_7-T_1		

222   *Biomechanical Approach*

Table 7.3—*continued*

LEFT					RIGHT	
				Examiner		
				Date		
		F I N G E R S	D.I.P.	Flexor Profundus 1st (median) C_8-T_1		
				Flexor Profundus 2nd (median) C_8-T_1		
				Flexor Profundus 3rd (ulnar) C_8-T_1		
				Flexor Profundus 4th (ulnar) C_8-T_1		
			5th MP	Flexor Digiti Minimi (ulnar) C_8-T_1		
				EXTENSION		
			M.P.	Extensor Digitorum 1st (radial) C_{7-8}		
				Extensor Digitorum 2nd (radial) C_{7-8}		
				Extensor Digitorum 3rd (radial) C_{7-8}		
				Extensor Digitorum 4th (radial) C_{7-8}		
				Extensor Digiti Minimi (radial) C_{7-8}		
		F I N G E R S		Lumbrical 1st (median) C_8-T_1		
				Lumbrical 2nd (median) C_8-T_1		
				Lumbrical 3rd (ulnar) C_8-T_1		
				Lumbrical 4th (ulnar) C_8-T_1		
				ABDUCTION		
				Dorsal Interosseus 1st (ulnar) C_8-T_1		
				Dorsal Interosseus 2nd (ulnar) C_8-T_1		
				Dorsal Interosseus 3rd (ulnar) C_8-T_1		
				Dorsal Interosseus 4th (ulnar) C_8-T_1		
				Abductor Digiti Minimi (ulnar) C_8-T_1		
				ADDUCTION		
				Palmar Interosseus 1st (ulnar) C_8-T_1		
				Palmar Interosseus 2nd (ulnar) C_8-T_1		
				Palmar Interosseus 3rd (ulnar) C_8-T_1		

Table 7.3—*continued*

LEFT					RIGHT	
			Examiner			
			Date			
			FLEXION			
			Flexor Pollicis Longus (median) C_8-T_1			
			Flexor Pollicis Brevis (median & ulnar) C_{6-8} & C_8-T_1			
			EXTENSION			
			Extensor Pollicis Longus (radial) C_{7-8}			
		T H U M B	Extensor Pollicis Brevis (radial) C_{7-8}			
			ABDUCTION			
			Abductor Pollicis Longus (radial) C_{7-8}			
			Abductor Pollicis Brevis (median) C_8-T_1			
			ADDUCTION			
			Adductor Pollicis (ulnar) C_8-T_1			
			OPPOSITION			
			Opponens Pollicis (median) C_8-T_1			
	5th		Opponens Digiti Minimi (ulnar) C_8-T_1			
			FLEXION			
			Iliopsoas (femoral) L_{2-3}			
			EXTENSION			
		H I P	Gluteus Maximus (inf. gluteal) L_5-S_2			
			ABDUCTION			
			Gluteus Medius (sup. gluteal) L_4-S_1			
			Gluteus Minimus (sup. gluteal) L_4-S_1			

Table 7.3—*continued*

				Examiner		
				Date		
		H I P	ADDUCTION			
			Adductor Magnus (obturator)L3-4 (sciatic)L4-S3			
			Adductor Longus (obturator) L3-4			
			Adductor Brevis (obturator) L3-4			
			EXTERNAL ROTATION			
			Gluteus Maximus (inf. gluteal) L5-S2			
			Six small external rotators L4-S2			
			INTERNAL ROTATION			
			Gluteus Medius (sup. gluteal) L4-S1			
			Gluteus Minimus (sup. gluteal) L4-S1			
		K N E E	FLEXION			
			Hamstrings (sciatic) L5-S2			
			EXTENSION			
			Quadriceps (femoral) L2-4			
		A N K L E	DORSIFLEXION			
			Tibialis Anterior (deep peroneal) L4-S1			
			Extensor Digitorum Longus (deep peroneal)L4-S1			
			Extensor Hallucis Longus (deep peroneal)L4-S1			
			PLANTAR FLEXION			
			Gastrocnemius (tibial) S1-2			
			Soleus (tibial) S.-2			
		F O O T	INVERSION			
			Tibialis Anterior (deep peroneal) L4-S1			
			Tibialis Posterior (tibial) L5-S1			
			EVERSION			
			Peroneus Longus (superficial peroneal)L4-S1			
			Peroneus Brevis (superficial peroneal)L4-S1			
			Peroneus Tertius (deep peroneal) L4-S1			

Innervations according to Lockhart.

Lockhart, Hamilton, Fyfe: Anatomy of the Human Body. Philadelphia:
    J. B. Lippincott, 1959.

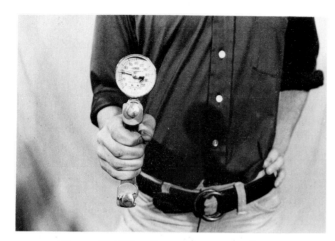

Figure 7.169 Grasp dynamometer.

Table 7.4
GRASP DYNAMOMETER NORMS IN POUNDS (Approx.)[a]

					Years			
		20	30	40	50	60	70	80
Male	R	125	120	115	100	95	85	80
	L	117	115	100	95	85	80	70
Female	R	64	60	57	55	51	50	48
	L	58	53	52	50	48	45	42

[a] N = 252, aged 18 to 84 years.

Table 7.5
TIP PINCH NORMS IN POUNDS (Approx.)[a]

					Years			
		20	30	40	50	60	70	80
Male	R	22.5	22	21	19.5	17.5	16.5	15.5
	L	21	20	18.5	17	16.5	15	14
Female	R	14	13	12.5	12	11	10.5	10
	L	13	12.5	12.0	11	10	9.5	9.0

Lateral Pinch Norms in Pounds (Approximately)[b]

					Years			
		20	30	40	50	60	70	80
Male	R	23.5	22.5	22	21	20	19.5	18.0
	L	22	21.4	20.5	20	19	18.0	17.0
Female	R	14.0	13.5	13	12.5	12	11.5	11.0
	L	13.5	13.0	12.5	12	11.5	11.0	10.5

Palmar Pinch in Pounds (Approximately)[c]

					Years			
		20	30	40	50	60	70	80
Male	R	23	21.5	19.5	18.5	17	15.5	14.5
	L	21	20	18	17	16	14.5	13.5
Female	R	15	14	13	12	11	9	8.5
	L	14	13	12	11	10	8	7

[a] N = 274, aged 20 to 98 years.
[b] N = 274, aged 20 to 98 years.
[c] N = 274, aged 20 to 98 years.

much force as he can two separate times with a 2- to 3-minute rest period between. The higher score is recorded[27] and compared to the patient's uninvolved hand or the norms for his age group to ascertain if he has a significant weakness.

The pinch meter measures the strength of pinch in pounds. Norms for tip pinch, lateral pinch, and palmar pinch using the Osco Pinch Meter were established on the same sample as the grasp norms were established.[27] Norms extrapolated from the Kellor article are included here (Table 7.5). However, these norms pertain to the older style Osco Pinch Meter. Since the original data were collected, the manufacturing of the Osco Pinch Meter has changed, and therefore these norms may not be valid for use with the new (colored finish) pinch meters. These newer meters seem to register a higher score than do the original ones for the same person. The calibration would need to be checked and new norms established if this pinch meter were used.

The standardized methods of measuring the three types of pinch for which norms were established are as follows.

Tip Pinch

The patient pinches the ends of the pinch meter between the tip of the pad of his thumb and the tip ends of his index and middle fingers (Fig. 7.170). He is

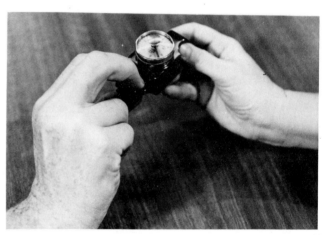

Figure 7.170 Pinch meter measuring tip pinch.

allowed one trial only, and the pounds attained are recorded.

Lateral Pinch

The patient pinches the pinch meter between the pad of his thumb and the lateral surface of his index finger (Fig. 7.171). He is allowed one trial only, and the pounds attained are recorded.

Palmar Pinch

The patient pinches the pinch meter between the pad of his thumb and the pads of his index and middle

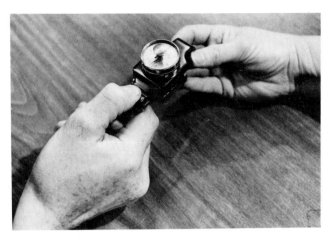

Figure 7.171 Pinch meter measuring lateral pinch.

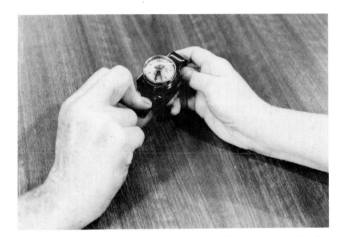

Figure 7.172 Pinch meter measuring palmar pinch.

fingers (Fig. 7.172). The score obtained on the first trial is recorded.

As when using any instrument to measure, the instrument must be set at zero to start and it must be calibrated. Dynamometers and pinch meters can be calibrated using a calibrated push-type spring scale in which the number of pounds of push against the compression part of the meter are registered on the spring scale and should correspond to the reading on the face of the meter. Calibration can also be done by placing known weights on, or suspending them from, the compression part of the meter.

Efforts to quantify other muscle strength measurements show promise for obtaining more objective test results. Edwards and Hyde[29] describe the use of a hand-held myometer for recording the force required to overcome a maximal voluntary contraction of muscle groups. The therapist offers the opposing force which must be stronger than the patient's effort. The use of a strain gauge is also described for measuring the force of a maximal voluntary contraction of the quadriceps. The maximal effort is registered on the gauge which is secured to the table and does not require a counterforce by the therapist. Electronic grasp and pinch meters are currently being used in

research; they require a recording device to obtain a readout of the strength obtained.

ENDURANCE

Endurance is the ability to sustain effort. Energy is needed for a person to produce the required intensity or rate of effort over a period of time necessary to complete a given exercise or activity. Length of time or duration of performance and the rate or intensity of the activity must both be considered when evaluating endurance. Factors influencing endurance may relate to muscle function, to oxygen supply from the cardiopulmonary system, or to combined impairment of muscle function and energy supply.[30] Anyone who suffers an illness or major trauma, and in fact anyone who is confined to bed for a few days, may experience generalized decrease of endurance. Friman[31] found that patients confined to bed with acute infectious diseases (*i.e.*, influenza and pneumonia) had reduced endurance capacity that did not return to full capacity until later than 4 months after the acute disease. Decreased endurance is inevitable if decreased cardiac function or decreased respiratory efficiency is a major symptom of the patient's diagnosis. Endurance of one muscle or a muscle group may be decreased due to localized trauma or immobilization; the muscles tire more easily. Patients with decreased muscle strength may require increased energy output to sustain a level of activity and may consequently have decreased endurance.

Other factors influencing fatigue have been under investigation. Asmussen[32] studied muscle fatigue and found evidence to support a "central" component to muscle fatigue in addition to the "peripheral" factors; "central" means primarily in the brain, whereas "peripheral" refers to the motor units. Subjects performed maximal dynamic muscle contractions to exhaustion using a finger or an arm ergograph. During 2-minute rest periods between exercise bouts, complete rest of these muscles was compared with rests of diverting light activities using different muscle or mental activity, such as counting. More work could be done after the diverting rest than after the complete rest. In explanation of this effect, it was proposed that during complete rest the input from fatigued muscles causes the reticular formation to inhibit voluntary efforts, whereas during diverting activity impulses to the reticular formation from the other body parts influence the reticular formation to facilitate voluntary efforts. Additionally, Asmussen studied the effect of having the eyes open or closed on the fatigue factor. An Alpha-rhythm on EEG indicates a lowered level of arousal: it is produced with the eyes closed due to central inhibition and disappears when the eyes are open. Subjects exercised to exhaustion with their eyes closed and then opened their eyes and were able to continue the work giving further support to the concept of a "central" component to fatigue. Clamann and Broecker[33] amplified EMG activity of the triceps, biceps, adductor pollicis, and first dorsal interosseous muscles during maintained maximal voluntary contraction and repeated contractions of low and high force to distinguish between the effects of fatigue on Type I (red tonic) and Type II (pale phasic) muscle fibers. Triceps and biceps have predominantly Type II fibers, adductor pollicis has Type I fibers, and in the first dorsal interosseus the fibers are equal. Type II fibers were found to fatigue more quickly than Type I fibers. Type II fibers fatigue during near maximal effort, whereas Type I fibers are difficult to fatigue at any level of force. Fiber type composition is somewhat variable in different individuals, and fatigue may help in the assessment of fiber type.

Activities are used for evaluation of muscle endurance. The amount of resistance and the time of performance or number of repetitions before the point of fatigue are recorded. Kottke[34] suggests the selection of a lightly resistive activity requiring 15 to 40% of maximal effort. DeLateur et al.[35] found that the amount of work, rate of work, and fatigue all contribute to increasing work capacity but that fatigue was the most important factor. If a low load is used it will take longer to reach the point of fatigue. Endurance can also be evaluated by determining the amount of time a patient can actively hold or maintain a position. Isometric holding, however, causes large increases in blood pressure and can stress the cardiopulmonary system.[36] Precautions regarding use of isometric exercise should be observed for cardiac patients and others for whom increased blood pressure is problematic. Time is also the measure of endurance for a splint or device. This type of endurance is often referred to as tolerance, e.g., wearing tolerance or sitting tolerance.

In addition to the fatigue of muscles the ability to sustain effort is influenced by a person's cardiopulmonary status. Lunsford[30] described the use of heart rate as an indicator of response to exercise that is easily evaluated by the therapist. Heart rate reflects the intensity of activity and is a good indicator of work capacity for patients with decreased endurance and a sound cardiopulmonary system. A resting pulse is taken after 5 minutes of sitting quietly and should be between 65 and 85 beats/min. Then, after exercise, the pulse is taken again; an increase in direct proportion to the increase in work load is expected. Activities that produce a heart rate that is 60 to 75% of maximal heart rate will produce a training effect and are ideal for endurance training for the cardiopulmonary system for patients with no cardiac problem. The formula 220 − Age = Maximum Heart Rate is generally used, and 60 to 75% of the result is calculated to determine the desired heart rate during activity. Heart rate is an easily done evaluation which helps to establish a treatment plan for increasing endurance.

SENSATION

Patients with disabilities which may affect peripheral sensation must be evaluated to determine the types and distribution of sensory loss or dysfunction. The procedures of this evaluation were discussed in Chapter 3.

FUNCTIONAL EVALUATION

Some therapists prefer to use evaluations which combine the several aspects of physical functioning in one evaluation and which relate these to activities of daily living. Such a test, "The Functional Motion Test," was devised by Zimmerman[37] for evaluation of the upper extremities of patients with lower motor neuron disturbances. The reader is referred to the source for the details of administration of this particular test.

References

1. Moore, M. L. Clinical assessment of joint motion. In *Therapeutic Exercise*, 3rd ed., edited by J. V. Basmajian. Baltimore: Williams & Wilkins, 1978.
2. Cole. T. M. Goniometry: The measurement of joint motion. In *Handbook of Physical Medicine and Rehabilitation*, 2nd ed., edited by F. H. Krusen, F. J. Kottke and P. M. Ellwood. Philadelphia: W. B. Saunders, 1971.
3. Gerhardt, J. J., and Russe, O. A. *International SFTR Method of Measuring and Recording Joint Motion*. Bern, Switzerland: Hans Huber Publishers, 1975.
4. American Academy of Orthopaedic Surgeons. *Joint Motion: Method of Measuring and Recording*. Chicago, 1965.
5. Mundale, M. O., Hislop, H. J., Rabideau, R. J., and Kottke, F. J. Evaluation of extension of the hip. *Arch. Phys. Med. Rehabil.*, 37: 75–80, 1956.
6. Kottke, F. J., and Kubicek, W. G. Relationship of the tilt of the pelvis to stable posture. *Arch. Phys. Med. Rehabil.*, 37: 81–90, 1956.
7. Clayson, S. J., Mundale, M. O., and Kottke, F. J. Goniometer adaptation for measuring hip extension. *Arch. Phys. Med. Rehabil.*, 47: 255–261, 1966.
8. Dworecka, F., et al. A practical approach to the evaluation of rheumatoid hand deformity. *Am. J. Orth. Surg.*, 1968.
9. Brown, M. E. Reheumatoid arthritic hands: Tactual visual approaches. *Am. J. Occup. Ther.*, 20(1): 17–23, 1966.
10. Regenos, E., and Chyatte, S. Joint range and deformity recorded by xerography. *J.A.P.T.A.*, 50(8): 190, 1970.
11. Wirta, R., and Taylor, D. Engineering Principles in Rehabilitation Medicine. In *Handbook of Physical Medicine and Rehabilitation*, 2nd ed., edited by F. H. Krusen, F. J. Kottke, and P. M. Ellwood. Philadelphia: W. B. Saunders, 1971.
12. Borden, R., and Colachis, S. Quantitative measurement of the good and normal ranges in muscle testing. *Phys. Ther.*, 48(8): 839–843, 1968.
13. Carlson, B. R. Relationship between isometric and isotonic strength. *Arch. Phys. Med. Rehabil.*, 51: 176–179, 1970.
14. Caldwell, L. S., Chaffin, D. B., Dukes-Dobos, F. N., Kroemer, K. H. E., Laubach, L. L., Snook, S. H., and Wasserman, D. E. A proposed standard procedure for static muscle strength testing. *Am. Ind. Hyg. Assoc. J.*, 35(4): 201–206, 1974.
15. Kendall, H. O., Kendall, F. P., and Wadsworth, G. E. *Muscles: Testing and Function*. Baltimore: Williams & Wilkins, 1971.
16. Daniels, L., and Worthingham, C. *Muscle Testing: Techniques of Manual Examination*, 3rd ed. Philadelphia: W. B. Saunders, 1972.
17. Nicholas, J. A., Sapega, A., Kraus, H., and Webb, J. N. Factors influencing manual muscle tests in physical therapy. *J. Bone Joint Surg.*, 60A(2): 186–190, 1978.
18. Brunnstrom, S. *Clinical Kinesiology*, 3rd ed. Philadelphia: F. A. Davis, 1972.
19. Basmajian, J. V. *Muscle Alive*, 3rd ed. Baltimore: Williams & Wilkins, 1974.
20. Long, C., and Brown, M. E. EMG kinesiology of the hand. Part III: Lumbricales and flexor digitorum profundus to the long finger. *Arch. Phys. Med. Rehabil.*, 43: 450–460, 1962.
21. Long, C. Intrinsic-extrinsic muscle control of the fingers. *J. Bone Joint Surg.*, 50A(5): 973–984, 1968.
22. Landsmeer, J. M. F., and Long, C. The mechanism of finger control based on electromyograms and location analysis. *Acta*

Anat. (Basel), *60:* 330–347, 1965.

23. Hines, T. Manual muscle examination. In *Therapeutic Exercise,* edited by S. Licht. New Haven: Elizabeth Licht, 1958.

24. Diekmeyer, G. Altered test position for hip extensor muscles. *Phys. Ther.* 58(11): 1379, 1978.

25. Salter, N. Muscle and joint measurement. In *Therapeutic Exercise,* edited by S. Licht. New Haven: Elizabeth Licht, 1958.

26. Granger, C. V. The clinical discernment of muscle weakness. *Arch. Phys. Med. Rehabil., 44:* 430–438, 1963.

27. Kellor, M., Frost, J., Silverberg, N., Iverson, I., and Cummings, R. Hand strength and dexterity. *Am. J. Occup. Ther.,* 25(2): 77–83, 1971.

28. Weiss, M. W., and Flatt, A. E. A pilot study of 198 normal children: Pinch strength and hand size in the growing hand. *Am. J. Occup. Ther.,* 25(1): 10–12, 1971.

29. Edwards, R. H. T., and Hyde, S. Methods of measuring muscle strength and fatigue. *Physiotherapy,* 13(2): 51–55, 1977.

30. Lunsford, B. R. Clinical indicators of endurance. *Phys. Ther.,* 58(6): 704–709, 1978.

31. Friman, G. Effect of acute infectious disease on human isometric muscle endurance. *Upsala J. Med. Sci.,* 83(2): 105–108, 1978.

32. Asmussen, E. Muscle fatigue. *Med. Sci. Sports,* 11(4): 313–321, 1979.

33. Clamann, H. P., and Broecker, K. T. Relation between force and fatigability of red and pale skeletal muscles in man. *Am. J. Phys. Med.,* 58(2): 70–85, 1979.

34. Kottke, F. Therapeutic exercise. In *Handbook of Physical Medicine and Rehabilitation,* 2nd ed., edited by F. H. Krusen, F. J. Kottke, and P. M. Ellwood. Philadelphia: W. B. Saunders, 1971.

35. DeLateur, B. J., Lehmann, J. F., and Giaconi, R. Mechanical work and fatigue: Their roles in the development of muscle work capacity. *Arch. Phys. Med. Rehabil., 57:* 319–324, 1976.

36. Whipp, B. J., and Phillips, E. E., Jr. Cardiopulmonary and metabolic responses to sustained isometric exercise. *Arch. Phys. Med. Rehabil., 51:* 398–402, 1970.

37. Zimmerman, M. E. The functional motion test as an evaluation tool for patients with lower motor neuron disturbances. *Am. J. Occup. Ther.,* 23(1): 49–56, 1969.

chapter

8

Treatment

Catherine A. Trombly, M.A., OTR

GOAL: TO PREVENT LIMITATION OF RANGE OF MOTION

Many range of motion limitations *can and should be prevented.* Patients who are unable to move their own joints, and for whom motion is not contraindicated, should receive passive range of motion exercises at least once a day. If edema exists, range of motion will be limited and contractures, due both to the lack of movement and to developing viscosity of the fluid, are a possibility. The edematous part should be elevated so that the fluid can drain back to the body. Active ranging is preferred because the contraction of the muscles will help pump the fluid out of the extremity. However, if AROM is not possible, PROM must be done.

Principles: Movement through Full Range of Motion; Positioning

The *methods* used for ranging (movement through full range of motion) include teaching the patient to actively move the joints that are involved or adjacent to an injury or passively moving the joints if the patient is paralyzed. In either case, the technique is the same. Each involved joint is moved from starting position to end position as described in range of motion evaluation in Chapter 7.[1] Exception: The hands of quadriplegic persons who will rely on tenodesis action for grasp must be ranged in the following manner to allow finger flexor tendons to develop necessary tightness for function. When flexing the fingers, the wrist must be fully extended, and when extending the fingers, the wrist must be fully flexed.

Positioning of joints to avoid development of deformities is essential. All potentially nonfunctional positions are avoided throughout the day and night. Positioning can be accomplished by the use of orthoses, pillows, rolled towels, positioning boards, etc. For example, when the patient is in bed, footboards may be used to prevent foot drop, and sandbags or trochanter rolls can be placed along the lateral aspect of the thigh to prevent hip external rotation.[2,3] Another example is suspension of the patient's edematous hand in a suspension sling.

Sometimes contractures and subsequent ankylosis are unavoidable due to the disease process. In these instances positioning, splinting, and bracing are used to ensure that ankylosis occurs in as nearly a functional position as possible.

GOAL: TO INCREASE PASSIVE RANGE OF MOTION

If the results of evaluation of passive range of motion indicate that limitations in joint motions are significant, *i.e.,* if they impair the patient's ability to function independently in life tasks or are likely to lead to deformity, then treatment may be indicated. Whereas some significant limitations of range of motion can be ameliorated or corrected by activity or exercise, some cannot. Problems which can be changed include contractures of soft tissue, *i.e.,* skin, muscle, tendon, ligament. Problems which cannot be changed include bony ankylosis or arthrodesis, long-standing contractures in which there are extensive fibrotic changes in soft tissue, and severe joint destruction with subluxation. Occupational therapy for limited range of motion problems which cannot be treated restoratively is rehabilitative in nature and focuses on providing techniques and/or equipment to compensate for the problems of limited range of motion, and is described in Part 6.

Principle: Stretch

It is important that stretch is done to the point of maximal stretch, defined as a few degrees beyond the point of discomfort, and held there for a few seconds. The stretching may be active or passive.

The patient controls the amount of stretch and force in active stretching, while the setup of the activity or exercise equipment controls the direction of force. By using activities that combine active stretch and minimal resistance to the contracting muscle, the patient can make instantaneous adjustments in the force of the stretch in response to pain by relaxing the contraction and moving away from the stretched position. Passive stretch, on the other hand, does not have the luxury of an internal feedback system, so that the force applied by an external force cannot be immediately adjusted by the patient or therapist to accommodate to small pain signals experienced by the patient. Nonetheless, passive stretch is usually more effective than active stretch because the therapist carefully ensures that each limited joint is stretched to the point of maximal stretch. When precautions are in effect, however, passive stretch must be done with extreme caution, and active stretch is preferable. Precautions are noted below.

Use of an electrogoniometer that provides feedback to the patient when he has achieved the desired limit of motion may increase the effectiveness of active stretching. A simple electrogoniometer that can be constructed by an occupational therapist has been described by Brown et al.[4] When used in combination with activity, effectiveness of treatment may be enhanced.

Active Stretching

At the limited joint, the patient contracts the muscles antagonistic to the contracture in order to stretch the contracture. For example, if there is a flexion contracture, the extensors must contract to pull against it. The patient controls the force, speed, extent, and direction of the stretch within his own tolerance for pain. It is the therapist's role to instruct the patient and to encourage him to frequently stretch the part correctly throughout the day, as well as during a treatment session.

Passive Stretching

An external force stretches the contracture at the limited joint. It is used when the patient does not have sufficient strength in the antagonist to do active stretching.

Methods to increase passive range of motion include orthoses that provide traction, manual stretching, joint mobilization techniques, exercise, and/or activities. All methods stretch the tissue beyond its customary limit of motion. The force, speed, direction, and extent of stretch must be controlled. Ballistic movements which are characterized by uncontrolled, forceful stretch at the end of range are avoided. The *force* must be enough to put tension on the tissue, but not enough to rupture the tissue. The *speed* should be slow to allow the tissue to gradually adjust. The *direction* of stretch is exactly opposite to the tightness. The *extent* of stretch is to the point of maximal stretch, defined above. Precautions are to be observed. Stretching tissue after it has been immobilized must

be done carefully. After prolonged immobilization or bed rest, osteoporosis can occur. Bone loses calcium, is more porous, and can be fractured more easily by tension or shear forces because there have been no compression forces on the bone to maintain its integrity.[5] Tendons and ligaments also biochemically change and lose tensile strength in the absence of motion and stress.[5] Muscle filaments which must slide during muscle contraction have not been sliding during immobilization; therefore, they lose the ability to slide, and the resultant adhesions of the filaments may be torn when stretched. Bed rest causes a decrease of blood pressure in the extremities which reduces the stress necessary for maintaining the strength of the collagen fibers of the vessel walls, and consequently blood vessels are weakened.[5] To reduce the effects of immobilization and bed rest the physician may prescribe weight bearing, isometric muscle contraction, or changing position in bed.

Inflammation of collagen tissues weakens the structure involved.[5] Collagen tissues include bone, cartilage, tendon, ligament, artery, fascia, dermis, and other connective tissues. Therefore, care must be taken not to cause stretch of inflamed tissues. If steroids are used in the treatment of inflammation, the therapist should be aware that possible side effects of these drugs include osteoporosis.

Sensory loss may prevent the patient from being aware of pain, thus permitting overstretching to occur unless the therapist pays particular attention to the tension of the tissues being stretched during manual stretching or activity. Overstretching causes internal bleeding with subsequent scar formation which may eventually ossify. An unfortunate common example of such ossification occurs in hip and elbow musculature of spinal cord-injured patients.

Orthotic devices that provide a continuous, gentle stretch (traction) are used to supplement gains made by means of exercise or activity as well as to provide a form of controlled, continuous, passive stretching. One such device is the Glove Flexion Mitt used to put a constant stretch on extensor contractures of the metacarpophalangeal and interphalangeal joints. An ordinary workman's glove is adapted by adding rubber bands to the fingertips which are anchored to the wrist.[6] Other orthoses are described in Chapter 12.

Manual stretching, a form of passive stretching, is done by the therapist. Ideally, the environment and the therapist are quiet and relaxed to encourage relaxation of the patient. The patient is informed about the process of manual stretching and that it involves tolerable pain. He is instructed that he is responsible for indicating when discomfort occurs in order for the procedure to be done properly. For stoic patients, the importance of this must be emphasized. Real pain would defeat the results of stretching, since relaxation of the tissue being stretched is required for an adequate result.[7] The therapist holds the extremity in such a way that the part is stabilized proximally to the joint and is moved distally to the joint in the exact plane of movement opposite to the tightness. The motions used in stretching are identical with the motions described in range of motion evaluation. The patient is encouraged to move the part with the therapist if he can, because during active motion the tight antagonistic muscles are reflexly programmed to relax, and therefore more motion may consequently be obtained. The therapist moves the part smoothly, slowly, and gently to the point of mild discomfort[7] which the patient indicates verbally or by facial expression. The therapist then moves the part a few degrees beyond the point of discomfort, and the part is held at this point, called the point of maximal stretch. The duration of the stretch when applied manually is usually only several seconds to a minute. It is clinically recognized that continuous stretching is most effective; however, gains are also noted using briefly held stretch. There are no research studies which specify the minimal amount of time required for effective stretching. Twenty seconds has been recommended for athletes who stretch their muscles before strenuous activity.[7]

There should be relief of discomfort immediately following release of stretch. Residual pain after stretching indicates that the stretch was too forceful and caused tearing of soft tissues or blood vessels.[8] During each treatment session, each joint with limitation of passive range of motion is gently stretched in the described manner several times to ensure achieving maximal stretch at least once. In order to maximize gains achieved by stretching it is necessary to stretch daily, because it has been determined by microscopic examination of connective tissue that the process involved in contracture formation begins in 1 day.[8] Gentle stretching that achieves small increments of gain over a period of time is more effective than vigorous stretching aimed at large gains quickly. As a protective mechanism, connective tissue resists quick, vigorous stretching, which is therefore ineffective or injurious.[8] The method of moving gently to the point of maximal stretch and holding this position allows connective tissue, having the property of plasticity, to adjust its length gradually over time.

In ligament or tendon tightness resulting from weakness of the shoulder musculature, it has been clinically demonstrated that pain, caused by the weight of the arm pulling on the rotator cuff muscles, can be reduced by approximating the head of the humerus into the glenoid fossa, while simultaneously ranging or stretching this joint. In ligament, muscle, or tendon tightness of the wrist, thumb, and fingers it has been clinically demonstrated that pain associated with stretching can be reduced by traction applied to each joint to separate the articular surfaces during stretching.[8]

Joint mobilization techniques are primarily used in physical therapy; however, the occupational therapist may find the techniques useful to increase range of motion in stiff hands and wrists.

Maitland[9] has described methods of joint manipulation and joint mobilization. He defines mobilization as passive movements that are done at such a speed that the patient could prevent the movement if he

chose. Two types of movement are included: (1) oscillatory movement (2 to 3 per second) of small or large amplitude applied anywhere in the range of motion; (2) sustained stretching with tiny amplitude oscillations at the limit of range. The oscillatory movements may be of the physiologic movements or accessory movements (also called "joint play", i.e., movement possible within a joint but not under voluntary control).

Manipulation is defined as either a sudden movement or thrust of small amplitude but of a speed too quick to allow the patient to prevent it, or a steady controlled stretch to break adhesions. Often manipulation is done under anesthesia and is never used without extensive special training.

Grades of movement have been defined to aid prescribing mobilization treatment and recording progress.

Grade I: Small amplitude movement performed at the beginning of the range.

Grade II: Large amplitude movement performed within the range but not reaching the limit of the range. If the movement is performed near the beginning of the range it is expressed as II−; if it is taken deeply into range yet not to the limit, it is expressed as II+.

Grade III: Large amplitude movement performed up to the limit of range. III− indicates a gentle approach to the limit, whereas III+ indicates movement that pushes vigorously into the limit.

Grade IV: Small amplitude movement performed at the limit of range. IV− and IV+ can be used to describe the vigor of the movement, as in the case of Grade III.

Treatment of stiff joints recommended by Maitland[9] includes small amplitude oscillatory movements done for approximately 2 minutes at the limit of range of the functionally limited physiologic movement. This is followed by small amplitude, strong stretching oscillatory movements of the accessory movements of the joint. These two types of movements are alternated until progress is achieved. If soreness develops, movement is changed to Grade II type. The reader is referred to Maitland's manual, *Peripheral Manipulation,*[9] for the details of this treatment method.

An exercise that has been found to be effective in increasing the passive range of motion of shortened tissue is the PNF technique called "hold/relax."[10] The "hold/relax" procedure involves a brief and maximal isometric contraction performed at the point of limitation. The tight muscle is contracted maximally and then relaxed. During the relaxation phase, the therapist moves the part in the direction opposite to the contraction into the new range. The "hold/relax" procedure may be repeated at each succeeding limit of range until a large gain in range is made. Example: if there were a contracture of elbow flexors, the elbow would be extended to its limit. The patient would be instructed to isometrically contract his flexors maximally, then relax, at which moment the therapist would smoothly extend the elbow into greater range until resistance is felt. The "hold/relax" procedure is repeated until increments of gain are achieved. The technique is neurophysiologically based on the hypothesis that after a motor unit contracts maximally, it is inhibited (relaxes) due to GTO influence. When a muscle contracts maximally, most or all motor units fire simultaneously, therefore stimulating all or most of the GTOs of that muscle with the effect of inhibiting all the active motor units, enabling the part to be gently moved to greater range.

The comparative effectiveness of passive stretch and "hold/relax" (isometric exercise) has been studied on young adult normal males. One study[10] found "hold/relax" to be the more effective procedure, and the other study[11] found no statistically significant difference between isometric contraction and passive stretch. Both treatments produced improved range of motion as compared to no treatment.[10] In a study of 30 young adult females, "contract/relax," an isotonic contraction against maximal resistance, was found superior to "hold/relax" in increasing range of motion; both improved range of motion as compared to no treatment.[12]

Activity used for increasing passive range of motion must provide a gentle active stretch by use of slow, repetitive isotonic contraction of the muscles opposite the contracture or by use of a prolonged passive stretched position of the tissue producing limitation. In both types of activity, the requirement is that the range be increased slightly beyond the patient's limitation. The use of activity for stretching is empirically based on the idea that a person involved in an interesting and purposeful activity will gain greater range because he is relaxed, not anticipating pain, is motivated to complete the task, and will be more likely to move as the activity demands. Therefore, the selected activity must be interesting to the patient and must intrinsically demand the correct motion. This means that the performance of the activity as it is set up for the patient must involve the desired motion, without unreasonable contrivance or the necessity for the patient to concentrate on the movement itself rather than the goal of the activity. Reasonable adaptations, however, are permissible and, in fact, may be necessary in order to elicit the desired motion. Creativity on the part of the therapist to devise appropriate adaptations is desirable, as long as the adaptation does not change the nature of the activity, put the patient in an awkward position, or cause him to perform unnatural movements. An example of an adaptation of an activity to provide active stretch of an elbow flexion contracture of a jig-saw puzzle enthusiast could be to require the patient to extend his elbow just beyond his comfortable range to reach for puzzle pieces.

Adaptations to activity can be made through the tools or equipment used in doing the activity. Equipment used in activities can provide traction (passive stretch) if resistance is provided by means of springs, weights, elastic material, or the weight of the tool. An example of how weights are used to adapt an activity can be seen in woodworking (sanding long boards such as used to make a book case). Each of the shelf boards are attached in turn to an inclined sanding frame. The patient tries to push the sander higher and higher which provides some stretch to the extensors. Weights are attached to the sander by suspending them from a rope through a pulley at the top of the incline, creating an upward force that stretches the extensors further (Fig. 8.1).

Adaptations made to adjust the size or location of handles of craft or recreational equipment can require the patient to move further into range actively. The size or location is gradually changed by the therapist as the patient improves.[13]

One cannot prescribe activity for specific purposes similar to the way a physician prescribes pills because each person moves in his own characteristic ways. The therapist must carefully monitor the patient's method of doing an activity and not assume that the activity, *per se*, will evoke the desired result in all persons. Two examples illustrate this. Pressing the weft of finger weaving using a passive hand and the force of shoulder extensors provides stretch to the finger flexors. Actively pressing the weft into place using finger flexion, on the other hand, stretches the finger extensors because the flexors contract. Both methods accomplish the same activity goal. The other example is similar: Pressing clay into a mold has been used successfully,

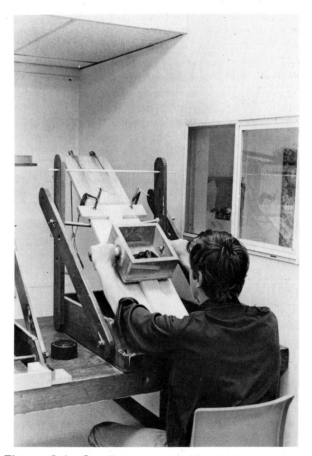

Figure 8.1 Sanding on an inclined plane using a bilateral sander with pulleys and weights attached.

in combination with other exercises, to stretch finger flexor tightness.[14] However, if the patient had actually pressed the clay into the mold using finger flexion instead of a passively held hand, then extensors would have been stretched. It is best to avoid the use of an activity which requires a motion that is habitual for the patient, but if done in this habitual manner, does not meet the therapy goal. Otherwise, the patient must concentrate on the new movement and will often revert back to the habitual method.

GOAL: TO INCREASE STRENGTH

If evaluation of the patient's strength reveals a significant limitation, one that prevents the person from carrying out his life tasks or which may lead to deformity, then treatment is aimed at gradually increasing the patient's strength. Weakness is potentially deforming if muscles on one side of a joint are weak in comparison to their antagonists.

Principle: Weak Muscle Is Overloaded to Limit of Its Capacity

Stated in more operational terms, stress is applied to the muscle or muscle group to the point of fatigue.[16] Parameters that may be manipulated to alter the stress on a muscle include *intensity* or load (resistance), *duration* of a held contraction or exercise period, *rate* or velocity of contraction (repetitions per period of time), and the *frequency* of exercise (exercise periods/day). Each parameter may be manipulated independently of one another. There may be precautionary reasons, for example, why the load should not be increased for a given patient. In that case, the therapist has the option of increasing one of the other parameters, for example, frequency (treatment twice daily), to thereby stress the muscle which will result in a strength gain. Strength is gained under stress because more motor units are recruited when the load is increased, or the speed of contraction is increased, or the muscle begins to tire. Strength is also gained when the muscle fibers hypertrophy in response to resistance.[5, 17]

Although research is limited, intensities as low as 50 to 67% of maximum appear to increase strength.[18, 19] Research reported to date has been done primarily on normal adults. The weight of the extremity itself is a load as are the weights of tools and the resistiveness of craft/work materials. Intensity can also be manipulated by adding a load (weights) to the extremity or by changing the length of the lever arm by changing the point where the load is applied to the limb.

The type of exercise, which reflects gradations of intensity from full assistance to full resistance, must be determined in designing a treatment program. The choice, based on the measured strength of the muscle(s), should require effort. The appropriate level of exercise for a patient who cannot move at all is *passive exercise* to maintain range of motion. Grading along the continuum of increasing resistance, *active assist-*

ive exercise is selected for muscles which grade Poor Minus (P−) and Fair Minus (F−). Gravity is eliminated during exercise of the P− muscle, but the F− muscle works against gravity by definition. Active assistive exercise means that the patient moves the part as much as he can for strengthening and is then assisted to complete the motion in order to maintain mobility. The motion may be completed by the therapist or by the force of therapeutic equipment. The next increment in the gradation of resistance is *active exercise*. The patient moves the part through full range of motion without assistance or outside resistance. Muscles which grade Poor (P) or Fair (F) would be exercised in this manner. Again, gravity would be eliminated for the P muscle, but not for the F muscle.

The plane of movement alters the manner in which a muscle functions because the influence of the force of gravity changes. In order to use tools, thereby permitting the use of activity in therapy, muscles must be able to take resistance. A fair muscle operating against gravity cannot take resistance. However, if this muscle is changed to a gravity-eliminated plane, resistance can be used. The plane of movement for a P muscle can also be switched to work against gravity, but it is obvious that this would put the muscle at a disadvantage. Finally, exercise becomes *active resistive*. Muscles which grade Poor Plus (P+), Fair Plus (F+), and Good (G−, G, G+) are exercised in this manner. Gravity is eliminated when exercising the P+ muscle. The amount of resistance applied increases with increasing strength.

Another factor that should be considered in designing a strengthening program is the type of muscle contraction to be required. Exercise to increase muscle strength can be accomplished by means of isotonic or isometric contraction. An isotonic contraction is one in which the muscle changes length while maintaining approximately the same tension. An isometric contraction is one in which the muscle maintains approximately the same length but changes tension. Isotonic contractions may be either concentric or eccentric. In concentric isotonic contraction, muscle fibers shorten; in eccentric isotonic contraction, muscle fibers lengthen to resist a force. In both concentric and eccentric contraction there is movement at the joint. In isometric contraction, muscle fibers shorten only enough to take up the slack but there is no joint motion. The examples will clarify the three types of contraction. Raising a mug of coffee to your mouth requires concentric contraction of the elbow flexors, whereas carefully lowering the mug requires eccentric contraction of the same muscle group. In operating a hand printing press (Fig. 8.2), concentric contraction of the shoulder extensors is used to pull the handle down and eccentric contraction of the same muscle group allows the handle to return gently to its starting position. Static or isometric contraction was used in maintaining the grasp on the handle of the printing press and on the mug in these examples.

When no movement of the joint is permitted, then isometric contraction is preferred. When hypertension

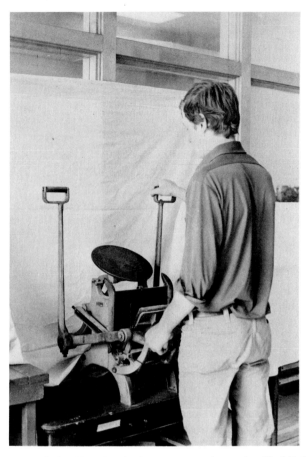

Figure 8.2 Hand printing press adapted with bilateral handles.

or cardiovascular conditions are problems for the patient, then isometric contraction should be avoided, since it has been found that isometric contraction of either small or large muscles increases the systolic and diastolic blood pressure and heart rate.[20] Downey and Darling[5] report the results of a study by Donald et al., in which sustained hand grip lasting 2 minutes and requiring 50% of maximal contraction increased the systolic blood pressure of a 27-year-old normal male from 100 mm Hg, to 165 mm Hg and increased his heart rate from 60 to 120 beats per minute.

If a person is required to use isometric contraction in his important daily life tasks, then treatment should utilize isometric contraction, because transfer of the effects of training is poor between isometric and isotonic training programs.[16, 18, 21, 22] DeLateur et al.,[16] in an elegantly designed study, found that ability gained in isometric training did transfer after several days of further isotonic training; however, ability gained in isotonic training did not transfer to the isometric task.

The effectiveness of concentric[23-25] and isometric[19, 21, 26-28] exercise to increase strength has been documented.

Force that can be generated during the three types of contraction decreases in this order: eccentric, isometric, and concentric.[29-31] In other words, more

weight can be lowered by a given muscle than can be lifted concentrically or held at any one point. A corollary is that less effort is exerted during lowering a given weight than is required to lift it. In comparing the relative effects of eccentric and concentric contractions, Mannheimer[32] reasoned that since more force is generated during eccentric contraction, strength gain should be greater using eccentric contraction. In his study of 26 normal male subjects, strength was gained faster by use of eccentric contractions, but there was no significant difference in the amount of strength gain after 1 month between the two types of contractions. Lawrence[33] found isotonic extension of the knee more effective than isometric for increasing strength of the quadriceps; however, the method of measuring gains (amount of weight that could be lifted through range once) was an isotonic measure and may have biased the outcome.

DeLateur et al.,[16] in a study comparing isotonic and isometric exercise of the quadriceps, found equal strengthening potential of the two types of exercise even with less than maximal resistance, as long as the muscle worked to the point of fatigue.

In terms of work (w = force × distance), a muscle doing an eccentric contraction is doing negative work, a muscle doing isometric contraction is doing no work, and one doing concentric contraction is doing positive work. Since negative work (meaning that work is being done to the muscle) is easier to do, i.e., less tension is required for the same load, it may be advantageous to start very weak muscles doing eccentric contraction.[22] The eccentric contraction should be a slow, *controlled*, lengthening in the direction of the pull of gravity. No research was found to support this hypothesis. Eccentric contraction is less stressful cardiovascularly[5, 22, 31] and thus would be a factor in choosing exercise for patients with cardiac or pulmonary conditions.

Isokinetic exercise has also been found effective to increase strength. Isokinetic exercise is dynamic concentric exercise to agonist and antagonist in which the rate of movement is controlled, that is, the same for each repetition.[8] Physical therapists use machines which deliver the correct rate of motion to the patient undergoing treatment. Some machines also vary the resistance to the motion to accommodate the differing tensions of the muscle at its different lengths throughout the motion. In this way, isokinetic exercise using such machines is similar to PNF in that both use the concept of accommodating maximal resistance throughout range. DeLateur et al.[25] found the same relative effectiveness of isokinetic and isotonic exercise and transfer of training was positive between them.

When an agonist muscle is significantly weaker than its antagonist, then an exercise or activity which requires the weaker muscle to contract concentrically and then eccentrically for the return motion may be more effective than one which requires reciprocal contraction of the agonist and antagonist. No research has been found to support this hypothesis. On the other hand, observations made incidental to the main question in electromyographic kinesiological studies show that the antagonist contracts synergistically (co-contracts) with the agonist as the load or velocity increases. One study,[34] in fact, established an increase in strength of antagonist due to exercise of the agonist, although the agonist gained proportionately more strength. In this study, the forearm muscles of 10 normal subjects were exercised using maximal eccentric contractions for an 8-week period.

Great intra- and intersubject differences have been seen electromyographically in the patterns of muscle contraction people use to accomplish the same goal.[35] In order for a particular treatment program to be effective for a particular person, careful monitoring, preferably using EMG biofeedback (see Chapter 11), should be done.

Methods by which strengthening can be achieved include exercise, activity, or a combination of both. The use of nonproduct-related exercise in occupational therapy is a source of continuing controversy. Exercise allows greater control over the intensity, rate, and duration. The therapist can grade any or all of the parameters more exactly. Improvement can be graphed and understood easily by the patient and others. Activity, on the other hand, provides interest, a motivator for some patients to endure the stress necessary to make gains. Those activities which can be adapted to provide some control over the parameters are chosen.

Weakness rarely exists in only one motion. If one activity involving several motions provided the correct amount of resistance for each of the motions needing strengthening, this activity would be ideal. Usually, however, the therapist must plan different activities within a given treatment period to strengthen all the weak muscles of a patient.

The therapist should plan several activities which would provide exercise to each motion to be strengthened and then allow the patient to select an activity of interest.

Isotonic activity should be characterized by repetition, movement to full range, and a means to gradually increase resistance (weight tool, change materials, etc.). Isometric activity should be characterized by a requirement to hold the contraction for increased periods of time and/or against increased load. Improvement is noted by the amount of work accomplished each work period.

Isometric Exercise and Activity

For muscles graded from Trace (T) strength, isometric contraction to increase the strength and passive exercise to maintain range of motion are most appropriate. Lawrence[36] reports successful case outcomes using two kinds of isometric exercise programs: *Progressive Prolonged Isometric Tension Method* and *Progressive Weighted Isometric Exercise Method*. The Prolonged Method is defined as holding the isometric contraction, at whatever level the patient is capable, for the longest period of time in 10 repetitions. The time of maximal contraction is determined by

trial and error during the 1st treatment day. The time is increased as the patient improves so that maximal effort is exerted to hold the contraction for 10 repetitions with a rest period between. The Weighted Method[27] requires the patient to hold a contraction against weight determined by the DeLorme method, described below, for a given period of time (30 or 45 seconds), with 15-second rest periods interspersed between the 10 repetitions.

Brief Maximal Isometric Exercise.[26] This has been found to be effective in increasing strength. A maximal isometric contraction is held for 6 seconds, once per day. Unfortunately it is difficult to detect without instrumentation whether the patient is exerting his maximal effort. Hislop[19] found that holding the contraction for 15 seconds twice per day was more effective than for lesser amounts of time. Maximal contraction was also more effective than the 67% suggested by Hettinger and Mueller.

Isometric contraction is achieved in activity by grasp of handles (the amount of grasp increases with increasingly resistive material that the tool is used against), stabilization of materials being worked on, or by positioning projects so that the limbs must maintain antigravity positions during the work.

Isotonic Assistive Exercise and Activity

Active assistive exercise can be accomplished manually. The patient moves the part as far as he can, and the therapist completes the motion. This is the method of choice for movements not easily exercised using equipment or activity. In Progressive Assistive Exercise (PAE), equipment is used to provide the minimal amount of weight required to complete the motion after the patient has moved as far as he can by means of muscle contraction. As the strength increases, the task is made more difficult by reducing the amount of weight, *i.e.*, the amount of assistance.[23]

The schedule for weight reduction is based on the Repetition Minimum which is determined by trial and error on the 1st day of treatment. The Repetition Minimum is the least amount of weight necessary to assist the limb to full range, 10 times. On the 2nd treatment day, the program begins using this schedule:

10 repetitions with 200% of Repetition Minimum, rest 2 to 4 minutes
10 repetitions with 150% of Repetition Minimum, rest 2 to 4 minutes
10 repetitions with 100% of Repetition Minimum

In other words, if 12 pounds are required to assist the patient to flex the shoulder through full range 10 times, the program would start out using 24 pounds, then 18, then 12.

The assistance is offered the muscle through the use of apparatus, such as counterbalanced sling or skate with weights and pulley attached. The antagonistic muscles must be strong enough to work against any weight used to assist the completion of motion by the weak muscles in order to return the apparatus to starting position. The therapeutic skate has free-moving ball bearings on the bottom of the skate to assist the patient to move more easily on a flat, smooth surface in a gravity-eliminated plane. The motions that can best be exercised by using this apparatus are shoulder-horizontal abduction and adduction and elbow flexion and extension. Assistance is achieved by use of weights hanging on a rope which passes through a pulley. Location of the pulley on the board provides guidance for the correct direction of movement (Fig. 8.3). The overhead counterbalanced sling suspension suspends (Fig. 8.4) the extremity from ropes that extend from the elbow and wrist cuffs to the overhead bar and finally to weights at the back of the apparatus. Antigravity motions of the proximal extremity, such as shoulder abduction, flexion, and external rotation, can be assisted. Using the springs on the Deltoid Aid cannot provide PAE because they can only be graded by knowing the compression force of each spring and by then selecting the correct number of springs to offer the desired assistance. However, the springs do provide momentum as an assistance to weak muscles and the springiness allows free motion so that patients with P− muscle strength can use the rebound of the spring to start motion in the opposite direction. Al-

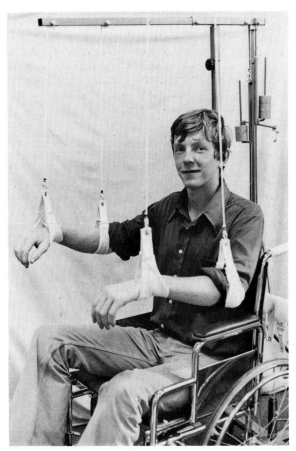

Figure 8.4 Deltoid Aid counterbalanced sling.

though weights are more easily gradable and therefore usually selected on this basis, springs are preferred during functional activities for very weak muscles and when weakness is present in all muscles around a joint.

Dynamic orthoses that assist motions provide active assistive exercise (see Chapter 12).

Few opportunities exist to provide assistive exercise by use of activity. Although a strong extremity can assist a weak one to do the gross, repetitive motions of an activity, the resistance offered by the activity itself must be low. Rolling dough or sanding using a bilateral sander would be too resistive for muscles requiring active assistive exercise, whereas polishing a smooth surface would be possible, but limited in scope. The beater of a floor loom can be weighted to provide progressively less assistance in the direction of weakness. If the elbow extensors are weak, returning the beater might be impossible without assistance of weights and pulley or springs which can be changed to be less assistive as the patient progresses.

Isotonic Active Exercise and Activity

Active exercise requires the patient to complete the range of motion without assistance or resistance. Activities are selected that allow these criteria to be met. For example, eating M & M candies which offers no resistance requires active motion of F elbow flexors. Contraction of the biceps in this case is alternately

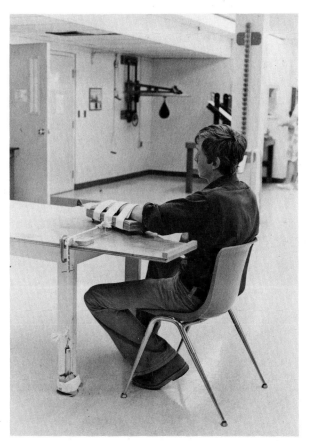

Figure 8.3 Skate with pulley and weight attached to resist horizontal adduction or assist horizontal abduction.

concentric and eccentric: the force against which the muscle works in both cases is that offered by the force of gravity on the lever arm (forearm and hand). An activity which demands contraction of the same muscle during both phases of a movement offers greater exercise potential than one in which return motion is accomplished by the antagonist muscles or by an outside force.

Since most activities require the use of a tool or other resistance, it is easier to find ways to strengthen F muscles if they are put on a gravity-eliminated plane where they can take resistance. For example, a F biceps on a gravity-eliminated plane could take enough resistance to function in a game of chess. In this example, when moving in a gravity-eliminated plane, the type of contraction of the biceps is concentric. Grading of this type of exercise could be accomplished by changing the rate of contraction, the duration, and/or frequency of exercise bouts.

Exercising underwater provides resistance to movement as well as buoyancy.[31] The buoyancy supports the limb. The amount of resistance offered by the water depends on the size of the limb or part being moved against the water; the larger the size, the greater the resistance.

Isotonic Active Resistive Exercise and Activity

Progressive Resistive Exercise (PRE). DeLorme organized an elaborate system of gradation of resistance to achieve maximal strength quickly.[37] The rationale for PRE was to provide a warm-up exercise period so that a greater maximal strength could be achieved. Studies compared the effectiveness of DeLorme's original technique to modified, less time-consuming versions and found them equally effective in attaining the same final outcome of increased strength. In the original technique the resistance was increased in increments of 10% of maximal resistance (Repetition Maximum or RM) up to 100% at 10 repetitions of each increment. Between each set of repetitions the patient rested 2 to 4 minutes. This was a time-consuming process. Two of the modifications found to be equally effective are presented here. The amount of weight the patient can carry 10 times through range of motion using his maximal effort is designated the 10 RM. Determination of 10 RM is done by trial and error: a load is selected which is anticipated to be maximal, and then weight is added or subtracted until 10 RM is established.[8] Jones[38] found that the trial and error method of determining the 10 RM is extremely reliable, even if the subject must lift a load 70 times to determine the 10 RM.

The DeLorme and Watkins modification[23] consists of 10 repetitions at 50% of 10 RM; 10 repetitions at 75% of 10 RM; and 10 repetitions at 100% of 10 RM. The McGovern and Luscombe modification[24] requires five repetitions at 50% of 10 RM and 10 repetitions at 100% of 10 RM. In either modification, between each set of repetitions, the patient rests for 2 to 4 minutes. This sequence is repeated once daily, 5 days per week. The weight is increased as strength improves.

Regressive Resistive Exercise (RRE). McGovern and Luscombe[24] reported a modified sequence of the original work of Zinovieff (Oxford technique) in which strength was increased as effectively using RRE as using PRE. The modification is: 10 repetitions at 100% of 10 RM; 10 repetitions at 75% of 10 RM; and 10 repetitions at 50% of 10 RM. The 10 RM is determined as described above for PRE. These researchers based this plan of regressive resistive exercise on the rationale that resistance should decrease as the muscle fatigues and contracts less effectively.

Overhead counterbalanced sling suspension was previously pictured (see Fig. 8.4) and described as a means of providing active assistive exercise for antigravity motions of the shoulder. It can also provide active resistive exercise to motions working against the pull of the weights or springs. The motions which can be resisted by this device are scapular depression, shoulder adduction, shoulder extension, and shoulder internal rotation. The overhead suspension can be positioned for use with patients in a semireclined position and is consequently often selected in the initial strengthening program for patients with quadriplegia and other conditions with proximal weakness for whom treatment begins before the patient has gained full sitting tolerance. The counterbalanced weights provide direct and easily gradable resistance through a large range of motion. The springs which

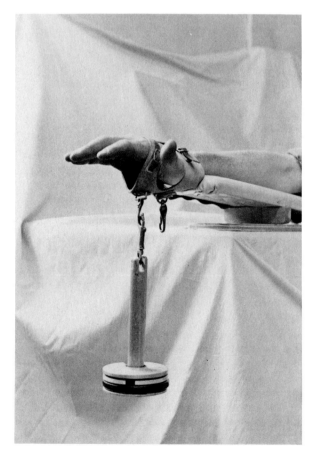

Figure 8.5 PRE for wrist extension.

can be used instead of the weights can be graded only by knowing the force of each spring and by selecting the appropriate number of springs. The skate, described above, can be set up to provide resistance to horizontal ab- or adduction or elbow flexion or extension through weights on a pulley or by use of a motor that puts a preselected amount of tension on the cable attached to the skate.[39]

Exercise of the wrist extensors of a C$_6$ quadriplegic person who will rely on tenodesis grasp may be done by supporting the forearm on an inclined board set at the edge of the table. The hand and wrist are free. A cuff is placed on the hand around the metacarpals to hold the weights (Fig. 8.5). In another example, exercise for a weak extensor digitorum may be accomplished with the forearm and hand supported on a table with the fingers free. Finger loops, to which weights are attached, are placed on each finger over the proximal phalanx (Fig. 8.6).

In occupational therapy, activities that involve repetitious movements and whose resistance can be graded in small increments can be used to provide active resistive exercise. One example is woodworking in which the weight of the sanding block or other tools can be graded (Fig. 8.7). Another example is a game in which the equipment or playing pieces can be changed to increase the resistance, such as grading balls from balloons to medicine balls or grading checkers from

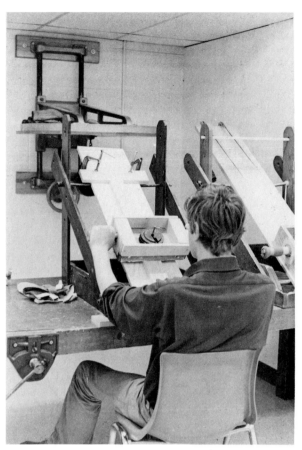

Figure 8.7 Sanding on an inclined plane using a bilateral sander with weights for resistance.

foam rubber pieces to lead pieces. A third example is weaving on a loom whose beater and/or harnesses can be weighted or otherwise adapted. A method of adapting a floor loom to provide PRE to shoulder depressor muscles has been devised. Although successful in increasing strength, the quality of the project suffered.[40] Some patients would not be tolerant of that and would therefore prefer to first do strengthening exercise and then do the weaving normally to increase endurance by using the newly acquired strength functionally.

GOAL: TO INCREASE ENDURANCE

Principle: Increased Duration at Less than 50% Maximal Intensity and Rate

Fatigue develops in a muscle fiber if insufficient recovery time is allowed for reabsorption of lactic acid. In ordinary daily activities which are lightly resistive, motor units contract asynchronously; after a motor unit contracts, it recovers to some degree while its fellow units take their turn to contract. Fatigue occurs slowly as contrasted to the rapidity of fatigue that occurs after maximal contraction in which many more units must contract simultaneously and do not have the opportunity to recover during the period of the contraction. Exercise for endurance, therefore, utilizes

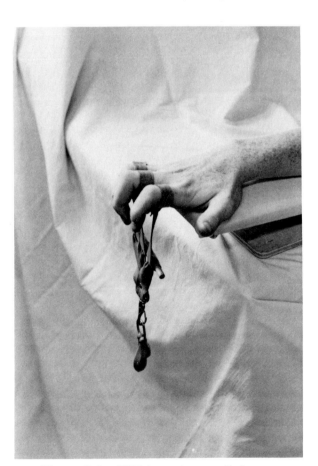

Figure 8.6 PRE for extensor digitorum.

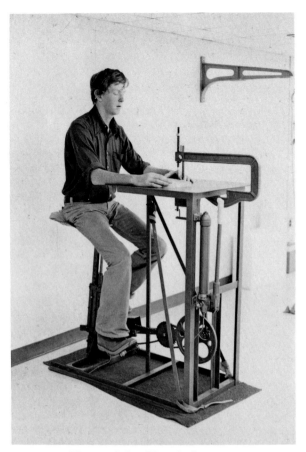

Figure 8.8 Bicycle jigsaw.

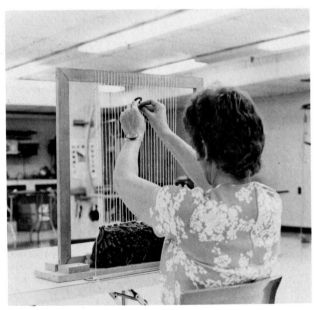

Figure 8.9 Turkish knot weaving.

of an isotonic contraction or length of time an isometric contraction is held. An interim method of upgrading the work output of the patient who is not ready to increase the duration is to increase the frequency of exercise or activity per day or per week.

Occupational therapy provides the patient with interest-sustaining activities which are gradable along the dimensions of time or repetition. As an example, a patient can operate a bicycle jigsaw, rather than a stationery bicycle, to increase both general endurance and specific endurance of lower extremity musculature while sawing a woodworking project of his choice (Fig. 8.8). This might encourage him to invest his effort longer than he might be willing to do for repetitious contraction exercise, such as lifting leg weights. As another example, a patient with severely low endurance can do light activities, such as mosaic tiles or turkish knotting (Fig. 8.9). The pieces completed each day can be counted, and progress can be easily measured by the therapist and the patient.

With the current emphasis on physical fitness in the USA, some persons prefer exercise to crafts. In that case, the person will want to continue beyond the PRE or RRE regime required to increase strength. The resistance can be reduced to less than 50% of 10 RM and the activity continued for a longer period of time.[8] A record of the time the patient can engage in the activity to the point of fatigue indicates changes in endurance. As the muscle increases in strength, the amount of resistance used in endurance activities will also increase.

Recalling that DeLateur *et al.*[16] found that strengthening occurred even with less than maximal resistance if a muscle worked to the point of fatigue, and recognizing that the ability to sustain effort requires less than maximal effort in order for metabolic recovery to occur, the relationship between activity to increase strength and activity to increase endurance can be clarified. When the objective of treatment is to increase endurance, less than maximal effort is required, but strengthening will also occur if the activity is repeated to the point of fatigue.

Programming for increasing endurance in patients with cardiac problems is discussed in Chapter 24.

References

1. Tookey, P., and Larson, C. *Range of Motion Exercise: Key to Joint Mobility.* Minneapolis: American Rehabilitation Foundation, 1968.
2. Bergstrom, D., and Coles, C. *Basic Positioning Procedures.* Minneapolis: Kenny Rehabilitation Institute, 1971.
3. Feinberg, J., and Andree, M. Dynamic foot splint for the Hoffman apparatus. *Am. J. Occup. Ther., 34*(1): 45, 1980.
4. Brown, D. M., DeBacher, G., and Basmajian, J. V. Feedback goniometers for hand rehabilitation. *Am. J. Occup. Ther., 33*(7): 458–463, 1979.
5. Downey, J., and Darling, R. *Physiological Basis of Rehabilitation Medicine.* Philadelphia: W. B. Saunders, 1971.
6. Heurich, M., and Polansky, S. An adaptation of the glove flexion mitt. *Am. J. Occup. Ther., 32*(2): 110–111, 1978.
7. Agre, J. C. Static stretching for athletes. *Arch. Phys. Med. Rehabil., 59*(11): 561, 1978.
8. Kottke, F. Therapeutic exercise. In *Handbook of Physical Medicine and Rehabilitation,* 2nd ed., edited by F. H. Krusen,

moderately fatiguing activity for progressively longer periods of time with intervals of rest to allow metabolic recovery.[8]

Activity or exercise used to increase endurance is graded by increasing the duration of the exercise period, which means increasing the number of repetitions

F. J. Kottke, and P. M. Ellwood. Philadelphia: W. B. Saunders, 1971.

9. Maitland, G. D. *Peripheral Manipulation*, 2nd ed. Boston: Butterworths, 1977.

10. Tanigawa, M. Comparison of the hold-relax procedure and passive mobilization on increasing muscle length. *Phys. Ther., 52*(7): 725–735, 1972.

11. Medeiros, J. M., *et al.* The influence of isometric exercise and passive stretch on hip joint motion. *Phys. Ther., 57*(5): 518–523, 1977.

12. Markos, P. Comparison of Hold-Relax and Contract-Relax and Contralateral Effects. Unpublished master's thesis, Boston University, 1977.

13. Maughan, I. V. Graduated supination-pronation attachments for table and floor looms. *Am. J. Occup. Ther., 16*(6): 285–286, 1962.

14. Eyler, R. Treatment of flexion contractures in occupational therapy. *Am. J. Occup. Ther., 19*(2): 86–88, 1965.

15. Hellebrandt, F. A. Application of the overload principle to muscle training in man. *Int. Rev. Phys. Med. Rehab.,* Oct.: 278–283, 1958.

16. DeLateur, B., *et al.* Isotonic versus isometric exercies: A double-shift transfer-of-training study. *Arch. Phys. Med. Rehabil., 53*(5): 212–216, 1972.

17. Barnard, R. J., Edgerton, V. R., and Peter, J. B. Effects of exercise on skeletal muscle. I. Biochemical and histochemical properties. *J. Appl. Physiol., 28:* 762–766, 1970.

18. Dons, B., Bollerup, K., Bonde-Petersen, F., and Hancke, S. The effect of weight-lifting exercise related to muscle fiber composition and muscle cross-sectional area in humans. *Eur. J. Appl. Physiol., 40:* 95–106, 1979.

19. Hislop, H. Quantitative changes in human muscular strength during isometric exercise. *Phys. Ther., 43*(1): 21–38, 1963.

20. Riendl, A. M., *et al.* Cardiovascular response of human subjects to isometric contraction of large and small muscle groups. *Proc. Soc. Exp. Biol. Med., 154:* 171–174, 1977.

21. Carlson, B. R. Relationship between isometric and isotonic strength. *Arch. Phys. Med. Rehabil., 51*(3): 176–179, 1970.

22. Rasch, P. J. The present status of negative (eccentric) exercise: A review. *Am. Correct. Ther. J., 28*(3): 77–94, 1974.

23. DeLorme, T. L., and Watkins, A. L. Technics of progressive resistance exercise. *Arch. Phys. Med. Rehabil., 29:* 263–273, 1948.

24. McGovern, R. E., and Luscombe, H. B. Useful modifications of progressive resistive exercise technique. *Arch. Phys. Med. Rehabil., 34:* 475–477, 1953.

25. DeLateur, B., *et al.* Comparison of effectiveness of isokinetic and isotonic exercise in quadriceps strengthening. *Arch. Phys. Med. Rehabil., 53:* 60–64, 1972.

26. Rose, D. L., *et al.* Effects of brief maximal exercise on the strength of the quadriceps femoris. *Arch. Phys. Med. Rehabil., 38:* 157–164, 1957.

27. Lawrence, M. S. Strengthening the quadriceps femoris: Progressive weighted isometric exercise method. *Phys. Ther. Rev., 40*(8): 577–584, 1960.

28. Hislop, H. Response of immobilized muscle to isometric exercise. *Phys. Ther., 44*(5): 339–347, 1964.

29. Doss, W., and Karpovich, P. A comparison of concentric, eccentric and isometric strength of the elbow flexors. *J. Appl. Physiol., 20*(2): 351–353, 1965.

30. Singh, M., and Karpovich, P. Isotonic and isometric forces of forearm flexors and extensors. *J. Appl. Physiol., 21:* 1435–1437, 1966.

31. Gowitzke, B. A., and Milner, M. *Understanding the Scientific Bases of Human Movement*, 2nd ed. Baltimore: Williams & Wilkins, 1980.

32. Mannheimer, J. A comparison of strength gain between concentric and eccentric contraction. *Phys. Ther., 49*(11): 1201–1207, 1969.

33. Lawrence, M. S. Comparative increase in muscle strength in the quadriceps femoris by isometric and isotonic exercise and effects on the contralateral muscle. *Phys. Ther., 42*(1): 15–20, 1962.

34. Singh, M., and Karpovich, P. Effect of eccentric training of agonists on antagonistic muscles. *J. Appl. Physiol., 23*(5): 742–745, 1967.

35. Hinson, M., and Rosentswieg, J. Comparative electromyographic values of isometric, isotonic, and isokinetic contraction. *Res. Q., 44*(1): 71–78, 1973.

36. Lawrence, M. S. Strengthening the quadriceps. Progressively prolonged isometric tension method. *Phys. Ther. Rev., 36*(10): 658–661, 1956.

37. DeLorme, T. Restoration of muscle power by heavy resistance exercises. *J. Bone Joint Surg., 27:* 645–667, 1945.

38. Jones, R. E. Reliability of the ten repetition maximum for assessing progressive resistance exercise. *J.A.P.T.A.* 42(10: 661–662, 1962.

39. Roemer, R. B., Culler, M. A., and Swartt, T. Automated upper extremity progressive resistive exercise system, *Am. J. Occup. Ther., 32*(2): 105–108, 1978.

40. Hultkrans, R., and Sandeen, A. Application of progressive resistive exercise to occupational therapy. *Am. J. Occup. Ther., 11*(4): 238–240, 1957.

Supplementary Reading

Arem, A. J., and Madden, J. W. Effects of stress on healing wounds. I. Intermittent noncyclical tension. *J. Surg. Res., 20:* 93–102, 1976.

Bell, C. C. Endurance, strength, and coordination exercise without cardiovascular or respiratory distress. *J. Natl. Med. Assoc., 71*(3): 265–270, 1979.

Chapman, E. A., deVries, H. A., and Swezey, R. Joint stiffness: Effects of exercise on young and old men. *J. Gerontol., 27*(2): 218–221, 1972.

Dontigny, R. L. Use of a sponge to improve hand strength and coordination. *Phys. Ther., 56*(5): 573, 1976.

Downer, A. H. Door frame exercise for tight shoulders. *Phys. Ther., 54*(3): 252–253, 1974.

Hellebrandt, F. A., and Houtz, S. J. Mechanisms of muscle training in man: Experimental demonstration of the overload principle. *Phys. Ther. Rev., 36*(6): 371–383, 1956.

Hygenic Corporation. *The Thera-Band Resistive Exerciser Instruction Book.* Akron, Ohio.

Johnson, B. L., and Adamczyk, J. W. A program of eccentric-concentric strength training. *Am. Correct. Ther. J.* 29(1): 13–16, 1975.

Johnson, M. M., and Bonner, C. D. Sling suspension techniques, demonstrating the use of a new portable frame. II. Methods of progression in an exercise program—the upper extremity. *Phys. Ther., 51*(10): 1092–1099, 1971.

Lesser, M. The effects of rhythmic exercise on the range of motion in older adults. *Am. Correct. Ther. J., 32*(4): 118–122, 1978.

Moffroid, M. T., and Whipple, R. H. Specificity of speed of exercise. *Phys. Ther., 50*(12): 1692–1700, 1970.

Moritani, T., and deVries, H. A. Potential for gross muscle hypertrophy in older men. *J. Gerontol., 35*(5): 672–682, 1980.

Petrofsky, J. S., *et al.* Comparison of physiological responses of women and men to isometric exercise. *J. Appl. Physiol., 38*(5): 863–868, 1975.

Pipes, T. Variable resistance versus constant resistance strength training in adult males. *Eur. J. Appl. Physiol., 39:* 27–35, 1978.

Rose, D. L., and Page, P. B. Conscious proprioception and increase in muscle strength. *Arch. Phys. Med. Rehabil., 50*(1): 6–10, 1969.

Vasudevan, S. V., and Melvin, J. L. Upper extremity edema control: Rationale of the techniques. *Am. J. Occup. Ther., 33*(8): 520–523, 1979.

Weeks, P. M., Wray, R. C., and Kuxhaus, M. The results of nonoperative management of stiff joints in the hand. *Plast. Reconstr. Surg., 61*(1): 58–63, 1978.

Zinovieff, A. N. Heavy-resistance exercises: The "Oxford technique." *Br. J. Phys. Med., 14:* 129–132, 1951.

PART FOUR

Activity

Activity is the medium of occupational therapy. One develops cognitive, perceptual, psychosocial, and motor skills through engagement in activity of interest and purpose. Anything that requires mental processing of data, physical manipulation of objects, or directed movement may be considered an activity. Any one activity used in therapy may offer the opportunity for skill development in cognition, perception, psychosocial function, and/or movement. Persons with physical disabilities will not only need to develop motor skills, but may also need to develop skills in other areas. However, since this book is focusing on the theory and practice of physical restoration, the sensorimotor components of activities are those with which this book is concerned. This is not to say that the other aspects of activity are unimportant, but to recognize that analysis of activity in each area of skill is based on an understanding of the theory and practice in that area.

Activities have intrinsic and potential therapeutic value. The therapist analyzes the activity to determine its intrinsic value and may adapt the activity to develop its potential value. Activity analysis and adaptation will be presented in this part.

chapter

9

Activity Selection and Analysis

Catherine A. Trombly, M.A., OTR

Activity of many kinds define human existence.[1] Activities are inherently important to the individual not only to fulfill basic needs and wants but also to achieve mastery and competence. Activity is the treatment occupational therapy offers to patients based on the hypothesis that activities can produce change away from dysfunctional and toward functional behavior.[1] The occupational therapist designs activities to apply the theories and treatment procedures given in chapters 5, 6, and 8. The use of purposeful activity makes treatment meaningful to the client and makes him his own co-therapist. No one can do occupational therapy to a person; the person must engage in the activity to benefit. However, the purpose of the activity may not be readily apparent to the client, and therefore the therapist must make the purpose explicit to him.

In this text, activities are defined not only as arts and crafts used traditionally in the practice of occupational therapy, but also as sports, games, vocational tasks, and exercise in which the attention is focused on the purpose of the exercise rather than the movement itself.

ACTIVITY SELECTION

The major function of the occupational therapist is to select the best activity to meet each goal of the patient's program. To select the best activity, the therapist identifies the patient's problem, the short-term goal that the activity is to effect, the theoretical approach and principle appropriate to the problem, and the person's interests and cognitive/psychosocial abilities.

Generally, activities used to increase physical function should be developmentally appropriate; be within the patient's capabilities; be gradable to progress the patient to the next higher level of function; involve, on a more or less selective basis, the muscles, motions, or joints being treated; be as repetitive as required to evoke the therapeutic benefit. The best activity is one which intrinsically demands the exact movement which has been determined to need improvement. Contrived methods of doing an ordinary activity may diminish the value of the activity in the eyes of the patient. Contrived methods also require the patient to constantly focus his attention directly on his movements rather than the end purpose of the activity. This, at the least, diminishes satisfaction and may even interfere with developing coordinated, smooth voluntary motion.

The activity selected should have a reasonable end goal or product. If the therapist chooses to strengthen shoulder flexors by the use of the activity of sanding wood, then the patient should sand pieces of something that become an end product. If the patient is not interested in the end product, perhaps the selection of activity is inappropriate. Some patients prefer "pure exercise" to other activity because of the value that is placed on exercise by the general public, or the doubt that a pleasurable activity is also therapeutic, or other reasons. In that case, the activity used in occupational therapy will be directed movement or exercise; it is of questionable value to require the outward appearance of productive activity when no product is involved. Sanding a board not intended to be used, riding a bicycle jig saw without sawing, screwing "millions" of screws into a board for no decorative or other purpose are all examples of poor activity selection.

Activity Characteristics

Some specific characteristics that an activity must have to be considered therapeutic for the goals listed below are the following.

Increase of Active Range of Motion

The activity must require that the part of the body being treated move to its limit repeatedly; the activity must be gradable, naturally or through adaptations (see Chapter 10), to demand greater amounts of movement as the patient's limit changes.

Increase of Passive Range of Motion

The activity must provide controlled stretch or traction to the part being treated for a defined period of time. See Chapter 8 for precautions.

Increase of Strength

The activity must stress the muscle up to its limits. Requiring the muscle to contract 10 times against maximal resistance is one way to stress it. Other methods will be found in Chapter 8, along with precautions. The activity should allow grading the increase of the stress as the patient's limit changes.

Increase of Endurance

The activity must be repetitious over a controlled number of times for a period of time. It should be resistive to 50% or less of maximal strength.

Increase of Coordination/Dexterity

The activity should allow as much range of motion as the patient can control; should be repetitious for practice; should allow grading from the point where the patient is able to function to a finer (more precise, accurate, faster) level.

Increase of Tone

The activity should offer exteroceptive, proprioceptive, and/or vestibular stimulation.

Decrease of Tone

The activity should be devoid of stimulation.

Increase of Stability (or Decrease of Mobility)

The activity should be developmentally correct; be resistive to axial or proximal limb musculature and/or demand weight bearing for a period of time (see Chapter 5 for a discussion on weight-bearing postures); be gradable to allow controlled movement after stability response is learned.

Increase of Mobility

The activity should be developmentally correct; offer little or no resistance; demand repeated full range of motion movements; be gradable to allow controlled movement of specific joints as the patient gains control (mobility at proximal joints with stability at distal ones and vice versa).

Examples of the use of activities to achieve therapeutic goals may be found throughout this book.

When deciding on a possible activity to use to increase physical function of a particular patient, other factors are important in the selection. The cognitive aspects of any activity must match the patient's capabilities. The number and complexity of the steps, the requirement for organization and sequencing of the steps or stimuli, and the amount of concentration and memory required are some of the cognitive factors of an activity to be considered. Some examples of perceptual factors to be considered are whether the activity requires the patient to distinguish figure from ground, position in space, or to construct from diagrams. The psychosocial aspects of an activity must be considered so that the patient may enjoy and benefit from the activity. Whether the activity must be done alone or may be done in a group; the length of time required to complete an activity; whether fine, detailed work or large movements are involved, and the ease with which errors can be corrected are some of the aspects of activity choice which may be psychologically important to patients.

Although the therapist has determined what seems to be the ideal therapeutic activity, it is inappropriate to assign any patient to a task without ascertaining his interests, discussing choices with him, and allowing him to select the activity of his choice from several which are equally effective. If he selects the activity, he is more likely to be committed to doing the activity as prescribed. Several activities may be required during one treatment session in order to work on several therapeutic goals simultaneously.

ACTIVITY ANALYSIS

The occupational therapist's job begins where the theoretical bases for improved movement leaves off; the therapist must translate these theories into activities appropriate for the individual client. Activity analysis is the process used to do that translation. Activity analysis is the process of closely examining activities to determine their components. The therapist who is skilled in analysis can more easily select the most therapeutically appropriate activity from those that are available and are of interest to the patient.

What the student therapist must do is to learn the process of activity analysis so that it becomes second nature. This takes practice. Students often ask why there isn't a book published with all activities analyzed and cross-referenced with disabilities so that activity prescription can be more like drug prescription. Perhaps that can be done in the decades to come when electromyographic analysis and computers will be used routinely. Right now it can't be done validly because any differences in the position or size of the patient, the relative position of the work to the patient, the tools, the materials, or the patient's manner of working may change the outcome of the analysis. The therapist must consider all these factors in the analysis.

Motor analysis of activities may be from a biomechanical or neurodevelopmental point of view.

Traditionally, analysis has been done by observing others or by doing the activity oneself while attending to what muscles should contract and relax, based on anatomical studies of muscles, joints, and bony levers. That method is used here, as it is still the most universal one. However, electromyographic kinesiological analyses of some exercises and activities have been done.[2-4]

Electromyography (EMG) is the process by which recordings of the electrical potentials produced by a contracting muscle are made for study. When a muscle is at rest no myopotentials are recorded. As the muscle contracts to maximum, the amplitude and frequency of the myopotentials increase proportionately. Electromyograms correlated to data from tracking devices which record the position of the monitored limb indicate which of the monitored muscles are working to what degree during performance of an activity. EMG studies have shown variability among subjects doing the same exercise; therefore, even by incorporating the newer EMG information into the analysis, the analysis will not be perfect for a particular patient because of individual differences in muscle action. If it is essential that a particular muscle of a particular patient be contracting to a certain level of activity, as may be the case when a tendon has been repaired; or if a certain muscle must be relaxing, as in the case of spastic hemiplegia, then it is best to monitor the muscle directly by using a small EMG monitor for biofeedback while the patient does the activity.

The results of one study[3] of low and high resistance activities made the following conclusions. In this study, the flexor profundus (FP), the extensor digitorum (ED), the dorsal interosseous I (DI), and the abductor pollicis brevis/opponens (ABD/OPP) were the only muscles monitored. The FP and ED were each more active as an antagonist during resisted activity than during unresisted activity when each was a prime mover. For instance, the extensor digitorum recruited 58% of maximum during resisted grasp while only <19% during opening the hand against no resistance. There was simultaneous contraction of agonist and antagonist even in low resistance activities in which skill or precision was involved. The size of the object grasped and released did not affect the level of activity of the FP or ED. There was increasing variability between subjects in the amount of output of the muscles as resistance increased from low to high; therefore, EMG biofeedback was recommended to ensure that the muscle under treatment is actually contracting to desired levels. The activities in which each muscle was most active (more than 50% of maximal output) by the most subjects (more than 50%) are listed in Table 9.1.

Unpublished data of EMGs taken on hemiplegic patients with active grasp but no voluntary finger extension indicate that while the patients were grasping maximally, a much greater electrical output (indicating recruitment of motor units) was seen in the extensor digitorum than would have been expected from observing the patients' ability to extend the fingers against no resistance.[5]

Some of these conclusions are contrary to our expectations based on anatomical studies or simple application of neurophysiological data to movement. Basmajian[2] reports other findings by electromyographers. It is recommended that therapists use published

Table 9.1
ACTIVITIES WHICH CALLED FORTH MORE THAN 50% OUTPUT IN FOUR HAND MUSCLES OF AT LEAST 50% OF THE 15 NORMAL SUBJECTS[a]

Muscles	Activities
Extensor digitorum	Extension game (lift Velcro checker off of Velcro board using finger extension); Theraplast donut (extend fingers and abduct thumb to spread a donut-shaped piece of Theraplast).
Flexor profundus	Closing the lid of a large jar; Theraplast grasp (grasp of a 2.5-cm cylinder of Theraplast and squeeze maximally); Theraplast donut and extension game.
Dorsal interosseous I	Theraplast grasp and Theraplast pinch (pinch a 2.5-cm ball of Theraplast between the pads of the thumb and index finger).
Abductor pollicis brevis/opponens	Opening and closing of a large jar lid; Theraplast pinch; Theraplast grasp; tip pinch game (lift Velcro checker off of Velcro board using tip pinch).

[a] From C. A. Trombly and J. M. Cole.[3]

EMG studies to assist in activity selection and analysis.

Biomechanical Analysis

The therapist begins the biomechanical analysis of the activity by *establishing the exact placement* of the selected tools and equipment in relation to the patient. Changes in the equipment, supplies, or placement change the demands of the activity; only analysis of a specific activity under specific circumstances is valid. The *steps of an activity are identified.* For example, the steps of hammering a nail are: (a) reach for and pick up the hammer; (b) carry the hammer to the start position; (c) pick up the nail; (d) place the nail; (e) hit the nail; and (f) return the hammer to the start position. Only c, d, and e would be analyzed; a, b, and f occur too infrequently to be therapeutic. *Each step is then subdivided into motions.* For example, hitting the nail can involve elbow flexion and extension or shoulder internal and external rotation, depending on the location of the nail. Wrist stabilization in extension and cylindrical grasp are also part of that step. The *range of each of these motions is estimated* by observation of the patient, another person, or the therapist himself, preferably in a mirror, while the activity is performed. Range can also be measured by using a goniometer in cases where the degrees of range of motion are crucial to the therapeutic effect. The *potential repetitions of each motion are noted.* Whether the activity is intrinsically unilateral, bilateral, or reciprocal also needs to be considered.

The *kind of contraction* for each motion is established by definition, *i.e.*, concentric, eccentric, isometric, or static. Each body part involved in the activity is observed to determine the kinds of contraction demanded by each muscle group for all of the motions involved in the activity. Each motion is further analyzed to determine *which muscle(s)* and *what minimal strength* are required based on anatomical, kinesiological, and electromyographical knowledge. The amount of work a muscle or muscle group is doing depends on the resistance. Resistance is determined by the pull of gravity on the limb and on the implements the patient may be using, which together act as the lever arm. The effect of a given amount of resistance can be altered by lengthening or shortening the lever arm. The longer the lever arm, the greater the force required to lift the resistance. The lever arm is lengthened or shortened by changing the location of the resistance, for example, application of the resistance at the end of the humerus rather than at the wrist. The lever arm can also be altered by "shortening or lengthening the limb"; for example, less resistance

Table 9.2
BIOMECHANICAL ACTIVITY ANALYSIS

Name of the Activity: _____

1. Describe how the person and the materials are positioned, especially in relation to one another:

_____

_____

_____

2. What precautions must be considered? _____

_____

3. What stabilization is necessary to do this activity? _____

_____

4. Analyze the activity using page two. What are its essential characteristics? _____

_____

_____

_____

5. How can this activity be graded to increase:
   a. Strength? _____

   b. PROM? _____

   c. Coordination? _____

   d. Endurance? _____

Steps in Activity and Motions in Each Step (do essential ones only) *e.g.,* *Step 1* Motions *Step 2* Motions	ROM	Prime Movers (Muscles)	Type of Contraction	Repetition	Gravity Assists/ Resists/ No Effect	Minimal Strength Necessary

Table 9.3
NEURODEVELOPMENTAL ACTIVITY ANALYSIS

1. Name of the activity _____
2. Describe how the person and the materials are positioned, especially in relation to one another.
3. What precautions must be considered?
4. Does this activity demand mobility, stability, distal stability with proximal mobility, or proximal stability with distal mobility?
5. What posture or ontogenetic pattern of motion is demanded by the activity?
6. Does this activity demand ballistic (too fast to allow correction via feedback; open loop) or guided (closed loop) movement?
7. Does the activity demand a response in synergistic patterns of the limbs or opposite to the synergies? Which synergy?
8. oes the activity demand movement of the whole limb or isolated control of single joints? Which ones?
9. What muscle groups are exercised?
10. Are these muscles activated reflexly; automatically in developmental patterns; or under voluntary control?
11. What *controlled* sensory stimulation is offered by the activity? To which muscle groups? Is the effect facilitatory or inhibitory?

Stimulation	Muscle group	⊕ or ⊖

12. Does the activity demand a cortical or subcortical response from the patient (attention to the movement *per se* or attention to the goal)?
13. Can this activity be adapted to progress the patient to the next level of development of motor control? How?
14. What short-term goals would be met by this activity (When would you choose to use this activity?)

is offered to hip flexion if the knee is flexed (limb shortened) than if it is extended.

Table 9.2 facilitates the analysis of activities using a biomechanical approach by structuring the components to be examined.

Neurodevelopmental Analysis

Neurodevelopmental analysis includes consideration of the developmental and neurophysiological aspects of activity. Adults with brain damage will need activities selected on the basis of development of voluntary motor skill. The neurophysiological aspects of activity refer to the sensory stimulation which it offers.

An activity is observed to determine which of the following characteristics may be present. A form, such as the one shown in Table 9.3, will guide the therapist in this analysis. Movements and positions involved in the activity are observed to determine if primitive reflexes are being reinforced or if the most desirable righting and equilibrium reactions are being encouraged. For example, if a patient were to reach out to the side to place or pick up an object while watching his hand placement, the asymmetric tonic neck reflex (ATNR) would be reinforced. A game of ball while sitting unsupported would encourage righting and equilibrium reactions.

Another characteristic to be observed is whether the activity demands stability and/or mobility responses and of which joints. For example, throwing a ball requires stability of the neck, trunk, and lower extremities and mobility of the throwing arm. Batting a baseball is an example of distal stability and proximal mobility of the upper extremity. The position in which the activity is done and/or the movements involved are noted for their developmental level according to known sequences. On this basis, the therapist selects activities which would be within the patient's capability but challenging to his development of motor control.

The amount of attention required in the performance of an activity and whether attention is directed toward the movement itself or toward the end goal is noted. There is more cortical control required when attention is directed to the movement itself.

Observation of the sensory stimuli offered by the activity is necessary because of the more-or-less empirically proven effects of sensation on movement. The kinds of sensation which the activity offers are noted and may include any or all of the following. Tactile stimulation is provided by various textures or contact with other surfaces. Temperature stimulation is provided by the environment or by contact with warm or cool objects or surfaces. Vestibular stimulation is offered by upsidedown or prone position, by acceleration, deceleration, or rotation or spinning movements of the head or whole body. Other proprioceptive stimulation is provided by resistance to movement, stretch of muscles, pressure, or vibration, in addition to movement and position. Visual, auditory, olfactory, and gustatory sensations offered by an activity are also noted.

References

1. Cynkin, S. *Occupational Therapy: Toward Health Through Activity*. Boston: Little, Brown and Company, 1979.
2. Basmajian, J. V. *Muscles Alive: Their Functions Revealed by Electromyography*, 4th ed. Baltimore: Williams & Wilkins, 1979.
3. Trombly, C. A., and Cole, J. M. Electromyographic study of four hand muscles during selected activities. *Am. J. Occup. Ther., 33*(7): 440–449, 1979.
4. Long, C. Intrinsic-extrinsic muscle control of the fingers. *J. Bone Joint Surg., 50*A: 573–584, 1968.
5. Trombly, C. A., and Quintana, L. A. Effects of exercise on finger extension of post-CVA patients. *Am. J. Occup. Ther.*, in press, 1982.

Supplementary Reading

Bissel, J. C., and Mailloux, Z. The use of crafts in occupational therapy for the physically disabled. *Am. J. Occup. Ther., 35*(6): 369–374, 1981.

Dicmonas, E. A. psychoneurophysiologically based activity analysis. In *Physical Disabilities Manual*, edited by B. C. Abreu. New York: Raven Press, 1981, pp. 201–223.

Hamill, C. M., and Oliver, R. C. *Therapeutic Activities for the Handicapped Elderly*. Gaithersburg, Md.: Aspen Systems Corporation, 1980.

chapter

10

Activity Adaptation

Catherine A. Trombly, M.A., OTR
Anna Deane Scott, M.Ed., OTR

Activity adaptation is the process of modifying a familiar craft/game/sport or other activity to accomplish a therapeutic goal. There are two reasons to adapt an activity in the treatment of the physically disabled. One is to modify the activity to make it therapeutic when ordinarily it would not be so in the unadapted form. Many examples of this can be seen in occupational therapy clinics. Some such examples are floor loom adaptations to provide exercise to muscles not usually involved in weaving[1]; wall checkers in which the board is painted on the wall and has pegs at each square to hold the enlarged checkers; and biofeedback units electronically coupled to switches to turn appliances on and off.

The other reason for adaptation is to graduate the exercise offered by the activity along therapeutic continua to accomplish goals. Although the same amount of assistance or resistance may be offered manually by the therapist while the patient performs an unadapted activity, adaptation is preferred because the resistance or assistance will be consistent over time; the patient can work independently and thereby have feelings of satisfaction; and, in cases where the patient is learning a new pattern of motion, the therapist would be an interference. One instance of adapting for exercise gradation is to change the size of the implements of the activity. To increase coordination, the activity must be graded along a continuum from gross, coarse movement to fine, accurate movement. Checkers and other board games lend themselves easily to such gradations; the board and pieces can be changed from large to small. The person who is a checker aficionado can continue a favorite game while continuing to benefit therapeutically.

The characteristics of a good adaptation are the following: The adaptation accomplishes the specific goal. The adaptation does not encourage or require odd movements or postures. Positioning must be rea-

sonable for the activity involved. The adaptation is soundly constructed and is not potentially dangerous to the patient. The adaptation does not require the patient to think in terms of the movement, *per se.* Adaptations must be such that they intrinsically demand a certain response by the patient, one that he does not have to concentrate on performing. Finally, it does not demean the patient; some rube goldberg adaptations seem ridiculous to the patient, and therefore he is embarrassed to use them.

When adapting activities, as with all therapeutic techniques, it is vital for the patient to understand the reason that an activity will be done in an adapted manner.

Principles of adaptation correspond to the treatment principles given in Chapters 5 and 8. Activity adaptations that implement these principles are described here.

POSITIONING THE TASK RELATIVE TO THE PERSON

The position of the person relative to the work to be done dictates the movement demanded by the activity. Adaptation by positioning refers to changes in incline of work surface, height of work surface, or placement of pieces to be added to the project (Figs. 10.1 to 10.3).

Activities which are usually done on a flat surface, such as fingerpainting, board games, sanding wood, or using the exercise skate, can be made more or less resistive by changing the incline of the surface. For example, if the surface is inclined down, forward and away from the patient, resistance is given to shoulder extension and elbow flexion. If the incline is up, resistance is given to shoulder flexion and elbow extension.

The standard horizontal work surface itself can be raised or lowered to make demands on certain muscle groups or to alter the effect of gravity. For example, a table raised to axilla height allows flexion and extension of the elbow on a gravity-eliminated plane. Another example is to lower the table surface to elbow

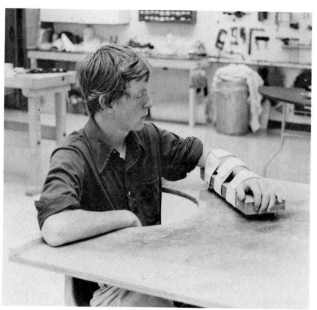

Figure 10.1 Skate and skateboard positioned at midchest level.

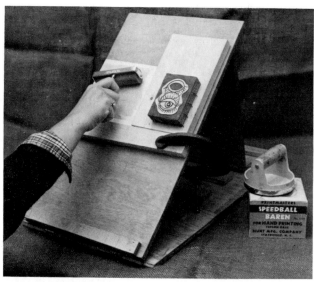

Figure 10.3 Block printing repositioned. Block is held in place by resting on nails below and to the right of the block. Height can be changed by moving the board C-clamped to the incline board.

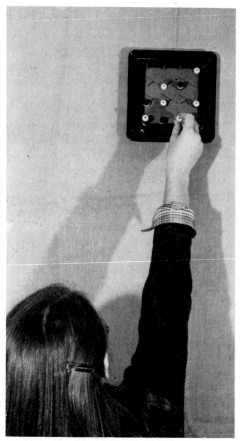

Figure 10.2 "Score Four" game mounted on the wall to require shoulder flexion and elbow extension.

height so that supination/pronation movements are evoked while eliminating shoulder rotation by allowing the upper arm to remain adducted during the process of moving items around on the table surface. Using a skate, if the skateboard is adjusted to axilla height, shoulder horizontal abduction or adduction can be resisted. If the table is adjusted waist high, shoulder external or internal rotation can be resisted.

Placing items such as mosaic tiles, pieces of yarn, beads, darts, bean bags, etc. in various locations changes the motion required to reach them when performing an activity in an otherwise standard manner. Placement may be high enough to encourage shoulder flexion or abduction; lateral to encourage shoulder rotation, trunk rotation, or horizontal motion; or low to encourage trunk flexion, or lateral trunk flexion.

Positioning can evoke responses within developmental patterns. For example, in sitting or side-sitting, placement of the pieces of an activity to one side will require that the person reach with one arm, stabilize with the other arm, and rotate the trunk to reach them. Activities requiring reaching for objects will evoke equilibrium responses.

ADDING WEIGHTS

The addition of weights adapts an activity to meet such goals as: increase of strength, promotion of co-contraction, increase of passive range of motion by stretch.

Some nonresistive activities can be made resistive by adding weights to the apparatus, directly or by use of pulleys, while others may be made resistive by adding weights to the person himself. For example, to resist shoulder extension and elbow flexion, weights can be suspended from pulleys attached across from the person on a flat or inclined surface with the weight lines running from each handle of a bilateral sanding block. The line of pull can be reversed to resist shoulder flexion and elbow extension by attaching the pulleys behind the person.

Resistance can be changed on all looms[2]; however, the floor looms lend themselves to more versatility in the application of the resistance. Weights can be added directly to the harnesses, treadles, or beater or can be added indirectly to the beater by the use of a pulley system (Fig. 10.4).

Weights can be attached directly to the person by means of weighted cuffs, as well as by pulley line attachments. For example, when using a weighted wrist cuff, leather lacing can become resistive to external rotation and elbow flexion. As another example, braid weaving can be made resistive to shoulder flexion by means of weights and pulleys attached over the back of the person's chair with the lines running to a cuff fastened around the person's humerus.

Tools also are weights and can be selected or adjusted to offer graded resistance. Some of the possibilites include the following. Hammers can be graded from light-weight tack hammers to heavy ball-peen or claw hammers. Weaving can be done on table looms, and as the patient gains range and/or strength, larger, heavier floor looms may be used.

ADDING SPRINGS AND RUBBERBANDS

Springs and rubber bands are means of adapting activity to increase strength or the cocontraction response through resistance, or to assist a weak muscle, or to stretch muscle and other soft tissue to increase passive range of motion. When offering resistance, the spring or rubber band is positioned so that its pull is opposite to the pull of motion of the target muscle group, whereas if used for assistance, they are set to pull in the same direction as the contracting muscle. Springs or rubber bands applied for the purpose of stretching are placed so the pull is against the tissue to be stretched (see Chapter 8 for precautions).

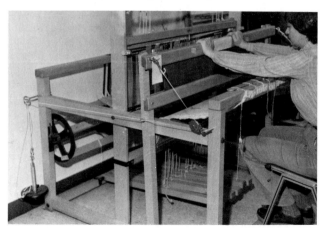

Figure 10.4 Floor loom adapted with weights and pulleys to resist elbow extension.

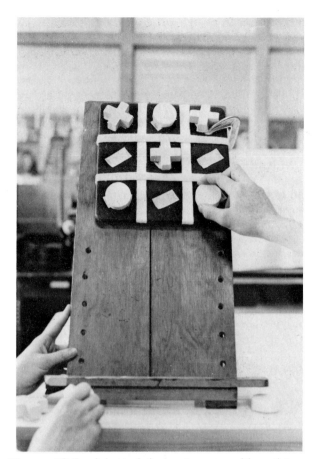

Figure 10.5 Adapted tic-tac-toe repositioned to require shoulder motions and size changed to accommodate poor coordination. The pieces are held in place with Velcro.

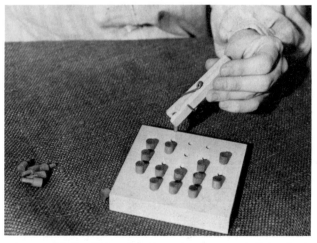

Figure 10.6 Game is played using a clothespin to move the pieces to strenghten pinch.

Springs of graduated tensions may be applied directly to the equipment. A beater of a floor loom can be made resistive to elbow extension or flexion by attaching springs either from the breast beam to the beater to resist elbow extension or from the beater to the castle, the center upright of the loom, to resist elbow flexion. A grip sander, which has springs in the handle, will resist finger flexion when the person squeezes to use it.[2]

Rubber bands can be added to smaller pieces of equipment and can be graded from thin and light tension to thick and heavy tension. For example, a rubber band can be wrapped around the pincer end of a spring-type clothespin to add resistance while it is used in games involving picking up small pieces.

When rubber bands or springs are used to create a force of resistance in one direction the return motion can involve passive stretch of the same muscle group during motion in the opposite direction, unless the person does an eccentric contraction of the resisted muscles to prevent the stretching pull. For example, if a spring is attached to a loom's beater to resist elbow flexion when the beater is pulled toward the person, on the return motion, the spring will pull into extension, thereby stretching the flexors unless the patient eccentrically contracts the flexors. Eccentric contraction would be desired as it would also exercise the weak flexors.

CHANGE OF MATERIALS OR TEXTURE OF MATERIALS

Gradation along the strengthening continuum may be accomplished by selection of material by type and also by variations of texture or density to change resistance. Coordination can be challenged by changing the material used to that of a finer, more delicate nature. Cutaneous stimulation changes as objects or surfaces which the person uses are more or less textured and has the effect of facilitating or inhibiting the muscles associated with the skin surface stimulated. Padding handles with textured material offers sensory stimulation to the finger flexors.

Resistance can be changed, for example, by starting a cutting project with tissue paper and then progressing to heavier materials, such as construction paper,

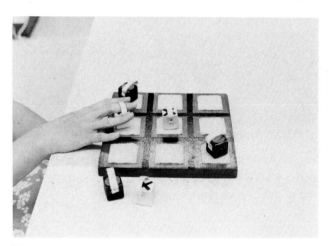

Figure 10.7 Adapted tic-tac-toe to exercise finger extensors; pieces are held by Velcro and require force to lift them.

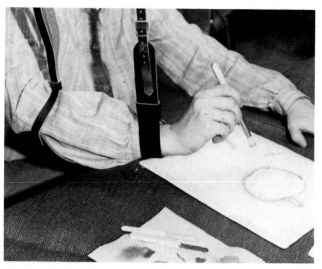

Figure 10.8 Stenciling is made possible by use of a suspension sling. Exercise to wrist extensors is obtained.

cloth, or leather. Proceeding in the opposite direction, increased coordination is required. Metal tooling can be graded for resistance by choosing materials in grades from thin aluminum to thick copper. Sandpaper is graded from extra fine to coarse, and resistance increases with the coarser grade. Mixing can be graded from making jello to scrambled eggs to biscuit batter, etc. Weaving may begin using rug roving and be graded toward fine linen threads as the patient progresses in coordination. By making balls from yarn or terry toweling, carpeting surfaces the person works on, etc., the therapist adapts the activity to increase sensory stimulation.

CHANGE OF THE SIZE OR SHAPE OF OBJECTS

Playing pieces of board games can be made a different size or shape than they standardly are and can therefore offer a therapeutic benefit that the standard objects would not. For example, checkers, which are usually flat pieces approximately 2.5 cm in diameter can be made cylindrical, square, cubes, or spheres and can range in size from tiny to as large as a person's reach permits.

By reducing the size or changing the shape of the pieces being worked on, the goal of increased dexterity and fine coordination is facilitated. Therapists creatively change sizes of craft materials, such as weaving thread, tiles, paint-by-number guidelines, ceramic pieces, etc., and recreational materials, such as puzzle pieces, chess men, target games, etc. to increase coordination. Tools are adapted by changing the size or shape of their handles or adding handles to tools that do not normally have them. The actual size of the tool used can be changed in which case tools offer more or less resistance. For example, saws range in size from small coping saws or hack saws to large crosscut or rip saws. Resistance of saws can also be graded by the number of teeth per inch on the blade; the lesser the number of teeth, the greater the resistance. Woodworking planes vary in size, and the amount of exposed blade can be adjusted to provide resistance. Scissors also vary in size, and the resistance can be increased by tightening the screw.

CHANGE OF METHOD OF DOING THE ACTIVITY

Bowling, basketball, and many other sports can be done from a seated position as opposed to the normal standing position. Change of rules adapts some sports to certain requirements of the physically disabled, such as track and field sports. Sewing and needlework, normally bilateral activities, can be made unilateral by adaptations which hold the material steady for the working hand. Holes can be punched in leather or packs of paper by use of a drill press in lieu of regular leather or paper punches. Block printing can be done in a hand- or foot-operated printing press rather than in a block printing press. Instead of foot races, crawling races can be done. Instead of rolling over on a therapy mat, rolling can be done on a shag rug to provide greater sensory stimulation.

Change of method is used both for exercise (Figs. 10.6 and 10.7) and for compensation (Fig. 10.8). By changing the method an activity is made possible when under ordinary circumstances it would not be possible because of the person's disability. This compensatory adaptation allows the therapist to offer activity of interest to the patient while at the same time accomplishing certain therapeutic goals.

References

1. Hultkrans, R., and Sandeen, A. Application of progressive resistive exercise to occupational therapy. *Am. J. Occup. Ther.,* *11*(4): 238–240, 1957.
2. Bellman, J. B., Myers, C., and Norton, C. G. *Therapeutic Devices 1956–1976 American Journal of Occupational Therapy.* Rockville, Md.: The American Occupational Therapy Association, 1977.

PART
FIVE

Biofeedback

Biofeedback refers to the process of making a subliminal sensory signal available to the patient in order that he might shape his own behavior. Feedback from bodily functions that are usually not in conscious awareness can be made manifest through the use of electronic equipment in order that the person can manipulate these functions voluntarily and know the result of his manipulation. Biofeedback devices have been developed which can make a person aware of the state of contraction of voluntary or involuntary muscles, joint position and small changes in joint motion, blood pressure, skin temperature, heart rate, and brain activity. These devices are being incorporated into therapeutic programs by occupational therapists, as well as other health professionals.

The following chapter will provide basic information concerning the use of electromyographic biofeedback (sensing muscle contraction) and electrogoniometric biofeedback (sensing joint position and motion). Electrogoniometric biofeedback is also called electrokinesiologic biofeedback or kinesthetic biofeedback. The student is referred to the voluminous literature available about biofeedback for additional information about other types of biofeedback.

chapter
11

Biofeedback as an Adjunct to Therapy

Catherine A. Trombly, M.A., OTR

Biofeedback provides knowledge to the patient about bodily functions of which he is otherwise not conscious and which he can then learn to control by knowing the effects of his efforts. Electromyographic (EMG) biofeedback is used to make the patient aware of the state of contraction of his muscles (Fig. 11.1). Electrogoniometric biofeedback is used to inform the patient of joint position or small increments of movement he may not notice (Fig. 11.2). Sometimes biofeedback treatment is limited to direct manipulation of the signal under voluntary effort. For example, the patient monitors his voluntary effort to contract or relax a muscle or to move a joint a certain amount. Preferably, biofeedback is used in conjunction with other therapeutic procedures that will enable the person to move successfully. The feedback makes both the patient and the therapist aware of the effects of the treatment procedures. Under certain circumstances, which will be discussed later, the information from some devices can also be used to record progress.

Poststroke or spinal cord-injured (incomplete) patients who have disturbed tactile or proprioceptive sensation which results in disturbed movement have been able to use biofeedback successfully. Biofeedback provides them with the afferent information which closes the otherwise open sensorimotor loop. A complete sensory motor circuit is necessary for coordinated motor control and motor learning. These patients can learn to inhibit spasticity and can relearn to move using biofeedback. For the patient with disturbed kinesthesis, but potentially useful motion, biofeedback combined with a knowledge of the end position of movement may help, through a recalibration or relearning process, to improve kinesthetic awareness. Biofeedback is also used for patients with intact sensation, such as patients with traumatic hand inju-

ries, tendon transfers, or peripheral nerve injuries. EMG biofeedback is particularly useful to these patients to make them aware of the results of their efforts to contract a 0 or T muscle. Electrogoniometric biofeedback enables the patient to see small increments of progress in control of P− and F− muscles by rewarding small gains in range of motion. Once motion is functional, the patient gets direct feedback from accomplishing goals, and a biofeedback device is no longer needed. The overall goal for all patients must be to wean them away from the machine and to use the motion gained functionally.

BIOFEEDBACK EQUIPMENT

All biofeedback devices have three visible parts: the transducer, the electronics box, and the output display (Fig. 11.3). The transducer is the part which senses the change in the parameter being measured. EMG transducers are electrodes, that is, small pieces of metal attached by wire to the electronics box. These electrodes pick up the tiny electrical signal that a muscle generates when it contracts and transmits the signal to be processed. The signal that is processed is the difference of electrical potential between the two electrodes. A difference of electrical potential is called voltage. The electrogoniometric transducer is a potentiometer, a type of variable resistor; when the position of one of its components (corresponding to the moveable arm of a goniometer) changes in relation to the rest of the device (corresponding to the stationary arm of a goniometer) the amount of resistance to the flow of electricity is changed. It can be set so that no electrical current flows at one limit of motion, e.g., extension, and so that full electrical current flows at the opposite limit of motion, i.e., flexion. The electric-

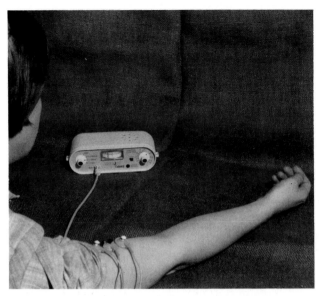

Figure 11.1 Electromyographic biofeedback using Cyborg J33 instrument.

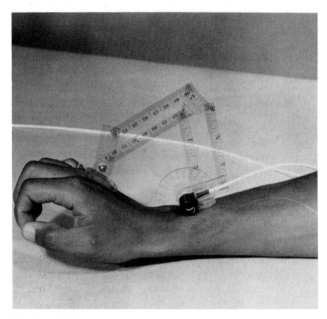

Figure 11.2 Electrogoniometric biofeedback. Elgon was designed and built by Gary de Bacher, Ph.D., Assistant Professor of Rehabilitation Medicine at Emory University and Rehabilitation Engineer at Center for Rehabilitation Medicine, Atlanta, Georgia.

ity that is spoken of comes from a battery or other source outside of the patient, in contrast to EMG which is electricity actually generated by the muscle itself.

The transducers must be placed absolutely exactly each time they are used with a certain patient if comparison of progress is to be made with any degree of reliability. Reliability will be discussed further relative to electrodes used in EMG biofeedback therapy.

The electronic box contains electrical circuits which amplify (enlarge), rectify (make all the same polarity; smooth), and integrate (collect, store, or sum)[1] the signal in preparation for its display. There may also be a level detector stage which can be set by the therapist so that only when the level of signal exceeds the set value will the display device be activated. The signal which is being processed is a voltage signal that is characterized by its *amplitude* (size), measured in volts, and its *frequency* (shape), measured in hertz (Hz) or cycles per second. The electronics box needs to be able to receive a very minute voltage signal and process and display it without distorting it too much. In order to do that, it must meet certain specifications. Electrogoniometric biofeedback devices are not yet commercially available; therefore, the engineer who builds the device makes it to meet the specific specifications of the therapist purchasing that unit. The engineer can work from the therapist's description of what is to be measured, how sensitive the unit must be, and what the limits need to be.

Specifications for EMG Biofeedback Equipment

The following are some specifications the therapist needs to pay attention to when purchasing or selecting equipment for EMG biofeedback.

Range

This specification refers to all the levels of input amplitude and frequency over which the device is expected to operate.[1] The specification sheet will state the range in amplitude in microvolts (μV = 1/1,000,000 V); for example, 1 to 500 μV. The desirable range level is 1 to 500 μV in order to detect output from a very weak or flaccid muscle and also to accommodate the huge bursts sometimes seen in spastic patients.[2] Frequency range is specified under terms such as "filters," "band pass width," or simply "frequency range" and is described below.

Frequency Range

The frequency range must be adequate to accommodate the major portion of the EMG signal. A range of 10 to 1,000 Hz will give a good representation of the EMG signal. Frequency does not refer to the repetition rate of motor unit firing but rather to the mathematical description of the wave form. If you were to visualize the output of one motor unit, it would have a characteristic shape which is composed of many frequencies of waveforms. Figure 11.4 schematically illustrates this concept. Figure 11.5 illustrates the effect of use of a 200-Hz low band-pass filter and a 20 Hz high band-pass filter. Frequencies less than 200 Hz but more than 20 Hz are passed, but those above or below those frequencies are not.

The filters cut out frequency components of the wave form of the signal below and above the values set by the high-pass and low-pass filters, respectively. These frequency components are said to be attenuated or suppressed.[1] Attenuation of the signal by the filters occurs at a certain rate called roll off, specified as

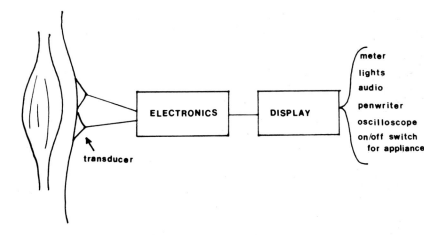

meter
lights
audio
penwriter
oscilloscope
on/off switch
for appliance

Figure 11.3 Biofeedback components.

transducer

ELECTRONICS

DISPLAY

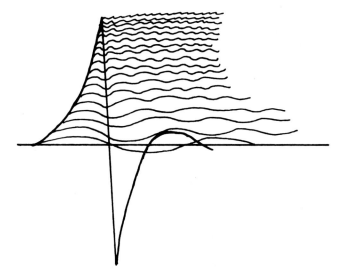

Figure 11.4 Conceptual illustration of frequency.

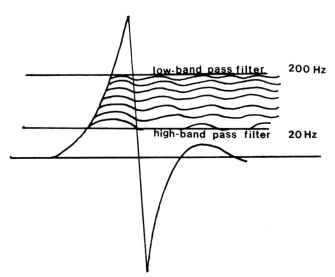

low-band pass filter   200 Hz

high-band pass filter   20 Hz

Figure 11.5 Conceptual illustration of the effects of filters.

decibels per octave. The higher the roll off, the more complete the attenuation. Roll off through the operational range of the unit should be low since attenuation is not wanted. However, in the case of a special filter, called a 60-Hz notch filter, the roll off should be high (30 db[1]) so the therapist knows that the signal is well attenuated. The 60-Hz notch filter is used to remove the 60-Hz interference caused by fluorescent lights, elevators, or other electrical equipment powered by house current. This interference could cause artifact in the output, and therefore the patient would be receiving false feedback. The notch filter also removes some of the adjacent frequencies to some degree. Some EMG biofeedback units have a frequency range of 100 to 1000 Hz; this eliminates the problem of 60 Hz artifact because frequencies lower than 100 are filtered out. However, a major portion of the EMG signal is also filtered out.

Sensitivity

This specification defines how small a variation of the signal can be reliably measured. It differs from range in that it is not concerned with absolute limits, but with the magnitude of change that can be detected.[1] The minimal value that can be detected is called the *resolution* of the device. Very high levels of sensitivity are not desirable because they can lead to instability and nonlinearity. Sensitivity values are listed as the smallest microvolt level detected.

Linearity

Linearity refers to the degree to which variations in the output of the instrument follow the variation in input. If linearity is not present over the whole range, it should be present over the most important segments of the signal.[1] Those are 10 to 250 μV.[3] Linearity is expressed as a percent of maximal range or of full scale deflection.[1]

Signal to Noise Ratio

This specifies the ratio of amplification of the signal in relationship to the amount of internal electronic signal (noise) that exists within the machine itself and is processed into the output. The signal to noise ratio should be at least 1000:1,[1] which means that the signal is processed 1,000 times more than the noise. Specifications may list this as microvolts of noise at a calibration of microvolts per centimeter, e.g., if there is 0.5 μV noise at a calibration of 10 μV/cm then a 10 μV signal seen at readout includes 5% noise.

Common Mode Rejection Ratio (CMRR)

This refers to how efficiently the differential amplifier amplifies the wanted signal vs. the unwanted, common, signal. Amplifiers used for electromyography are *differential* amplifiers, that is, they process that part of the signal which is different from the signal held in common; therefore, they are less likely to process non-EMG signal, such as 60 Hz (household current). The higher the CMRR, the better because the more likely the wanted signal is processed vs. the unwanted. 100,000:1 CMRR means there is a 100,000 chance that the wanted signal is processed vs. 1 chance that the common signal will be processed.

Input Impedance

The input impedance (resistance) of the differential amplifier should be very high, at least 10 times greater than the electrode impedance. Surface electrodes, properly applied, have impedances of up to 10 kilohms.[1]

The display of the signal can take many forms. One type of display is the direct sound and the picture of the raw (unrectified) electrical signal, such as seen on the cathode ray oscilloscope of a clinical electromyograph. Or that EMG signal or output of an electrogoniometer can be recorded on a paper using a polygraph. Other types of display include buzzers of various types, lights that turn on and off or turn on in sequence as the effort increases, or meters. One particularly motivating type of display for children is the use of a switching unit which turns equipment on and off or keeps the equipment running for as long as the patient maintains the effort. It can be reversed also to keep the equipment running as long as no unwanted signal is detected, e.g., for use with control of spasticity. Any type of equipment can be attached to the switching unit: radio, TV, record player, toy train, etc. The rectified signal can also be displayed on the TV viewing screen of a computer and when it reaches correct levels can be rewarded by whatever the computer is programmed to offer. Of course, most occupational therapists do not yet have access to such sophisticated equipment. The selection of the type of display is usually limited in any OT department, but there is always a choice between audio or visual displays. Some patients may know which type of feedback would be most meaningful to them; others may need to discover it by trial and error. If the patient is confused by one or the other, it, of course, should not be used.

It is very helpful if the therapist has access to an oscilloscope to monitor the EMG signal at least from

time to time. The signal from a feedback device does not differentiate between a signal from many small and moderate sized motor unit potentials or a signal from one or two huge units firing repeatedly, nor between the signal and 60-Hz artifact.[4, 5]

ELECTROGONIOMETRIC BIOFEEDBACK

Electrogoniometric biofeedback is more useful and effective than EMG biofeedback when increased range of motion is the goal.[6] The EMG output does not linearly relate to joint angle and therefore is not helpful in learning movement, only in learning specific muscle contraction[4, 7] or relaxation. EMG does not relate to joint angle for two reasons: (1) Different amounts of tension are required in a muscle depending on the limb's relation to gravity, e.g., more tension is needed in the biceps to hold a position at 90° of elbow flexion than 120°. (2) Tension is a composite of motor unit activity, seen in EMG, and viscoelastic properties in the muscle tissue. The more tissue tension generated by stretch or lengthening of the muscle tissue, the less motor unit activity needed to get the same amount of tension.[8]

The electrogoniometer is a device which measures joint angle electronically. It is fastened over the bones adjacent to the joint being monitored, using straps, tape, electrode collars,[4] or rubber contact cement, if the person is not allergic or hairy. A potentiometer is the transducer, and it is mounted on the goniometer so that its wiper arm moves in relation to movement at the joint. When applying the electrogoniometer to the person, it is important that the axis of the potentiometer be aligned with the axis of joint motion. In the case of use of a parallel linkage goniometer (see Figs. 7.87 and 11.2), the device needs to be aligned so the hinge in the linkages nearest the joint is located directly above the joint.

The signal that is being picked up for processing is a voltage signal, having an amplitude from 0 to the full voltage of the battery or electrical source being used in the device. The frequency of the signal is 0 Hz because the source voltage is DC (direct current), which means the magnitude and polarity remain fixed with relation to time.[1]

The processing can be as relatively simple as the use of the current to directly operate the display.[6] The signal can be displayed on a meter, by switching on a light, over a speaker, on a strip recorder,[9] on a computer viewer, or by turning equipment off and on.

Electrogoniometers are not yet commercially available and must be purchased from engineers or rehabilitation engineering centers. One engineer has devised a simple goniometer that can be constructed by the occupational therapist; plans are available from him.[6]

Training

The procedures found useful in training persons using electrogoniometric biofeedback are the following:[6]

1. Patient's AROM and PROM are measured using

a standard goniometer, and these baseline measurements are recorded. The patient must have some pain-free AROM to use the electrogoniometric feedback to advantage.

2. The dysfunctional joint, or a key joint if many are dysfunctional, is selected, and the electrogoniometer is carefully positioned over it as described above.

3. The target angle or threshold is set by the therapist. For the first session, this should be an easily attainable angle that the patient can successfully achieve. Concentration and voluntary effort are used by the patient. The therapist encourages. The session should last no more than 10 to 15 minutes, as tolerated, with the person working at his own pace and with ample rest periods. Using biofeedback to achieve certain goals takes full concentration and is tiring.

4. Later sessions can increase in duration and frequency, as tolerated. The target angle is changed in small increments so that the goal is always achieved at each session.

5. As the range of motion increases, the feedback can be used in combination with therapeutic activities to maintain motivation.

ELECTROMYOGRAPHIC BIOFEEDBACK

When a muscle fiber depolarizes in response to a neural impulse, a small electrical charge or voltage is generated (Fig. 11.6). Each motor unit is composed of many fibers which fire more or less simultaneously when the motor nerve to that unit activates it. If many motor units depolarize at the same time, their signals add together, and the amplitude of the signal that is produced is larger as an indication of that summation. When no contraction of extrafusal muscle is occurring (when the muscle is at rest), no signal is generated. The EMG signal is an AC (alternating current) signal, that is, it reverses polarity periodically and is constantly changing in magnitude.[1]

Physicians have studied these signals for many years, using a process called clinical electromyography, to detect and/or diagnose neuromuscular diseases. Marinacci and Horande[10] very cleverly figured that viewing this information could be therapeutic to persons relearning to control their muscular output.

Electrodes, the transducer. are used to pick up the signal. Surface electrodes are small metal discs. Any metal can be used, but the electrical conductivity of some metals are better than others. Most surface electrodes in use today are silver-silver chloride (Ag-AgCl) electrodes. The chloriding of the silver provides a more stable ionic transmission between the electrode and the electrolyte (electrode gel). Electrodes convert ionic potentials into electronic potentials.[1]

It is important to know conceptually how the signal is picked up so that the importance of careful application of the electrodes is understood and adhered to for accuracy of the signal. The electrons move away from the muscle, through the saline of the tissues, toward the surface of the body, as well as deeper into the body. The body is a volume conductor, that is,

electrical signals (electrons) are conducted throughout its volume. This is different from a wire which conducts electrons along its length. The skin has a dead, horny layer which in effect is a resistor. A resistor is an electrical component that resists the flow of electrons. This layer needs to be removed or reduced for good electron conductance. One way to reduce the resistance is to rub the skin with rough material (gauze pad) and then rub a little electrode gel into the skin. Electrode gel is also put into the cup of the electrode housing. When the electrode is placed over the skin where the gel (electrolyte) was rubbed in, the electrons move from body saline to gel on the skin, to gel in the electrode cup, to the metal electrode, and up the wires. There is also an exchange of ions between the gel and the metal electrode, that is, there is an inherent voltage of the electrode due to this electrode-electrolyte interface.[1] This is a DC voltage, and as long as the electrode remains stationary on the skin, this voltage does not interfere with the bioelectric signal. The electronics box has a component in it called a capacitor which does not conduct DC signals, and they are therefore stopped before they enter the processing section. However, if the electrode moves because it isn't taped down well, then the DC signal begins fluctuating, and the capacitor sees it as an AC signal, accepts it, and sends it on for processing. Or, if the electrodes are different in size or composition, or the resistances are different due to incomplete skin preparation or a dirty electrode, then instead of the differential amplifier receiving a common level of interference (ambient) signal from each electrode, it receives different levels from each, and therefore the interference is not all cancelled out. What happens then is

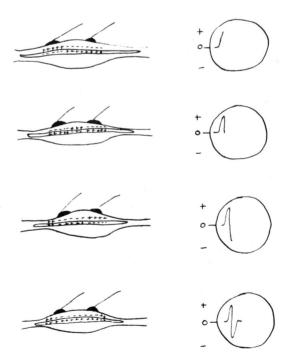

Figure 11.6 Schematic of how the EMG signal is generated by the muscle.

that this artifact becomes part of the signal and gives false information to the patient. The high input impedance of the biofeedback unit will allow the CMRR to account for the inevitable small differences in electrode impedances.

EMG signal of one motor unit has an amplitude of 0 at rest to approximately 250 μV^3 for a large motor unit; many units firing simultaneously may result in a voltage of 1000 μV or higher. The frequency components of the wave form of the EMG signal of one unit are up to approximately 10,000 Hz, but a machine that accepts up to 1,000 Hz will produce a good signal for biofeedback. For diagnostic EMG, a true picture of the signal is necessary; therefore, the physician uses an oscilloscope with a very high frequency capability that faithfully reproduces the peaks of the signal. The biofeedback machine with its limited frequency range still gives accurate information about whether the muscle is or is not contracting, and whether it is contracting more or less than previously.

Even though the EMG signal does go to a low frequency of 1 Hz, the low frequency filter switch is usually set to 3 or 10 Hz to eliminate the chance of getting slowly fluctuating DC signals into the processed signal.

Although some biofeedback machines are simply on-off types (signal reaches criteria and display come on), most biofeedback machines have a control to change the level of signal (threshold) needed in order for the display to be activated. This is an important feature that allows the therapist to shape the patient's response so that improvement is necessary to obtain the reward of the display. This is an operant conditioning principle: A response that only approximates the final performance is rewarded at first, then as that is learned, only an improved response is rewarded, and so on, until the final level of performance is reached. There may be two controls, one to select a broad range of microvolt values, such as 10 to 100 μV or 100 to 1,000 μV, and one to select fine gradations within the broad range. Obviously, shaping the response is easily done using these knobs in combination.

Patient Selection

The patient must be able to understand the relationship between his effort and the feedback. This does not necessarily automatically exclude all receptive aphasics and mentally retarded patients. No definitive studies have been done to determine with significant reliability which patients are best treated and which are not by use of biofeedback. Wolf et al.[11] found that while proprioceptive loss greatly impaired recovery of limb function, receptive aphasia only reduced chances of recovery of function slightly. Age, sex, side affected by stroke, amount of previous rehabilitation, or number of biofeedback treatments were not significantly correlated with outcome. Greenberg and Fowler[12] found similar results.

There is also much variability seen electromyographically in a person's muscle output during similar motions. This is especially true of persons with neuromuscular dysfunction. Therefore, if a patient fails to benefit on the first try, another try is justified.

Electrode Selection

For reasons mentioned above, the electrodes should be of the same material and should be clean. Size makes a difference both in the amount of signal that is picked up (Fig. 11.7) and the resistance (impedance) they offer. Large electrodes have more metal surface which enables the electrons to flow easier and therefore offer less resistance than small electrodes. Electrode impedance and input impedance of the machine need to be compatible ($\geq 1:10$). High impedance of electrode and/or skin resistance in relation to input impedance results in attenuated EMG signals and increased noise levels.[1, 2]

Electrode Placement

The muscle that is to be trained is carefully palpated to determine its margins. The electrodes will be placed in line with the axis of motion. The reason for this is that the signal is a difference between what each electrode "sees." Theoretically the wave of depolarization passes down the parallel muscle fibers equally. If the electrodes are perpendicular to the muscle, little potential difference is seen (Fig. 11.8).

The spacing of the electrodes determines the size and specificity of the signal. Closely placed electrodes pick up signals more superficially and from a more circumscribed area than do widely spaced electrodes (Fig. 11.9). To reeducate a weak muscle, it may be preferable to space the electrodes apart, but still within the boundaries of the muscle, i.e., not on tendon, in order to pick up whatever signals may be generated by this muscle and its synergists. To relax spasticity, close spacing will reduce the area and consequently increase the likelihood of success.

One of the electrodes (reference) can also be placed

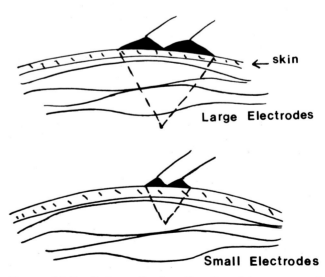

Figure 11.7 Schematic denoting the pick-up area of different sized electrodes.

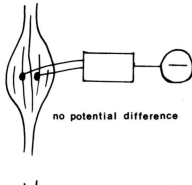

no potential difference

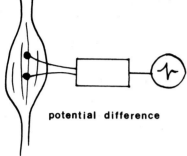

potential difference

Figure 11.8 Schematic to show need for electrode placement along muscle axis.

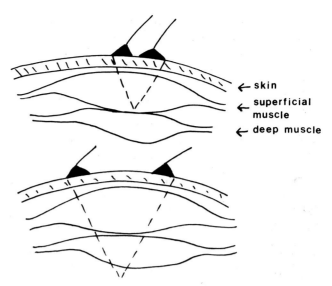

← skin

← superficial muscle

← deep muscle

Figure 11.9 Electrode placement affects pick-up of signals.

over bone (no signal) and recording done from the other (active) electrode (monopolar recording). This enhances the signal because the potential difference is greater than between two electrodes placed on the muscle, each having some level of signal. This set-up would be used for reeducation, rather than for reducing spasticity.

The ground electrode can be located over a bony prominence, on the ear lobe, or an equal distance between, or to the side of, the active and reference electrodes. Follow the manufacturer's direction. The ground electrode is better termed the common electrode. It is the electrode which tells the differential amplifier to cancel out all signals seen by it in common with the other two electrodes. Therefore, ambient signals from fluorescent lights, etc. which are seen by all three electrodes are not processed. This electrode does not "ground" the person to prevent shock.

Electrode Application

1. If the patient is hairy, the hair is shaved off.
2. The skin is rubbed with gauze and alcohol to remove body oil and the layer of dead skin cells. When the site is reddened, it is ready. Do not cause an abrasion. Some gel can be rubbed into the skin in distinct areas. It cannot communicate between the sites because it will short-circuit (stop) the signal.
3. While the alcohol is drying, the electrode is prepared. This process is described for Beckman* electrodes. An adhesive electrode collar with its protective ring is peeled off the backing and placed exactly

---

* Beckman Instruments, Inc., Schiller Park, Ill. 60176.

around the bottom of the plastic rim of the electrode. The cup of the electrode is filled with electrolyte, and a straight edge paper is used to level the gel in the cup. The remaining gel is inspected for bubbles and, if found, these are broken. Bubbles cause artifact due to the disturbance of the electrode-electrolyte interface. The electrode with its leveled amount of gel is attached to the skin after removing the protective ring from the collar. The periphery of the electrode is pressed into place before the center to prevent oozing of the gel. Oozing causes short circuiting and/or poor attachment.

4. It is useful to tape the lead (wire) near the electrode to the skin. Also if the patient is going to move during the treatment, the leads should be taped in place to prevent them from swinging, which causes artifact.

Electrodes should be carefully handled because breaks can easily occur in the leads, which of course makes them inoperative. The circuit is open because of the break, and therefore a 60-Hz signal may be all that is processed. An intact electrode registers 0 ohms when tested using an ohm meter. To test, one lead of the ohm meter is placed on the electrode and the other on the plug.

Training

Although there is no universally correct method, some procedures used in training persons using electromyographic biofeedback are:

1. The patient is oriented to the apparatus and procedure. A trial, using a nondysfunctional limb, allows the patient to understand the treatment and begin to determine strategies for achieving the goal with the impaired limb.
2. Baseline level of activity of the monitored muscle is determined. This level is found by adjusting the

settings until no signal is produced but would be if the dial were turned the slightest amount.

3. The threshold goal is set by the therapist so that the patient must reach the goal to gain correct feedback. If the muscle is being reeducated, the baseline level is low; the goal is to get greater output, and therefore the threshold is set a small increment greater than baseline in order to get feedback. If the muscle is being inhibited, the baseline is high; the goal is to decrease output; therefore, the threshold is set a small amount below baseline. Feedback in this case is to turn off the signal, unless the machine is equipped with a special arrangement by which absence of signal turns the feedback display on. This example may clarify:

Goal	Baseline	Threshold	Feedback
Reeducate	10 μV	15 μV	Display "on"
Decrease spasticity	20 μV	15 μV	Display "off"

4. For brief treatment periods, the patient follows a treatment protocol appropriate for the goal.

Goal: Reeducation of Muscle Contraction

These techniques are appropriate for weak (0 or T) or flaccid muscles. The electrodes are large and are spaced apart but within the muscle's limits. As the patient improves, the spacing and size are reduced.[12] The target threshold is set above baseline level.

The patient is encouraged to contract, and facilitation techniques are used. Especially useful techniques are the tonic reflexes, tapping, and vibration. Vibration, unfortunately, introduces an artifact similar to 60-Hz artifact into the output due to the electromagnetic forces generated by the available vibrators. This is a time when an oscilloscope would help distinguish between artifact and signal. Kelly et al.[13] have outlined specific electrode placements and procedures to elicit contraction of almost all upper extremity motions of hemiplegic patients.

As the patient achieves success, the threshold is raised. When movement begins to occur, the EMG feedback is removed. Depending on the circumstances, electrogoniometric feedback may be appropriate for further treatment.

Goal: Reduction of Spasticity[4, 14]

The atmosphere should be relaxing. The therapist uses a soothing voice. The electrodes may be small and should be closely spaced. The target threshold is set below baseline level. The patient is encouraged to relax to turn off the signal. Relaxation methods such as imagery (imagining soothing scenes), Jacobson's relaxation techniques, and contract/relax are some techniques used. The best position for each patient to achieve relaxation is determined and used.

The patient seeks to maintain the silence of the signal for as long as possible. Then relaxation is maintained despite contraction of the opposite extremity, arousal, or mental effort (counting backward, for example). When relaxation can be achieved in various

positions under these conditions, relaxation during elicitation of the static and dynamic stretch reflexes is the next goal. After this is achieved fairly well, relaxation during unresisted contraction of the antagonist is aimed for.

At each stage of recovery of control, the patient needs to be weaned from the feedback before he is progressed on to the next level. Weaning involves making the feedback unavailable to him, but under the monitoring of the therapist, for as long as he can maintain an acceptable level of inhibition.

Measuring Success

The microvolt level of the machine can be used to register the success of EMG biofeedback for the patient from day to day only if the same, cleaned electrodes are replaced exactly as previously and if the skin is prepared exactly as before[4] so that the skin resistance is the same. Then differences will still be seen which are measurement error. Whenever electrodes are removed and then replaced, they are possibly sampling a different population of motor units which changes the amplitude of the signal. Whenever the electrode-electrolyte interface changes, there is a potential alteration of the processing of the signal by the differential amplifier.

Measurement of the difference from the beginning to the end of a treatment period is an accurate reflection of the gains made at that session. Gains so noted can be compared validly and reliably from day to day.

The gains achieved during electrogoniometric biofeedback can be determined by comparing the degrees of range of motion gained within one treatment session to those gained in another. The absolute improvement in range cannot accurately be determined from one treatment period to the next, unless the electrogoniometer is reapplied exactly each time and calibrated exactly the same each time.

Middaugh[15] and Middaugh and Miller[16] have determined in controlled, counterbalanced studies of EMG biofeedback and no biofeedback that significant improvement of function resulted from the use of EMG biofeedback for normal, hemiparetic, and peripheral nerve lesion subjects.

Other effectiveness studies have been included in the chapters on treatment of specific disabilities.

EMG biofeedback is also being used in conjunction with functional electrical stimulation for good benefits.[17]

References

1. Cohen B. A. Basic biofeedback electronics for the clinician. In *Biofeedback—Principles and Practice for Clinicians*, edited by J. V. Basmajian. Baltimore: Williams & Wilkins, 1979.
2. Baker, M. P., and Wolf, S. L. Biofeedback strategies in the physical therapy clinic. In *Biofeedback—Principles and Practice for Clinicians*, edited by J. V. Basmajian. Baltimore: Williams & Wilkins, 1979.
3. Basmajian, J. V. *Muscles Alive: Their Functions Revealed by Electromyography*, 4th ed. Baltimore: Williams & Wilkins, 1979.
4. De Bacher, G. Biofeedback in spasticity control. In *Biofeedback—Principles and Practice for Clinicians*, edited by J. V.

Basmajian. Baltimore: Williams & Wilkins, 1979.
5. Regenos, E. M., and Wolf, S. L. Involuntary single motor unit discharges in spastic muscles during EMG biofeedback training. *Arch. Phys. Med. Rehabil., 60:* 72-73, 1979.
6. Brown, D. M., DeBacher, G., and Basmajian, J. V. Feedback goniometers for hand rehabilitation. *Am. J. Occup. Ther., 33:* 58-463, 1979.
7. Harris, F. A. Exteroceptive feedback of position and movement in remediation for disorders of coordination. In *Behavioral Psychology in Rehabilitation Medicine: Clinical Applications,* edited by L. P. Ince. Baltimore: Williams & Wilkins, 1980.
8. Long, C., Thomas D., and Crochetiere, W. J. Viscoelastic factors in hand control. *Excerpta Med. Int. Congr. Ser.* Proceedings of the IVth International Congress of Physical Medicine, Paris, September 6-11. no. 107: 440-445, 1964.
9. Morris, A. F., and Brown, M. Electronic training devices for hand rehabilitation. *Am. J. Occup. Ther., 30*(6): 376-379, 1976.
10. Marinacci, A. A., and Horande, M. Electromyogram in neuro-muscular re-education. *Bull. Los Angeles Neurol. Soc., 25:* 57-71, 1960.
11. Wolf, S. L., Baker, M. P., and Kelly, J. L. EMG biofeedback in stroke: Effect of patient characteristics. *Arch. Phys. Med. Rehabil., 60:* 96-102, 1979.
12. Greenberg, S., and Fowler, R. S. Kinesthetic biofeedback: A treatment modality for elbow range of motion in hemiplegia. *Am. J. Occup. Ther., 34*(11): 738-743, 1980.
13. Kelly, J. L., Baker, M. P., and Wolf, S. L. Procedures for EMG biofeedback training in involved upper extremities of hemiplegic patients. *Phys. Ther., 59:* 1500-1507, 1979.
14. Brown, D. M., and Nahai, F. Biofeedback strategies of the occupational therapist in total hand rehabilitation. In *Biofeed-back—Principles and Practice for Clinicians,* edited by J. V. Basmajian. Baltimore: William & Wilkins, 1979.
15. Middaugh, S. J. EMG feedback as muscle reeducation technique. A controlled study. *Phys. Ther., 58:* 15-22, 1978.
16. Middaugh, S. J., and Miller, M. C. Electromyographic feedback: Effect on voluntary muscle contractions in paretic subjects. *Arch. Phys. Med. Rehabil., 61:* 24-29, 1980.
17. Bowman, B. R., Baker, L. L., and Waters, R. L. Positional feedback and electrical stimulation: An automated treatment for the hemiplegic wrist. *Arch. Phys. Med. Rehabil., 60:* 497-501, 1979.

Supplementary Reading

Basmajian, J. V., Biofeedback in therapeutic exercise. In *Therapeutic Exercise,* 3rd ed, edited by J. V. Basmajian. Baltimore: Williams & Wilkins, 1978.

Basmajian, J. V. Introduction: Principles and background. In *Biofeedback—Principles & Practice for Clinicians,* edited by J. V. Basmajian. Baltimore: Williams & Wilkins, 1979.

Basmajian, J. V., and Blumenstein, R. *Electrode Placement in EMG Biofeedback.* Baltimore: Williams & Wilkins, 1980.

Bernstein, D. A., and Borkovec, T. D. *Progressive Relaxation Training: A Manual for the Helping Professions.* Champaign, Ill.: Research Press, 1973.

Hurd, W. W., Pegram, V., and Nepumuceno, C. Comparison of actual and simulated EMG biofeedback in the treatment of hemiplegic patients. *Am. J. Phys. Med., 59*(2): 73-82, 1980.

Thomas, D., and Long, C. Electrogoniometer for the fingers: Kinesiologic tracking device. *Am. J. Med. Electronics, 3:* 96-100, 1964.

PART SIX

Orthotics

Orthotics refers to that part of rehabilitation which focuses on the fitting, construction, and training to use special devices that can be applied to a patient to substitute for a lost function. The certified orthotist is an expert in the fit and construction of all types of permanent orthoses.

Occupational therapists specialize in the adaptive use of the upper extremities in occupational performance tasks. Physical therapists specialize in ambulation and gait training. It has therefore developed that occupational therapists have taken a major responsibility for the checkout, training, and in some cases, the design and construction of orthoses for the upper extremities, whereas physical therapists have taken the responsibility for checkout and training of trunk and lower extremity orthoses.

Rehabilitation engineers are developing electronic aids and orthoses for the severely disabled. The further growth of the field of Rehabilitation Engineering and the use of electronics in rehabilitation and in everyday life in the next decades will make a more satisfying life-style available to severely disabled persons. Occupational therapists will increasingly need to become familiar with basic electronic information, just as the engineers are learning medical and rehabilitation information, in order to competently incorporate these devices into planning for patients' increased independence in occupational performance tasks.

Part Six has been divided into three chapters: one on the purposes and types of orthoses, one on the materials and methods of construction of temporary orthoses, and one on wheelchair measurement and prescription. Whether the physical therapist, occupational therapist, or both take responsibility for wheelchair prescription seems to be according to the tradition of the particular rehabilitation center.

chapter

12

Orthoses: The Purposes and Types

Catherine A. Trombly, M.A., OTR

An orthosis is a device added to a person's body to substitute for absent motor power, to restore function, to assist weak muscles, to position or immobilize a part, or to correct deformities.[1] Orthoses for the hands are sometimes called splints.

There are two basic classifications of orthoses: static and dynamic. Static devices have no moving parts, whereas dynamic devices have moving parts. Movement in dynamic splints may be provided by another body part, battery-operated motors, gas-operated devices, elastics, springs, pulleys, or electrically stimulated muscle.

The same orthosis may fulfill several functions. For example, a dynamic splint that provides prehension function also positions the paralyzed thumb in a useful position and one which prevents deformity. Therefore, although orthoses are listed here in certain categories as common examples of those categories, it is not meant that that function is their only function. This representative sampling of orthoses is also not meant to be exhaustive. The reader is referred to the references for additional information.

ORTHOSES TO SUPPORT, POSITION, OR IMMOBILIZE A PART

When a patient lacks the ability to hold a part in a functional position, is developing spasticity, or has suffered soft tissue injury which may result in deformity as healing progresses, such as in the case of burns, orthoses to maintain a functional position are needed. During acute episodes of rheumatoid arthritis or other instances when rest or immobilization of a joint is required, supportive types of splints may be used.

These types of splints are often worn all day, all night, or both, in order to provide the best benefit.

However, in every case, the splint is removed several times a day for gentle passive range of motion exercises to maintain the patient's mobility.

Some common examples of these kinds of orthoses are as follows.

Proximal Supports

The *suspension sling* is a device which supports the upper extremity with cuffs that fit under the elbow and wrist. These cuffs are suspended from a spring attached overhead. Suspension slings can be used unilaterally or bilaterally. Some are designed for suspension from a rod that attaches to the wheelchair (Fig. 12.1), some attach to a trunk corset, some are mounted on floor stands, and others are suspended directly from the ceiling. Regardless of how the sling is suspended, the distance between the point of suspension and the cuffs should be as far as is practical, because the longer the pendulum, the wider the arc of motion and, consequently, the longer the relatively flat section of the arc. Movement is easier for the patient in the flatter area of the arc because the resistance offered by the inclined ends of the arc is eliminated or minimized.

Arm slings to prevent shoulder subluxation in patients with brachial plexus injuries,[2] polymyositis,[3] hemiplegia,[4] and other similar disabilities have been developed by therapists. Some support and immobilize the whole arm[2] whereas others support only the shoulder and leave the rest of the arm free for function[3, 4] (Fig. 12.2). Instructions for constructions of these slings can be found in the original articles.

Some slings are commercially available. In using these, the therapist must not only check for size and comfort, but must also be sure the sling does not prevent function the patient has and should use or create new problems for the patient, such as edema in

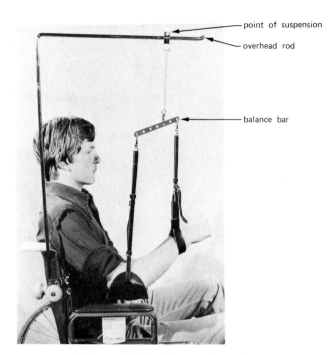

Figure 12.1 Suspension sling.

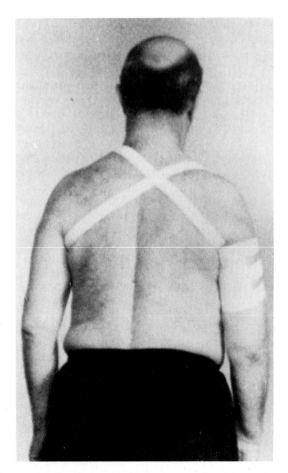

Figure 12.2 Arm sling to support shoulder. (Reproduced with permission from B. Bobath.[4])

the dependent hand, or increase disability by positioning in patterns of spasticity, or pull the head of the humerus out of the glenoid fossa. Basmajian[5] concluded from anatomical and electromyographic studies that subluxation occurs due to weakness of the supraspinatus and other rotator cuff muscles combined with a relative abduciton of the humerus which neutralizes the locking mechanism offered by the upward slant of the glenoid fossa.[5] Subluxation of the head of the humerus can occur easily in a very weak shoulder.

Wheelchair arm boards are an alternative to the use of a sling for a wheelchair-bound patient. They are specially constructed arm rests (Fig. 12.3). Some designs have been published.[4, 6-7] The arm board is attached over the regular wheelchair arm rest and is usually approximately 10 to 12 cm wide, is padded, and may have straps to hold the arm in place. Some have special sections to hold the hand in a particular position.[4] The arm board is preferred to a sling because it allows the humeral head to approximate the glenoid fossa at an angle, its more natural position, and it supports the hand so that edema is less likely to occur. The sling would be preferred while patients were ambulating, of course.

An alternative to an arm board is the use of a wheelchair lapboard. This provides all the advantages of the arm board plus allows the arm to be positioned forward to pull the scapular forward, a position of choice for hemiplegic patients.[4] Clear plexiglass lapboards allow the patient to visualize his whole body. Lapboards do make independent wheelchair propulsion difficult, however.

Distal Supports: Hand Splints

Volar wrist cock-up (Fig. 12.4) supports the wrist in a position of 20–30° of dorsiflexion. The person for whom a wrist cock-up splint would be appropriate would have use of the fingers. This splint can be made of plaster of Paris bandage, plastic, or metal. It is a simple splint which extends from the distal palmar crease, over the wrist, to approximately two-thirds the

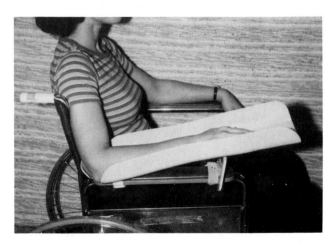

Figure 12.3 One type of wheelchair armboard.

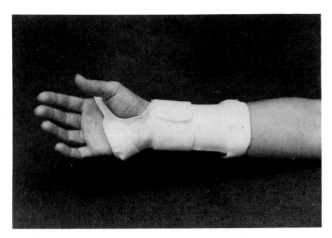

Figure 12.4 One style of volar cock-up splint.

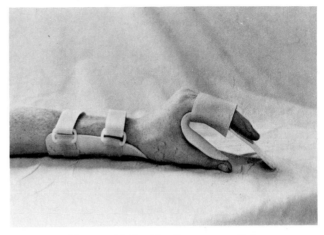

Figure 12.5 Resting pan splint.

length of the forearm. Small hands do not require such a long splint because that amount of leverage offered by the forearm piece is not needed for the light weight of the small hand. The palmar piece is trimmed to avoid interfering with the thenar eminence and is molded to the palm to support the arches of the hand.

Resting pan (Fig. 12.5) is chosen for patients who lack use of the fingers and who need support of both the wrist and the fingers. It is designed to hold the wrist, fingers, and thumb in the functional position. This splint may be a volar or dorsal splint, depending upon the patient's needs. The design of this splint is such that exact fit is not required, and therefore commercially made resting pans are satisfactory. The commercial splints can be adjusted if necessary by spot heating the plastic material. It is time-saving to have a stock of these splints already made especially in the case of need to use for burn patients where time is of the essence and a splint cannot be formed directly on the newly burned skin anyway.

A variation of the resting pan has been devised to splint the burned hand after primary excision and early skin grafting.[8] The splint is made prior to surgery. A large circular piece of splint material is added to the finger part of the splint to act as an outrigger. Dress hooks are cemented to the fingernails of the patient and rubber bands attached to them and stretched to the perimeter of the circular piece to hold the fingers abducted and partially flexed at the metacarpophalangeal (MP) joints, and extended at the proximal interphalangeal (PIP) and distal interphalangeal (DIP) joints.

Long and short opponens splints (Figs. 12.6 to 12.8) are designed to support the thumb in an abducted and opposed position. The long opponens hand splint also supports the wrist. These splints would be used for patients with finger use; however, either splint may be adapted by adding a platform support to support the fingers. A lightweight wire and foam volar wrist and thumb splint is commercially available.[9] It may be ordered by size and adjusted to fit most patients satisfactorily.

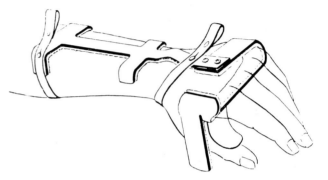

Figure 12.6 Long opponens splint. (Reproduced with permission from C. Long.[1])

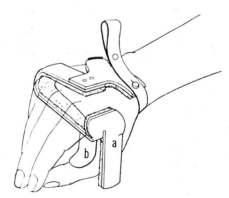

Figure 12.7 Short opponens splint. *a*, opponens bar; *b*, C-bar. (Reproduced with permission from C. Long.[1])

Finger stabilizer splint (Fig. 12.9) is the name given to a variety of splints designed to stabilize one or more joints of a finger. These splints are commercially available and can be adjusted to hold the finger in a flexed or extended position.

Spasticity reduction splint (Fig. 12.10) is another variation of the resting pan. It has been devised to reduce flexor spasticity.[10] The splint is molded to provide 30° of wrist extension, 45° of MP flexion, full

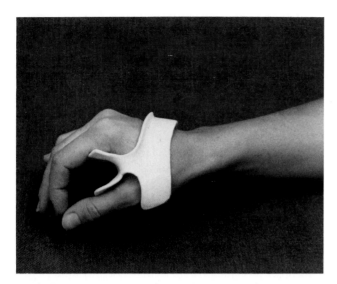

Figure 12.8 Short opponens splint made from Orthoplast.

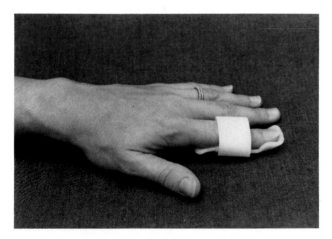

Figure 12.9 One type of finger stabilizer splint. This one immobilizes the PIP and DIP joints.

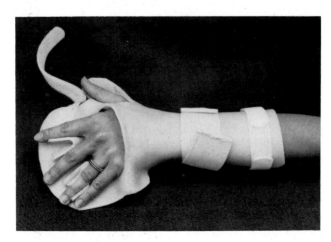

Figure 12.10 Spasticity reduction splint.

IP extension, finger abduction, and thumb extension and abduction. This position duplicates a suggested reflex-inhibiting pattern of Bobath. No data on the effectiveness of this splint in reducing spasticity has been published.

In a study of 10 hemiplegic patients, Kaplan[11] reported increased free range of motion (decreased spasticity) at the wrist and fingers following maintained splinting of the affected arm into maximal extension.[11] The wrist was hyperextended to approximately 90° and the fingers and thumb to 0°. The fingers were adducted. This dorsal splint, with textured lining for sensory stimulation, was worn at least 8 hours per day as tolerated by the patient.

Finger abduction splint for the spastic hand (Fig. 12.11) utilizes Bobath's reflex-inhibiting pattern theory. Originally, the splint was constructed of a block of foam with holes punched through the foam to allow insertion of the fingers and thumb in an abducted position.[4] A more permanent splint has been designed for the same purpose using low temperature splinting materials.[12]

Zislis[13] demonstrated electromyographically on one poststroke patient a decrease in finger flexor activity when a volar splint that held the fingers extended and abducted was used as compared to a dorsal splint which maintained the fingers adducted and extended. The thumb was not included in either splint; the wrist was held in neutral position in both.

Orthokinetic splint for the spastic hemiplegic was developed by A. Joy Huss and uses ideas from Rood as its theoretical base: a firm surface in the palm of the hand will inhibit the extrinsic flexor muscles, and tactile stimulation of the extensor surface of the forearm will facilitate extensor tone. The hand and forearm pieces are made of low temperature plastics. The hand piece is shaped into a cone; the larger end of the cone is ulnar-directed. The forearm shell extends two-thirds of the length of the forearm from approximately 3 cm from the wrist crease. The cone is attached to the forearm piece by two side supports that are bent

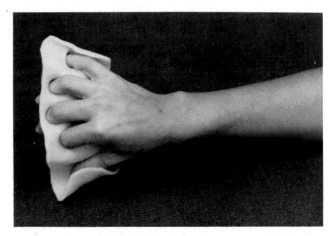

Figure 12.11 Finger abduction splint for the spastic hand.

to follow the contour of the hand laterally. The side supports are attached loosely, using rivets so that the wrist is free to move. The forearm piece is secured to the patient using elastic bandage for straps (orthokinetic cuff).[14] No data on effectiveness has been published.

ORTHOSES TO CORRECT DEFORMITIES

Static and dynamic orthoses, including hand splints, are used to provide prolonged stretch to correct deformities. The orthosis is adjusted to provide stretch of the tissue to the point at which the patient indicates discomfort rather than at the point of maximal stretch, which would result in intolerable pain if prolonged. As in manual stretching, gentle pressure over a long time is preferred to forceful stretching used to achieve fast gains. Wearing time of the orthosis is gradually increased as the patient tolerates the device. The importance of wearing the device must be emphasized to the patient. Daily adjustments of the splints are made as the tissue adjusts to each new position. It is advantageous if the orthosis is easily adjustable. After wearing tolerance has increased to several hours it might be preferable for the patient to wear the device at night when he is asleep, freeing the part for active use during the day. If sleep is interrupted due to discomfort from the splint, the force is too great.[1]

Splints designed to correct or prevent scarring secondary to burns must provide firm, even pressure over the entire surface. These splints are worn constantly except for the brief period needed for hygiene.

The following orthoses were selected to illustrate the principles involved in increasing range of motion or preventing scarring. Others are available, or the therapist may need to design one to suit a particular patient's unique problem.

Proximal Correction

Shoulder abduction splint, also called the airplane splint, (Fig. 12.12) is designed to maintain or increase range of motion in shoulder abduction. It is usually made of metal and can be adjusted to allow internal or external rotation, as well as change the degree of abduction of the shoulder. It may be made from plaster or plastics if an orthotist is unavailable. If these materials are used, however, readjustment of the abduction angle is difficult.

Neck extension splint (Fig. 22.1), also called the conformer neck splint, is used for patients whose neck has been burned to hold the neck extended and to prevent the fusion of the chin to the chest during the healing process.[16, 17] It can also be used to reduce the thickness of scar tissue through the constant, uniform pressure offered against the developing scar tissue.

The transparent face mask has been used successfully to prevent hypertrophic scarring of facial tissue after deep, partial or full thickness thermal injury.[18] The mask is made of cellulose acetate butyrate (Uvex), a high temperature plastic. Directions for making the negative and positive molds and the mask are published.

Turnbuckle splint for elbow flexion contractures (Fig. 12.13) has been used successfully in 12 of 15 patients on whom it was researched.[19] The average increase in range of motion was 43°; the average reduction of deformity was 37°. It is constructed by an orthotist and utilizes a turnbuckle on the lateral aspect of a hinged elbow brace to exert the force towards extension.

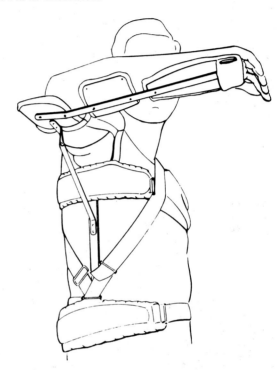

Figure 12.12 Airplane splint. (Reproduced with permission from C. Long.[1])

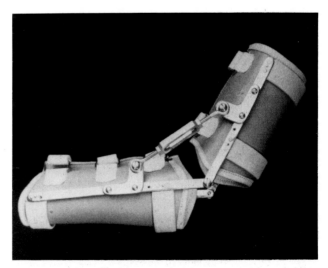

Figure 12.13 Turnbuckle splint for elbow flexion contractures. (Reproduced with permission from D. P. Green and H. McCoy.[19])

Elbow flexion-extension braces[15] are useful to correct elbow contractures. To increase elbow flexion, a threaded bar and wing nut are mounted on the uprights of an elbow brace which allow easy adjustment to increase the pull into flexion (Fig. 12.14).

To increase elbow extension, force is exerted by elastic webbing which is mounted to the elbow brace and passes over a bowed fulcrum located posteriorly to the elbow joint (Fig. 12.15). This force may be adjusted by shortening the webbing.

Distal Correction

Spring cock-up splint to force the wrist into dorsiflexion[20] (Fig. 12.16) provides a gentle force toward wrist hyperextension to stretch the wrist flexors while permitting some active wrist flexion against the spring steel support. It may be combined with an outrigger to allow finger flexion traction, as pictured.

Metacarpophalangeal flexion splint with outrigger (Fig. 12.17) can be easily constructed using thermoplastics. Finger loops are placed over the proximal

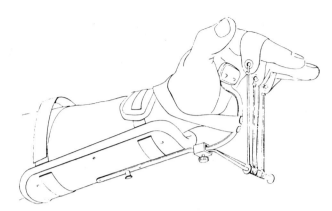

Figure 12.16 Bunnell spring cock-up splint with outrigger and metacarpophalangeal flexion traction. (Reproduced with permission from S. Licht: *Orthotics Etcetera*. New Haven, Conn., Elizabeth Licht, 1966.)

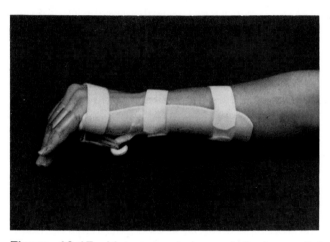

Figure 12.17 Metacarpophalangeal flexion splint with outrigger.

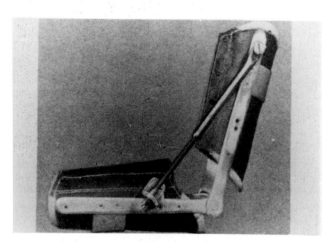

Figure 12.14 Forced flexion elbow brace. (Reproduced with permission from J. W. Edwards.[15])

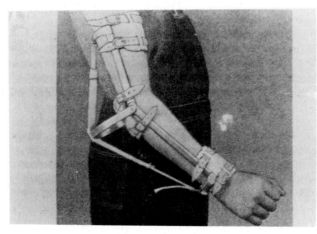

Figure 12.15 Elastic traction brace for elbow flexion contracture (to force extension). (Reproduced with permission from J. W. Edwards.[15])

phalanges and attach via rubber bands to a volar outrigger. The angle of pull of the rubber bands must be perpendicular to the proximal phalanges. This angle may be obtained by attaching the rubber bands directly to an outrigger or by the use of a pulley system.

Wrist deviation splint,[1] a modified volar cock-up splint, has a free-moving wrist joint which permits wrist deviation. Force is exerted by the use of a rubber band located on either the ulnar side to stretch out the radial deviators or on the radial side to stretch out the ulnar deviators. The more typical deformity is ulnar deviation; therefore, the rubber band is located as pictured in Fig. 12.18. This splint can also be used to assist weak radial or ulnar deviator muscles.

Adjustable metacarpophalangeal flexion control[21] (Fig. 12.19) is a padded metal bar which extends across the dorsal surface of the proximal phalanges. It can be attached to a long opponens hand splint by wing nuts. These wing nuts allow daily fine adjustment to slowly stretch out a metacarpophalangeal extension contracture. This splint is chosen to maintain daily gains of manual stretching of this contracture because adjustments can be so easily made in small increments.

Glove flexion mitt is a splint used to force the fingers into flexion.[22] It has sometimes been used as exercise equipment to resist finger extension. The splint is made from a cotton gardener's glove. Rubber bands are attached between the fingertips and a button secured at the wrist. Directions for construction of an adaptation of the mitt for a patient whose impairment is limited to less than all fingers has been published.[23]

Bunnell knuckle bender splint[1] (Fig. 12.20) is commercially available in several sizes. It provides effective dynamic pull into metacarpophalangeal flexion by

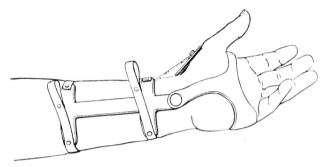

Figure 12.18 Wrist deviation splint. (Reproduced with permission from C. Long.[1])

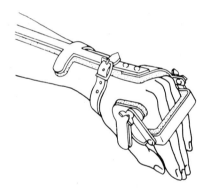

Figure 12.19 Adjustable metacarpophalangeal flexion control. (Reproduced with permission from M. Anderson.[21])

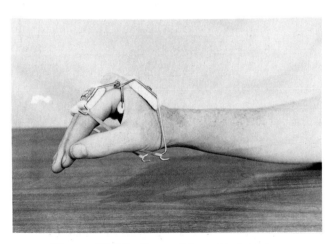

Figure 12.20 Bunnell knuckle bender.

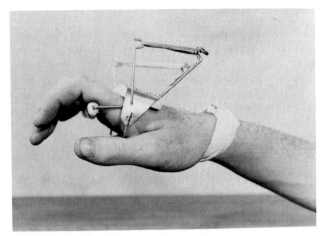

Figure 12.21 Bunnell reverse knuckle bender.

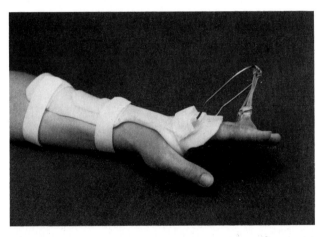

Figure 12.22 Interphalangeal extension splint with lumbrical bar.

means of rubber bands which can be adjusted easily. All fingers are forced into the same degree of flexion, whereas the metacarpophalangeal flexion splint with outrigger is used when one or more of the fingers need more or less force. The reverse knuckle bender (Fig. 12.21) forces the metacarpophalangeal joints into extension.

Interphalangeal extension splint with lumbrical bar[21] (Fig. 12.22) has a lumbrical bar which prohibits metacarpophalangeal hyperextension while a dorsal outrigger provides attachment for finger loops and rubber bands which exert a rotary force at an angle of 90° to the interphalangeal joints to pull the fingers into extension.

Spring safety pin splint[24] (Fig. 12.23) is commercially available and uses spring steel wires to force a finger into extension.

Finger knuckle bender[24] is a commercially available splint that works on the same principle as the knuckle bender for metacarpophalangeal joints, except that this one forces flexion of one proximal interphalangeal joint only. Reverse finger knuckle benders (Fig. 12.24) are also available for extension of the proximal interphalangeal joints.

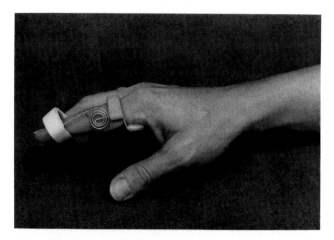

Figure 12.23 Spring safety pin splint.

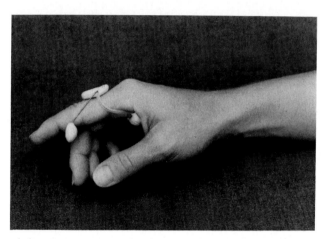

Figure 12.24 Reverse finger knuckle bender.

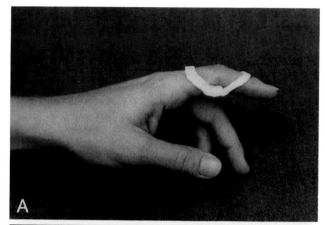

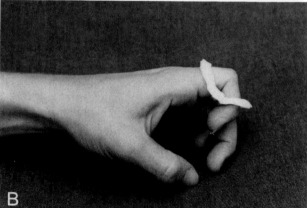

Figure 12.25 Finger splint for swan neck deformity. *A.* Prevents hyperextension of PIP joint. *B.* Allows flexion.

Fingernail splint utilizes dress hooks which are cemented to the dorsal surfaces of the fingernails. Rubber bands extend from these hooks to an outrigger to pull all joints of the fingers into flexion or extension.[25] The length and location of the outrigger controls the direction and extent of pull. This type of splint may be used for burn patients and others for whom skin contact is contraindicated.

Finger tubular splint is a type of splint which surrounds the finger in a tube of plastic. They are easily constructed from bits of thermoplastic splinting material. By using the splint one way, swan neck deformity can be prevented or corrected, since the splint will prevent PIP hyperextension. By reversing the splint, boutonnière deformity is prevented (Fig. 12.25).

Foot drop splint (Fig. 12.26) is used when a person is confined to bed and lacks the ability to keep his feet dorsiflexed; plantar flexion contractures often develop. Foot drop splints are made to hold the foot perpendicular to the leg, as if the patient were standing up straight. The newer thermoplastic materials lend themselves nicely to this application.

ORTHOSES TO RESTORE FUNCTION

Orthoses which assist weak muscles or substitute for absent motor power may enable functional activities to be performed more easily by the patient. Some common examples of these orthoses are described here.

Often the use of orthoses that enable the patient to move to do activities will contribute to an increase in strength and endurance. The need for the orthosis or a modification of it should be reevaluted over time. Patients with degenerating diseases should be reevaluated regularly so that they can be provided with devices that will allow as much independence as possible. The need for increased orthoses is a psychologically critical time for the patient, and attention should be given to the mourning process.

Residual weakness of the upper extremity that results in an inability to move the limb effectively to orient the hand to objects or an inability to pinch or grasp the object can be particularly compensated for by the use of permanent orthoses. For a permanent orthosis to be useful to the patient, he must accept it, value it, and incorporate it into his body image. A

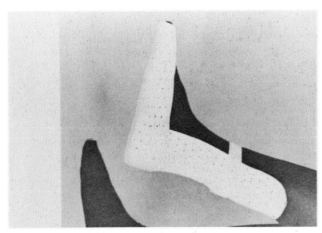

Figure 12.26 Orthoplast splint to prevent foot-drop. (Reproduced with permission from Johnson & Johnson.)

prime prerequisite to acceptance is that the device allow the patient to do something *he wants to do* which he cannot do without the orthosis.[26] Other factors that increase the likelihood of acceptance are mechanical reliability, cosmesis, ease of application and control, and thorough training to the point of automaticity of control.

The principles of orthotic training were borrowed from the field of prosthetics and include check out of the fit and mechanical aspects of the orthosis; instruction in the names of the parts, the care of the orthosis, how to put it on and remove it; controls training; and use training. Repetition and the opportunity for use of the device under varying circumstances are essential aspects of orthotic training.

Proximal Function

The *suspension sling* (Fig. 12.1) can be adjusted to assist certain movements of the upper extremities. Remember that whenever a motion is assisted, its opposite is resisted. For example, the patient must have relatively strong shoulder horizontal abductor muscles if the suspension sling is adjusted to assist weak shoulder horizontal adductors. Motions which can be assisted using an overhead suspension sling are shoulder horizontal abduction and adduction, shoulder external and internal rotation, shoulder abduction, and elbow flexion and extension. Adjustments to assist weak muscles are made to parts of the suspension sling as follows:

Motion Assisted by Suspension Sling	*Adjustment*
Shoulder motions:	
Horizontal abduction	The overhead rod is rotated laterally, that is, the top part of the rod is turned out away from the patient, which carries the suspended arm out toward horizontal abduction.
Horizontal adduction	The overhead rod is rotated medially, that is, the top part of the rod is turned in toward the patient. The suspended arm is thereby carried in toward horizontal adduction.
Abduction	The distance between the spring and the overhead rod is shortened to pull the arm into abduction.

Some adjustments are made by moving the position of the cuffs on the balance bar.

External rotation	The cuffs are moved back on the bar to shift the weight toward the elbow.
Internal rotation	The cuffs are moved forward on the balance bar to shift the weight toward the hand.
Elbow motions:	
Flexion	The point of suspension is moved backward on the overhead rod, which puts the hand back toward the patient's face.
Extension	The point of suspension is moved forward on the overhead rod, which puts the hand out away from the patient's face.

Each ajustment may be made in as small an increment as is just necessary to assist the patient's motion.

Mobile Arm Supports (MAS)

This term, once inclusive of suspension arm slings and feeders, now refers only to feeders. Their former name was ball-bearing forearm orthoses (BFO). MAS are frictionless arm supports that are usually mounted on a wheelchair but also may extend from a waist belt for ambulatory patients. They utilize the principle of the inclined plane in which gravity causes movement when something is inclined away from horizontal. They assist weak shoulder and elbow muscles to place the hand in space as needed. Adjustments are made to individually tailor the assistance of the MAS for each person's disability.

The neutral set up and adjustments for a Rancho Los Amigos type mobile arm support are described here. The Georgia Warm Springs feeder (Fig. 12.27) is very similar to the Rancho one (Fig. 12.28) with two exceptions, the proximal ball-bearing wheelchair bracket assembly and the rocker arm assembly. The bracket of the Georgia Warm Springs feeder is adjustable and the rocker arm assembly is offset which allows unimpeded vertical motions. The Michigan feeder (see Fig. 12.29) allows more minute adjustment of the position of the proximal ball-bearing and the rocker assembly. The Michigan rocker assembly allows adjustment in the Z coordinate of movement (up and down) which allows the therapist to match the axis of the motion of the forearm trough to the exact axis of the bulk of the forearm, thereby enabling a weaker patient to use the feeder effectively.

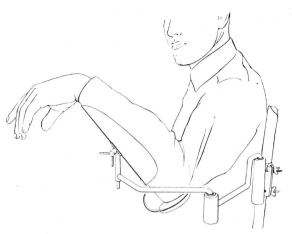

Figure 12.27 Georgia Warm Springs feeder (mobile arm support). (Reproduced with permission from C. Long.[1])

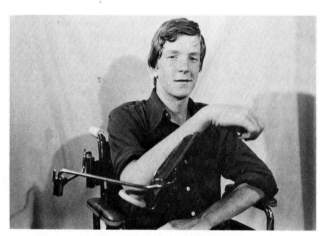

Figure 12.28 Rancho mobile arm support.

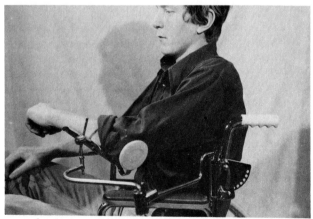

Figure 12.29 Michigan feeder (mobile arm support).

Adjustment of Mobile Arm Supports. The principles of setup and balancing described below generally apply to all designs of mobile arm supports, although the exact methods of adjusting the pieces are slightly different.

Neutral set up of the MAS is sufficient for the patient who has generalized, balanced weakness throughout the upper extremity. Modifications of this neutral setup must be made for patients with other patterns of weakness. Many therapists prefer to adjust the MAS initially into neutral position before proceeding to make modifications in the balance as required by the patient's pattern of weakness.

A properly balanced MAS will hold the patient's forearm in a position of 45° from the horizontal of the lapboard without any effort on the patient's part. The upper arm will be held in approximately 45° of combined shoulder abduction and flexion.

In order for MAS to be fitted to the patient, he ought to be able to sit for 1 hour. He must be able to sit upright at 90 or 95° and have good lateral trunk stability which may be provided by corsets, seat adaptations, braces, or restraints if he does not have it actively. MAS cannot be used in bed or when the patient is semireclined in his wheelchair. He can use suspension slings in these positions, however.

The patient must have some source of power to operate the MAS, although some external power can be added for very weak patients. If the patient is too weak to operate a feeder, the alternate orthosis is the Rancho Electric Arm described below.

Passive range of motion (PROM) must be within normal limits in order to obtain the most benefit from the MAS. Limited range of motion combined with very limited strength precludes the use of feeders in most cases. Incoordination or poor head or trunk control are contraindications for the use of MAS.

If the patient wears a hand splint, this is put on *before* beginning to balance the feeders. All screws, nuts, etc. *must be secured* to prevent slipping of the MAS while the patient is attempting to use it, even during fitting. It may be necessary to put tape or other friction material on the wheelchair upright before applying the bracket in order to prevent the bracket from slipping down under the weight of the patient's arm.

Parts, Functions, and Adjustments of Mobile Arm Supports. Ball-bearing Feeder Bracket Assembly (Fig. 12.30). The bracket is the piece that attaches to the wheelchair upright. The ball-bearing assembly is the piece that fits into the bracket and holds the proximal ball-bearing rings.

This assembly determines the height of the feeder in relation to the patient's body. Neutral = set at a height equal to midhumerus. Raise to enable the patient to get his hand to his mouth or for the elbow dial of the trough to clear the lapboard. Lower the bracket if the patient's shoulders are pushed into elevation. The height of the patient's seat cushion affects this setting. This assembly holds the proximal swivel arm. Be sure the proximal arm is pushed all the way down into the ball bearing until the first 90° angle of the proximal arm rests against the top of the ball bearing to prevent pushing the bottom ball bearing out. This assembly also determines the horizontal motion at the shoulder. Neutral = set the ball bearing perpendicular to the floor so that the proximal arm, when inserted, neither falls forward nor backward. Move the bracket out (posteriorly around the wheelchair upright) to assist horizontal abduction; move it in (anteriorly around the upright) to assist horizontal adduction. There is a right and left assembly: the bevel for the screwhead indicates the back of the bracket.

The Rancho assembly requires that the patient sit upright, whereas the Georgia Warm Springs or Michigan types allow 5 to 10° of recline of the wheelchair back.

Proximal Swivel Arm (Fig. 12.31). This piece corresponds to the humerus; it permits humeral motion. The proximal swivel arm holds the distal swivel arm in the distal ball bearing. The distal ball bearing may be angled down to assist elbow extension or upward to assist elbow flexion. The patient's permanent feeders will be angled by the orthotist; there is an adjustable

proximal arm available for trial purposes (Fig. 12.32). The proximal arms are interchangeable unless adapted, in which case the right and left one must be marked.

Elevating Proximal Arm (Fig. 12.33). The elevating proximal arm is a component which may be selected in lieu of the standard proximal arm. This component is used to assist a weak (F−)deltoid. A strong rubber band assists the weak deltoid muscle to abduct and flex the shoulder, thus allowing the hand to be brought toward the head.

Distal Swivel Arm (Fig. 12.34). This piece corresponds to the forearm; it permits elbow motion in the horizontal plane. It supports the rocker arm assembly and feeder trough. Right and left distal swivel arms differ; to distinguish them, hold the solid end in your hand, the arm should angle in toward you in both cases (R or L). The hollow post at the distal end of the arm may need to be cut lower if the patient is

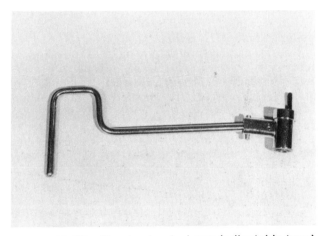

Figure 12.32 Proximal swivel arm (adjustable type).

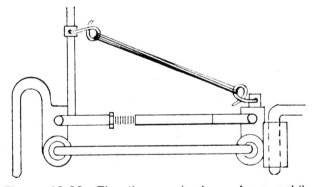

Figure 12.33 Elevating proximal arm for a mobile arm support. (Reproduced with permission from C. Long.[1])

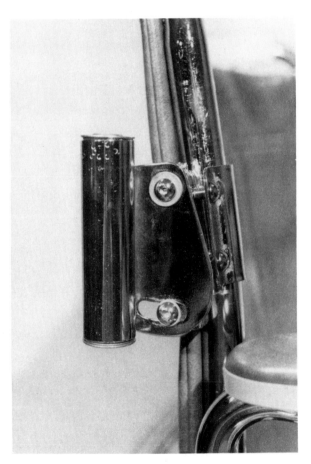

Figure 12.30 Ball-bearing feeder bracket assembly (Rancho type).

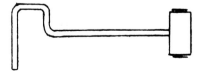

Figure 12.31 Proximal swivel arm.

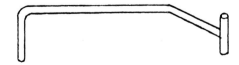

Figure 12.34 Distal swivel arm.

having trouble inwardly rotating. The curvature of the distal arm occasionally may need to be different than standard for a particular patient to allow the elbow dial of the trough to clear the distal arm during vertical motion. The orthotist will do this. Be sure the patient is using a proper motion pattern before you take the problem to the orthotist. The length of the distal arm, like the proximal arm, is standard; however, an unusually small or large patient may need special length arms. The distal ball bearing should be located directly opposite the patient's elbow; not behind the elbow nor in front of it.

Post (Fig. 12.35). The post provides added height at the distal end of the distal arm for specific activities. This part must be added by another person whenever it is needed; therefore, an effort should be made to balance the feeders without using this. If one must be used permanently, the orthotist can make the permanent post of the distal arm higher to alleviate the need for this piece.

Horizontal Stop (Fig. 12.36). The horizontal stop limits horizontal motion to within the patient's controllable limits. The horizontal stop can also be used to transfer motion from the shoulder to the elbow by applying it at the proximal ball bearing to prevent horizontal abduction; this will result in elbow extension when the patient attempts horizontal abduction. It can be used to transfer power from moving the distal part of the feeder to moving the whole feeder by applying it at the distal ball bearing. It is used when the patient lacks shoulder power. The horizontal stop is usually applied to the ball bearing on the outside—to limit horizontal abduction or extension rather than adduction or flexion. Neutral setup is no stop.

Rocker Arm Assemblies. Five will be described here; any one of these may be used on any MAS setup.

1. Rancho type (Fig. 12.37) permits vertical motion of the feeder trough. It swivels to produce added

horizontal motion at the elbow. Right or left are indistinguishable. The trough is attached to this part which is inserted into the distal end of the distal swivel arm.

2. Georgia Warm Springs type (Fig. 12.38) provides an offset which permits the elbow dial of the trough to clear the distal arm. The functions listed above for the Rancho type are also offered. The right and left differ; when inserted into the distal arm, the assembly should angle toward the patient.

3. Michigan type (Fig. 12.39) allows, in addition to the features of the two assemblies noted above, adjustment in the Z axis (vertical) and thereby allows the pivot point to be located directly opposite the

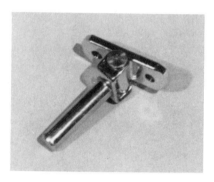

Figure 12.37   Rancho type rocker arm assembly.

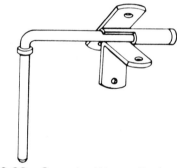

Figure 12.38   Georgia Warm Springs type offset rocker arm assembly.

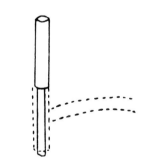

Figure 12.35   The post.

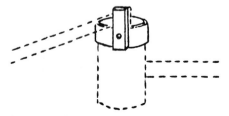

Figure 12.36   The horizontal stop.

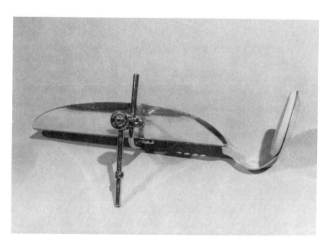

Figure 12.39   Michigan type rocker arm assembly attached to trough.

center of gravity of the forearm. A weak patient is more easily able to use this type.

4. Modular adjustment mechanism (Fig. 12.40) improves on the Rancho type assembly by alleviating the need for unscrewing the assembly when making proximal/distal adjustments on the trough.[27]

5. Supinator assist (Fig. 12.41) is a special rocker arm assembly which provides mechanical supination during flexion, actually humeral external rotation, and reciprocal pronation during internal rotation. The amount of supination-pronation can be controlled by limiting the length of the wire loop. The supinator assist can be mounted onto a Rancho or offset rocker assembly. Right and left differ: the wire loop is on the side toward the patient.

Vertical Stop (Fig. 12.42). The vertical stop is attached to the offset rocker assembly to limit vertical motion. It keeps the motion within the controllable limits of the patient. It may be used to limit both up and down motions or only one or the other by adjusting the screws. Neutral set up = no stop.

Troughs. Two types will be described. (1) Trough with elbow dial (Fig. 12.43). The length of the trough is 2 inches less than the distance from the olecranon to the head of the ulna. The distal end is flared. The motion of the wrist should not be impeded. The distal lip of the trough should not limit circulation in the patient's hand. The trough supports the forearm. It is possible to adjust the location of the trough on the

rocker assembly to assist either internal rotation (hand heavy—move the trough forward on the rocker assembly) or external rotation (elbow heavy—move the trough backward on the rocker assembly). For neutral setting, set the trough on the rocker assembly so that the forearm rests at an angle of 45° in relation to the lapboard. The elbow dial can be bent to provide fine adjustments to assist internal or external rotation. Sometimes the dial restricts elbow extension, although it offers good stable elbow support. In neutral setup, the elbow dial is in line with the center line of the trough. Right and left troughs differ: the angle of the dial indicates the difference—the dial angles in slightly toward the patient.

(2) The "flying saucer" feeder trough (Fig. 12.44) supports the forearm. It is used in cases where the patient has active elbow flexion and external rotation of the humerus and does not need the vertical motion. This part supplants both the trough and the rocker arm assembly.

Once the MAS is assembled, always mark the location of pieces in relation to one another before making changes during the balancing so that it is easy to return to the previous position, which may prove to be the better adjustment after all. When the MAS is finally balanced, erase all extraneous marks, re-mark

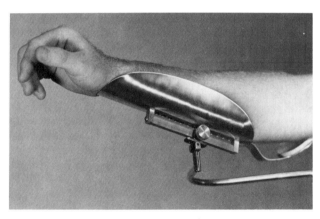

Figure 12.40 Modular adjustment mechanism attached to Rancho rocker arm assembly. (Reproduced with permission from W. E. Drew and P. H. Stern.[27])

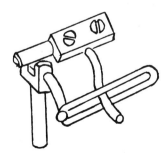

Figure 12.41 Supinator assist.

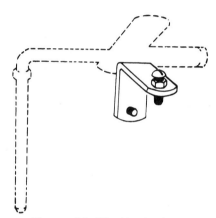

Figure 12.42 Vertical stop.

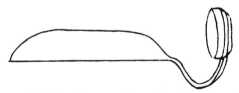

Figure 12.43 Forearm trough with elbow dial.

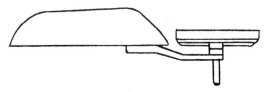

Figure 12.44 "Flying saucer" forearm trough for feeder.

all final positions in case the MAS are knocked out of adjustment and need to be rebalanced. Be sure all screws are *tight*.

Movement Patterns and Equipment Adjustments to Achieve Motion in Mobile Arm Supports. It is preferable to instruct the patient in movement patterns to achieve certain motions in the neutrally adjusted mobile arm supports. However, as is frequently the case, the patient may be too weak to be able to do these motions. In that case the equipment can be adjusted to assist the motions which are weakest. It is not advisable to require the patient to practice the motions a long time before making the equipment adjustments because he will become discouraged and may reject the orthosis. The movement patterns and the equipment adjustments are not listed here in any order of preference. One motion, or one adjustment, may be all that is necessary; or for greater effect a combination of two or more motions, two or more adjustments, or a combination of a motion plus an adjustment may be necessary for the extremely weak patient. Use only the movement patterns and adjustments which are completely safe for the patient, use the least energy, most nearly approximate normal or acceptable movement, and which are most effective. The process of discovery of the correct combination is one of trial and error. The patient should not be allowed to become fatigued in the process, however, because fatigue invalidates the adjustments. The movement patterns listed below are adapted from a manual once available from Georgia Warm Springs Rehabilitation Center.

DESIRED MOTION: HAND TO MOUTH

Instructions for Movement Patterns

1. Depress your shoulder while adducting your humerus.
2. Externally rotate your shoulder.
3. Bend laterally toward the same side that the MAS you want to move is on.
4. Shift your body weight toward the side that the MAS you want to move is on (only if enough strength to regain balance).
5. Straighten up or lean back in the chair.
6. Rotate your trunk toward the side the MAS that you want to move is on.
7. Tilt or turn your head toward the MAS that you want to move.
8. Press the elbow dial against a friction pad placed on the lapboard near the waist by depressing your scapula. This may cause enough supination to aim the eating utensil toward your mouth.

Equipment Adjustment

1. Move rocker assembly forward on trough. (Make "elbow heavy.")
2. Turn ball-bearing bracket assembly toward individual.
3. Adjust the proximal swivel arm up.
4. Position the anterior vertical stop to decrease internal rotation.
5. Raise the ball-bearing bracket assembly on the wheelchair upright.

6. Adapt the utensil's length or angle.
7. Raise the trough by use of a post.
8. Lower the posterior vertical stop under the trough to permit additional shoulder external rotation.

DESIRED MOTION: HAND TO TABLE

Instructions for Movement Patterns

1. Elevate and internally rotate your shoulder to lower the hand.
2. Roll the shoulder forward which encourages horizontal adduction with shoulder flexion, internal rotation, and elbow extension.
3. Laterally bend toward the side opposite to the MAS that you want to move.
4. Shift your body weight to the side opposite the MAS that you want to move is on if your balance can be regained.
5. Rotate your trunk toward the side opposite from MAS that you want to move.
6. Tilt or turn your head away from the MAS that you want to move.

Equipment Adjustment

1. Move the rocker assembly further back on the trough ("hand heavy").
2. Turn the ball-bearing bracket assembly backward, away from individual.
3. Adjust the proximal swivel arm down.
4. Position the anterior vertical stop under the trough to allow more elbow extension (internal rotation).
5. Lower the ball-bearing feeder bracket assembly on the wheelchair upright.
6. Lower the trough by removing the post or cutting down the distal channel into which the rocker arm assembly fits.

DESIRED MOTION: HORIZONTAL ABDUCTION

Instructions for Movement Patterns

1. Shift your body weight toward the side that the orthosis you want to move is on.
2. Rotate your trunk toward the side that the orthosis you want to move is on.
3. Turn your head briskly toward the orthosis.

Equipment Adjustment

1. Rotate the ball-bearing bracket assembly on the wheelchair upright backward, away from the individual.
2. Shorten the proximal swivel arm.

DESIRED MOTION: HORIZONTAL ADDUCTION

Instructions for Movement Pattern

1. Shift your body weight away from the side the orthosis you want to move is on.
2. Rotate your body away from the side the orthosis you want to move is on.
3. Turn your head briskly away from the orthosis.

Equipment Adjustment

1. Rotate the ball-bearing bracket assembly on the wheelchair upright forward, toward the individual.
2. Lengthen the proximal swivel arm.

Checkout and Training for Mobile Arm Supports. Checkout of the mobile arm support may be done using the form shown in Table 12.1.

The patient will not be able to put on his MAS independently but must instruct others in their proper application. Patients can remove them by lifting their arms slightly and the MAS move away. The MAS, except for the ball-bearing bracket assembly, is removed when the wheelchair is stored. Care must be taken that the bracket assembly does not get knocked out of alignment when the chair is put into the car or when the patient is wheeled through doorways because this will change the entire balance of the MAS.

Controls training involves having the patient move the MAS as far as he can *horizontally* from side to side and then from front to back. If the patient needs much practice in order to do these motions effortlessly, then activities requiring horizontal motions, such as drawing with felt-tipped pens, turning large-sized magazine pages, playing board games, etc. offer some stimulation to the exercise. The patient learns to control first one feeder, then the other. Both are usually worn for balance, but if the patient is tall and has lateral instability he may be more stable if his non-training arm is out of the feeder and resting on the lapboard. Next, *vertical* motions are learned, first out to the side which is easiest, then in front of the face, then at any point within his horizontal range. Games that require picking up of playing pieces and movement in space are interesting exercises for the patient.

Use training is not initiated before the patient has excellent control of the feeders *and* his hand splint if he has one. Use training activities will include feeding, grooming, use of telephone, typewriter, calculators, and other electronic devices, page turning, and possibly writing and drawing.

The Rancho Electric Arm

The Rancho Electric Arm (See Fig. 12.45) is a full upper extremity orthosis which fastens to the wheelchair. It is used for very weak patients and allows movement in five degrees of freedom: shoulder flexion-

Table 12.1
CHECK-OUT SHEET FOR MOBILE ARM SUPPORTS[a]

Patient's Name ——————————————————————— Type Feeder (R) ——

Date Fitted ————————————————————————— (L) ——

I. Patient's position in wheel chair

Yes	No	Is patient able to sit up straight?
Yes	No	Are hips well back in chair?
Yes	No	Is spine in good vertical alignment?
Yes	No	Does patient have lateral trunk stability?
Yes	No	Is chair seat adequate for comfort and stability?
Yes	No	If patient wears hand splints, does he have them on?
Yes	No	Does patient meet requirements for passive ROM and coordination?

II. Mechanical Check-out

Yes	No	Are all screws tight?
Yes	No	Is bracket tight on wheelchair?
Yes	No	Are all joints freely movable?
Yes	No	Is proximal arm all the way down into the bracket?
Yes	No	Is bracket at proper height so shoulders are not forced into elevation?
Yes	No	Does elbow dial clear lapboard when trough is in "up" position?
Yes	No	Is patient's hand (in "up" position) as close to mouth as possible?
Yes	No	Can patient obtain maximal active reach?
Yes	No	Is feeder trough short enough to allow wrist flexion or to prevent pressure on blood vessels?
Yes	No	Are trough edges rolled so that they do not contact forearm?
Yes	No	Is elbow secure and comfortable in elbow support?
Yes	No	In vertical motion, does the dial clear the distal arm?

III. Control check-out

Yes	No	Can patient control motion of proximal arm from either extreme?
Yes	No	Can patient control motion of distal arm from either extreme?
Yes	No	Can patient control vertical motion from either extreme?
Yes	No	Have stops been applied to limit range within controllable limits if necessary?

[a] Devised by staff at Rancho Los Amigos Hospital, Downey, Calif.

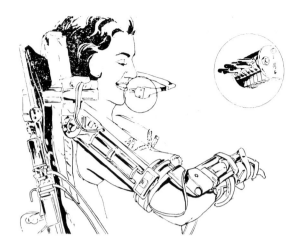

Figure 12.45 Rancho electric arm orthesis with detail of the seven bidirectional tongue switches. (Reproduced with permission from S. Licht: *Orthotics Etcetera*. New Haven, Conn., Elizabeth Licht., 1966.)

extension, shoulder abduction-adduction, shoulder internal and external rotation, elbow flexion and extension, and forearm pronation and supination. Electric motors supply the power. An externally powered hand splint is also usually worn to provide prehension. The arm is controlled by a bank of seven pairs of microswitches mounted on a stand near the face. Each pair of microswitches controls one degree of freedom of the arm. Additionally there is one set for prehension and also one set for moving the control box toward and away from the face. The patient must consciously program each movement by moving each joint in sequence so that he may move the end point of this system (the hand) into the desired position.

Range of motion and sitting requirements for the Rancho Arm are similar to those for a MAS. A myoelectric X-Y-Z control system was developed for the Rancho Arm which allows the patient to concentrate on moving the hand horizontally toward or away from himself (Y), back or forth horizontally (X), or vertically up or down (Z).[28] The patient controls this system myoelectrically by contracting or relaxing three different muscles plus whatever muscle is used to control prehension of the hand splint.

In either case the extensive controls training required makes this orthosis warranted only when the patient is so weak that he is unable to use a mobile arm support adapted with elevating proximal arm and/or motorized distal arm.

Pronator Lively Splint for C$_5$ Tetraplegic Arm (Fig. 12.46)

This splint provides active elbow extension through the use of coiled springs mounted at the elbow joint and pronation through the use of specially designed springs. The assisted arm movement enables the C$_5$ spinal cord-injured patient to use a prehension splint functionally and is an alternative to MAS for those patients with good shoulder musculature.[29]

Distal Function: Hand Splints

The following dynamic splints were selected to illustrate orthoses used to assist weakness and to increase strength. Assistance may be given to a motion by use of rubber bands which are adjusted so that after the patient has moved as far as he can, the rubber band completes the motion. Assistance can also be provided by use of springs or coiled wire. The weak muscle is strengthened by actively moving the part as far as it can before the assisting mechanism completes the motion. The opposing muscles may also be strengthened if they are required to work against the elastic, wires, or springs.

Long Opponens Hand Splint with Action Wrist and Dorsiflexion Assist (Fig. 12.47)

This is a dorsal splint which supports the thumb and assists the weak wrist extensors by way of the rubber band which extends from the proximal band of the splint to the hand piece.

Thomas Dorsal Outrigger (Fig. 12.48)

This device substitutes for lost or weak metacarpophalangeal extension while supporting the weak wrist of the patient with radial nerve paralysis. An outrigger from which a narrow rod or dowel is suspended by an elastic is used to assist these muscles. A thumb extension assist can be added if the thumb extensor muscles are also weak. This splint is commercially available in

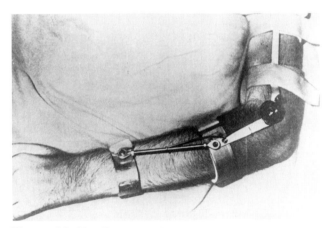

Figure 12.46 Pronator lively splint for C$_5$ tetraplegic arm. (Reproduced with permission from D. Abraham et al.[29])

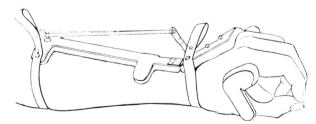

Figure 12.47 Long opponens hand splint with action wrist and dorsiflexion assist. (Reproduced with permission from C. Long.[1])

The criteria of fi[t]
hand splints. In a
smoothly and all
as large objects.
coincide with the
pophalangeal joi[nt]
tate independent[ly]

The patient v[...]
remove his own [...]
until he is able t[...]
is important bec[...]
such as propellin[...]
quickly put on a[...]
as just one more [...]

Controls train[...]
move, and releas[...]
weights, and cru[...]
1½ inches (2.5 t[...]
semirough textu[...]
tient's skill inc[...]
smoothness, flatt[...]
per cups, fresh j[...]
cils, metal or gla[...]
for a person wi[...]
objects, the obj[...]
partially overha[...]
soft surface, suc[...]
rubber to allow t[...]
prehension, whic[...]
mally used to [...]
absence of active [...]
the patient com[...]
tate at the shou[...]
the patient has p[...]
fine control of [...]
training will be [...]

Use training [...]
tional performan[...]
splint, how thes[...]
if metal or glass [...]
to provide fricti[...]
problem it is p[...]
large size secre[...]
thumb post to [...]
of any object th[...]
the strength of g[...]
extremity. A p[...]
(grams) is used [...]
when using a pr[...]

Wrist-Drive[n]
desis). The thu[...]
splinted as desc[...]
located at the [...]
joint to allow fin[...]
at the exact axis [...]
wrist movement [...]
active wrist ext[...]
cause the powe[...]
prehension thro[...]
This splint aug[...]
patient has and[...]

the Bunnell series, although the design idea is used for handmade splints.

Metacarpophalangeal Extension Assist (Fig. 12.49)

The metacarpophalangeal extension assist is a dorsal outrigger from which plastic cuffs are suspended by way of rubber bands which support the fingers individually to assist weak metacarpophalangeal extension. The pull of the rubber bands must be perpendicular to the proximal phalanx in order for the full benefit of the pull to be applied in moving the finger around the axis of the joint, rather than applying traction or compression forces on the joint. The tension of the rubber bands is adjusted to complete the extension motion while allowing the patient to actively extend and flex to his limits. This orthotic design may also be used to increase range of motion of the fingers when there is a flexor contracture by increasing the tension of the rubber bands to stretch the fingers into extension.

Low Profile Dorsal Dynamic Splint

This splint is designed to support the wrist and assist the weak finger extensors of patients with radial nerve injuries. The fingers are supported by elastic

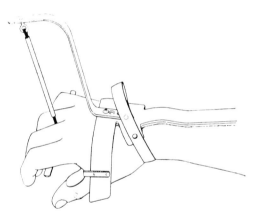

Figure 12.48 Thomas dorsal outrigger. (Reproduced with permission from C. Long.[1])

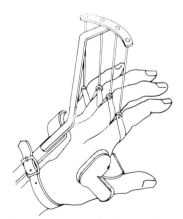

Figure 12.49 Metacarpophalangeal extension assist. (Reproduced with permission from M. Anderson.[21])

slings attached to wire prongs that lie close to the extended fingers. The splint allows active finger flexion. This splint has the advantage of being less cumbersome than splints with outriggers. Directions for construction are published by Sellers.[30]

Thumb Abduction Assist (Fig. 12.50)

This is a splint in which a spring wire outrigger extends from the palmar piece to abduct the thumb (Fig. 12.50*A*). If the location of the outrigger were moved dorsally the thumb could be assisted into extension (Fig. 12.50*B*).

First Dorsal Interosseus Assist (Fig. 12.51)

This assist may be an attachment added to a metal short opponens hand splint or may be an integral part of the design of a plastic splint. The assist is made from spring steel wire with a cuff attached to it that slips over the index finger to assist that finger toward abduction (function of the first dorsal interosseous muscle), thereby increasing the effectiveness of pinch.

Metacarpophalangeal Stop or Lumbrical Bar (Fig. 12.52)

The bar is attached to a hand splint dorsally and exerts a force over the proximal phalanges to hold the metacarpophalangeal joints into slight flexion. The

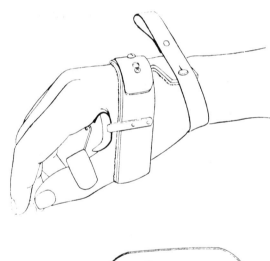

A

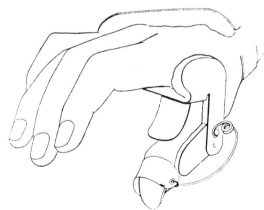

B

Figure 12.50 *A.* Thumb abduction assist. *B.* Thumb extension assist. (Reproduced with permission from C. Long.[1])

Figure 12
duced wi

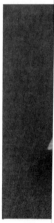

Figure 1
ponens s

force of
to the i
bar prev
that res
The bar
all or se

Rancho F

This (
principl
deviatio
allowing
used for
arthritis
bands a
either c
carpoph

Flexor H

Palm
is provi
factors:
abducti
phalang
are post

Power to drive hand splints can be obtained from any of the following:

1. A small rotary motor that runs forward, backward, and holds when stopped. One end of a cable is attached to the motor and the other end of the cable is attached to the bar that extends from the finger piece of the splint (Fig. 12.56). As the cable is pulled in by the motor, the fingers are flexed and pinch against the thumb. As the cable is reeled out, the spring pulls the fingers into extension. The patient can control the extent of the opening by turning the motor on and off more or less quickly. Some motors are proportional and operate fast or slow, depending upon the force the patient exerts on the control switch.

2. Electrical stimulation of a patient's muscle over which he has no control.[32] When the electrical stimulation is on, the muscle contracts and when the stimulation ceases the muscle relaxes. The opposite motion, usually flexion, is accomplished by a spring. Originally, this type of splint seemed to have limited value for quadriplegics because the stimulated muscle rapidly fatigued. This fatigue phenomenon occurred when the finger extensor muscles were repetitively stimulated with enough voltage to overcome the strong pull of the spring that is needed for the pinch used in daily tasks (3 to 4 pounds) and these muscles lost their ability to continue to contract. Stimulating the flexor muscles instead of the extensor was not a satisfactory solution; fatigue developed due to the prolonged tetany needed for maintained holding. This problem seems to have been overcome by using a program of electrically induced exercise and by utilizing a sequential stimulation technique. Contractions that are strong, fatigue-resistant, smooth, and have controllable strength have been produced.[33]

Functional Electrical Stimulation (FES) has been under study.[34] FES is defined as a neural prosthetic technique that utilizes stimulation of neural tissue for inward information transfer.[34] In FES, the motor point is stimulated, thereby efficiently activating the muscle

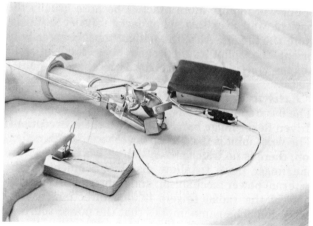

Figure 12.56 Flexor hinge hand splint externally powered by battery-driven motor with microswitch control.

through its neural mechanism. Fatigue is not a problem. The electrical stimulus causes an afferent and both a peripheral and a central efferent wave of depolarization. FES has been used successfully to provide correct walking patterns in children with cerebral palsy and in hemiplegics. After many repetitions, the walking pattern seems to be relearned. FES is also used to attempt to restore finger extension in hemiparetic patients; however, carryover of function after a period of FES training has not been as successful to date.[35, 36] This is probably because for learning to occur, the afferent-central efferent loop must be completed, which it is for stepping motions since they are probably organized subcortically. However, finger extension is cortically directed, and the afferent input stops at the level of the lesion, never to reach the central efferent part of the loop.[35]

No exoskeletal support, *i.e.*, flexor hinge hand splint or brace is used with FES. The idea of enabling a paraplegic to walk using multichannel FES is being tested.[37, 38]

3. An "artificial muscle" (Fig. 12.57) is made of a tubular, helically woven nylon sleeve covering a leak-proof rubber bladder. When gas (carbon dioxide) is allowed to flow into the bladder it enlarges as a balloon would; however, the constraint of the helical weave of the sleeve causes the ends of the "muscle" to move closer together as the circumference increases. When the gas is released, the "muscle" gets thin and long again. A Chinese finger trap operates on the same principle. The end of the "muscle" is attached to the finger piece and causes the fingers to flex when it is distended, while a spring causes extension when the tension in the "muscle" is reduced.

The *control transducer* of the externally powered splint is operated by a part of the patient's body over which he has voluntary control, where he has normal sensation, and which does not activate the transducer accidentally during habitual motions. For A C_4, C_5 quadriplegic this means upper trapezius-, tongue-, or chin-operated controls. If shoulder elevation is to be

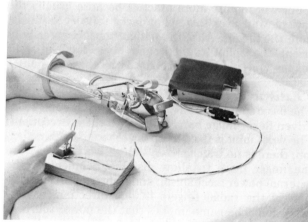

Figure 12.57 "Artificial muscle" driven flexor hinge hand splint. (Reproduced with permission from C. Long.[1])

used, the opposite shoulder is usually chosen to reduce the likelihood of associated unintentional activation. Spotty muscle weakness such as occurs in polio may preserve control sites in the lower extremities if none exist in the upper body.

The motor can be controlled by microswitches which require about 1 ounce of pressure to activate (Fig. 12.56). These microswitches may be mounted over the patient's shoulder so he can elevate or retract the shoulder to touch and activate them (Fig. 12.58), or near his face so his tongue can press them, or in a joy-stick arrangement which can be controlled by the chin pushing on the stick, or in any other position where the patient can exert voluntary pressure. The microswitches must be mounted so that the patient can activate two switches—forward and reverse—for each motor. The motor can also be controlled by myoelectric signals which when amplified can electronically switch the motor.[39, 40] The electrical activity of the voluntarily contracting control muscle is picked up using surface electrodes. Forward and reverse directions of the motor are achieved by using a low amplitude signal to switch forward and a high amplitude signal to switch backward or vice versa instead of using two muscles like the two switches mentioned above.

Voice activation of the motor is a possible, but as yet unreliable, method of control because extraneous noise also activates the motor.

In electrical stimulation splints, the flow of electrical stimulation can be controlled by myoelectric signals or by a potentiometer, which is an electrical component which increases or decreases the resistance to the flow of electricity as the armature is moved, or by a switch. The switch or potentiometer can be arranged so they can be controlled by shoulder elevation or any other movement the patient can control.

The "artificial muscle" (also known as the McKibben muscle after the physicist who invented it) is controlled by a three-position valve: when the stem of the valve is pushed all the way in, the gas flows to activate the "muscle"; when released, the valve holds the gas in place, and the fingers remain in whatever position they were (Fig. 12.59). When the stem of the valve is pushed half way in, the gas is allowed to escape, which deflates the "muscle." The gas can be allowed to escape in short, quick spurts, thus opening

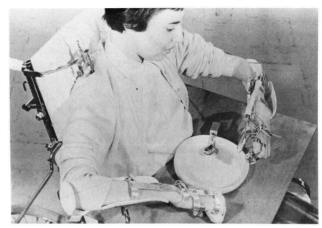

Figure 12.59 Patient using an artificial muscle-powered flexor hinge hand splint on left hand with control valve mounted over right shoulder, activated by scapular elevation. (Photograph used with permission of Doris Brennan.)

the fingers a little at a time; this is called feathering the valve.

Check-out of Externally Powered Hand Splints. The check-out involves all that has been cited for the two other flexor hinge hand splints above. In addition, the reliability of the control mechanism must be carefully checked: the signal used to close the splint must always close the splint and always work with the same amount of pressure of the control site. A too short cable or "muscle" or too much tension in the springs may impede pinch of thin paper and should be adjusted. Adjustments would need to be made also if large (2-inch) items could not be grasped. A stop can be incorporated into this splint to prevent excessive pressure on the fingertips in closed position; however, it should still allow holding paper or playing cards if the patient needs to do this.

Rarely will a patient who needs this type of splint be able to put it on and off by himself. However, he should be able to clearly instruct another and should receive supervised practice in giving this instruction. He must also instruct others in the care and recharging of the power unit. Battery-powered splints (motor, electrical stimulation) can be charged overnight using the charger that comes with the unit. The CO_2 gas bottle refill may need to be obtained from the orthotist; fire station supply houses or bottling plants have CO_2 and often are willing to fill the empty bottle, but the proper adapter must be obtained from an orthotist. A full 12-inch bottle of CO_2 lasts about 3 weeks if the splint is opened and closed once every 5 minutes, 8 hours per day. This amount of use is rare since the splint is opened and closed once to grasp something which is then usually held; no gas is used during the holding phase.

All hand splints should be treated like fine jewelry: washed, polished, and stored where they cannot be bent or misaligned. An out-of-kilter hand splint is dangerous; at the very least it exerts pressure which

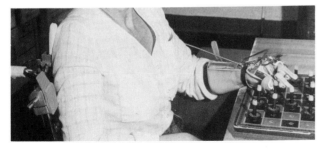

Figure 12.58 Microswitch activation of motor-driven flexor hinge hand splint via shoulder retraction.

can cause decubiti and at worst can cause undesired forces on the joints.

Controls training must be thoroughly completed before use training is attempted to decrease the inevitable frustration. Controls training begins with observation of the effect of the control motion on the hand splint.[41, 42] The hand splint may be on the patient's hand, but if it cannot be seen easily, the splint is best mounted some other place so the patient can watch it while simultaneously feeling his controlling movement. Once the effect of the control motion is learned, the patient begins the same practice of picking up, moving, and releasing various objects as described above for the other flexor hinge hand splints. A good test of the patient's automaticity of control of the splint is to have him pick up on signal a 1-inch cube that has been placed on a premarked spot and to release it into a small box placed 6 to 8 inches away. The time in tenths of seconds is recorded. This is repeated 20 or so times, and the mean and the standard deviation is computed (see page 297). A low standard deviation indicates consistency of operation, a sign of skill. Tasks attempted during use training will be limited by the patient's disability. Adaptations will probably be necessary to accomplish these, and the reader is referred to the chapter on spinal cord injury for specifics.

Electronic Control Units

Electronic controls are available for electric wheelchairs. The occupational therapist is the professional who usually does the check-out, controls, and use training if the patient has these controls.

Electronic devices are available to allow a severely paralyzed person to control electrical apparatus in his environment. Examples of such apparatus include television, television channel selector, radio, nurse call, lamp, adjustable bed, special telephone, intercom, etc.[43] The person uses the motion he has available to operate a switch or a "sip and puff" type control transducer. Again, the occupational therapist does the check-out and training for this orthosis. Training aids are available for both types of transducers.[43, 44] It is as important that the control units be reliable and that the patient have mastery of the controls for these units as it is for any complicated orthosis.

References

1. Long, C. Upper limb orthotics. In *Orthotics Etcetera*, 2nd ed., edited by J. B. Redford. Baltimore: Williams & Wilkins, 1980.
2. DeVore, G. L. A sling to prevent a subluxed shoulder. *Am. J. Occup. Ther.*, 24(5): 580–581, 1970.
3. Neal, M. R., and Williamson, J. Collar sling for bilateral shoulder subluxation. *Am. J. Occup. Ther.*, 34(6): 400–401, 1980.
4. Bobath, B. *Adult Hemiplegia: Evaluation and Treatment*, 2nd ed. London: Heinemann Medical Books, 1979.
5. Basmajian, J. V. *Muscles Alive: Their Functions Revealed by Electromyography*, 4th ed. Baltimore: Williams & Wilkins, 1979.
6. Goold, N. J. A versatile wheelchair armrest attachment. *Am. J. Occup. Ther.*, 30(8): 502–504, 1976.
7. Salo, R. E. A hammock wheelchair armrest. *Am. J. Occup. Ther.*, 32(8): 525, 1978.
8. Fishwick, G. M., and Tobin, D. G. Splinting the burned hand with primary excision and early grafting. *Am. J. Occup. Ther.*, 32(3): 182–183, 1978.
9. Barber, L. *LMB Wire-Foam: The Gentle Splints.* Catalogue, LMB Hand Rehab Products, San Luis Obispo, Calif.
10. Snook, J. H. Spasticity reduction splint. *Am. J. Occup. Ther.*, 33(10): 648–651, 1979.
11. Kaplan, N. Effect of splinting on reflex inhibition and sensorimotor stimulation in treatment of spasticity. *Arch. Phys. Med. Rehabil.*, 43(11): 565–569, 1962.
12. Doubilet, L., and Polkow, L. S. Theory and design of a finger abduction splint for the spastic hand. *Am. J. Occup. Ther.*, 31(5): 320–322, 1977.
13. Zislis, J. Splinting of the hand in a spastic hemiplegic. *Arch. Phys. Med. Rehabil.*, 45(1): 41–43, 1964.
14. Kiel, J. L. Making the dynamic orthokinetic wrist splint for flexor spasticity in hand and wrist. In *Sensorimotor Evaluation and Treatment Procedures for Allied Health Personnel*, 2nd ed, edited by S. D. Farber and A. J. Huss. Indianapolis: Indiana University Foundation, 1974.
15. Edwards, J. W. *Orthopaedic Appliances Atlas*, Vol. 1. Ann Arbor: Edwards Brothers, 1952.
16. Making the least of burn scars. *Emergency Med.*, 4: 24–45, 1972.
17. Larson, D. *The Prevention and Correction of Burn Scar Contracture and Hypertrophy.* Galveston, Tex., Shriner's Burn Institute, University of Texas Medical Branch, 1973.
18. Rivers, E. A., Strate, R. G., and Salem, L. D. The transparent face mask. *Am. J. Occup. Ther.*, 33(2): 108–113, 1979.
19. Green, D. P., and McCoy, H. Turnbuckle orthotic correction of elbow-flexion contractures after acute injuries. *J. Bone. Joint Surg.*, 61A(7): 1092–1095, 1979.
20. Bunnell, S. *Surgery of the Hand*, 2nd ed. Philadelphia: J. B. Lippincott, 1948.
21. Anderson, M. *Upper Extremity Orthotics.* Springfield, Ill.: Charles C Thomas, 1965.
22. Malick, M. H. *Manual on Dynamic Hand Splinting with Thermoplastic Materials.* New York: ABC Inc., 1974.
23. Heurich, M., and Polansky, S. An adaptation of the glove flexion mitt. *Am. J. Occup. Ther.*, 32(2): 110–111, 1978.
24. Bunnell, S. *Surgery of the Hand*, 3rd ed. Philadelphia: J. B. Lippincott, 1956.
25. Von Prince, K., Cureri, W., and Pruitt, B. Application of fingernail hooks in splinting burned hands. *Am. J. Occup. Ther.*, 24(8): 556–559, 1970.
26. Nichols, P. J. R., et al. The value of flexor hinge hand splints. *Prosthet. Orthot. Int.*, 2(2): 86–94, 1978.
27. Drew, W. E., and Stern, P. H. Modular adjustment mechanism for the balanced forearm orthosis. *Arch. Phys. Med. Rehabil.*, 60(2): 81, 1979.
28. Zebo, T., Long, C., and Beard, J. Myoelectric control of the Rancho electric arm. In *Proceedings of the Annual Conference on Engineering in Medicine and Biology*, Vol. 10, (26B2), Houston, November, 1968. Arlington, Va.: The Alliance for Engineering in Medicine and Biology, 1968.
29. Abraham, D., Shrosbree, M. B., and Key, A. G. A functional splint for the C_5 tetraplegic arm. *Paraplegia*, 17: 198–203, 1979–80.
30. Sellers, J. A low-profile dorsal dynamic splint. *Am. J. Occup. Ther.*, 34(3): 213, 1980.
31. McKenzie, M. The ratchet handsplint. *Am. J. Occup. Ther.*, 27(8): 477–479, 1973.
32. Long, C., and Masciarelli, V. An electrophysiological splint for the hand. *Arch. Phys. Med. Rehabil.*, 44(9): 499–503, 1963.
33. Peckham, P. H., and Mortimer, J. T. Restoration of hand function in the quadriplegic through electrical stimulation. In *Functional Electrical Stimulation*, edited by F. T. Hambrecht and J. B. Reswick. New York: Marcel Dekker, 1977.
34. Hambrecht, F. T., and Reswick, J. B. (eds) *Functional Electrical Stimulation.* New York: Marcel Dekker, 1977.
35. Gracanin, F. Functional electrical stimulation in control of mo-

tor output and movements. In *Contemporary Clinical Neurophysiology* edited by W. A. Cobb and H. Van Duijn. Amsterdam: Elsevier, 1978.

36. Vodovnik, L., Kralj, A., Stanic, U., Acimovic, R., and Gros, N. Recent applications of functional electrical stimulation to stroke patients in Ljubljana. *Clin. Orthop.*, 131: 64–70, 1978.
37. Vodovnik, L., and Grobelnik, S. Multichannel functional electrical stimulation—facts and expectations. *Prosthet. Orthot. Int.*, 1: 43–46, 1977.
38. Kralj, A., Bajd, T., and Turk, R. Electrical stimulation providing functional use of paraplegic patient muscles. *Med. Prog. Technol.*, 7: 3–9, 1980.
39. Trombly, C., Prentke, E., and Long, C. Myoelectrically controlled electric torque motor for the flexor hinge hand splint. *Orthop. Prosthet. Appl. J.*, 21: 39–43, 1967.
40. Silverstein, F., French, J., and Siebens, A. A myoelectric hand splint. *Am. J. Occup. Ther.*, 28(2): 99–101, 1974.
41. Trombly, C. Principles of operant conditioning related to orthotic training of quadriplegic patients. *Am. J. Occup. Ther.*, 20(5): 217–220, 1966.
42. Trombly, C. Myoelectric control of orthotic devices for the severely paralyzed. *Am. J. Occup. Ther.*, 22(5): 385–389, 1968.
43. Catalogue, *Electronic Aids for the Severely Handicapped.* Shreve, Ohio, Prentke-Romich Company, 1982.
44. Fried, P., and Balick, J. Sip and puff control evaluator and trainer. *Am. J. Occup. Ther.*, 32(6): 398, 1978.

Supplementary Reading

Anderson, M. *Upper Extremity Orthotics*, 3rd ed. Springfield, Ill.: Charles C Thomas, 1974.

Engen, T. J. Accomplishments in modern orthotic patient management—indications for the future. *Orthot. Prosthet.*, 33: 3–9, 1979.

Fess, E. E., Gettle, K. S., and Strickland, J. W. *Hand Splinting: Principles and Methods.* St. Louis: C. V. Mosby, 1981.

Huddleston, O. L., Henderson, W., and Campbell, J. The static night splint. *Am. J. Occup. Ther.*, 12(5): 245–246, 1958.

Jamison, S. L., and Dayhoff, N. E. A hard hand positioning device to decrease wrist and finger hypertonicity: A sensorimotor approach for the patient with nonprogressive brain damage. *Nurs. Res.*, 29(5): 285–289, 1980.

Nichols, P. J. R., Peach, S. L., Haworth, R. J., and Ennis, J. The value of flexor hinge hand splints. *Pros. Orthot. Int.*, 2(2): 86–94, 1978.

Peterson, L. T. Neurological considerations in splinting spastic extremities, Tech. form 4-126. Menomonee Falls, Wis, Rolyan Medical Products.

Pollock, D., and Sell, H. Myoelectric control sites in the high-level quadriplegic patient. *Arch. Phys. Med. Rehabil.*, 59(5): 217–220, 1978.

Reswick, J. B., and Simoes, N. Application of engineering principles in management of spinal cord injury patients. *Clin. Orthop.*, 112 (October): 124–129, 1975.

chapter

13

The Materials and Methods of Construction of Temporary Orthoses

Catherine A. Trombly, M.A., OTR

Orthoses used in the treatment of weakness or limited range of motion for the purpose of assisting, positioning, or correcting are often considered temporary in nature and are more typically made by the occupational therapist from plastic materials than by the orthotist. Orthoses used to restore function are usually needed on a permanent basis and are machined from metals by the certified orthotist. Unfortunately, the supply of certified orthotists does not yet meet the demand, and the therapist may find it necessary to make the intricate metal splints that substitute for function. Anderson[1] graphically demonstrates this process; however, it is recommended that if the therapist is to have this duty, he or she should enroll in a postgraduate course offered at New York University, Northwestern University, or the University of California at Los Angeles (UCLA) for advanced training in the fitting, fabrication, check-out, and training related to permanent orthoses.

HAND SPLINT CONSTRUCTION BY THE OCCUPATIONAL THERAPIST

Selecting the Splint Design

To decide whether a hand splint is needed and what type is required, the therapist examines the patient's hand to determine why the hand either is not operating functionally to provide grasp and prehension or is not being held in a functional position at rest. The functional position of the hand is 15 to 30° of wrist dorsiflexion, neutral to slight ulnar deviation of the

wrist, partial flexion of the metacarpophalangeal and interphalangeal joints of the fingers and thumb, and thumb abduction and opposition. At rest, the normal hand assumes this position due to the balance of biomechanical forces that is brought about by the shape of the joints and the viscoelastic properties of the ligaments, tendons, skin, and innervated muscles. Changes in any of these factors will result in a hand problem that may require a hand splint.

The ideal goal of hand splinting is to restore or preserve normal hand function. To determine what splint design will be necessary to achieve the desired result, the therapist applies corrective forces manually to the patient's hand. While applying these forces the therapist notes how much and where force is needed to put the hand into a functional position or to assist it to move in functional grasp and prehension patterns. The therapist must remember that a relationship exists between the position of the wrist and the position and operation of the fingers due to tenodesis effect. This is an important fact to remember when deciding whether to make a short hand splint or one that crosses and supports the wrist. Both grasp and release should be at least potentially permitted by the position of the wrist in the splint. By splinting only the wrist or only the fingers of a patient with flexor spasticity, spasticity, or at least increased flexion, of the unsplinted joint will occur.

Once the therapist has the design parameters of the hand splint in mind, he can use a standard splint design for which patterns exist[2-6] or adapt a standard design to fit the particular problem or design a new splint and make the pattern for the patient's unique problem.

Fitting the Pattern (Figs. 13.1 to 13.4)

For each splint made, the pattern will have to be fitted to the particular person. Standard patterns almost never fit perfectly. There are two stages to the fitting process: gross adaptation of the pattern to the particular hand and final adjustment. Gross adaptation, or sizing, of the pattern is done directly on the hand or on the nonaffected hand.

To draw the pattern on the hand, a paper towel is placed over the entire surface of the hand and arm that the splint is meant to cover. The pattern is drawn free-hand to fit the contour of the hand which is palpated beneath the paper towel. If the therapist finds it difficult to draw the contour of the splint free-hand, he or she may use the too small or too large patterns available in the books cited as references to

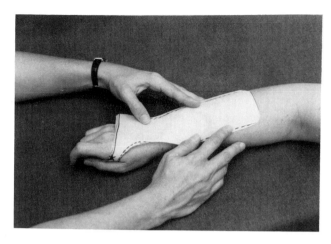

Figure 13.3 Paper pattern is fitted to the patient's hand.

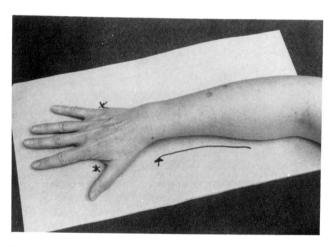

Figure 13.1 Important points of fit are marked onto paper pattern.

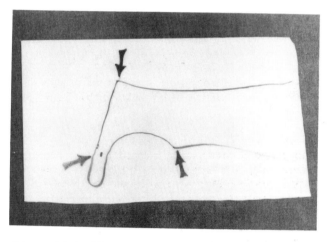

Figure 13.4 The pattern is transferred to the material (Aquaplast).

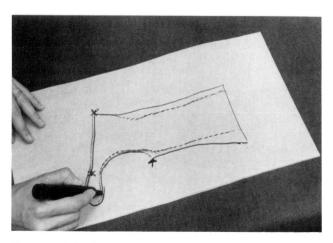

Figure 13.2 The pattern is drawn onto the paper to fit the tracing of the patient's hand.

this chapter and change the size by adding to or trimming away the pattern until it fits without altering the basic shape of the pattern.

If the hand splint is simple, such as a resting pan, an alternate method of sizing the pattern is to trace the outline of the patient's hand onto a flat piece of paper. On this drawing is indicated the location of the patient's joints. Then, the outline of the splint pattern is drawn over the drawing of the hand, meeting the landmarks of the hand as it should. This is a two-dimensional process, and extra length in parts that wrap around must be added to allow not only for the thickness of the material but also for the thickness of the hand. Final sizing is done by cutting the pattern out of paper towelling, dampening it, and smoothing it onto the patient's hand.

Final adjustment of the pattern is done by dampening the paper towel pattern to help it conform to the hand and by carefully checking the fit at every point both with the hand stationary and when the fingers and wrist are gently moved if movement is meant to take place. Extra material is snipped away or tucks made, and lacking material is added until the final pattern is perfected. The thickness of the material to be used must be allowed for in the paper pattern; any part that wraps around must be longer by twice the thickness of the material.

Because of the need to apply correct forces and to make the orthosis comfortable and safe, certain recommendations for fitting hand splints have evolved. These criteria of fit are also used during the check-out process to be described later.

Recommended Criteria of Fit of a Hand Splint

1. Any splint follows the contours of the hand and arm as closely as possible.

2. A wrist splint extends two-thirds the length of the forearm for proper leverage. It does not interfere with elbow motion.

3. A wrist splint holds the wrist in neutral position or in 15 to 30° of dorsiflexion, depending upon the patient's condition and the purpose of the splint.

4. For stability, the width of the forearm piece of wrist splints usually extends from the lateral to the medial midline of the forearm.

5. Bony prominences are kept free from pressure either by not covering them or by pushing out space above them.

6. Except in special circumstances, volar hand splints must allow 90° of metacarpophalangeal flexion and therefore not extend beyond the distal palmar crease.

7. Allowance is made in dorsal hand splints for padding over the metacarpal area because of the need to protect superficial bones and tendons.

8. Because a splint should not unnecessarily restrict motion that the patient has, the ideal length of a short hand splint is that it extend on the dorsum of the hand from the most distal wrist crease to a diagonal line drawn over the dorsum of the hand proximal to the metacarpophalangeal joints and connecting the ends of the volar palmar creases. This length will prevent restriction of motion at the wrist and at the metacarpophalangeal joints.

9. The longitudinal and palmar arches are maintained.

10. The fingers are in a functional position.

11. Finger and thumb pieces are long enough to give adequate support but not so long as to interfere with pinch or cause pressure on opposing fingertips.

12. Tight, narrow, encircling parts and straps are avoided; wide straps distribute the pressure over a greater area.

13. The thumb is in a position of function: abduction and opposition.

14. The splint does not restrict the thenar eminence, which would thereby restrict motion.

15. There is no indication of reddened pressure areas 20 minutes after removal of the hand splint that has been worn for ½ hour.

Selection of Material

Materials commonly used by occupational therapists include plaster of Paris bandage and low, moderate, and high temperature plastics. Each type will be discussed in turn; the advantages and disadvantages of each can be judged by the reader on the basis of the properties of each and the methods required to work with each. This is not a comprehensive list of available materials. The reader is referred to Malick[3, 6] and to rehabilitation supply house catalogues and conference displays for the latest materials as they are developed.

High temperature plastics become soft and can be formed when they are heated in the oven to about 300 to 350°F[3] (149 to 177°C). Because they are so hot when malleable, these plastics must be formed on a mold. These materials are strong and rigid when cooled; therefore, splint designs having more delicate parts can be used. Royalite, Plastazote, and Kydex are examples of this type of material. Royalite comes in a variety of colors. Preformed resting hand and wrist splints made of this material are commercially available. Plastazote is a light-weight, strong, but soft, material that looks foamy but is actually a closed cell material and therefore water-resistant. Plastazote (foamed cross-linked polyethylene) comes in various densities and colors. Kydex is similar to Royalite except that it stays malleable for a longer period when heated and is available in colors of flesh beige to parchment.[6]

Moderate temperature plastics are heated to 170 to 225°F (77 to 107°C) in the oven or in hot water prior to forming.[3] These plastics can be formed directly on a patient if his limb is carefully protected with layers of dry stockinet. This padding decreases the exactness of the fit, however. Bioplastic is an example of this kind of plastic. It is a smooth, pink, rigid material.

Low temperature plastics are heated to 140 to 170°F (60 to 77°C) in hot water before forming directly onto the patient after a momentary pause to allow some air-cooling.[3] They can be reheated and adjusted if an error is made. Orthoplast, Aquaplast, Kay Splint, and Polyform are examples of these plastics. Orthoplast is a white, waxy, smooth or perforated material that is elastic when hot. It fuses to itself when hot, which is desirable when adding pieces but which ruins the splint if it happens accidently. Polyform[6] is a whitish-beige, waxy surfaced material which is self-adhering when hot, rigid when cool, nontoxic, and biodegradable. It has a critical working temperature range of 140 to 167°F; below 140°F it will not soften enough to be workable and above 167°F it will become too pliable, sticky, and stretched out.[5] Kay Splint is similar to Polyform. It is flesh-colored recyclable material. Regular Kay Splint is used for rigidity, and Kay Splint isoprene is used when strength and flexibility are required. Both types come in smooth or perforated sheets. Aquaplast is an off-white material that molds easily—"drapes onto the skin"—when warm. A less pliable version is available, called Green Stripe Aquaplast. Both types are equally rigid when cool.[7] Aquaplast is transparent when warm which allows immediate correction of pressure areas. It fuses to itself and other materials unless they are lubricated or wet and cool. Polyform, Kay Splint, and Aquaplast are more stretchy than Orthoplast, and therefore some therapists prefer them for molding outriggers and other intricate parts or small finger splints. Splints made of low temperature plastics lose their shape if left in hot cars, submerged in hot water, or left near radiators. In time, the cumulative effects of body heat may also loosen the fit.

Plaster of Paris does not require heating to form it, but in the process of curing, heat is generated; therefore, the patient's skin must be protected. Splints are made from plaster of Paris bandage, a gauze material impregnated with plaster of Paris. It requires 2 to 12 hours of drying time. It is not washable as the other materials are unless the splint has been treated by painting it with varnish or enamel. It is comparably very inexpensive, so plaster bandage is often chosen when a splint needs frequent modification. Wires for outriggers and reinforcement are easily added.

Splintmaking Procedures (Figs. 13.5 to 13.14)

After the splint design has been selected, the pattern fitted to the patient, and the material selected to best suit both the purpose of the splint and the skill of the therapist, the procedures listed below for the material selected are followed for the actual construction of the splint.

Royalite (Uniroyal, Inc.) and Kydex (Rohm & Haas). *Marking the Pattern onto the Material.* Any writing instrument may be used. Sharp curves must be notched because Royalite does not stretch and Kydex has only a limited stretch characteristic when heated.

Cutting. A jig saw or band saw may be used.

Reinforcing. This is not necessary because these are very strong and rigid materials.

Finishing Edges. Sand or file the edges using a power sander, sand paper, or a wood file. The edges may also be buffed using a machine buffer.

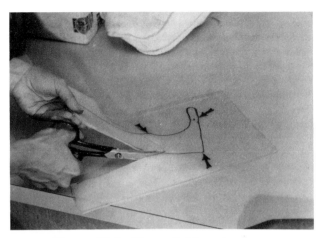

Figure 13.6 The splint is cut out.

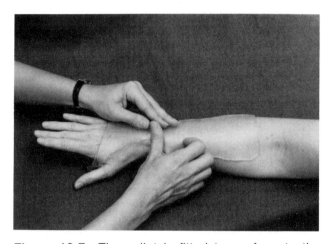

Figure 13.7 The splint is fitted to conform to the contours of the forearm.

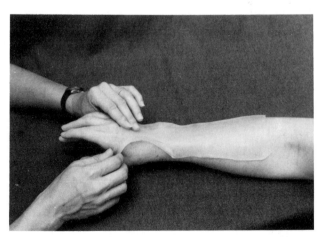

Figure 13.8 The splint is fitted to the contours of the hand.

Adding Straps. Prior to shaping the Royalite or Kydex, holes are drilled for the rivets that will hold the straps on. Straps are made from 1-inch (2.5-cm) wide cotton webbing and fastened with a Velcro clo-

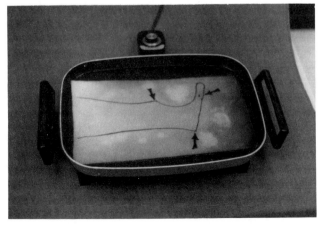

Figure 13.5 Aquaplast is warmed before cutting.

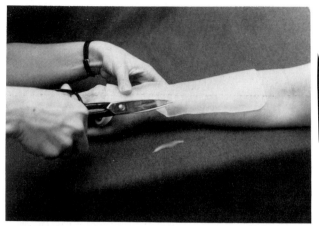

Figure 13.9 Adjustments are made as necessary by snipping off excess material.

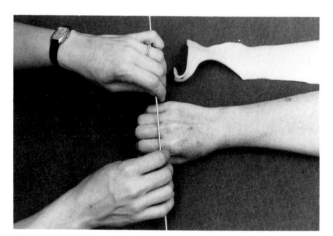

Figure 13.10 The width of the outrigger is measured.

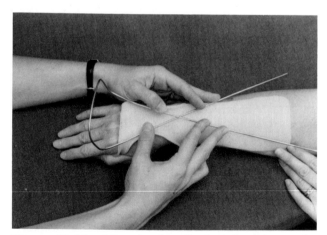

Figure 13.11 After shaping, the length of the outrigger is measured.

sure. A 1- to 2-inch (2.5 to 5 cm) strip of the hook part of the Velcro is glued or riveted to the outside of the splint after the splint is shaped, and a similar sized strip of the soft part of the Velcro is glued and sewn to

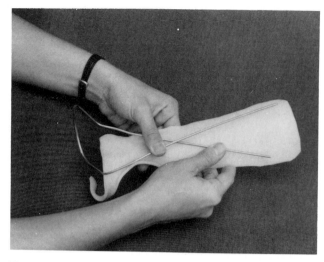

Figure 13.12 After cutting, the fit of the outrigger is rechecked.

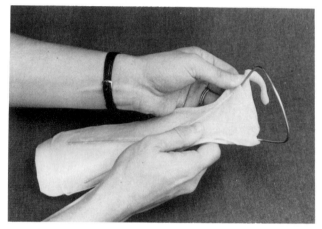

Figure 13.13 The reinforcement piece of Aquaplast is added to hold the outrigger in place.

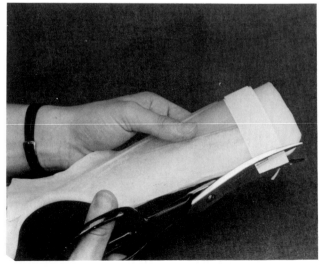

Figure 13.14 Straps are added and trimmed.

the strap. In this way only the soft part comes into contact with the patient's skin. The closure is usually located on the radial side of the splint since it is easier for the patient to fasten. Attach the straps using rivets after the splint is shaped. A rounded anvil may be necessary to use as a striking surface if the strap is added to a curved area: the rivet must be hit so it is smooth on the inside of the splint to prevent irritation to the patient's skin. Straps may also be added using contact cement or self-adhesive Velcro.

Adding Outriggers. Outriggers are extensions added to splints. They are used to suspend rubber bands with finger cuffs attached to them to support or stretch the fingers or thumb into certain positions. The outrigger must be angled in such a way as to allow the rubber band to approach the finger at a 90° angle (see Fig. 13.11). Outriggers of Royalite, Kydex, or aluminum may be added using rivets. The holes for the rivets are drilled prior to shaping.

Shaping. Place the cut-out splint on a flat surface such as a board or a cookie sheet. Heat the Royalite in a 300°F (149°C) oven or the Kydex in a 350°F (177°C) oven for several minutes to soften the material in preparation for shaping; bubbling indicates over-heating. Use potholder mitts while forming the hot material over a wooden or a plaster of Paris mold of the patient's hand. These materials set into shape as they cool, which happens very quickly for Royalite and a little less quickly for Kydex.

Plastazote (Bakelite Xylonite, Ltd.).[8, 9] *Marking the Pattern onto the Material.* Use a pencil to mark the pattern. Plastazote comes in 2- to 30-mm thicknesses. The usual thickness chosen for neck collars and arm splints is 9 mm. This thickness need not be taken into consideration when preparing the paper pattern because the material expands approximately 25 mm/30 cm when heated.

Cutting. A sharp knife or scissors may be used to cut the cold material.

Reinforcing. Two sheets of Plastazote placed one on top of the other in a 140°C (248°F) oven will laminate. A piece of solid low density polyethylene sheeting can be inserted between the layers before fusion for added strength.

Finishing Edges. A very sharp knife is used for trimming; an emery wheel or no. 1 glass paper is used for smoothing. Warm water and detergent wash marks off.

Adding Straps. Rivets or double stick tape are used to attach the straps.

Shaping. A layer of closely fitting stockinet is placed on the patient. The splint is placed on a board covered with the easy release paper provided with the material or dusted with French chalk and put into a 140°C oven (284°F) for a period of time that is twelve times (in seconds) the thickness (in millimeters). It must not be heated above 160°C (320°F). The material cools quickly. The surface temperature is checked before applying it to the patient. Mold it directly on the patient, who has been protected with stockinet, by gently stretching it to fit the contours. Plastazote sets

in the same amount of time it takes to heat it and may be removed from the patient after 2 to 3 minutes. It is cooled thoroughly before finishing.

Bioplastic (Smalley & Bates, Inc.). *Marking the Pattern onto the Material.* A grease crayon marks and erases easily from Bioplastic. This material is brittle and therefore a pattern cannot have notches or small, sharp curves because the material will crack and split at these points.

Cutting. Use a coping or jig saw when the material is cool or scissors when it is hot.

Reinforcing. Although it is not usually necessary to reinforce Bioplastic, aluminum or Bioplastic strips can be riveted to this material.

Finishing Edges. Sand the edges by hand using a fine sandpaper when it is cool or scrape with the blade of scissors when it is warm.

Adding Straps. Self-adhesive Velcro and/or rivets can be used to attach the strap to the splint. The holes for the rivets are drilled most easily before the splint is shaped. Use a hand drill and place the hole in from the edge of the splint to avoid cracking this brittle material. The strap itself is made as described in the directions for Royalite.

Adding Outriggers. Outriggers of aluminum may be added using rivets.

Shaping. To soften the material for shaping, place the cut-out piece of Bioplastic on a flat surface and heat in a 170°F (77°C) oven, or use 170°F water (dry the splint before applying it to the patient, however), or use a heat gun to heat small splints or certain areas of a larger splint. Protect the patient's limb from burns by putting several layers of stockinet on the patient before shaping the splint on him. Hold the entire splint in place until it cools and hardens, which happens quickly.

Orthoplast (Johnson & Johnson). *Marking the Pattern onto the Material.* Use a grease crayon. Ball point pen ink cannot be removed and a pencil will not mark. The pattern must not have slender, delicate parts because such parts will require excessive reinforcement to be strong enough, which will make the splint unacceptably bulky.

Cutting. Scissors are used to cut the material after it is heated for a few moments in hot water. Long strokes are made with the scissors in order to get as smooth an edge as possible.

Reinforcing. Several methods may be used:

1. A strip of Orthoplast can be fused to the as yet unformed splint by heating both pieces and firmly pressing them together at exactly the place where the reinforcement is desired. You cannot separate fused Orthoplast. On the other hand, dirty Orthoplast will not bond.

2. For added strength, an aluminum strip or wire may be embedded between the two pieces of Orthoplast before they are fused.

3. A soda straw may be placed between the two pieces of Orthoplast before they are fused so that the reinforcing Orthoplast piece becomes semitubular and therefore stronger than a flat piece.

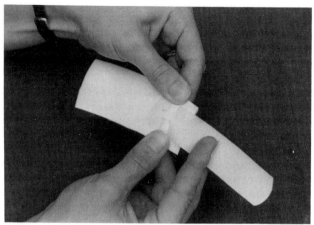

Figure 13.15 Orthoplast strap applied to a scrap piece using self-bonding method.

4. Edges can be "hemmed," that is, folded over to add strength. This method gives a finished look if done very neatly.

Finishing Edges. Soften the Orthoplast edges with a bonding iron and smooth the edges with the iron or with a finger. Folded edges need no further finishing.

Adding Straps. There are several methods by which straps can be added to an Orthoplast splint. One way is to use contact cement to hold the strap and the hook part of Velcro on. Another way is to use a leather punch to punch holes in the splint where rivets will be used to hold on the straps. A third way is unique to Orthoplast and Polyform because of their self-bonding characteristic: the straps are attached using strips or buttons of Orthoplast in the following manner (Fig. 13.15). A narrow (approximately 3-mm or ⅛-inch) strip of Orthoplast is cut one and a half times as long as the strap is wide. For example, if the strap is 1 inch wide, the little Orthoplast strip will be about 1½ inches long. Two large holes are punched in the webbing strap, and it is aligned onto the splint in the desired location. A bonding iron is used to heat a small area adjacent to the edge of the strap, then one end of the little strip of Orthoplast is heated and bonded there next to the strap. In the same manner, the little strip is bonded to the underlying Orthoplast first in one hole of the strap, then in the other, then on the far edge. Self-adhesive Velcro may also be used.

Adding Outriggers. Wire, aluminum, or Royalite outriggers can be added to Orthoplast by embedding the ends between layers of Orthoplast and fusing them there. This must be done before the splint is actually shaped. The outrigger may be also riveted for strength. Very short outriggers can be made of doubled Orthoplast fused together and can be attached by fusion. Orthoplast is too weak to be used for longer outriggers. If the splint is already formed, the small Orthoplast outrigger may be attached by spot heating the splint at the desired location and fusing the hot outrigger to it, or the outrigger can be added using rivets.

Shaping. Heat the Orthoplast in 140 to 170°F (60 to 77°C) water. Remove the Orthoplast from the hot water by using tongs. Dry it or expose it to the air momentarily to cool it to a reasonable temperature before forming it directly on the patient. Smooth and hold the entire splint until it cools and hardens, which may be speeded up by immersing the splinted hand in cool water or ice water. Immersion in ice water produces physiological effects in a person; therefore if the splint is to be cooled using ice water, remove it gently from the patient after a few moments when it has begun to firm up, then put it in the ice water. A large splint should be loosely wrapped in ace bandage or should have a piece of close-fitting stockinet placed over it to help hold it in proper contour during the cooling and hardening process. Orthoplast is very elastic and molds very well in convex and concave curves if repeatedly smoothed over curved areas.

Polyform (Rolyan Medical Products, Inc.)[5] and KaySplint. *Marking the Pattern onto the Material.* A pen or scratch awl may be used on cold Polyform. A fingernail will mark soft Polyform.

Cutting. Scissors are used to cut the material after it has been warmed for 20 to 25 seconds in water that is 150 to 160°F (66 to 71°C). Care must be taken to prevent this highly self-adhering material from fusing during the cutting process. Rose pruners or a saw can be used to cut unheated Polyform.

Reinforcing. Press together two dry pieces of properly heated Polyform and they will fuse. Aluminum or wire strips may be added between the fused layers for added support, although this may be rarely necessary due to the rigidity of the cooled material. The edges can be "hemmed" or rolled over for reinforcement and for a finished look.

Finishing Edges. Heated edges can be smoothed with the finger, the edges can be rolled, or cold Polyform can be filed, sanded or buffed.

Adding Straps. This can be done in the same ways as described for Orthoplast.

Adding Outriggers. Aluminum outriggers can be added by riveting them or embedding them between layers of Polyform from which the clear coating is scraped off and which are then fused together. Outriggers made of doubled over and fused Polyform are probably rigid enough to be used to support weak digits. The Polyform outrigger adheres to a Polyform splint best if both it and the part to which it is being attached are dry and hot. Polyform will not stick to Orthoplast, polyethylene, polypropylene, wax paper, human skin, or hair.

Shaping. The best method for softening Polyform for shaping is to use heated water. The recommended temperature range for ⅛-inch Polyform is 150 to 160°F (66 to 71°C). Do not lay it on the bottom of a pan because if it overheats, it will stick. A heat gun can be used to heat small areas. Overheating causes the material to become sticky. If this should happen, lay it on a flat surface to cool slightly. The material can be formed directly on the patient. It stretches and follows concave and convex contours easily. This property makes it a useful material to use to make adapted handles on utensils or tools. Scrap pieces can be used for this purpose.

Aquaplast (WFR Corp.).[2, 7] Use regular for small splints and Green Stripe for large ones. The therapist's hands must be wet at all times when working on warm Aquaplast.

Marking the Pattern onto the Material. The wet pattern is simply placed under the transparent material, and the splint is cut out according to the pattern. Or, a grease pencil can be used to trace the pattern onto the material.

Cutting. The splint design can be cut using long-bladed shears when the material is warm, but hazy and no longer sticky. A piece the size of the splint should be cut from the stock when the material is cold by using a razor-blade knife to score the material and then breaking off the piece. A band saw or heavy shears can also be used when the material is cold.

Reinforcing. Regular Aquaplast can be used for reinforcement. Heat the reinforcement in water until it is transparent; spot heat the splint where the attachment is to be made; apply the reinforcement piece and feather the edges with a wet finger. A bond will not occur if there is grease on the material.

Finishing Edges. Use a potato peeler or leather edger to bevel the edges. Then, dip the edge into hot water and polish it with the heel of the hand. Quench in cold water to set the new, smooth edge. Edges can also be hemmed over within the 1st minute after being removed from the hot water.

Adding Straps. To attach a patch of hook Velcro spot heat the splint where the patch is to be applied, while at the same time softening a thin strip of Aquaplast. Place the patch over the heated spot, wet your fingers, and stretch the thin strip around the patch, overlapping the edge all around, and press it down firmly. To attach a strap, cut notches on both edges of the strap near the end to be attached to the splint. Spot heat the splint where the strap is to go, while warming a patch of Aquaplast of a size large enough to cover the end of the strap. With a wet finger, press the soft patch around the end of the strap and into the notches to bond the strap to the splint. Self-adhesive Velcro can also be used.

Adding Outriggers. Outriggers are attached in the same manner that reinforcements are. Both surfaces must be hot; dry heat forms the most secure bonds. Rivets may also be used.

Shaping. Heat in 140°F (60°C) water just until the material becomes transparent. An Aquaplast Frypan Guard *must* be used to prevent the Aquaplast from sticking to the pan when hot. When soft, lift the Aquaplast out of the hot water on the Frypan Guard mesh. Place it, mesh side down, on a terry towel. Wet your hands to handle the material. The patient's arm must also be wet with water and then the slightly cooled (about 30 seconds) Aquaplast can be molded directly. Mold into and around concave and convex surfaces. It will cling to the limb when stretched.

Aquaplast shrinks 2% as it cools and will become too tight around bony prominences unless spread slightly as it cools. As Aquaplast cools, the splint will lift from the skin, signifying it is rigid enough to remove without deforming.

Hinges. Hinges can be formed between two pieces of Aquaplast (or other splinting material) using rivets by making the holes slightly larger than the rivet post. The rivet is hammered until it is secure, but not tight, and the pieces may still move freely.

Plaster of Paris Bandage. To make a slab-type splint from plaster of Paris bandage, cut strips equal to the length of the pattern. Enough strips are cut to make 8 to 10 layers. The number of layers needed depends upon the amount of support required. The pattern is drawn on the bandage using a pencil and may be cut out with large scissors. Any outriggers or straps should then be made because they will be embedded in the plaster as the splint is formed. Outriggers can be made from coat hangers or from brass welding rod that will not rust. The part of the outrigger which will be embedded in the splint must conform to the shape of the part to be splinted. If the outrigger rod is round rather than flat, the part to be embedded should be flattened or serpentined so that it will not rotate between the layers of plaster bandage.

Allowing extra length, place a close-fitting tubular stockinet bandage over the part of the patient's limb to be splinted. Then dip half of the plaster layers in lukewarm water one at a time; cooler water slows down setting time and warmer water speeds up setting time. Gently squeeze out the bandage until it just stops dripping; more water slows down setting time and less water speeds up setting time. Next, place the bandage over the part to be splinted, for example, the anterior wrist, palm, and forearm when making a cock-up splint, making sure the pattern of the strip conforms as it should. Smooth it with the fingers to spread the plaster particles into the gauze bandage. Apply several layers in this manner.

The stockinet should be trimmed to within ½ to ¾ of an inch from the edge of the plaster and folded up onto the plaster bandage to form a "hem." Wetting the stockinet will hold it to the plaster as it is turned up. If outriggers or reinforcing aluminum strips are to be added to the basic splint, these should now be added by attaching the outrigger with small strips of wet plaster bandage which are looped over the metal rod and pressed onto the plaster; small squares of plaster bandage also help reinforce and secure the outrigger. Next, lay the straps across the splint at the proper locations. Now wet, squeeze, and smooth the remaining plaster layers and place them on the splint to cover the stockinet edges, outriggers, and straps. Additional plaster strips should be placed near strap edges and to cover any edges which are uneven. Sprinkle talcum powder and rub it into the splint surface to obtain a smooth, shiny surface.

Note. The curing process of plaster produces heat and causes slight shrinking. If the patient is sensitive to heat, several layers of stockinet must be used. The splint may be carefully removed from the patient for the curing and drying process as soon as the shape has been set.

Making a Mold of Patient's Hand. In order to make a mold that can be used to form a splint made of the high temperature materials, it is necessary to make a negative mold first, then a positive mold. The process of making a palmar mold of the hand and forearm will be described. This type of mold can be used to form a resting pan, wrist cock-up, or other volar splints which do not have circumferential parts. The same process may be used to make a dorsal mold, of course. The process for making a mold of the entire hand or forearm, that is, one that encircles these parts, is complicated and will not be included here. The reader is referred to Malick.[3, 6]

Negative Plaster of Paris Palmar Mold.[3] Cut three or four pieces of plaster of Paris bandage long enough to extend from the patient's fingertips to approximately 1 inch (2.5 cm) below the elbow. Cut a 4- to 5-inch (10 to 12.5-cm) slit in the end of each piece of the bandage approximately 1½ inches (3.7 cm) from the side edge of the bandage; this will allow the thumb to be positioned in abduction. Apply mineral oil or petroleum jelly to the entire area to be covered by the plaster bandage. Loosely roll up the first piece of plaster bandage and dip it into a bowl of lukewarm water. Holding the rolled bandage by two ends, gently squeeze excess water out but do not wring it so hard that much of the plaster is squeezed out. Unroll the bandage strip, place it over the forearm and hand of the patient, and smooth it carefully to eliminate wrinkles and to work the plaster into the bandage. The patient's limb must be held in a functional position while this mold is being made.

Repeat with the remaining pieces of bandage, making certain to smooth each carefully so that the layers of bandage will adhere to each other.

The limb is held in the functional position until the plaster hardens. Fast-setting plaster bandage sets in about 5 minutes.

Mark vertical lines on each side of the cast using a ruler and indelible pencil and indicate the width that the cast edges should be separated at these points; these lines and measurements are used to realign the cast should it become distorted in the process of removing it from the patient or pouring the positive mold.

Slide the patient's hand out of the mold. Realign the mold according to the markings and maintain this position by using narrow strips of plaster bandage to bridge the open side of the mold.

Negative Mold from Alginate Dental Impression Material.[11] When exact fit over contoured areas is important, this method may be preferred to use of plaster bandage described above.

Apply petroleum jelly over the entire area to be molded. The Alginate (Jeltrate) is prepared in a flexible bowl using cold water by quickly spatulating the mixture against the side of the bowl to eliminate bubbles. It is poured over the part to be molded. It would be helpful to place the hand and arm in a plastic dishpan that has one end cut out to accommodate the arm that must be held flat in position. The excess material could then be easily discarded. After the Alginate sets, reinforce it with at least four layers of plaster bandage which are smoothed into the impression contours. After the plaster bandage begins to set, the patient moves or contracts the muscles to help break the vacuum to remove the mold. The ends are covered with plaster bandage to form a "bowl" shape to receive the plaster of Paris that will be used to make the positive mold.

Positive Mold. Place strips of plaster bandage over the finger, thumb, and elbow edges of the negative mold to make the mold a container which will hold the plaster when poured. Use a brush to coat the inside of the negative mold with a substance such as liquid green soap which will allow the positive mold to be separated from the negative mold.

Mix plaster of Paris in a flexible bowl or in a waxed milk carton by placing about 2 cups of water into the bowl and slowly adding and mixing plaster until it is of the consistency of cake batter.

Pour the plaster into the negative mold, gently shaking and tapping the negative mold to eliminate air bubbles. Add more plaster to fill the mold and tap again. Insert a metal rod lengthwise into the thumb section to reinforce it and a larger rod or dowel into the length of the whole mold. These rods protrude from the mold and allow it to be held securely in a vise when later using the positive mold for shaping the high temperature plastics.

Allow the plaster to set. *Do not pour excess plaster into a sink drain; it will harden there.* After it has set up in the bowl, which will be the clue also that the mold is ready for the next step, get it out of the bowl by flexing the sides of the bowl and dispose of it in the trash.

Gently remove the positive mold from the negative one by removing the narrow strips of bandage that were used to bridge the width of the negative mold and by spreading the sides of the negative mold as you extract the positive. Be careful not to damage the more delicate thumb part.

Smooth any ridges by using a file, sandpaper, or a piece of wire mesh screening. After the plaster has dried for about ½ hour, sand it smooth. Allow to dry overnight before using it.

CHECK-OUT OF THE SPLINT

It is the responsibility of the occupational therapist to check out the fit of any upper extremity orthosis or any splint which he or she has made. The check-out is the process of examining the fit, function, and reliability of the orthosis. The check-out is done prior to establishing a wearing schedule and prior to either controls or use training. Periodic recheck of the orthosis may be necessary for those patients who wear the orthosis on a permanent or long-term basis.

Table 13.1
CHECK-OUT FOR HAND SPLINTS

		General Considerations
Yes	No	Is the splint on the patient correctly?
Yes	No	Does this splint needlessly immobilize a joint?
Yes	No	If the splint, or parts of it, immobilizes a joint, is the splint removed periodically and the joints moved through passive range of motion?
Yes	No	Does this splint actually accomplish the function for which it was intended?
Yes	No	Does this splint cover the least amount of skin area to permit tactile sensation, but also provide good distribution of force over sufficiently large areas?
Yes	No	After wearing the splint for ½ hour does the patient have reddened areas?
Yes	No	Do these disappear within 15 to 20 minutes?
Yes	No	Is the splint cosmetically acceptable to the patient?
Yes	No	*Traction Splints* If elastics are used, do they pull perpendicularly to the part as they should?
Yes	No	Is the tension in the elastics exactly right (just enough to provide a small force beyond that needed to pull the part to the limit of range of motion)?
Yes	No	If this is a static traction splint, is the force just enough to push slightly beyond the limit of range of motion?
Yes	No	Is the traction force distributed over as large an area as possible?
Yes	No	Is the force adjusted periodically to keep up with the changes in the patient's limits of range of motion?
Yes	No	Has a wearing schedule been established?
Yes	No	*Externally Powered Hand Splints* Is the splint mechanism reliable? If not, what seems to be the problem?
Yes	No	Is the control located at a site over which the patient has voluntary control, has sensation, and which does not trigger the control accidentally during habitual movements?
Yes	No	Does the control work reliably, i.e., the same signal repeatedly causes same response?
Yes	No	Can the patient operate the controls with the splint held in any position?
Yes	No	Can the patient put it on by himself or clearly instruct another in its application?
Yes	No	Is the power source ready for use? When does it get refilled or recharged _____ By whom? ____How? _____
Yes	No	Does the splint prevent the patient from doing any functional activity he can otherwise do? What? _____Why? _____
Yes Yes Yes Yes Yes Yes	No No No No No No	Can the patient pick up correctly: Squashable things (paper cup, marshmallow, cotton, etc.) Glass or metal objects Thin things (cards, paper, checkers) Small things (pencil, dice) Eating utensils Large things (beer can, cup, razor)
		As an indication of the patient's level of learning to control the orthosis, what is the reaction time? It can be figured in the following manner: 1. Find the average time, in tenths of seconds, of 20 trials of picking up and releasing a 1-inch cube on command. The cube is placed at same place each time; the patient starts from same position each time; and cube is released into a small box which is consistently positioned. 2. Consistency of reaction time can be measured figuring the standard deviation. The lower the deviation, the more consistent the performance and therefore an indication of learning. A formula for standard deviation is: $$SD = \sqrt{\frac{\sum x^2}{N - 1}}$$ Where $\sum$ = sum, x = difference between each score and the mean, and N = number of trials.

chapter

14

Wheelchair Measurement and Prescription

Anna Deane Scott, M.Ed., OTR

It is essential that a wheelchair be correctly prescribed to meet the needs of the patient. It must be the type that offers the support required, is the correct size for comfort and prevention of decubiti, and has the features and accessories needed for safety and maximal independence.

TYPE

Electric Wheelchair

An electric wheelchair is selected for high level quadriplegic individuals and for others who are unable to propel a standard wheelchair or would use excessive energy. Some models are small and maneuverable with a molded or cushioned seat and a center bar control stick.[1] Others are similar to a standard wheelchair with a power drive control box located in the left or right side near the arm rest (Fig. 14.1). A stick on top of the box is held and pushed in the direction the patient wishes the chair to move. The speed can be proportional to adjust speed in relation to the pressure applied to the stick with a solid state control or preselected by a microswitch control to preset the speed if the user would have difficulty controlling a proportional speed.[2] For persons unable to use a hand or finger control, a power-driven chair can be operated with mouth (puff and sip controls), foot, chin, or other control.[3] The choice depends on remaining function— for example, vital capacity and control of mouth for puff and sip or head control for chin use.

Standard Wheelchair (Fig. 14.2)

A standard wheelchair is selected if a person is able to propel the wheelchair independently. There are

three frame types to consider when selecting a standard wheelchair. The outdoor frame which has the large wheels in the back with front casters is the most frequently appropriate. The outdoor frame is the most maneuverable, easiest to propel, and allows the tilt needed for curbs.[4] An amputee frame is designed for the lower extremity amputee; the rear axle is offset

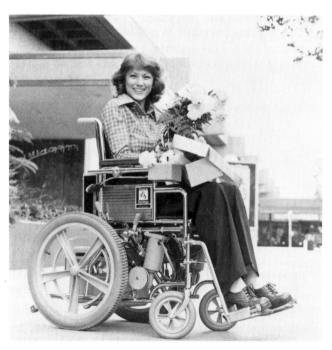

Figure 14.1 Electric wheelchair. (Reproduced with permission from Everest & Jennings, Inc., Los Angeles, California.)

behind the large rear wheels. This design accommodates to the fact that the person's weight is distributed further back in the wheelchair and prevents the chair from tipping over backwards. The amputee frame can be ordered with or without footrests, depending on whether or not artificial limbs are worn.[5] An indoor frame is least often selected; it has the large wheels in the front with back casters. Occasionally people prefer or need this chair for indoor use if reaching rear wheels is difficult due to limited range of motion. It rolls over door sills and rug edges more easily but is impractical for curbs and restricts access for transfers.[2, 4]

Frame construction is selected to suit the expected activity level of the user. Heavy duty construction is for rugged use by heavy or overweight people. A lightweight chair is half the weight of a standard chair and requires less energy to propel or to lift in and out of a car; it is for moderately active people. An active duty lightweight chair combines heavy duty bracing and durability with lightweight metals to provide a chair for very active people when rugged use and maneuverability are both desirable.[2, 4] There are also frame constructions for special uses. The sportsman model has a lower back and safety features for active use in competitive sports.[2] An outdoor frame in standard or lightweight construction is available with a lower seat height for the hemiplegic patient who uses one leg to assist in propeling the wheelchair.[4] A one-arm drive chair has both handrims on the same side so that the two wheels can be controlled simultaneously or individually by a person who operates the chair with one arm.[2]

Postural Supports

For patients who cannot assume an upright posture in a wheelchair or who need the back reclined at times to change position, a semireclining or fully reclining back with an extension for head support may be needed.[4]

There are inserts and attachments for wheelchairs as well as chairs of unique design available for special problems. Postura is a support system with components that provide additional adjustments and postural supports for persons with severe disabilities and is especially useful for many patients in nursing homes. The modular supports include a headrest, lateral trunk supports, side cushions, an abduction wedge (a triangular cushion to keep the knees separated), a leg rest cradle for full support of both legs, an adjustable depth seat, and an inclinable seat that shifts weight toward the back of the seat. When postural supports are required wheelchairs with semireclining or fully reclining backs are most often selected, although the components can also be used on a wheelchair with a fixed back and detachable arms.[6]

SIZE

The wheelchair size is determined by measuring the patient and then selecting a wheelchair that will fit. The patient is seated in a wheelchair, in a straight

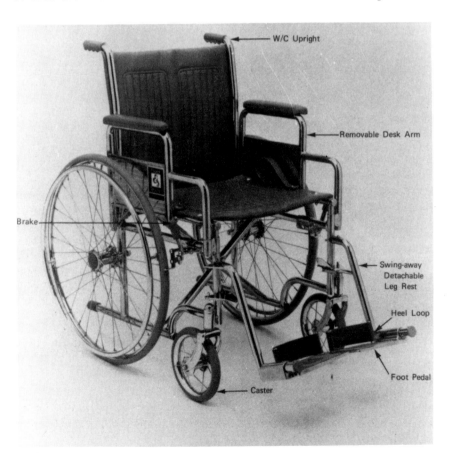

Figure 14.2 Standard wheelchair. (Reproduced with permission from Everest & Jennings, Inc., Los Angeles, California.)

back chair, or on the edge of a raised mat, and measurements are taken using a tape measure.

Seat Width

This measurement is taken across the hips or thighs at the widest part and should include the width of braces if worn. Then 5 cm (2 inches) are added to allow for a 2.5 cm (1 inch) clearance on each side. This width will prevent rubbing against the side panels and allow for ease of transfers, while keeping the chair as narrow as possible for ease of propulsion and accessibility through doorways.

Seat Depth

This measurement is taken from behind the buttocks along the thigh to the bend behind the knee. Then 5 cm to 7.5 cm (2 to 3 inches) are subtracted to avoid having the seat upholstery press into the popliteal area while still having enough depth to support the thighs and distribute the weight.

Seat Height

Leg length is measured from under the distal thigh to the heel of the shoe. The seat height needed is determined by adding 5 cm (2 inches) to the leg length measurement. This will allow a 5-cm (2 inch) clearance from the footrests to the floor so the footrests will clear thresholds, inclines, and uneven surfaces. If a seat cushion is to be used it will raise the height of the seat. A cushion is often used, and for many people it is all that is needed to raise the seat height enough for the footrests to be adjusted for adequate clearance. Special seat heights are available for unusually tall individuals. In addition to having a 5-cm (2 inch) minimal floor clearance the footrests should be adjusted so that the patient's distal thigh is approximately 2.5 cm (1 inch) above the front of the seat upholstery or cushion to avoid pressure under the distal thigh. It is important that the footrests be no higher than necessary to achieve this distal thigh clearance or the patient's weight will be unevenly distributed in the chair, causing more pressure to be placed over the ischial tuberosities, a prime site of decubiti.

Arm Rest Height

Arm height is measured from the seat to the elbow which is flexed to 90°. Then 2.5 cm (1 inch) is added to determine the height of the arm rest. This height supports the arms comfortably without encouraging slouching if too low or elevation of the scapulae if too high. Use of a seat cushion would also affect this measurement.

Back Height

Measurement is taken from the seat to the axilla. Then 10 cm (4 inches) are subtracted from this measurement to determine the height of the back upholstery. The current trend is to lower the back height to increase arm freedom and functional capabilities when trunk strength is sufficient to permit reduced back support.

These measurements are then compared to the sizes of standard models designed to meet the needs of the majority of people, and a wheelchair of the correct size for the individual patient is selected (Table 14.1). If custom modifications are required for any dimension these can be specified but are expensive.

FEATURES AND ACCESSORIES[2, 4, 5]

Many features and accessories can be selected for a standard wheelchair according to the needs of the patient. Consideration should be given to the choice of types of casters, arm styles, footrests or leg rests, and accessories for safety or special needs.

Casters

Casters are the small wheels located in front on the outdoor frame wheelchair; there is a choice of 5-inch or 8-inch diameter. Casters that are 8 inches in diameter are most frequently selected because they are stable and roll more easily over a variety of surfaces. Caster locks are available for the 8-inch casters to prevent rotation of the casters during transfers. Casters which are set forward are available for increased stability. Rubber bumpers can be ordered to cover the axle of the 8-inch casters for ankle protection if one or both legs are used to propel the chair.

Arm Rests

Wheelchair arms may be fixed as a permanent part of the chair or detachable, so that the arms may be removed for transfers. The wheelchair with fixed arms is lighter and narrower than the detachable arm wheelchair but requires front transfers from the chair. An offset fixed arm is constructed so that the arm comes up just beside the seat frame rather than straight up from the seat edge and consequently adds 4.4 cm (1¾ inches) to the seat width without adding to the width of the wheelchair, thus keeping it narrow. Detachable arms are necessary for depression or sliding board transfers. They add 3.75 cm (1½ inches) to the width of the wheelchair. Wrap-around detachable arms are constructed to avoid adding to the width of the wheelchair, but the ability to exchange or reverse the arms is sacrificed. A desk arm style is available in the offset fixed or detachable arms; the arm is low in front with a smaller padded area at the back for an arm rest. The cutout allows the wheelchair to be rolled under the edge of a table or desk to enable the person to move closer to these surfaces. Locks for the detachable arm rests prevent them from being inadvertently detached when used for leverage by the patient who may pull on the arm rest to assist in changing position or when the wheelchair is lifted in and out of the car. An adjustable height feature is available in all detachable arm styles. This is particularly useful when a variety of cushions may be used or for severe disabilities when the height of the arms may need to be adjusted as trunk stability changes.

Table 14.1
STANDARD DIMENSIONS[a]

Standard Dimensions[b]	Seat Width (inches)	Seat Depth (inches)	Seat Height (inches)	Arm Height (inches)	Back Height (inches)
Adult Designed for full grown adults of average size and build.	18 (45.72 cm)	16 (40.64 cm)	20 (50.80 cm)	10 (25.40 cm)	16½ (41.91 cm)
Narrow Adult For relatively slender full grown adults. Combines dimensions of both Adult and Junior models.	16 (40.64 cm)	16 (40.64 cm)	20 (50.80 cm)	10 (25.40 cm)	16½ (41.91 cm)
Slim Adult Designed for the thin tall adult or youth.	14 (35.56 cm)	16 (40.64 cm)	20 (50.80 cm)	10 (25.40 cm)	16½ (41.91 cm)
Junior[c] For full grown adults with smaller than average body size.	16 (40.64 cm)	16 (40.64 cm)	18½ (46.99 cm)	10 (25.40 cm)	16½ (41.91 cm)
Low Seat For shorter persons who desire a lower seat height or for persons who propel chair with foot.	18 (45.72 cm)	16 (40.64 cm)	17½ (44.45 cm)	10 (25.40 cm)	16½ (41.91 cm)
Kid or 13-inch Junior[c] Designed for children between 9 and 12 years of age.	16 (40.64 cm)	13 (33.02 cm)	18½ (46.99 cm)	8½ (21.59 cm)	16 (40.64 cm)
Growing Chair[c] For children between 6 and 8. A 13-inch Junior model with special features. Upholstery and footrest can be changed as the child grows so chair will serve for several years.	14 (35.56 cm)	11½ (29.21 cm)	20 (50.80 cm)	6½ (16.51 cm)	14½ (36.83 cm)
Child's Chair	14 (35.56 cm)	11½ (29.21 cm)	18¾ (47.62 cm)	8½ (21.59 cm)	16½ (41.91 cm)
Tiny Tot-Hi	12	11½	19½	6	17½
Tiny Tot-Lo For children from 4 to 6 years of age. Scaled to size, the "Hi" and "Lo" feature determines the seat height most functional for either attendant or patient.	12 (30.48 cm) (30.48 cm)	11½ (29.21 cm) (29.21 cm)	17 (49.53 cm) (43.18 cm)	6 (15.24 cm) (15.24 cm)	17½ (44.45 cm) (44.45 cm)
Pre-School Pediatric Designed for children 2 to 4 years of age.	10 (25.40 cm)	8 (20.32 cm)	19½ (49.53 cm)	5 (12.70 cm)	15 (38.10 cm)

[a] Reproduced with permission from *Measuring the Patient.* Los Angeles, Calif.: Everest & Jennings, Inc., 1979.
[b] *Note:* Heavy duty chairs of extra width are available up to 24 inches (60 cm) and will still fold. Caution should be taken to investigate seat height for this type of chair.
[c] Dimensions are for detachable arm chairs. Refer to Catalog for complete dimensions.

Footrests

Footrests may be nondetachable or detachable. Swinging detachable footrests permit closer access to the bed, toilet, or other surfaces. Detachable footrests are essential for a forward transfer into the tub or for other transfers where a side approach is not possible and the footrest would prevent getting close to the transfer surface. Elevating legrests are needed if the chair is a reclining one or if the patient's disability requires elevation of one or both legs. The legrest has a padded support for the leg in addition to the foot plate so that the leg is supported when the height of elevation is adjusted. Elevating leg rests may be ordered nonremovable or they may be swinging detachable if approach to surfaces, transfers, or ease of fitting the chair into a car are important.

Tire Types

Wheels and casters are available in solid, semipneumatic, or pneumatic. Pneumatic tires are air-filled similar to a bicycle tire; they give a cushioned ride for outdoor use over rough ground. Pneumatic tires, however, make the wheelchair difficult to push and they are subject to flat tires. Semipneumatic tires also soften the ride and increase the difficulty of chair propulsion, but the tires are not inflated and will not go flat. If the wheelchair is primarily used indoors or on paved surfaces solid tires are adequate.

Footplates

Footplates are standard on all wheelchairs, but additional features or accessories may be selected. Size variations are available to extend the width of the pedal forward or backward. Plastic coated footplates, heel loops, or metal heel rests are ordered if the person's feet have a tendency to slide off of the pedals. Toe loops or ankle straps may be needed for patients with excessive clonus, spasms, or involuntary movements in order to keep their feet on the pedals. Pop-up footplates have a spring action that offers an assist to tipping up the pedals. Footplates can be ordered with an angle adjustment for providing foot support when the angle of the ankle is a problem. Several styles of heel straps or a leg rest panel may be attached across the footrest uprights behind both heels or calves to assist in keeping the legs in position on the footrests.

Specialized Accessories

Other accessories may be needed for safety, convenience, or special needs. A *Grade-Aid* is an accessory that attaches under the brake for use going up inclines. It releases when the chair is pushed forward and stops against the wheel between pushes to prevent the wheelchair from losing ground by rolling backwards as the patient propels the wheelchair forward up a ramp or incline. The *Grade-Aid* is disengaged when the chair is on a level or downhill surface. *Brake lever extensions* permit locking and unlocking the brakes when the patient cannot reach down to the standard sized levers. For weak patients the increased lever arm length reduces the force required. An extension for the brake on the involved side is often ordered for a hemiplegic patient for ease in reaching the opposite brake with the noninvolved hand. If tipping the wheelchair forward is a likely hazard a *forward stabilizer* can be attached in front of the caster to stop against the floor if the chair tips forward. Also *antitipping devices* can be attached to the projections at the rear of the wheelchair frame to extend them and angle them toward the floor to prevent the wheelchair from tipping backwards. A *cane or crutch holder* is available for the back of the wheelchair so that canes or crutches may be carried conveniently when using the chair. A *"Quad" release* ("Lever-Ease" or "Cam Ease") for swinging detachable footrests or leg rests has an easier release mechanism than the standard and is for quadriplegic patients or others with limited hand use. *Reduce-a-Width* is a crank handled device that attaches to one side of the wheelchair arm and seat; the handle can be turned to reduce the wheel-

chair width temporarily for passage through a narrow doorway. Special *handrims* may be needed by a patient with weak or absent grasp. Friction to assist weak grasp is provided by plastic coated handrims or rubber handrim covers. If grasp is very weak or absent the wheelchair can be propelled by pushing the palms against projections on the handrims; these include knobs spaced around the rim or rubber-tipped projections extending vertically or obliquely from the handrim. Choice of the type of projections should take into consideration the fact that some projections add up to 10 cm (4 inches) to the wheelchair width. A *seat belt* is advisable for patients with excessive involuntary movement, severe spasms, or any problem that would make falling out of the wheelchair a possible hazard during functional activities or if the chair stopped suddenly. Items available for special posture or positioning needs are a *solid seat*, a *solid* or *padded back*, and a *body positioner* for lateral trunk support. A *zippered* or *detachable back* is available when a transfer in and out of the back of the wheelchair is required. A *carrying pocket* fits across the back of the wheelchair and is useful for books or other items. *Antifolding devices* are available for theft prevention; they prevent the wheelchair from folding and thus make it difficult to transport the chair.

SEAT CUSHIONS

A seat cushion may be ordered for comfort and is necessary for patients with loss or impairment of sensation to assist in prevention of decubiti. Many cushions are available, and all types relieve some pressure on the ischial tuberosities and distribute pressure on the buttocks and posterior thighs. Seat cushions currently available are: (a) gel cushions which are filled with a substance that shifts to conform to the seat contour and thereby distributes pressure more evenly; (b) air or water-filled cushions that offer a surface that can shift to vary the support; (c) latex foam rubber cushions that absorb some pressure and are of a thickness and density that will not compress fully under the weight of the patient; (d) alternating pressure pads which have channels that fill with air and a compressor to shift the air in and out of the channels alternately to relieve and redistribute pressure.

Several effectiveness studies have been conducted to compare various types of cushions. Decubiti are a result of pressure which reduces blood flow to a skin area and thus causes necrosis of tissue in that area with subsequent ulceration. Souther et al.[9] used a surface pressure manometer to compare ishial tuberosity pressure of subjects using 11 different cushions, including all types of commercially available cushions except the alternating pressure pad. Cushions with a mean pressure that was significantly less than the pressure obtained when sitting in a wheelchair with no cushion were the following: the Jobst Hydro-Float cushion ($p < 0.01$), the Jobst Hydro-Float pad ($p < 0.01$), the Bye-Bye Decubiti ($p < 0.05$), and the

2-inch latex foam rubber pad ($p < 0.05$). All cushions were helpful in reducing pressure, but none reduced mean pressure to less than capillary pressure (32 mm Hg.). Therefore, use of a seat cushion is helpful, but must be accompanied by changing position and proper skin care. DeLateur et al.[10] studied the effects of seven different cushions on hyperemia of the skin by measuring the duration of the skin redness of paralyzed patients after they sat for 30 minutes on each of the cushions. There was no significant difference found among the cushions, and some hyperemia was found using all types of cushions. This study lent further support to the need for regular position change or push-ups several times an hour as a supplement to the use of a wheelchair cushion. The Jobst Hydro-Float Cushion was found to vary in performance and "bottomed out"; the correct amount of water in the cushion was the performance variable. Footrest height was important to cushion effectiveness in both of these studies; footrests needed to be adjusted to distribute pressure evenly along the thighs and buttocks. Fisher et al.[11] studied the effect of various wheelchair cushions on skin temperature because an increase in temperature is a secondary factor contributing to tissue breakdown. Five cushions including foam rubber, gel, and the Jobst water flotation cushion were studied with normal subjects sitting for 30 minutes on each cushion. Surface temperature thermistors were taped under the ischial tuberosities and posterior thighs; graphic recordings and a printout of temperature readings were obtained. Skin temperatures decreased significantly on the water flotation cushion, remained the same on the gel cushions, and increased significantly on the foam rubber cushions. Fisher and Kosiak[12] studied the effectiveness of the ROHO cushion, a newer cushion not included in the previous studies. The ROHO cushion is lightweight, washable, and comfortably stable, but no significant difference in resting pressure or temperature change was found between the ROHO cushion and a 4-inch foam rubber cushion. Ma et al.[13] found that a cutout board placed under a 2 or 3-inch foam rubber or T-foam cushion reduced pressure over the ischial tuberosities significantly more than use of a foam cushion alone, although not below capillary pressure. The board is ⅝ inch plywood with a posterior cutout made to fit individual measurements. The ischial tuberosities must be cleared but without extra width so that weight can be distributed over a broad area of the buttocks and thighs. The cutout area and the anterior edge should be rounded; the posterior corners are notched to fit the back uprights of the wheelchair (Fig. 14.3). Measurements are taken with the patient lying prone on a firm, padded table. The height from the surface to the coccyx is measured between the legs, and 4 inches are added to determine the depth of the cutout. The lateral edges of the ischial tuberosities are found by palpation, and 2 inches are added to determine the width of the cutout. Seat depth and width are measured to determine the overall size of the board. Garber et al.[14] used a Pressure Evaluation Pad with transducers that reg-

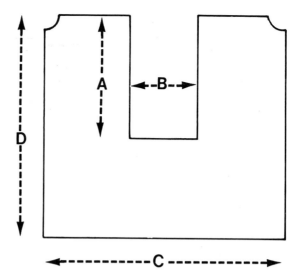

Figure 14.3 Cutout board to be placed under a foam cushion. See text for procedures to derive measurements for A, B, C, and D. (Reproduced with permission from D. M. Ma.[13])

istered pressure which was displayed in a corresponding grid pattern on a lighted panel. Six cushions were evaluated with spinal cord-injured patients. The ROHO cushion and the Scimedics foam cushion with a "U"-shaped cutout registered the most pressure; the Temper Foam cushion registered the least pressure. Individual variation, however, was considerable and it was recommended that an evaluation of pressure be used in selecting the best cushion for each patient.

It seems that any cushion is better than none, that individual variation in pressure distribution influences the effectiveness of different cushions, and that no cushion can prevent decubiti unless pressure is also relieved several times an hour by a change of position in the wheelchair.

References

1. *Amigo, "The Friendly Wheelchair".* Bridgeport, Mich.: Amigo Sales.
2. *Premier Catalog.* Los Angeles, Calif.: Everest & Jennings, 1977.
3. *Disability Analysis.* Los Angeles, Calif.: Everest & Jennings, 1978.
4. *Modification & Accessory Analysis.* Los Angeles, Calif.: Everest & Jennings, 1979.
5. *The Wheelchair Catalog.* Los Angeles, Calif.: Everest & Jennings, 1980.
6. *Posture Position Equipment.* Los Angeles, Calif.: Everest & Jennings.
7. *Measuring the Patient.* Los Angeles, Calif.: Everest & Jennings, 1979.
8. *Wheelchair Prescription.* Los Angeles, Calif.: Everest & Jennings, 1978.
9. Souther, S. G., Carr, D., and Vistnes, L. M. Wheelchair cushions to reduce pressure under bony prominences. *Arch. Phys. Med. Rehabil., 55:* 460–464, 1974.
10. DeLateur, B. J., Berni, R. B., Hongladarom, T., and Giaconi, R. Wheelchair cushions designed to prevent pressure sores: An

evaluation. *Arch. Phys. Med. Rehabil.*, *57:* 129–135, 1976.

11. Fisher, S. V., Szymke, T. E., Apte, S. Y., and Kosiak, M. Wheelchair cushion effect on skin temperature. *Arch. Phys. Med. Rehabil.*, *59:* 68–72, 1978.

12. Fisher, S. V., and Kosiak, M. Pressure distribution and skin temperature effect of the ROHO wheelchair balloon cushion. *Arch. Phys. Med. Rehabil.*, *60:* 70–71, 1979.

13. Ma, D. M., Chu, D. S., and Davis, S. Pressure relief under the ishial tuberosities and sacrum using a cutout board. *Arch. Phys. Med. Rehabil.*, *57:* 352–354, 1976.

14. Garber, S. L., Krouskop, T. A., and Carter, R. E. A system for clinically evaluating wheelchair pressure—relief cushions. *Am. J. Occup. Ther.*, *32*(9)*:* 565–570, 1978.

Supplementary Reading

Care and Service. Los Angeles, Calif.: Everest & Jennings, 1976.

Garber, S. L. A classification of wheelchair seating. *Am. J. Occup. Ther.*, *33*(10)*:* 652–654, 1979.

Glaser, R. M. *et al.* An exercise test to evaluate fitness for wheelchair activity. *Paraplegia*, *16*(4)*:* 341–349, 1978–79.

Rehabilitation and Patient Aids. Los Angeles, Calif.: Everest & Jennings.

Reswick, J. B., and Simoes, N. Application of engineering principles in management of spinal cord injury patients. *Clin. Orthop.*, *112*(October)*:* 124–129, 1975.

Safety and Handling. Los Angeles, Calif.: Everest & Jennings, 1976.

PART
SEVEN

Application of Neurodevelopmental Approach

Hemiplegia, some often-seen central nervous system degenerative diseases and closed head trauma have been selected as representative diagnoses for application of this approach. Their selection is not meant to exclude the application of this approach to any problem of central nervous system disease or trauma.

chapter
15

Stroke

Catherine A. Trombly, M.A., OTR

Stroke is the common term for cerebrovascular accident (CVA). As a result of the CVA, the patient may be paralyzed (hemiplegic) or weak (hemiparetic) on the side of the body opposite to the site of the stroke. Neurological deficits of all types may occur in addition to the motor signs. The exact site and extent of the lesion in the brain determines which neurological deficits will manifest poststroke.[1]

Although this chapter will focus on the therapy designed for stroke patients, many of the same neurological manifestations occur due to trauma or tumor and can be treated similarly.

INCIDENCE

Stroke is the largest single diagnosis seen by the occupational therapist in clinics for the treatment of the adult physically disabled. Mossman[1] summarized studies of incidence of stroke in the United States. It is estimated that 170 to 190 per 100,000 persons suffer CVAs each year. The incidence of stroke increases with age.

ETIOLOGY

Thrombosis, or total occlusion of a blood vessel due to atherosclerosis, is the most common cause of CVA, an estimated 38 to 75%,[1] depending on the study. The next most common cause is hemorrhage which is usually secondary to hypertension. Hemorrhage more likely results in death during the 1st month post onset.[1] Embolism, a moving clot which blocks a vessel, and subarachnoid hemorrhage account for a small number of strokes. There is a greater tendency for those who have suffered an embolitic stoke, and to a lesser degree a thrombotic stroke, to have a recurrence within 5 years.[1]

SYMPTOMS OF STROKE

Strokes cause anoxic damage to nervous tissue.[1] Symptoms vary depending on which artery is affected. Functions subserved by the affected areas are either temporarily disrupted or lost depending upon the etiology and extent of nervous tissue damaged. The symptoms of damage to the major arteries are presented below.[1-3] If the occlusion or hemorrhage affects only a small branch of one of these major arteries, then the symptoms would reflect only loss of the function controlled by the area affected. If collateral circulation is established or resorption of edema occurs, recovery reflects this. The middle cerebral artery is the most vulnerable to stroke.

Middle Cerebral Artery

Contralateral hemiplegia and sensory loss, especially affecting the face, tongue, and upper extremity, results from a disruption of the flow of blood in this artery. Other symptoms may include: contralateral homonymous hemianopsia; cortical sensory disturbance with loss of spatial and discriminative sensibility which results in mislocation of stimuli or extinction of stimuli; and expressive aphasia and/or receptive aphasia. Aphasia occurs when the left hemisphere is damaged in right-handed persons and two-thirds of left-handed persons; one-third of left-handed persons suffer aphasia when their right hemisphere is damaged.[4]

Anterior Cerebral Artery

Following occlusion or hemorrhage of this artery, the lower extremity is more involved than the upper extremity. There is sensory loss of the cortical type, especially of the lower extremity. Aphasia and apraxia may result if the artery on the left side of the brain is involved. Confusion, homolateral amaurosis (blindness), and occasionally a grasp reflex of the upper extremity may occur.[2, 3]

Internal Carotid Arteries

Each internal carotid artery branches to form the anterior and middle cerebral arteries of one hemisphere of the brain. Occlusion of the carotid artery would result in symptoms of both middle and anterior artery damage.

Posterior Cerebral Artery

If only the posterior cerebral artery of one hemisphere is involved, the symptoms may include: contralateral homonymous hemianopsia with macular sparing, visual agnosia, visual memory disturbance, homolateral cerebellar ataxia, dysphonia, dysphagia, Horner's syndrome, facial paralysis, and contralateral loss of pain and temperature sensibility. If the pyramidal tract is involved, a contralateral hemiplegia will occur.

Basilar Artery

The basilar artery divides to form the two posterior cerebral arteries. This system serves the brain stem, cerebellum, medial and inferior aspects of the temporal lobe, the occipital lobe, and the thalamus. Since not all tracts have crossed in areas served by the artery, ipsilateral and contralateral signs can be mixed. Damage can result in any of the following: hemiplegia, quadriplegia, ipsilateral ataxia, thalamic syndrome (pain), contralateral disturbances in touch, pain, temperature awareness, burning pain, contralateral cerebellar asynergia, and tremor.

PROGNOSIS

Prognosis for recovery of function is greater in the young patient, possibly because of the greater plasticity of the young brain or the generally better physical condition of the young. Traumatic head injury causing damage to an extent similar to that caused by a CVA portends greater hope of recovery over a longer period of time than that expected in a post-CVA patient, possibly because the blood vessels are not diseased, and collateral circulation can be established more effectively.

Heart disease, obesity, peripheral vascular disease, and hypertension are all common in patients who have cardiovascular disease and all mitigate against optimal functional recovery. These concomitant diseases decrease the person's ability to expend the energy necessary to be functional.[5] Being independent in spite of a physical handicap requires much more energy than that required of a normal person.

It is estimated that of those patients who survive 2 to 5 years poststroke, 40 to 60% become independent; 10 to 25% remain dependent, and the rest become partially dependent.[1]

Rate of recovery of function is influenced by etiology. The posthemorrhagic stroke patient, if he survives, is very ill and may have bilateral signs initially, but recovery continues over a long time as the edema subsides. On the other hand, the most significant recovery that a postocclusion stroke patient will make will occur within 3 months[1] and plateau at 6 months.[6]

Accurate prediction of function or rate of return in a given stroke patient is not possible due to variability of anatomy and extent of brain damage; differences in types of cerebrovascular insult; in learning ability; in premorbid personality and intelligence; and differences in motivation. However, estimates of final goal can be made based on the observations collected over time. With regard to motor recovery, those patients with good sensation, minimal spasticity, and adequate selective motor control and no fixed flexion contractures have been shown to make the greatest improvements in functional abilities.[7] However, if the patient does not have a concept of his affected side and cannot localize any stimuli to the affected side, the outlook for independent use of the extremity is poor.[7] Fine motor coordination requires intact sensation. If motor control is very good, but sensation is partially lost, the limb will be used assistively only.[7]

The least likely motor function to recover is finger extension.[8] It is probably the most cortically controlled upper extremity function.[9, 10]

PROCESS OF RECOVERY

Recovery from brain damage does not seem to occur due to time, *per se*, but rather what happens during the time. Spontaneous recovery of function may occur in a stroke patient because edema subsides or nonfunctional but viable neurons reactivate.[1, 11] Recovery may also occur due to neuronal sprouting, reorganization of the cell bodies, or stimulation.[11] Brodal[12] suggests a process of recovery of motor function: (1) muscle fibers belonging to the motor units that have retained their central connections hypertrophy due to demands of exercise; (2) terminal endings of preserved corticospinal and other central fibers form new terminals which occupy the synaptic sites on motoneurons vacated by the dead fibers. However, Brodal points out, the latter process results in considerable diminution of specificity and a loss of old motor patterns since, for example, a rubrospinal fiber may occupy the synaptic site formerly occupied by a corticospinal neuron. Motor patterns need to be relearned because of this, but they are never regained to the level prior to the stroke, especially those patterns involving distal muscles.[12]

Another process underlying recovery of function may be the development by the patient of alternate behavior strategies to solve behavioral tasks. By using different brain areas and different problem-solving strategies, the patient is sometimes able to succeed so well in tasks that only very careful testing will reveal that the disability still exists.[13] An example of this is the recovery of manipulospatial skills (stereognosis) via use of verbal strategy and deduction (self-cueing of characteristics of the object and deduction of the identity from a limited array). The patient seems to discover these strategies himself if he is clever[13]; therapists try to teach these substitutive strategies to those who do not discover them.

OCCUPATIONAL THERAPY EVALUATION OF THE POSTSTROKE PATIENT

The occupational therapist treats the sensorimotor, perceptual, and cognitive deficits of the stroke patient in order to increase independent functioning in occupational performance tasks. During evaluation, therefore, the therapist must determine which occupational performance tasks the patient realistically can expect to be able to do, what tasks he can now do, and what the status of sensation, tone, motor control, perception, and cognition are. Additionally, information concerning other factors that affect the ability of the person to progress or learn must be gathered. Examples are visual field cuts, emotional status, concomitant disease, passive range of motion, and level of adaptation to the stroke by the patient and this family.

Each stroke patient has his own combination of disabilities. Careful evaluation must be done to reveal the deficits and their probable interrelatedness before a treatment plan can be formulated.

One writer states that paralysis alone may not account for a particular patient's incapacity and may even contribute little to it. The overriding defect may actually be a change in intellect or some potentially reversible "neurophysiological disturbance."[14]

Because treatment of the stroke patient is complicated and because progress can only be made if all aspects of the patient's disability are taken into consideration, an evaluation form that incorporates everything helps in treatment planning. Such evaluation forms are usually developed by each occupational therapy department to reflect its philosophy regarding treatment of the stroke patient. Some evaluations have been published.[7]

Many of the evaluations used for stroke patients have already been described in earlier chapters. Any special consideration concerning the administration of the tests to this special population will be pointed out in the subsections of this chapter. Also, those evaluations which are unique to persons who have suffered a stroke will be described.

LANGUAGE AND SPEECH DISTURBANCES

Aphasia is a disturbance of language, of the symbolic use of the spoken or written word. Expressive aphasia or Broca's aphasia is the inability to say what one desires to say due to a lesion in the anterior speech cortex.[15] A patient with expressive aphasia may be able to sing or speak in other automatic ways, such as praying.[16] A person who learned English as a second language may be aphasic for English but able to speak his native language. Usually, however, the patient is aphasic in both languages. Agraphia is the inability to write what one wishes to. An expressive aphasic person may have agraphia also. Receptive aphasia or Wernicke's aphasia is the inability to understand spoken language due to a lesion in the posterior speech cortex. A combination of receptive (sensory) and expressive (motor) aphasia is called global aphasia.[3] Alexia is the inability to understand written symbols or language and therefore the inability to read.

Dysarthria is a slurring of speech due to paralysis or incoordination of the speech musculature. The patient is able to understand and express symbolic language.

The speech pathologist evaluates these functions. The occupational therapist needs information concerning the patient's language function in order to evaluate, instruct, or communicate with the patient effectively. When the opportunity arises, the occupational therapist should reinforce speech therapy. This is important because of the value of language to the person. In this, the occupational therapist is guided by the speech therapist. Reinforcement of speech therapy involves requiring verbal or written responses of the patient at the level of which he is capable.

Talking loudly to the aphasic patient is not useful and may even be more confusing. Also, displaying annoyance or frustration at being unable to communicate with the patient is nontherapeutic. Providing nonstressful opportunities for communication is an adjunct to the patient's progress. One method of reducing the stress of communication is to phrase questions so that the patient has only to answer by "yes" or "no" rather than by a descriptive phrase.

EVALUATION AND TREATMENT OF THE MOTOR DEFICIT

The basic motor deficits are changes in neuromuscular tone (positive symptoms) and the lack of automatic, background movement and/or skilled movement (negative symptoms). The motor problem is not one of weakness due to disuse or atrophy, as is the case in lower motor neuron disease or orthopedic conditions. The problem is a loss of ability to move each joint in isolation or to direct the limb in other than stereotyped reflex-based movement. It is as if the person cannot generate the proper motor program to meet the environmental demand.

Brodal,[12] writing about his own stroke, described the negative motor symptoms. He observed that the "power of will" needed to make a severely paretic muscle contract was considerable, whereas if the muscle was able to generate even about half of its potential tension, only slight mental effort was needed.[12]

EMG analysis of 16 patients with upper motor neuron lesions (12 CVAs) and 8 normals led Sahrmann and Norton[17] to the conclusion that "impairment of movement is not due to antagonist stretch reflexes, but rather to limited and prolonged recruitment of agonist contraction and delayed cessation of agonist contraction at the termination of movement,"[17] *i.e.,* lack of voluntary control.

The negative symptoms seem to be the overriding deficit. Therapy is a matter of relearning motor patterns on a continuum from reflex to voluntary isolated movements rather than strengthening of muscles, *per se.* Bobath[18] states that a stroke patient loses his memory of his former sensorimotor patterns and that therapy should be aimed at helping the person reexperience the feelings of normal movement, without the interference of spasticity and without excessive effort, in order to rebuild a memory of normal movement. Rehabilitation is a learning process, and if the patient is capable of receiving and interpreting the sensory input, then motor skills can be relearned. Acquisition of motor skill requires much repetition.[19] Redevelopment of motor control should not be done in the abstract. That is, newly relearned patterns of movement should be part of activities of daily living and practiced in that context.[18]

Secondary motor deficits that may occur as a result of the paralysis and spasticity include subluxation of the shoulder and contractures. Shoulder-hand syndrome (reflex sympathetic dystrophy) which may lead to a frozen shoulder may also occur.[19]

Evaluation of Changes in Tone

Methods of evaluating tone have been described. Notice should also be made of the changes in tone due to effort (usually increases), to the rate of passive movement (the faster the movement, the more likely the stretch reflex will be elicited), to temperature, to emotion or stress, and to the various attitudinal reflexes.[20] If any of these affect the level of tone, then care must be taken during reevaluation that the testing is done in a standardized manner in order to yield reliable data.[20]

Therapy for Hypertonus

If tone is excessive, movement may be prevented if the muscles opposite to the spastic ones are also weak. Excessive tone is inhibited using the previously described procedures. Not mentioned before is the inflatable splint that Johnstone has developed which holds the shoulder in external rotation with the elbow, wrist, and fingers extended and the thumb abducted (RIP of Bobath). It is used while working on movement reeducation at the shoulder. Use of the splint is followed by weight bearing on the limb.[21]

As mentioned in Chapter 11, EMG biofeedback can be used to decrease spasticity. The limb in which spasticity has been decreased via EMG biofeedback should be used functionally to reinforce the learning.

Increased tone should not be indiscriminantly inhibited. Some patients rely on their spasticity and hyperactive postural reflexes for function[22]; however, these are usually patients with long-standing spasticity who relearned functional tasks in spite of the spasticity.

Therapy for Hypotonus

If tone is low, movement may not occur because too few motor units are sufficiently excited in response to supraspinal commands since they lack this background of excitation. In the case of hypotonia, therapists use various sensory stimulation techniques to facilitate the motor neurons; these have been described previously. Reports of studies of the effects of

some of these stimuli on hemiplegic patients are included here. Using the TVR (tonic vibration reflex) as a background of excitation, Matyas and Spicer[23] demonstrated electromyographically the effectiveness of 15 seconds of cutaneous stimulation (fast brushing) on the recruitment of motor units in the stimulated muscles (quadriceps) of 12 hemiplegic patients. The effects were immediate as opposed to a 30-second or 30-minute delay suggested by Rood.[23]

Although not tested statistically, a therapeutic program that included vestibular stimulation (rotation in a chair) seemed to result in better scores of standing balance and ambulation in the parallel bars than did a program similar except for the vestibular stimulation.[24]

Norton and Sahrmann,[25] in a study of 25 hemiparetic patients, demonstrated that motor unit recruitment is enhanced by a combination of stretch and voluntary effort to use the muscle as compared to either method alone. The stretch stimulus was offered as resistance to retard an ongoing movement. Effort alone produced more motor unit activity than stretch alone did. However, the level of recruitment for the combined stimuli was still less than that obtained in normals for effort alone, thereby demonstrating the negative symptom of hemiplegia.[25]

A sling, designed by Mary Jo Winsinky, RPT, can be used to facilitate the elbow extensors via stretch and resistance offered by the surgical tubing strap as the patient walks. It also inhibits finger flexion, and possibly the whole flexion pattern, by use of a cone in the hand. To construct this sling, the cone is placed on a length of surgical latex that is long enough to loop over the patient's shoulder while he holds the cone in his hand and has his elbow flexed to 90° or less. A knot is made in the tubing, and it is pushed inside of the cone out of view. The cone can be made of thermoplastic splinting material or be the spool from weaving thread. The large end of the cone is worn ulnarward, and the tubing crosses under the axilla if the sling is applied correctly (Fig. 15.1). It may be necessary to fasten the tubing onto the shoulder and to strap the hand onto the cone.[26]

Evaluation of Motor Control

The natural course of return of function is from proximal to distal and from mass, patterned, undifferentiated movement to fine, isolated movement. The recovery process can unpredictably stop at any point. It is usual that most patients will not regain full function of the upper extremity, especially of skilled hand function. These patients usually prefer to use the affected upper extremity as the assistive extremity. The recovery process follows this sequence as outlined by Brunnstrom:[27]

1. Flaccidity or lack of muscle tone. The stretch reflexes may not be elicited or may be elicited only by repetitive, rapidly applied stimuli.

2. Spasticity develops in the antigravity muscles.

3. Movement occurs in patterns called synergies. Synergistic movement is stereotyped whole limb

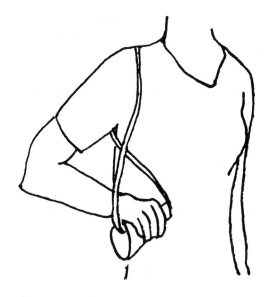

Figure 15.1 A sling to facilitate the elbow extensors.

movement which occurs first reflexly than in response to an effort to move. The flexor synergy usually develops before the extensor synergy. In the upper extremity, the flexor synergy is composed of scapular retraction and elevation; shoulder abduction and external rotation; elbow flexion, the strongest component; forearm supination; and wrist and finger flexion.

The lower extremity flexor synergy is composed of hip flexion, the strongest component; hip abduction and external rotation; knee flexion; dorsiflexion and inversion of the ankle; and dorsiflexion of the toes.

The extensor synergy of the upper extremity is composed of scapular protraction; shoulder adduction and internal rotation; elbow extension; forearm pronation; wrist and fingers are held in variable postures, usually flexion. The lower extremity extensor synergy is composed of hip adduction, knee extension, and plantar flexion of the ankle with inversion. Internal rotation, extension of the hip, and plantar flexion of the toes are also components.

It is good prognostic sign if the patient uses his affected limbs spontaneously, even if they move only in patterned motion.

4. As improvement continues, the patient becomes increasingly able to fractionate the mass patterns and finally to isolate motions at one joint. At this time usually all traces of spasticity have disappeared.

This sequence of recovery was also confirmed by Fugl-Meyer et al[28] in a longitudinal study of 20 hemiplegic patients followed from the 1st week of stroke to 1 year post stroke.

The evaluation of motor control may be made using Brunnstrom's[27] or Bobath's[29] procedures and scoring methods (see Chapter 6). Fugl-Meyer and others[28] have published a standardized method of evaluating physical performance; it quantifies Brunnstrom's procedure. Because the detail is too extensive to include here, the reader is referred to the original source for this useful evaluation.

Additionally, it will be helpful for treatment planning if other aspects of the patient's motor abilities are evaluated such as:

Is there a difference in the patient's ability to do automatic vs. voluntary movement? Does the patient automatically adjust to disturbance of balance? Do proximal segments (neck, trunk, shoulder, hip) stabilize to provide firm support for movement of the distal parts? Is the patient able to do a habitual movement sequence but not a new sequence of movement? Is the patient able to initiate a rapid, ballistic movement, although he may not complete it due to spasticity of the antagonists?

Is the patient able to do simple repetitive movements? Are sequenced movements that are related to the body, such as brushing the teeth, possible? Are movements requiring interaction with objects in space possible?

Answers to these questions can direct the therapist to the starting point of a therapeutic exercise program and can give the therapist clues as to the essential problem underlying the motor deficit. Whereas in the past, spasticity was considered *the* major motor problem, it may not be so. Enhanced performance is not necessarily directly related to reduction of spasticity.[30] Improved function following exercise and BFT, but no significant change in spasticity as measured by EMG, was observed in 20 hemiplegic patients. A few other studies that point to programming/learning/perceptual problems are included here to stimulate thinking along these lines.

In a study of 45 hemiplegic patient's ability to do three simple hand tasks, the right hemiplegics (left CVA) made significantly more perseverative errors than left hemiplegics. Kimura[31] concluded that it doesn't seem to be the ordering of movement *per se* which is particularly dependent on the left hemisphere but rather the ability to change to another movement. One might tentatively conclude that the right hemiplegic has no problem using a stored program but does have trouble accessing programs to meet environmental demand. Kimura states that compared to right hemisphere damage, left hemisphere damage causes impairment in acquisition and subsequent performance of a motor skill which involves several changes in limb and hand posture.[31] The most common errors are perseverative and hesitance errors unrelated to task. Ballistic, programmed movements (speed of tapping) and sequencing (ordering errors) were not problems for the left hemisphere-damaged patients.[31]

The less a series of movements depends on external guidance, *e.g.*, visual, the more likely it is to involve reference to a more autonomous internal system of control (programmed). Newly learned skills are guided externally, but if the guidance is constant, with practice the movement becomes automatic.[31, 32]

Cerebral blood flow studies are beginning to clarify the loci of cortical control of certain functions. Simple repetitive voluntary movements only activate the primary sensorimotor area. More complex motor patterns having a sequential component that are executed in intrapersonal space (movement performed with the body or extremities as the reference system) require participation of the supplemental motor areas also. Movements in extrapersonal space also require the parietal lobes for the integration of information concerning spatial coordinates in the external world.[33]

Treatment of Motor Control Deficits

Therapy is aimed at decreasing spasticity and increasing voluntary movement with special emphasis on movement or postures controlled by muscles antagonistic to the spastic muscles.[34] Usually this means decreasing or preventing flexor/adductor spasticity and increasing the likelihood of contraction of the extensor/abductor muscle groups. Once the muscles begin to contract fairly predictably, old movement patterns may be relearned and new ones developed.

The neurodevelopmental approaches outlined in Chapter 6 are used. Neurodevelopmental techniques cannot overcome an anatomical block if such exists but are chosen on the basis that physiological blocks caused by nonuse of existing nerve and muscle tissue can be overcome.[35] The Bobath and Rood approaches emphasize the importance of weight bearing not only to increase extensor muscle participation, but also to decrease flexor spasticity.[35] Brunnstrom[27] uses weight bearing and resistance to extensor patterns to improve the extensor output. All seem to start the patient in the roll over developmental pattern if he is seen soon after the stroke and has not learned to do this. This pattern is both functionally important to the patient and also begins to break up patterns of spasticity if trunk rotation is incorporated.[27, 29, 35]

Practices used by physical educators in teaching motor skills to potential athletes may also be applicable, although so far untested in the reeducation of a person with an acquired motor disability. Short bouts of intensive practice followed by rest periods are preferable to long practice sessions. Brodal states from personal experience that it is exhausting to the stroke patient to expend the mental energy necessary to contract the paretic muscles.[12] It helps the patient who is unable to move to be moved passively in the motion that he is trying to produce actively. It gives him sensory information about the range and goal of the movement. This probably lets him access his memory for the correct program to be used.[12] Teaching the right hemiplegic to move at a natural pace rather than teaching him to move slowly at first may be beneficial to the recovery of automatic (well learned) voluntary movements. Decreased speed of learned movement may interrupt the automatic progression of movement needed to carry out a whole task, even though there is no problem with initiating the task. This may be similar to reciting a poem and forgetting it midway; to go on, the person has to start at the beginning of the chain of responses.[12] Other treatments include biofeedback (BFT) and functional electrical stimulation (FES). These treatments provide concentration on practice in repeating the movements and confirmation of successful performance. All or some of these factors

may be essential in motor relearning, whether using therapeutic exercise or electronic devices.

Electromyographic biofeedback presents an opportunity for a patient to know the result of his effort to perform a certain contraction. By combining this knowledge of results (KR) with proprioceptive sensations and visual observation of movement, if movement occurs, the patient can redevelop motor patterns.[36]

Greenberg and Fowler[37] tested the hypothesis that if a hemiplegic patient received correct sensory monitoring of a volitional motion, via electrogoniometric biofeedback, the motor act would be reproducible. Half of 20 subjects were treated 8 times over 4 weeks with feedback, and the other half were treated using Brunnstrom-based exercises and functional activities. Both groups made equal gains in active elbow extension, suggesting that perhaps the specificity of the feedback is not as important as the practice.

Hurd et al.[38] concluded from their study of EMG biofeedback, placebo EMG biofeedback (the feedback signal was generated by the therapist unbeknownst to the patient), and no feedback that since there was a significant difference between the performance of the groups receiving biofeedback and those not, but no difference in the performance between the true and placebo BFT groups, biofeedback (true or placebo) was effective in increasing the conscious awareness and control of specific muscle groups.

Long lasting improvement of motor control seems to occur with greater frequency in the lower extremity than in the upper extremity. In one follow-up study of 34 hemiplegic patients who had achieved success (complete restoration of function) or moderate success (some functional use) via BFT the year before, no deterioration of function occurred in 19 of 28 upper and 20 of 26 lower extremities.[39] Knowledge of results (KR) is considered to be potent in reducing movement error. However, some persons have difficulty in processing the KR into appropriate response strategies[32]; therefore, additional emphasis needs to be placed on the initiation of movement, such as may be done through use of facilitation techniques and verbal cueing, along with biofeedback therapy. Techniques of BFT to facilitate weak muscles are listed in Chapter 11.

Functional electrical stimulation (FES) is "electrical stimulation of muscle, both smooth and striated, deprived of nervous control with a view to providing muscular contraction to produce a functionally useful movement."[40]

Afferent FES seems to be a viable method of making possible "a selective, repetitive and reproducible programmed input of information activating reflex mechanisms indispensible in organizing the motor activity and movement"[40] which are lost or diminished in patients with upper motor neuron lesions. Following a period of FES, movements are sometimes relearned. Upper extremity function, especially distal function, is more cortically controlled as compared to gait and lower extremity functions which seem to be organized at a lower neurological level[40] and are therefore less likely to be improved. In a feasibility study of a 2-channel FES unit for the upper extremities, five of eight patients showed functional improvement with the orthosis, and after 2 months, three of five showed evidence of relearning elbow extension, but not finger extension. It was concluded that elbow extension and hand opening are the movements that when stimulated give the best functional improvement in hemiplegic patients and that voluntary control was improved following use of FES.[41] Transcutaneous electrical stimulation to the wrist and finger extensor muscles of hemiplegic patients has been used in lieu of passive ranging to prevent or correct finger and wrist flexor contractures secondary to spasticity. Two groups were treated in a 30-minute, 3 times per week for 4-week program. In one group without contractures (N = 9) all maintained their range of motion. In the other group with contractures (N = 7) a statistically significant increase in range of motion was recorded. During 2 months of passive exercise, after electrical stimulation was discontinued, there was a loss of the increased range.[42] FES has been found useful in increasing strength of muscles antagonistic to spastic ones and in increasing range of motion. Three ½-hour periods of passive cyclical (7 seconds on; 10 seconds off) electrical stimulation 7 days a week for 4 weeks to the extensor muscles of 16 hemiplegic patients resulted in gains of passive range and strength of contraction of wrist and finger extensors, but no definite trend of reduction in spasticity or changes in sensation were seen.[41]

Secondary Motor Deficits

Subluxation of the Shoulder

Subluxation of the glenohumeral joint occurs secondary to paralysis of the scapulohumeral and/or scapular muscles. One hypothesis is that the weakness of the supraspinatus combined with the normal dependent position of the arm is the cause of the subluxation; this hypothesis is based on a study that correlated lack of EMG of the supraspinatus with radiographic evidence of subluxation.[43] This study lead to the conclusion that loading of the glenohumeral joint should be avoided as long as the affected limb is flaccid.[43]

Slings, arm boards, and lapboard wheelchair trays are all used to provide a positive upward force to the hemiplegic shoulder. Choice depends on the needs of each patient and the characteristics of each support.[44] Some examples are listed here. Fitted slings support the arm close to the body. Many designs exist.[44-46] One supportive design consists of elbow and wrist cuffs connected by 2-inch webbing that extends from the elbow cuff, over the affected shoulder, across the back, under the affected arm to the wrist cuff, around the wrist cuff up the front of the chest and over the unaffected shoulder, across the back to the elbow cuff under the affect arm. The webbing makes a figure-of-

eight on the patient's back. The crossed areas are permanently sewn, as is the webbing to the cuffs. Stabilizing pieces are added behind the elbow and between the elbow and wrist straps in front (Fig. 15.2). Needless to say, the ward staff and patient need careful instruction in applying this sling correctly.

The type of sling that binds the humerus close to the chest wall may not be appropriate because the head of the humerus seems to be forced out of the glenoid fossa when the humerus is so adducted. An alternate sling choice is the Bobath roll which is a roll of soft foam rubber that fits under the axilla and holds the arm abducted slightly, which therefore orients the humeral head more directly into the glenoid fossa while supporting the joint.[29] The patient wears the sling when he is up ambulating or in his wheelchair. This sling can be constructed as follows: an 8- to 10-inch wide piece of foam rubber is rolled up jelly-roll fashion and secured. An ace bandage is used to hold the roll in place under the axilla. The ace bandage is passed through the center of the roll, over the patient's chest and opposite shoulder, under his opposite axilla, then over the same shoulder again and across the back to connect with the other end at the foam roll under the affected axilla (figure of eight). Care must be taken when using this sling that the humerus is not displaced laterally[29] or that the radial nerve is not compressed.

The use of a humeral cuff suspended by a figure-of-eight harness, similar to that used for upper extremity prostheses, to support the humerus while allowing use of the extremity is also suggested by the Bobaths.[29]

Some therapists[47, 48] attach an arm board to the arm of the patient's wheelchair which supports the arm in about 45° of abduction and also supports the wrist and fingers in a functional position. The arm board

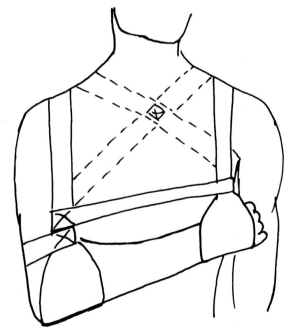

Figure 15.2 A sling to support a flaccid shoulder.

may be made out of plexiglass, royalite, or padded wood; some conform to the contour of the patient's arm and hand.

Use of a lapboard is suggested, since it may not only support the shoulder but also encourages weight bearing and compression of the glenohumeral joint. It puts the limb within the vision of the patient which may contribute to awareness. Use of the lapboard also allows positioning out of the typical hemiplegic posture. The lapboard also seems "more natural and less a badge of disability" than a sling.[49]

Basmajian[50] describes the "locking mechanism" by which the head of the humerus, through gravity, remains locked in contact with the upwardly facing glenoid fossa in normal shoulders. Based on the hypothesis that loss of the locking mechanism is the basis for subluxation, it is suggested that a treatment goal should be improvement of mobility of the scapula with emphasis on restoring the normal orientation of the glenoid fossa which is upward, forward, and lateral.[51] The hemiplegic orientation of the glenoid fossa is downward, backward, and medial due to scapular retraction and downward rotation which are part of the common spastic pattern.

Prevention of Contractures

Contractures are detrimental to function and hygiene and are therefore to be avoided. Certain pain-free ranges of motion are required at each joint to allow accomplishment of self-care activities.[7]

Contractures develop when limbs remain in one position. The hemiplegic who develops contractures usually develops them in the typical hemiplegic pattern: shoulder adduction and internal rotation, elbow flexion, forearm pronation, wrist and finger flexion.

Contractures are prevented by (1) passive range of motion of the limb at least once daily, preferably more often and (2) positioning opposite to the typical deformity.[5]

Self-administration of passive range of motion exercises is often taught to patients in group classes. Care must be taken that the motions are done correctly, especially at the shoulder. Forcefully abducting the arm above horizontal without externally rotating the humerus can result in a rotator cuff tear because the tissue is jammed between the greater tuberosity of the humerus and the acromion. This tear is usually the cause of shoulder pain in hemiplegics and often results in a frozen shoulder because the patient refuses to move it.[52, 53] Najenson and his colleagues[52] x-rayed 32 hemiplegic patients with severe shoulder pain and found evidence of rotator cuff injury in all. They recommended that ranging be done only by properly trained professionals and that overhead pulleys, used in some clinics to provide self-ranging of the shoulder, not be used because external rotation does not occur and the force may be too great. Pain is a sign of too strenuous and improper movement of the joint which has lost its active rotational component.[53]

Positioning is used to maintain the limb in "antispastic" position or in functional positions. Bob-ath[29] recommends positioning the upper extremity so that the scapula is forward, the elbow, wrist, and fingers are extended, and the fingers and thumb abducted.

Another recommendation is that instead of sitting with the wrist and fingers flexed in the lap, a typical posture, the patient hold his hands folded with the fingers interlocked, and therefore abducted, which is a reflex-inhibiting pattern.[29]

Splinting is used to position limbs; however, splinting of the spastic hand is controversial. A recent poll of 100 registered therapists concerning their practice of splinting the hemiplegic hand resulted in no clear direction or rationale for whether or not splinting should be used or what type should be used at various stages of recovery.[54] Some therapists choose volar splints; others choose dorsal splints, fearing the effects of sensory stimulation of the flexor surface and hoping to use the sensory stimulation of the dorsal surface to facilitate extension. One pilot study found that volar splinting did tend to increase spasticity, whereas dorsal splinting tended to decrease it in hemiplegic patients.[55] Zislis[56] compared the effects of dorsal and ventral splints which held the fingers extended and the wrist in neutral to decrease spasticity in one hemiplegic patient. The fingers were abducted in the ventral splint and adducted in the dorsal splint, which clouds the comparison. Electromyography demonstrated the decrease in motor unit output of the spastic flexors using the ventral splint and the increase using the dorsal splint. Kaplan[57] studied the effects of long-term application of a dorsal splint which held the hand in full extension (wrist 90° dorsiflexion, fingers and thumb at full extension) to decrease spasticity and increase function in 10 hemiplegic patients. The results show a trend toward improvement. Louis[58] hypothesized that a light-weight, snugly fitting hand splint will decrease or eliminate the tactile stimulation, whereas when tactile stimulation is desired to increase tone of certain muscles lying under the splint, a heavier, looser splint covering a greater amount of skin area was recommended. Rood theorized that pressure over the tendons of a muscle are inhibitory due to the tension created on the GTOs and Pacinian corpuscles. This is the basis for incorporating a cone into some splint designs.

A spastic patient, or potentially spastic patient, if splinted at all, must have a splint that incorporates both the wrist and the fingers because the effect of splinting one part of the spastic hand in extension is to cause flexion contractures of the unsplinted part.

Splint designs for the hemiplegic hand include the dorsal or volar resting pans (Fig. 12.5), the orthokinetic splint, and the finger abduction splints (Figs. 12.10 and 12.11).

Serial casting of spastic limbs is developing as a treatment choice for stroke patients. By replacing the casts, the limb is pulled more and more away from the spastic posture with each application, and greater range and function are obtained. There is some evidence that prolonged immobilization (3 months with removal for washing and free movement twice daily) of the limb in a position of full stretch will decrease the spasticity, increase the range of free movement, and increase the tone of the antagonists (except in cases of wrist and finger extensors).[59] Pain and skin damage may occur during prolonged immobilization, unless the device is well constructed and the condition of the limb frequently monitored.[59] Plaster of Paris was found to erode the skin,[59] and therefore the newer plastic materials may be preferable.

Other Motor Goals

Another complication is shoulder-hand syndrome which manifests by pain in the shoulder and hand, as well as nonpitting edema of the hand. Treatment is to decrease both the edema and pain and to increase passive movement[19] using the principles listed in Chapter 8 for increasing range of motion.

At first, the patient's endurance may be too low for function. If no cardiac contraindications exist against increased activity, endurance may be improved by using principles outlined in Chapter 8.

When the patient has gained voluntary control of isolated movement, strengtheninng of weak muscles may be done using the methods of the biomechanical approach listed in Chapter 8.

The unaffected upper extremity may require therapy to increase strength and coordination. The unaffected upper extremity must now become the preferred, dextrous one. The need to retrain skill in the right hand of left hemiplegics is not often stressed, since the right hand is most often the dominant one and considered "normal." However, Bell et al.[60] report severe disability in hand skill of left hemiplegics using their "normal" right hand as compared to right hemiplegics using their normal nondominant left hand. The latter scored in the low normal range.

Methods to increase coordination and dexterity of the unaffected upper extremity follow the principle of selecting activities which the patient is just able to do coordinately (quickly and accurately) and then grading the activities to require increased amounts of speed and/or accuracy.

If a change of hand preference is involved, considerable time will be spent in writing training if the patient is not agraphic. The paper is stabilized so the lower corner is about at the midline of the patient. Writing practice begins with "Palmar Method" exercises of continuous circles and progresses to connected up and down strokes. These exercises are done using first large strokes and a large pencil or crayon if necessary, then the stroke and writing tools are graded smaller and smaller. Later, the alphabet and words are practiced. The patient should at least be able to sign his name before this therapy is discontinued.

Precautions Related to Exercise

Cardiac problems are not uncommon in stroke patients. During treatment the therapist should attend to signs of cardiac distress such as dizziness, diaphoresis, shortness of breath, excessive fatigue, or chest pain and should discontinue therapy if any of these are noted. Therapy should be modified for patients with cardiac symptoms to include warm up and cool down exercise. Resistive exercise should be avoided.[61] In those patients with cardiac precautions, heart rate and rhythm, noted by palpation, and blood pressure measurement should be made during rest and during or within 15 seconds of cessation of activity to note the patient's response to exercise. If any of the following occur, therapy is discontinued and the physician notified.[61]

1. Decreased systolic blood pressure with increasing activity.
2. Diastolic blood pressure greater than 110 mm Hg.
3. Combination of decreased systolic and increased diastolic pressure with activity.
4. Decreased heart rate with activity.
5. More than 5 missed beats per minute during or immediately after activity. (Missed beats are premature ventricular contractions or PVCs.)
6. More than 10 missed beats/minute at rest.

EVALUATION AND TREATMENT OF THE SENSORY DEFICIT

Sensory losses have major significance in affecting the degree of recovery. Another significance is their association with less easily recognized parietal lobe syndromes of gross unilateral neglect, spatial and body disorientation, and bilateral apraxia, all of which are serious impediments to rehabilitation success.[62]

Sensory evaluation is found in Chapter 3. When evaluating a hemiplegic patient's sensation, the uninvolved limbs should be evaluated to gauge expected levels of response for the involved extremities. There is some evidence, however, that the so-called normal extremities are actually also involved to a lesser degree following a CVA.[63]

In testing sensation of a person who has expressive aphasia, it is necessary to establish a means of communication with the patient. This may be a nod of the head or other facial expression[64] or the use of two distinct sounds within the capability of the patient to mean "yes" or "no." When it is necessary to name an object, as in testing for stereognosis, the patient with expressive aphasia may be presented with a small array of objects from which he selects the stimulus object. The degree of discrimination can be tested by making the objects in the array more or less similar. Sensory testing of a patient with receptive aphasia is questionably valid. Be sure that the person's ability to understand is not overestimated.[65] A method to check the level of understanding is to say one thing and gesture another. How the patient responds will give you a clue to his understanding.[65]

Therapy for Sensory Losses or Disturbances

Some attempts at sensory retraining have been made by therapists who used such techniques as rubbing the limb vigorously with terry toweling while the patient watches[62] before repetitively moving the limb. Another technique, used to improve stereognosis, involved having the patient feel the object first with the eyes occluded and then with the eyes open for immediate feedback and reinforcement. One group who used this method had limited success in increasing manual dexterity of patients with cortical sensory disturbances, but their patients failed to learn to use the arm spontaneously, as had been hoped.[66]

Most therapists attempt to teach the patient to compensate visually for lost sensation. The patient is also taught to remind himself in some way of the location of his anaesthetic extremities. If he is capable, he is taught to use a mental checklist that includes locating the anaesthetic limb before moving. Noisy bracelets on the wrist or ankle provide an auditory reminder. Success is limited if the patient is hemianoptic or confused. Distractible patients are often unable to structure sensory input. Marmo[67] advocates that therapy include not only elimination of stimuli, but also gradual reintroduction of stimuli as the patient is able to assimilate it because it is unfunctional to require an environment free of stimuli.

EVALUATION AND TREATMENT OF VISUAL DISTURBANCES

The most common visual disturbances are hemianopsia and impaired depth perception. Hemianopsia is a visual field defect in which the patient is unable to see part of his visual field while looking straight ahead. Right homonymous hemianopsia means that the patient has lost the perception of vision in the nasal half of the right eye and the temporal half of the left eye and is unable to see to the right of midline.[1]

Hemianopsia may be tested in several ways. Two commonly used tests are:

1. Draw a horizontal line on a blackboard. With the patient positioned in exact center of the line and with his head held so that he looks straight ahead, give him the chalk and ask him to bisect the line.

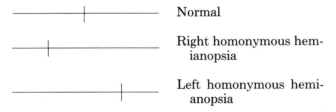

Normal

Right homonymous hemianopsia

Left homonymous hemianopsia

2. Stand in front of the patient who is looking straight ahead so that he will not compensate for the loss by turning his head. Hold two new pencils at the 180° limits of peripheral vision. Keep your arms and hands down below his level of vision so that he does not get extra cues by watching your arms. Simultaneously move the pencils in an arc toward the patient's midline. He is to indicate when he sees each of them. To rule out the possibility that the patient is extinguishing one stimulus, test only the defective side

again to confirm the defect. A patient with brain damage may have discriminative sensory loss and perceptual deficits which allow him to perceive only one stimulus of a similar nature at one time.

When hemianopsia is combined with sensory loss of the affected side, the patient may neglect the side altogether. However, he may also do this in the absence of these two symptoms due to a malfunction in the central processing system of the right parietal lobe.[68] This is a perceptual deficit termed unilateral neglect. The patient ignores personal and extrapersonal space on the left side and does not as readily learn to compensate as does a person with only left homonymous hemianopsia.[69]

Depth perception can be tested by holding two pencils in front of the patient's face at eye level and at different distances. Slowly move one toward the other until the patient indicates when they are parallel with each other. Another way to test depth perception is to place one block farther away from another on a table which is raised to approximately eye level to eliminate the cues obtained from looking down on the blocks, and to ask the patient to identify which is closer.

Therapy is aimed at retraining the patient to scan his environment. Visual deficits which are not complicated by sensory/perceptual deficits are often overcome with training. Compensation for hemianopsia may be taught be reminding the patient to turn his head to view the scene on his affected side or by having the patient do activities that require him to turn his head in order to complete them. Exercises which require motor crossing of the midline often force and also reinforce visual crossing of the midline.[62] Examples of such activities include weaving on a floor loom, ironing, reading aloud, making a puzzle with some prominent pieces placed on the hemianoptic side, or playing a board game that forces scanning for pieces or place for the next move. If the patient has certain perceptual deficits, however, he will not do the activities properly and will be unaware of errors so that self-correction of his performance will not happen.

Practice in compensating for disturbances of depth perception occurs intrinsically in activities of daily living, homemaking, and other therapy. Imperceived, an object which is in the way will be knocked over and is immediate negative reinforcement. Exercises to practice depth perception may be done if necessary. An example is to place a container at the patient's arm reach at about waist level and to have him put objects into the container. Gradually raise the level of the container to eye level as the patient improves. Pouring from container to container, needle threading, and games with tall pieces, such as chess, are all interesting drills.

EVALUATION AND TREATMENT OF PERCEPTUAL DEFICITS

Patients with perceptual losses exhibit an inability to get around in their world and/or to manipulate the components of their environment for normal functioning. The right hemisphere in most people appears to be responsible for spatial perception, an ability acquired during the 1st decade of life.[15, 70] Patients with right hemisphere damage exhibit a disorientation or an inability to relate to present and absent (previously seen) space.[64, 68, 71] They have disturbed body image, topographical disorientation, disturbed position-in-space perception, disturbed depth perception, dressing apraxia, constructional apraxia, and possibly a disturbance of recognition of faces.[64]

Evaluation of cognitive/perceptual function needs to be fine grained in the case of a patient seeking reemployment in a job which requires normal cognitive/perceptual abilities. For patients with lesser goals, the evaluation and treatment can be more coarse.

The OTR is the rehabilitation professional to whom sensory-perceptual deficits are assigned for remediation and compensation to permit greater independence in occupational performance tasks. Unfortunately, the minimal cognitive/perceptual requirements for these tasks have not been identified. This seems to result in too little or too much therapy aimed at improved perception.

Anderson and Choy[68] recommend that therapy aimed at remediation of perceptual deficits (body image, space perception, unilateral neglect) be done prior to training in activities of daily living (ADL). These defects correlate highly with failure to progress in rehabilitation.[68] Lorenze and Cancro[72] found that patients who did poorly on the Block Design and Object Assembly subtests of the WAIS (Weschler Adult Intelligence Scale), taken as a measure of perceptual organization, also did poorly in ADL despite intensive rehabilitation. All remained dependent. These patients were left hemiplegics; their verbal IQs were average or above.

Whether to treat the adult patient's perceptual deficits neurophysiologically or through the use of compensatory education remains a question. Fox[73] used cutaneous stimulation on 39 adult hemiplegics in an attempt to improve their perception of stereognosis, finger gnosis, graphesthesia, and other perceptual-discriminative sensory abilities and found some limited success, especially in the improvement of finger gnosis. Anderson and Choy[68] report positive results from a therapy program aimed at increasing awareness of body image, space perception, and unilateral neglect in hemiplegic patients with parietal lobe damage secondary to suffering a CVA. They have detailed an entire program which essentially combines sensory (cutaneous) stimulation with activities to direct the patient's attention to the part stimulated. In addition to sensory stimulation, they used movement, the use of the uninvolved arm as a helper and guide, puzzles, paper and pencil exercises, and a great amount of practice. No statistics were included in their report to indicate the significance of the success.

Marmo[67] advocates a program of controlled stimulation to minimize stress for brain-damaged patients and to reorient the patient to his body image. She suggests the use of cutaneous stimulation of the entire body, rolling from side to side, lying prone, vestibular stimulation, all with the aim of increasing the patient's awareness of his body and decreasing his disorientation.

Other therapists prefer to structure the environment to increase the patient's success. An example of this is to suggest that a patient with figure-ground deficit use sheets of contrasting color on the bed so that there will be less difficulty making the bed.

Some teach the patient attack skills. Some of these are the use of cues to chain an activity, *i.e.*, one step of an activity cues the next; organizational methods using logical, sequential thinking to group things according to color, shape, size, function, etc.; the use of categorizing skills in which the patient cognitively describes the object to himself in order to categorize it, *i.e.*, "this object has three angles and three straight sides; it is therefore a triangle"; and the use of verbal memory by which the patient learns a verbal sequence and cues himself to perform sequential tasks by repeating the sequence aloud.

Specific deficits seen in the hemiplegic patient, their evaluation, and treatment suggestions are noted below.

Body Image

A deficit of body image perception is the inability to perceive the location and relationship of body parts. Body scheme is a more correct term for this dysfunction, as the term body image includes the visual and mental memory one has of his body and a representation that includes the feelings one has about his body, rather than an exact picture of the physical structure.[69]

Evaluation includes such tests as (a) pointing to body parts on request, (b) answering questions about the relationship of body parts, *e.g.*, "Are your fingers closer to your wrist or your elbow?" (c) drawing a person, and (d) assembling a puzzle of a person with the pieces cut to represent anatomical parts. The reader is referred to Siev and Freishtat[69] for details of administering and scoring these and other perceptual tests used with adult hemiplegic patients. A test for body scheme that discriminates between neurologically and nonneurologically impaired adults was developed by MacDonald,[74] and the reader is referred to the reference for the directions for that test.

The patient with a body scheme disturbance may experience difficulty in dressing or in transferring or ambulating safely because he lacks awareness of the relationship of his body to the environment.

The goal of therapy to improve body image is to increase the awareness of spatial relations and attention to the affected side.[68] Methods are to ask the patient to identify the part of the body touched and to mimic positions that the therapist assumes.[68]

Figure-Ground

The stroke patient may have difficulty distinguishing figure from background. The patient may evidence this deficit functionally by being unable to do such things as locate a white towel lying on top of a white sheet, locate buttons visually on a printed dress or shirt, or find an item in a jumbled array. The Ayres' Figure-Ground Test, a subtest of the Southern California Sensory Integrative Tests,* presents a design to the patient in which the outlines of three common objects or geometric designs are embedded. The patient must select the correct figures from six pictured choices. This test has norms for children only; however, Siev and Freishtat[69] report limited normative data for adults aged 20 to 59 years.

Topographical Orientation

This is the ability to find one's route with or without the use of maps.[74] A person who has parietal lobe damage of the right hemisphere cannot follow maps using visual or haptic (tactual-kinesthetic) cues. The patient seems unable to make and retain in memory appropriate symbols or to be able to manipulate them.

Evaluation of this deficit is often by clinical observation: can the patient find his way from his room to other known areas at the rehabilitation center? Teuber[71] reports a more objective test developed by himself and other researchers. It consists of placing a patient in a square room, the floor of which is marked with nine equidistant dots and one wall marked to indicate north. The patient is given "maps" one at a time which he may not reorient as he moves through the maze as directed by the map. The map consists of nine dots, a start and an end position and an indication of northward direction. Some are visual maps; others are tactual maps made of raised nails and string and hung around his neck so the map is on his chest within each reach but cannot be seen.[71]

Position in Space and Spatial Relations

A person with disturbance of position-in-space perception is unable to deal with spatial concepts such as above, below, behind, etc. Disturbed perception of spatial relations does not allow the patient to perceive the position of objects in relation to himself or to other objects. Again the Southern California Sensory Integrative Test has subtests to measure these abilities with norms for children only. Other tests include the Bender Visual Motor Gestalt Test, the Cross test and Positioning Blocks.[69]

Therapeutic exercises suggested by Anderson and Choy[68] include having the patient hold onto a dowel with both hands while the therapist assists him to move in various directions to cross the midline. Next, the patient moves without assistance, and finally he moves following the lead of a moving target.[68]

---

* Ayres, A. J. *Southern California Kinesthesia and Tactile Perception Tests.* Beverly Hills, Calif.: Western Psychological Services, 1966.

Apraxia

This is the inability to perform purposive or complex movements, despite intact mobility, sensation, and coordination.[14] There may be a disconnection between the idea of movement and its motor execution; this is called ideomotor apraxia.[14] The patient may be able to execute the motion automatically, yet not on command. For example, the patient is unable to "blow" on command but blows out a match placed in front of his face.

Or, the patient may have a defect in actually handling and using objects, which is ideational apraxia.[14] Ideational apraxia limits the patient further, as he is unable to execute the act automatically.

Goodglass and Kaplan[16] describe a test of apraxia in which the patient is asked to demonstrate universally known movements such as "Show me how you would pretend to brush your teeth with a toothbrush." When the patient does not pretend to hold the brush, he would be instructed to try again as though he were really holding the implement in his hand. If this does not modify the performance, the examiner demonstrates and invites the patient to imitate. The ability to correct performance on verbal instructions is counterindicative of apraxia, while the inability to change even after demonstration is typical of the apraxic patient. The reader is referred to the original source for the complete test.

Whole body movements may be preserved in apraxic patients who are unable to do individual limb movement.[75] Other types of apraxia include: dressing apraxia, which is the inability of the patient to dress himself properly. The evaluation is by clinical observation. The patient with dressing apraxia will be unable to self-correct.[91] Constructional apraxia is the inability to copy, draw, or construct designs in either two or three dimensions.[69] Constructional apraxia limits the patient's ability to manipulate his environment effectively. Patients with right hemisphere damage seem to lack the visual-spatial ability to do the task,[14,64,69] whereas patients with left hemisphere damage seem to lack the analytical, logical planning ability or the ability to sequence movement to do the construction task.[14]

Two-dimensional constructional apraxia is tested using design copying. The patient draws the design presented or constructs it from matchsticks. Three-dimensional constructional apraxia is tested using blocks. The patient is asked to copy increasingly more difficult three-dimensional block designs.[69]

The basis of apraxia is uncertain and may reflect a number of factors such as: the loss of the capacity to permit automatic performance of movements organized at the spinal level; inability to move in response to command if movement is language-dependent; defective kinesthetic memory; inadequate feedback system; and failure to process information at a normal speed.[14] Successful treatment of apraxia may occur with more accurate diagnosis; there is a need for more discriminating tests.[14]

Treatment methods that are suggested include: moving the person passively,[12, 14, 68] especially in gross patterns of posture and movement rather than isolated muscle function.[14] Speak to the patient in short sentences and state information about the movement just prior to moving him.[68] Chain movements together into a function whole.[68] Increase sensory input to increase awareness of activity in the affected limbs.[14]

Verticality

The hemiplegic patient may misperceive verticality when environmental clues are eliminated.[76] When asked to place an illuminated line in a vertical position in a dark room, the patient stops about "ten minutes to twelve."When asked to line up the line with the horizontal, the patient stops about "twenty minutes to nine." He can correct this if the lights are on because he can then use visual cues of verticality.

Teuber[71] postulates that perception of verticality depends upon "corollary discharge," which is a simultaneous discharge of neural impulses to the peripheral effectors and to the sensory systems preparing them for changes that will occur in verticality as a result of intended movement. This "corollary discharge" and subsequent adjustment in the perception of verticality depend on the integrity of the basal ganglia and the frontal lobes. An absence of self-produced movement, and hence no "corollary discharge," prevents reorganization of visual-motor function.[71, 77]

Agnosia

The patient may suffer agnosia, or the inability to recognize familiar objects.[3, 69] Tactile agnosia (astereognosis) is the inability to identify objects by touch. Visual agnosia involves inability to recognize objects or faces, although visual acuity is intact. Visual-spatial agnosia is the inability to perceive spatial relationships between objects or between self and object. Auditory agnosia is the inability to recognize sounds or words.

Visual agnosia is tested by asking the patient to name or demonstrate the use of familiar objects. The method for testing stereognosis was described in Chapter 3. Visual-spatial agnosia is related to spatial relations, topographic orientation, and depth perception and is tested by use of tests described for these disorders. Auditory agnosia is usually tested by the speech pathologist; however, an estimation of the patient's ability in this area may be made by having the patient identify sound, e.g., a bell, a piano, animal noises, etc.

Unilateral Neglect of Space and Body

Unilateral neglect is a perceptual deficit usually associated with right brain damage. The person with a serious neglect problem behaves as if he were selectively ignoring all that happens on the impaired side.[65] Tests of this function include cancelling certain letters out of lines of typed material, draw a man, draw a clock, copy a flower, copy a house, and reading aloud.[69]

Suggested therapy to increase awareness of the neglected space is to force the attention across the midline.[68] The therapist stimulates the neglected limbs using ice or tactile stimuli while the patient watches; then the patient applies the stimuli himself. Exercise using the uninvolved arm to assist movement across the midline is used.[68] Tasks that are sufficiently compelling to cause the head to turn to view the objects are presented.[78] An initial target on the neglected side can be provided to act as an anchoring point, e.g., a prominent red line at the start of a reading or writing line or on the side of a food tray.[78] Left hemiplegics should be paced to slow down and talk themselves through the activity to cue themselves to remember to turn their heads to scan.

Compensatorily, avoid isolating the patient by orienting his involved side toward the action in the room, which he will then be unaware of; and arrange the environment for function and safety.[65]

DIFFERENCES IN RIGHT AND LEFT HEMISPHERES

The patient with unilateral brain damage does not necessarily have to lose the capacity to do certain functional tasks: he may be able to relearn them using the information processing system that remains to him. Each half of the brain attends to different aspects of the same experience. Stroke patients have difficulty attending to rehabilitation tasks of different types: left hemiplegics have a primary problem with information processed through the visual modality, whereas the right hemiplegic has a primary problem with processing through the auditory modality.[80]

The right cerebral hemisphere is especially involved in visual-spatial perception and mental operations involving distance. There seems to be a diffuse processing of information which is integrated for immediate use, a process that describes what some call intuition. This is in contrast to the sequential processing of information that seems typical of the left hemisphere.[64] The patient with right hemisphere damage may tend to omit or minimize problems: drawings are marked with omissions, contradictions, and rigidity. The patient tends to perform a task too quickly and not to pay attention to detail. Pantomime and demonstrated instructions confuse him, but he can understand oral or written instructions.[4, 65, 79]

The left cerebral hemisphere is involved in analytical, logical thinking and in symbolic functions or language, concepts, ideas, and numbers. Even a nonaphasic person with left hemisphere damage may have these difficulties.[4, 58] Such a patient notes the existence of a problem and performs tasks very slowly in an effort to perform correctly. His performance of visual-spatial tasks is free from error, usually. The patient may have trouble receiving and understanding oral instructions but understands pantomime.[4, 59, 76]

Information processing proceeds through two stages: 1. Short-term memory (STM) registers the information temporarily until it is shifted to long-term memory (LTM). Information in STM is subject to decay unless it is attended to by a process such as verbal rehearsal. 2. The information from STM goes to LTM where it is more permanent. Patients with left hemisphere damage lack the language ability to sustain auditory information long enough in STM to get it to LTM, whereas right hemispheric damage interferes with STM handling of visual stimuli.[80]

Right hemiplegic patients (left hemisphere damage) should be encouraged to persist in performing a task, although they require more than the normal amount of time. They need frequent specific feedback that they are proceeding correctly.[65]

Left hemiplegic patients (right hemisphere damage) need to be slowed down and their attention focused in order to improve the quality of their performance.[14]

OTHER DEFICITS SEEN AS A RESULT OF BRAIN DAMAGE

Two general indicators of brain damage are the inability to persist in a motor task and perseveration. The patient, when asked to maintain his gaze, keep his eyes closed, hold out his tongue, or similar motor tasks, cannot do it for as long as a normal person can. Perseveration, on the other hand, is a continuation of a response after the stimulus has been removed. For example, the patient writes the same letter over and over, says the same word or phrase repeatedly, or does the same motion repeatedly without purpose or after the stimulus has been changed.

Brain damage causes a deficiency in learning efficiency in which there is difficulty in receiving and processing incoming information, assimilating or retaining information, associating new information with previous information, or retrieving information from memory in order to effect behavior.

Memory may be disturbed. Patients with left hemisphere damage have reduced memory for language and numbers, whereas patients with right cerebral damage lose memory for tasks involving position and movement.[64, 65, 70] Learning rate is reduced. Each patient will have a particular learning requirement depending upon the site of the lesion. Patients with difficulties with auditory retention spans may be able to remember short messages but not longer ones. Remote memory or learning is more likely to be preserved than immediate memory or recall. Patients with disturbed recent memory find it difficult to learn new things.

Quick tests of concentration and memory are to ask the patient to serially subtract sevens from one hundred,[3] taking into account educational level, or to ask the patient to repeat a telephone number told to him by the examiner. For patients with any brain damage, instruction should be brief, concrete, and standardized. Delivering one instruction at a time may be necessary for some patients.

If the patient cannot understand verbal, written, or gestured communication he may be able to understand demonstration in which the therapist moves his limbs to accomplish one part of the task; he is then immediately requested to repeat it alone.[67] This may be combined with backward chaining to teach a task that has many steps, such as putting on one's shirt. The therapist moves the patient through the complete activity repeatedly, then does it again through each step until they reach the last one, at which point the patient completes the task alone. Then they stop two steps from the end and the patient completes the two steps, etc. until the patient can do the entire activity from start to finish.

Task conditions influence the success of a brain-damaged person in performing a task. In a normal person, for example, peripheral stimuli facilitate performance, whereas in brain-damaged persons they may impede it.[76] If a patient seems to be having difficulty completing a task, the task conditions could be modified by reducing the stimuli in the environment to the point that the patient is able to perform successfully. Gradually over time as the task becomes learned the stimuli should be reinstated if possible. The patient needs to be able to perform in natural situations rather than be dependent on adapted ones.[76]

The patient may be emotionally labile.[4, 65] He may cry, laugh, or express anger unprovocated by events in the external environment or to a greater degree than warranted. He needs to be told that lability is a symptom of the stroke, reassured that he is not mentally ill, and assured that his control will improve in time. In the meantime, interrupting the behavior will be helpful—call the patient's name, clap, or ask a question and the emotional behavior due to organic lesion will stop, as opposed to emotional behavior that reflects true feeling which won't be stopped so easily.[65]

OCCUPATIONAL PERFORMANCE TASKS

The patient's ability to perform the self-care, recreational, and vocational tasks which he hopes to continue postrehabilitation are evaluated using the methods described in Chapter 23 of this book. The self-care evaluation is usually administered early in the patient's rehabilitation. The other evaluations are done as the improvement of the patient warrants them. All aspects of daily life in which the patient intends to engage postdischarge should be evaluated prior to the patient's discharge in order to ensure that the patient can do them successfully and safely.

Increase in independent self-care, as well as vocational and recreational pursuits, is an essential goal. Part 8 of this book describes the compensatory methods by which persons with the use of only one side of their body may be independent. Other sources of adapted techniques are listed in the references.

The patient must practice to learn these techniques because activities of daily living (ADL) tasks, thought habitual, are actually new tasks due to the condition.[80]

Employment

Ability to achieve independence in self-care, younger age, greater education, stable marital status, and cognitive capacities, such as higher intelligence, point to a greater likelihood of returning to work in general.[81] In particular, the variables that differentiate those that return to work from those that don't are: right hemiplegia—verbal-cognitive and communicative deficits; left hemiplegia—ambulation, use of affected upper extremity, and nonverbal abstract reasoning, such as measured by the Block Design subtest of the WAIS.[81]

FAMILY AND COMMUNITY REINTEGRATION

The hemiplegic patient, as with any patient who has suffered a change in his physical abilities, will need to be assisted to make a healthy emotional adjustment. His family will also need this help. In addition to supportive therapy, family group education and therapy sessions have been used in some rehabilitation centers.[82] Topics of discussion include how to communicate with an aphasic patient, how to modify the environment or task to augment functional performance, sexual counselling that focuses on coping processes within the partnership, which have been found to be the real cause for major changes in the sex life of married couples poststroke,[83] and other topics of concern. These sessions are a rehabilitation team effort; the occupational therapist contributes to the discussion about the topics of which he/she is most informed.

Prior to discharge, the patient needs to be reintegrated into his community at the level at which he will function in it. The family can share this responsibility with the rehabilitation team under their guidance as part of the family group education sessions.

EFFECTIVENESS OF THERAPY

No definitive studies have been done to establish the effects of specific therapeutic procedures in improving the function of poststroke patients. A few studies have reported effectiveness of certain treatments in improving the motor performance of patients who have suffered a stroke. A limited study of the hypothesized neurophysiological effects of activities on the finger extensor muscles of hemiparetic patients indicated that following 2 weeks of treatment, there was an increase in strength following light, unresisted extension, static grasp of handles with large surfaces, and a heavily resistive extensor movement.[84] The light activity caused loss of strength to a small degree immediately following treatment on the first few days. The resisted extension activity caused large losses of strength following treatment on the first days, but in both cases a trend toward increased strength developed toward the end of the 2-week period. These limited data suggest the need to further study the expected and actual effects of activity on the development of increased motor control of hemiplegic patients. Perhaps the usual avoidance of maximally resisted grasp and advocacy of resisted and unresisted extension are not the most effective approaches.

Stern et al.[85] report that no significant difference was found in a comparison of neuromuscular reedu-cation techniques with a regular, control program of therapy that did not include these techniques. The hemiplegic patient sample was randomly assigned to one of these two programs. Both groups improved in lower extremity strength, overall mobility, and functional abilities.[85]

Inaba et al.[86] reported a study in which three groups of patients of a homogeneous population were randomly assigned to one of three treatment groups. Group I received functional physical therapy and selective stretching; Group II received active exercise in addition to the treatment Group I received; Group III received progressive resistive exercise in addition to the treatment also given Group I. After 1 month of treatment, PRE in mass extension pattern of the lower extremities (Group III) was shown to significantly contribute to early increase of lower extremity function in hemiplegics; however, after 2 months no difference was seen in the functional level of the three groups.[86]

Andrews[87] reports the use of electromyographic biofeedback with 20 patients with spastic and flaccid musculature. Needle electrodes were placed in the nonfunctioning biceps or triceps. Immediate results were obtained in the first 10 cases; in the last 10 cases three failed to achieve control by the end of the 5-minute period, which was Andrews[3] criterion for success.

Johnson and Garton[88] used electromyographic biofeedback to teach 10 hemiplegic patients, of at least 1 year poststroke, to voluntarily control the paralyzed tibialis anterior muscle. Indwelling electrodes were used during the initial training. The patients were sent home with a portable unit and used surface electrodes. The patients practiced at home for 30 minutes twice daily for 2 to 16 weeks. All patients gained at least one grade of manual muscle testing; seven obtained grades of fair plus or above, whereas prior to training nine patients had zero to poor grades. One might question their method of measuring voluntary control, but one cannot question an increase in strength of contraction.

In a study by Brudny et al.[89] of the use of electromyographic biofeedback to increase the voluntary control of the affected upper extremity of 39 hemiparetic patients, 60% of the patients gained function enough to be classified as being able to do prehension and/or to use the extremity assistively. The significant functional gains persisted in 50% of the patients who were reevaluated 3 months to 3 years after the completion of biofeedback training. Seven of the patients who did not maintain functional gains were nevertheless able to use the limb voluntarily; these patients demonstrated a greater degree of sensory loss.

CONCLUSION

A choice must be made whether to concentrate on compensatory rehabilitation of the stroke patient or treatment aimed at restoration of motor control in preparation for function. Too often the choice is made based on a blanket policy of treatment of poststroke patients, rather than the differences among the patients[3] status, goals, and prognosis. It is Bobath's opinion that should the compensatory choice be made too early, the effectiveness of restorative treatment is lessened since the patient learns unilateral habits of movement. She believes that preferential use of the sound side of the body for weight bearing and functional tasks increases the spasticity, making development of normalized motor control less possible.[18]

The type of rehabilitation program will be influenced by the patient's age, type of stroke, and resultant prognosis for life and recovery. The rehabilitative approach of proven benefit[90] may be best for some patients, whereas the greater time, expense, and effort required by the neurodevelopmental approach directed at the recovery of perceptual and/or sensorimotor functions, and as yet unproven, may be warranted for the younger stroke patient.

One view is that in order to develop versatility in a patient, the underlying sensorimotor processes that result in dependence must be attacked and that stereotyped performance will result from "splinter skill training" of self-care skills directly. The other view is that functional activity training results in success at a faster rate and is therefore more economical and more satisfying to the patient who again feels competent. The different approaches represent a controversy that needs clinical research to resolve.

In either case, the goal is to improve independence in occupational performance tasks and hence to improve the quality of life.

References

1. Mossman, P. L. *A Problem Oriented Approach to Stroke Rehabilitation.* Springfield, Ill.: Charles C Thomas, 1976.
2. Bannister, R. *Brain's Clinical Neurology*, 4th ed. New York: Oxford University Press, 1973.
3. Levenson, C. Rehabilitation of the stroke hemiplegia patient. In *Handbook of Physical Medicine and Rehabilitation*, 2nd ed., edited by F. H. Krusen, F. J. Kottke, and P. M. Ellwood. Philadelphia: W. B. Saunders, 1971.
4. Fordyce, W. Psychological assessment and management. In *Handbook of Physical Medicine and Rehabilitation*, 2nd ed., edited by F. H. Krusen, F. J. Kottke, and P. M. Ellwood. Philadelphia: W. B. Saunders, 1971.
5. McCollough, N. C. The role of the orthopedia surgeon in the treatment of stroke. *Orthop. Clin. North Am.*, 9(2): 305–324, 1978.
6. Moskowitz, E., Lightbody, F., and Freitag, N. Long term follow-up of the poststroke patient. *Arch. Phys. Med. Rehabil.*, 53(4): 167–172, 1972.
7. Caldwell, C. B., Wilson, D. J., and Braun, R. M. Evaluation and treatment of the upper extremity in the hemiplegic stroke patient. *Clin. Orthop.*, 63: 69–93, 1969.
8. Shah, S. K. Volition following hemplegia. *Arch. Phys. Med. Rehabil.*, 61(11): 523–528, 1980.
9. Lawrence, D., and Kuypers, H. Pyramidal and non-pyramidal pathways in monkeys: Anatomical and functional correlation. *Science*, 148(May 14): 973–975, 1965.
10. Brinkman, J., and Kuypers, H. Splitbrain monkeys: Cerebral control of ipsilateral and contralateral arm, hand and finger movements. *Science*, 176(May 5): 536–538, 1972.
11. Braun, J. J. Time and recovery from brain damage. In *Recovery from Brain Damage: Research and Theory*, edited by S. Finger. New York: Plenum, 1978.
12. Brodal, A. Self-observations and neuro-anatomical considerations after a stroke. *Brain*, 96: 675–694, 1973.
13. Gazzaniga, M. S. Is seeing believing: Notes on clinical recovery. In *Recovery from Brain Damage: Research and Theory*, edited by S. Finger. New York: Plenum Press, 1978.
14. Non-paralytic Motor Dysfunction after Strokes. *Br. Med. J.*, 1(6121): 1165–1166, 1978.
15. Penfield, W. Speech, perception and the uncommitted cortex. In *Brain and Conscious Experience*, edited by J. C. Eccles. New York: Springer-Verlag, 1966.
16. Goodglass, H., and Kaplan, E. *The Assessment of Aphasia and Related Disorders.* Philadelphia: Lea & Febiger, 1972.
17. Sahrmann, S. A., and Norton, B. J. The relationship of voluntary movement to spasticity in the upper motor neuron syndrome. *Ann. Neurol.*, 2: 460–465, 1977.
18. Bobath, B. Treatment of adult hemiplegia. *Physiotherapy*, 63(10): 310–313, 1977.
19. Swenson, J. R. Therapeutic exercise in hemiplegia. In *Therapeutic Exercise*, 3rd. ed., edited by J. V. Basmajian. Baltimore: Williams & Wilkins, 1978.
20. Brennan, J. B. Clinical method of assessing tonus and voluntary movement in hemiplegia. *Br. Med. J.*, 1(March 21): 767–768, 1959.
21. Johnstone, M. Inflatable splint for the hemiplegic arm. *Physiotherapy*, 61(12): 377, 1975.
22. Anderson, T. P., and Kottke, F. J. Stroke rehabilitation: A reconsideration of some common attitudes. *Arch. Phys. Med. Rehabil.*, 59(4): 175–181, 1978.
23. Matyas, T. A., and Spicer, S. D. Facilitation of the tonic vibration reflex (TVR) by cutaneous stimulation in hemiplegics. *Am. J. Phys. Med.*, 59(6): 280–287, 1980.
24. Fiebert, I. M., and Brown, E. Vestibular stimulation to improve ambulation after a cerebral vascular accident. *Phys. Ther.*, 59(4): 423–426, 1979.
25. Norton, B. J., and Sahrmann, S. A. Reflex and voluntary electromyographic activity in patients with hemiparesis. *Phys. Ther.*, 58(8): 951–955, 1978.
26. Farber, S. D., and Huss, A. J. *Sensorimotor Evaluation and Treatment Methods for Allied Health Personnel*, 2nd. ed. Indianapolis: The Indiana University Foundation, 1974.
27. Brunnstrom, S. *Movement Therapy in Hemiplegia.* New York: Harper & Row, 1970.
28. Fugl-Meyer, A. R., *et al.* The Post stroke hemiplegic patient. I. A method for evaluation of physical performance. *Scand. J. Rehabil. Med.*, 7: 13–31, 1975.
29. Bobath, B. *Adult Hemiplegia: Evaluation and Treatment*, 2nd ed. London: Heinemann Medical Books, 1978.
30. Takebe, K., *et al.* Biofeedback treatment of foot drop after stroke compared with standard rehabilitation techniques (Part 2): Effects on nerve conduction velocity and spasticity. *Arch. Phys. Med. Rehabil.*, 57(1): 9–11, 1976.
31. Kimura, D. Acquisition of a motor skill after left-hemispheric damage. *Brain*, 100: 527–542, 1977.
32. Newell, K. M. Knowledge of results and motor learning. *J. Mot. Behav.*, 6(4): 235–244, 1974.
33. Roland, P. E. Quantitative assessment of cortical motor dysfunction by measurement of the regional cerebral blood flow. *Scand. J. Rehabil. Med.*, Suppl. 7: 27–41, 1980.
34. Jones, R. F. Stroke rehabilitation. Part II. Special consideration. *Med. J. Aust.*, 2(21): 799–801, 1975.
35. Goff, B. The application of recent advances in neurophysiology to Miss M. Rood's concept of neuromuscular facilitation. *Physiotherapy*, 58: 409–415, 1972.
36. Nafpliotis, H. Electromyographic feedback to improve ankle dorsiflexion, wrist extension, and hand grasp. *Phys. Ther.*, 56(7): 821–825, 1976.
37. Greenberg, S., and Fowler, R. S. Kinesthetic biofeedback: A treatment modality for elbow range of motion in hemiplegia. *Am. J. Occup. Ther.*, 34(11): 738–743, 1980.
38. Hurd, W. W., Pegram, V., and Nepomucens, C. Comparison of actual and simulated EMG biofeedback in the treatment of hemiplegic patients. *Am. J. Phys. Med.*, 59(2): 73–82, 1980.
39. Wolf, S. L., Baker, M. P., and Kelly, J. L. EMG biofeedback in stroke: A 1-year follow-up on the effect of patient characteristics. *Arch. Phys. Med. Rehabil.*, 61(8): 351–354, 1980.

40. Gracanin, F. Functional electrical stimulation in control of motor output and movements. *Contemp. Clin. Neurophysiol. (EEG Suppl No. 34)*: 355–368, 1978.

41. Merlette, R., Acimovic, R., Grobelnik, S., and Cvilak, G. Electrophysiological orthosis for the upper extremity in hemiplegia: Feasibility study. *Arch. Phys. Med. Rehabil.*, 56(12): 507–573, 1975.

42. Baker, L. L., Yeh, C., Wilson, D., and Waters, R. L. Electrical stimulation of wrist and fingers for hemiplegia patients. *Phys. Ther.*, 59(12): 1495–1499, 1979.

43. Chaco, J. and Wolf, E. Subluxation of the glenohumeral joint in hemiplegia. *Am. J. Phys. Med.*, 50(3): 139–143, 1971.

44. Smith, R. O., and Okamoto, G. A. Checklist for the prescription of slings for the hemiplegic patient. *Am. J. Occup. Ther.*, 35(2): 91–95, 1981.

45. DeVore, G., and Denny, E. A sling to prevent a subluxed shoulder. *Am. J. Occup. Ther.*, 24(8): 580–581, 1970.

46. Steverson, B. The Steverson sling for the flaccid hemiplegic. *Am. J. Occup. Ther.*, 27(1): 44–46, 1973.

47. Ferreri, J., and Tumminelli, J. A swivel cockup splint-type armtrough. *Am. J. Occup. Ther.*, 28(6): 359, 1974.

48. Iveson, E., Phillips, M., and Ream, W. D. A removable armtrough for wheelchair patients, *Am. J. Occup. Ther.*, (5): 269, 1972.

49. Enstrom, J., and Davies, J. Labboard modification to help support a flaccid upper extremity. *Phys. Ther.*, 60(6): 795–796, 1980.

50. Basmajian, J. V. *Muscles Alives: Their Functions Revealed by Electromyography.* 4th ed. Baltimore: Williams & Wilkins, 1979.

51. Basmajian, J. V., Regenos, E. M., and Baker, M. P. Rehabilitating stroke patients with biofeedback, *Geriatrics*, 32: 85–88, 1977.

52. Najenson, T., Yacubovich, E., and Pikielni, S. S. Rotator cuff injury in shoulder joints of hemiplegic patients. *Scand. J. Rehab. Med.*, 3: 131–137, 1971.

53. Jensen, E. M. The hemiplegic shoulder. *Scand. J. Rehab. Med.*, Suppl. 7: 113–119, 1980.

54. Neuhaus, B. E., *et al.* A survey of rationales for and against hand splinting in hemiplegia. *Am. J. Occup. Ther.*, 35(2): 83–90, 1981.

55. Charait, S. A comparison of volar and dorsal splinting of the hemiplegic hand. *Am. J. Occup. Ther.*, 22(4): 319–321, 1968.

56. Zislis, J. M. Splinting of hand in a spastic hemiplegic patient. *Arch. Phys. Med. Rehabil.*, 45(1): 41–43, 1964.

57. Kaplan, N. Effect of splinting on reflex inhibition and sensorimotor stimulation in treatment of spasticity. *Arch. Phys. Med. Rehabil.*, 43(11): 565–569, 1962.

58. Louis, W. Hand splinting: Effect on the afferent system. *Am. J. Occup. Ther.*, 16(3): 144, 1962.

59. Brennan, J. B. Response to stretch of hypertonic muscle groups in hemiplegia. *Br. Med. J.*, 1(5136): 1507–1507, 1959.

60. Bell, E., Jurek, K., and Wilson, T. Hand skill measurement: A gauge for treatment. *Am. J. Occup. Ther.*, 30(2): 80–86, 1976.

61. Baumgarten, J. Hands on: Stroke importance of physiological screening to occupational therapy assessment. *Physical Disabilities Specialty Section Newsletter*, 3(3): 1–2, 1980. Rockville, Md., American Occupational Therapy Association.

62. Anderson, E. K. Sensory impairments in hemiplegia. *Arch. Phys. Med. Rehabil.*, 52(7): 293–297, 1971.

63. Gersten, J., Jung, A., and Brooks, C. Perceptual deficits in patients with left and right hemiparesis. *Am. J. Phys. Med.*, 51: 79–85, 1972.

64. Ornstein, R. *The Psychology of Consciousness.* San Francisco: W. H. Freeman, 1972.

65. Fowler, R. S., and Fordyce, W. E. Stroke: Why do they behave that way? (50-035-A) Dallas: American Heart Association, 1974.

66. Vinograd, A., Taylor, E., and Grossman, S. Sensory retraining of the hemiplegic hand. *Am. J. Occup. Ther.*, 16(5): 246–250, 1962.

67. Marmo, N. A new look at the brain damaged adult. *Am. J. Occup. Ther.*, 28(4): 205, 1974.

68. Anderson, E., and Choy, E. Parietal lobe syndromes in hemiplegia: A program for treatment. *Am. J. Occup. Ther.*, 24(1): 13–18, 1970.

69. Siev, E., and Freishtat, B. *Perceptual Dysfunction in the Adult Stroke Patient.* Thorofare, N.J.: Charles B. Slack, 1976.

70. Nemec, R. E. Effects of controlled background interference on test performance by right and left hemiplegics. *J. Consult. Clin. Psychol.*, 46(2): 294–297, 1978.

71. Teuber, H. L. Alterations of perceptions after brain injury. In *Brain and Conscious Experience.*, edited by J. C. Eccles. New York: Springer-Verlag, 1966.

72. Lorenze, E. J., and Cancro, R. Dysfunction in visual perception with hemiplegia: Its relation to activities of daily living. *Arch. Phys. Med. Rehabil.*, 43: 514–517, 1962.

73. Fox, J. Cutaneous stimulation: Effects on selected tests of perception. *Am. J. Occup. Ther.*, 18(2): 53–55, 1964.

74. MacDonald, J. C. An investigation of body scheme in adults with cerebral vascular accidents. *Am. J. Occup. Ther.*, 14(2): 75–79, 1960.

75. Geschwind, N. Disconnection syndromes in animals and man. Part II. *Brain*, 88: 585–644, 1965.

76. Diller, L. Perceptual and intellectual problems in hemiplegia: Implications for rehabilitation. *Med. Clin. North. Am.*, 53(3): 575–583, 1969.

77. Hein, A., and Held, R. A neural model for labile sensorimotor coordination. In *Biological Prototypes and Synthetic Systems Proceedings*, Vol. I, edited by E. Bernard and M. R. Kare. New York: Plenum, 1962.

78. Weinberg, J. *et al.* Visual scanning training effect on reading-related tasks in acquired right brain damage. *Arch. Phys. Med. Rehabil.*, 58(11): 479–486, 1977.

79. Fordyce, W. E., and Jones, R. H. The efficacy of oral and pantomime instructions for hemiplegic patients. *Arch. Phys. Med. Rehabil.*, 47(10): 676–680, 1966.

80. Diller, L., and Weinberg, J. Differential aspects of attention in brain-damaged persons. *Percept. Mot. Skills*, 35: 71–81, 1972.

81. Weisbroth, S., Esibill, N., and Zuger, R. R. Factors in the vocational success of hemiplegic patients. *Arch. Phys. Med. Rehabil.*, 52(10): 441–446, 486, 1971.

82. Bouchard, V. C. Hemiplegic exercise and discussion group. *Am. J. Occup. Ther.*, 26(7): 330–331, 1972.

83. Fugl-Meyer, A. R., and Joasko, L. Post-stroke hemiplegia and sexual intercourse. *Scand. J. Rehab. Med.* Suppl 7: 158–166, 1980.

84. Trombly, C. Effects of selected activities on finger extension of adult hemiplegic patients. *Am. J. Occup. Ther.*, 18(6): 233–239, 1964.

85. Stern, P. H. *et al.* Effects of facilitation exercise techniques in stroke rehabilitation. *Arch. Phys. Med. Rehabil.*, 51(9): 526–531, 1970.

86. Inaba, M., *et al.* Effectiveness of functional training, active exercise, and resistive exercise for patients with hemiplegia. *Phys. Ther.*, 53(1): 28–35, 1973.

87. Andrews, J. M. Neuromuscular re-education of the hemiplegic with the aid of the electromyograph. *Arch. Phys. Med. Rehabil.*, 45(10): 530–532, 1964.

88. Johnson, H., and Garton, W. H. Muscle re-education in hemiplegia by use of electromyographic device. *Arch. Phys. Med. Rehabil.*, 54(7): 320–322, 1973.

89. Brudny, J., *et al.* EMG feedback therapy: Review of treatment of 114 patients. *Arch. Phys. Med. Rehabil.*, 57(2): 55–61, 1976.

90. Lehmann, J. F., *et al.* Stroke: Does rehabilitation affect outcome? *Arch. Phys. Med. Rehabil.*, 56(9): 375–382, 1975.

Supplementary Reading

Brinkmann, J. R., and Hoskins, T. A. Physical conditioning and altered self-concept in rehabilitated hemiplegic patients. *Phys. Ther.*, 59(7): 859–865, 1979.

Cailliet, R. *The Shoulder in Hemiplegia.* Philadelphia: F. A. Davis, 1980.

Goldman, H. Improvement of double simultaneous stimulation perception in hemiplegic patients. *Arch. Phys. Med. Rehabil.*, 47(1): 681–687, 1966.

Haaland, K. Y., Porch, B. E., and Delaney, H. D. Limb apraxia and motor performance. *Brain Language*, 9: 315–323, 1980.

Heilman, K. M., Schwartz, H. D., and Geschwind, N. Defective motor learning in ideomotor apraxia. *Neurology, 25*: 1018–1020, 1975.

Heilman, K. M., and Valenstein, E. Mechanisms underlying hemispatial neglect. *Ann. Neurol., 5*(2): 166–170, 1979.

Johnstone, M. *Restoration Of Function in the Stroke Patient.* New York: Churchill Livingstone (Longman Group Ltd.), 1978.

Keane, W. Occupational therapy for the hemiplegic patient. *Nurs. Mirror,* Aug. 9: 69–73, 1974.

Lehmann, J. F. Lower limb orthotics. In *Orthotics Etcetera*, 2nd ed. edited by J. B. Redford. Baltimore: Williams & Wilkins, 1980.

Luria, A. R. *The Man with A Shattered World.* New York: Basic Books, 1972.

Parent, L. H. (ed). *Cerebral Vascular Accident and Brain Damage 1947-1976: American Journal of Occupational Therapy.* Rockville, Md.: American Occupational Therapy Association, 1978.

Schultz, D. W. Despite hemiplegia, dentist returns to practice, thanks to innovative NYU program. *N.Y.S. Dental J.,* October: 335–337, 1978.

Strike Back at Stroke (50-024-A). *Up and Around* (50-026-A). *Do it Yourself Again* (50-005-A). Dallas: American Heart Association.

Taylor, M., Schaeffer, J. N., Blumenthal, F. S., and Grisell, J. L. Perceptual training in patients with left hemiplegia. *Arch. Phys. Med. Rehabil., 52*(4): 163–169, 1971.

Warren, M. Relationship of constructional apraxia and body scheme disorders to dressing performance in adult CVA. *Am. J. Occup. Ther., 35*(7): 431–437, 1981.

Wilson, D. J. Training for daily living: Occupational therapy in rehabilitation of patients with CVA. *Qual. Rev. Bull., 4*(11): 12–14, 1978.

Wilson, D., and Caldwell, C. B. Central control insufficiency III. Disturbed motor control and sensation: A treatment approach emphasizing upper extremity orthoses. *Phys. Ther., 58*(3): 313–320, 1978.

Yu, J. Functional recovery with and without training following brain damage in experimental animals: A review. *Arch. Phys. Med. Rehabil., 57*(1): 38–41, 1976.

chapter

16

Degenerative Diseases

Anna Deane Scott, M.Ed., OTR

Degenerative diseases involve pathology which leads to progressive disability. This chapter will describe the evaluation and treatment of representative degenerative diseases commonly seen in rehabilitation programs. Multiple sclerosis is representative of diseases in which cerebellar signs of ataxia and intention tremor are often prominent. Parkinson's disease is representative of basal ganglia disorders with rigidity and resting tremor. Amyotrophic lateral sclerosis is representative of lower motor neuron diseases in which muscle weakness is the outstanding problem.

Evaluation is done to determine the deficits in each area of function. Periodic reevaluations are done in order to determine any changes. In these disorders, changes tend to be declines in function, except that there may be gains initially when treatment begins. The goal of treatment is to delay the degenerative effects of the disease and to maintain a level of function. Treatment is directed toward management of existing symptoms, prevention of deformity, and compensation for lost abilities to maintain independence in occupational performance tasks.

MULTIPLE SCLEROSIS

Multiple sclerosis, or disseminated sclerosis, involves patches of demyelination in the white matter of the brain and/or spinal cord followed by the overgrowth of glial cells which form sclerotic plaques creating focal lesions of the central nervous system. It usually begins between the ages of 20 and 40 years. Although the cause remains unknown, some related factors have been identified and much of the current literature reflects continuing research efforts to identify the cause.[1] Multiple sclerosis is more prevalent in Canada, northern Europe, and northern United States. There is a familial tendency to develop the disease, but the explanation for this appears to be common exposure to an environmental factor rather

than heredity.[2] Some precipitating factors include influenza and upper respiratory tract infections, pregnancy, surgery, tooth extraction, and electric shock. Current theories regarding etiology suggest that multiple sclerosis could be a rare sequel of a childhood viral infection, because patients with multiple sclerosis have a high antibody titer to measles and herpes viruses.[1] It is suspected that a virus in childhood with a long latency period is activated by a secondary factor later in life and that multiple sclerosis is an autoimmune reaction which attacks the myelin.[2, 3] However, there is still not enough evidence to confirm either a viral cause or that multiple sclerosis is an autoimmune reaction.[1, 2]

The disease may have an acute onset with several focal lesions in a short time (visual field defects, double vision, numbness of the face or parts of the extremities, weakness of a lower extremity) or the onset may be subacute, usually involving slowly progressive lower extremity weakness and sensory loss with a spastic and ataxic gait. Lesions continue to develop after onset and are predominantly located in the brain stem, where cranial nerve nuclei and motor and sensory pathways can be affected; in the fasciculus cuneatus, causing losses of proprioception and stereognosis; and in the cerebellum, resulting in problems of incoordination. The course of the disease may be acute or malignant with rapid decline of function, or it may progress slowly. Remissions and relapses are a feature of the disease, and the intervals between episodes are highly variable.[1]

Symptoms depend on the location of the plaques or areas of demyelination, but some symptoms are more common. Motor weakness with spastic paraparesis may progress to paraplegia. Spinal cord involvement affects the lower extremities more than the upper extremities. Decreased position sense and response to vibration, numbness, and paresthesia are frequently seen. Visual impairment may include optic neuritis, decreased acuity, blurring and, occasionally, field defects. Brain stem involvement also contributes to visual problems of diplopia and nystagmus as well as bulbar problems of dysarthria and dysphagia. Ataxia may be related to posterior column or cerebellar involvement. With cerebellar involvement intention tremor and dysmetria frequently occur. There may be bladder retention, urgency or incontinence, but bowel incontinence is less often a problem.[2, 4] Cerebral signs of hemiparesis, convulsions, aphasia, and homonymous hemianopsia[5] may be seen, as well as frontal lobe signs of mild dementia with loss of judgment and loss of recent memory.[4] Fink and Houser[6] found that intellectual loss in multiple sclerosis, particularly in the areas of memory and abstract reasoning, was directly correlated with physical loss. Emotional lability with sudden laughter or crying may occur, or denial may be evidenced by lack of awareness of symptoms, by euphoria as a form of denial, or by withdrawal.[7] Others who are more aware may be anxious, depressed, or irritable.

Evaluation

Evaluation must be carefully done and possible symptoms inquired for, because the patients are often "peculiarly unhelpful" and may pay little attention to focal symptoms as a result of denial. Euphoria may cause a sense of well-being with resultant lack of recognition of changes in physical status.[1] Evaluation includes determination of muscle strength, range of motion, endurance, sensation, muscle tone, balance and coordination, visual field, swallowing, memory and judgment, psychological reactions, and functional performance of daily life tasks. Specific evaluation procedures are described in chapters on evaluation throughout this book or may be found in other chapters by using the index. Fatigue should be avoided[1] during both evaluation and treatment because relapses are related to anxiety and exhaustion.[8] Rests during evaluation and the avoidance of unnecessary changes in position will help prevent fatigue and ensure valid and reliable evaluation results.[9]

Many rating scales have been devised to record the degree of disability in multiple sclerosis. These scales aid in evaluation, reevaluation, predicting the course of the disease or the prognosis, determining effectiveness of treatment in delaying progression of disability, and in comparison of patients with diverse symptoms by use of a numerical score.

The McAlpine and Compston grading scale for recording the degree of disability in multiple sclerosis is as follows.

Grade 1: Unrestricted. Without restriction of activity for normal employment and domestic life but not necessarily symptom free.

Grade 2: Restricted. Able to walk unaided for up to ½ mile and able to use public transportation.

Grade 3: Markedly Restricted. Capable of moving out of doors with difficulty for up to a ¼ mile, usually with the aid of sticks, often unable to use public transportation.

Grade 4: Mobile at Home. Able to move with difficulty about the house with support from furniture; unable to climb stairs.

Grade 5: Immobile at Home. Confined to a chair or wheelchair.

Grade 6: Bedridden. Required assistance for nearly all activities.

This categorization is useful, but is unsatisfactory for noting small changes which do not result in a change of grade.[8]

Kurtzke[10, 11] developed a more detailed scale with 10 grades based on scores in eight functional systems. The Disability Status Scale is a composite of performance in the eight functional areas. The reader is referred to the original articles for the more detailed charts of the functional systems and grading criteria. An adapted form of the Disability Status Scale[10, 11] is as follows.

Disability Status Scale in Multiple Sclerosis

0—Normal neurologic examination
1—No disability and minimal signs, such as Babinski sign or vibratory decrease
2—Minimal disability, for example, slight weakness or mild gait, sensory, visual-motor disturbance
3—Moderate disability though fully ambulatory (for example, monoparesis, moderate ataxia, or combinations of lesser dysfunctions)
4—Relatively severe disability, though fully ambulatory and able to be self-sufficient and up and about for some 12 hours a day
5—Disability severe enough to preclude ability to work a full day without special provisions. Maximal motor function: walking unaided no more than several blocks
6—Assistance (canes, crutches, or braces) required for walking
7—Restricted to wheelchair but able to wheel self and enter and leave chair alone
8—Restricted to bed but with effective use of arms
9—Totally helpless bed patient
10—Death due to multiple sclerosis

Kurtzke et al.[12] studied the medical records of 476 patients with a definite diagnosis of multiple sclerosis and 51 patients with a probable diagnosis and used the Disability Status Scale to establish early predictors of the later course of the disease. Symptoms at onset were not predictive of the later course of the disease, but the status 5 years after onset was found to be highly predictive. Pyramidal and cerebellar scores were the most significant predictors of the later course of multiple sclerosis together with the number of functional systems affected. Patients with pyramidal and cerebellar signs at 5 years after onset showed severe impairment at 10 and 15 years after onset, and involvement of these two systems is indicative of a poor prognosis.

Other evaluation scales have been devised to meet the requirements of different settings. Pedersen[13] described a rating scale that is simple to use and to localize defects. Areas of evaluation include mental state, visual function, sphincter function, upper extremities, lower extremities, and personal efficiency. Fog[14] devised a numerical rating scale in which a point value is given for each sign on the scale and an overall score is determined.

Because so many areas of function are involved in multiple sclerosis, evaluation is a team effort including the neurologist, urologist, psychologist, and therapists in each discipline. The occupational therapist evaluates upper extremity function and areas of occupational performance.

Interpretation of evaluation results enables the therapist to describe deficits and list problems. It is also important to recognize assets which can be used in training the patient to compensate for losses and to maintain a level of functioning.

Treatment

As in evaluation, treatment planning for patients with multiple sclerosis is also a team effort because of the many areas of involvement. Treatment goals must be realistic and directed toward relief of the debilitating effects of existing problems, prevention of additional problems such as deformities or decubiti, and maintenance of a level of function by means of compensatory aids and techniques.

It is important to avoid muscle fatigue, which can lead to decreased muscle strength. Avoidance of fatigue will influence the scheduling of treatment by all members of the team in a rehabilitation setting. Fatigue is more evident in the afternoon, when a rest period may be advisable.[8] Increased body temperature due to infections, sun, or heat must also be avoided because exacerbation of the disease process can result.[15] Psychological support is important in all rehabilitation programs,[15] and it has been noted that patients with multiple sclerosis respond favorably to the interest and encouragement involved in all therapy.[8] For acute exacerbations the treatment of choice is essentially no treatment with complete bedrest and avoidance of all exertion.[16]

Decreased muscle strength resulting from the disease process cannot be significantly improved and is often associated with spasticity, but decreased strength resulting from disuse can be increased.[15] Activities to increase muscle strength follow the principles of maximal resistance or less than maximal resistance to stress the muscle. In multiple sclerosis, however, fatigue must be strictly avoided, and this precaution is observed in selecting and supervising both the resistance and duration of activities. When physicians and physical therapists consider braces for lower extremity weakness, weight of metal braces must be considered. Plastic materials offer lightweight support[15] of assistance to ambulation for some patients.

Spasticity is a significant problem for which many therapeutic measures have been tried but for which there is no universally effective treatment. Physicians have prescribed Valium and have found it to be effective in some cases.[15] Nerve blocking agents have been used by others, but Block and Kester[15] report little success with this means. Daily active or passive range

of motion through the full range at each joint[15, 16] with gentle stretching of tight muscles[9] together with splinting to maintain range or provide a slight stretch[16] are the currently used therapeutic means of preventing contractures from muscle weakness and/or spasticity.

Prevention of decubiti is another important goal of treatment. Trauma, heat, cold, and especially pressure should be avoided on skin areas where there is sensory loss. Changing position at least every 2 hours is recommended.[15] A wheelchair cushion relieves some pressure, and push-ups in the wheelchair provide a change of position.[16] Turning in bed[16] or use of a water bed if decubiti are present are suggested.[15]

Compensation for problems of incoordination include a wide base of support in standing, and a weighted cane or walker[15] may be recommended by the physical therapist. For the upper extremity, weight cuffs may slow down extraneous movement.[15] Stabilizing the proximal extremity to help gain distal control may be effective. The upper arms can be held against the sides of the body or against the sides of the wheelchair, or the elbows can be rested on the table with hands free and efforts toward controlled movement limited to the distal part. Another means of stability is to hold one wrist with the other hand for fine activities such as writing. Hewer et al.[17] studied the effect of the use of a weighted wrist cuff on 50 patients with intention tremor due to a variety of neurological diagnoses. They found a therapeutic benefit from reduction of intention tremor in 36% of the patients. The amount of weight used was between 480 gm (1 lb.) and 600 gm (1 lb. 5 oz.) with the amount increased in proportion to the severity of the tremor. Increased weight above an optimum value produced no further decrease in tremor, increased tremor in some patients, reduced limb function when there was weakness, and increased fatigue even when there was no weakness. Chase et al.[18] studied the effect of cooling an intention tremor in 13 patients and found that cooling the extensor surface of the forearm markedly reduced intention tremor in eight of these patients. A 0° C water bottle was applied on the extensor surface between 7 and 30 minutes. One patient, after 30 minutes of cooling, was tremor free for 30 minutes. Neither cooling the flexor surface nor warming either surface reduced tremor, and warming of the extensor surface increased tremor in almost half of the patients tested.

Mobility and transfers are also important problem areas to consider when planning treatment. Mobility in bed includes learning to turn over in bed and to come to a sitting position. Side rails or a rope attached to the end of the bed may be helpful. A standard wheelchair may need a high back, a reclining back, or projections on the wheel rims or, for the severely disabled, an electric wheelchair may need to be selected. Transfers are practiced to maintain a level of independence and to encourage some standing if lower extremity involvement permits weight bearing or walking short distances. Bathroom transfers may be difficult or hazardous. When lower extremities are weak or spastic, a raised toilet seat makes it easier to get up from sitting. Grab bars assist in the safety of transfers, and a tub seat or shower stall chair is often essential. For severe disabilities a mechanical lift may be needed by family members to transfer the patient.[15]

Aids are available to assist the patient in compensating for deficits that limit independence in self-care. Weighted utensils for eating may reduce the effects of tremor if incoordination is a problem. Built up handles are useful if grasp is weak.[15] Adapted or specially designed clothing or shoes, a reacher[15], and practice in dressing techniques may be helpful. Other aids to independence may be needed for problems in writing, phoning, page turning, or other activities of interest or importance to the patient. When limitations are more severe, the use of mechanical aids increases and environmental controls for television, radio, lights, and other electronic devices may be needed.[15]

Independence out of the home can be assisted by car hand controls. The possibility of decreased judgment resulting from euphoria and denial must be considered when evaluating the patient's safety for driving. If the degree of disability does not permit the patient to continue work in the same occupation, prevocational exploration will be necessary. If job retraining is required,[15] the rehabilitation counselor may be able to obtain funding through the state department of vocational rehabilitation.

Other problems are varied and require efforts of different team members. For speech and swallowing problems, some improvement can be expected from resistive exercises to the muscles of the face, neck, and tongue. Speech therapy has been successful in increasing volume and promoting clearer pronunciation.[15] Encouragement regarding speaking is helpful as well as recognition that the effort of speaking may be tiring.[16] For diplopia a patch over one eye is suggested to eliminate the problem of a double image; this is functionally beneficial, even at the sacrifice of depth perception.[15, 16] Nursing is primarily responsible for bladder and bowel programming. The social worker, psychologist, or others may work with family support groups[15] and patient groups where sharing of experiences and reactions with others is beneficial.[16] Sexual problems are frequently found with spinal cord involvement. Sexual counseling should be available for those who desire it. Informing the patient's spouse of the effects of the disease and compensatory methods for sexual satisfaction are suggested.[16]

Abrams[9] reported increases in muscle strength, endurance, range of motion, and the performance of daily life tasks of many patients in a group of 100 patients with multiple sclerosis treated at Wilmington Medical Center for 3 weeks of hospitalization. The magnitude of the change and results of follow-up to note long term effects were not reported. The physical therapy program included hydrotherapy to relax muscles and to assist active exercise of weak muscles, although a temperature above body temperature was avoided because it is fatiguing; passive stretching to increase range of motion; active coordination exercises to correct poor habits of posture and gait, including

use of the stationary bicycle; training in transfers and ambulation with bracing as needed; breathing exercises; and resistive exercises for increasing strength. Patients were discharged with a home program to help maintain gains. In the hospital and at home, frequent rest periods were emphasized to avoid fatigue.

Many theories on etiology have been proposed, but none have as yet been proven.[16] One treatment program based on a theoretical concept of causality is described by Russell and Palfrey,[8] who reported positive results utilizing a program of rest and exercise (R.E.P.) in the treatment of multiple sclerosis. The program is based on the hypotheses that circulatory insufficiency in the white matter of the brain and spinal cord causes or influences the formation of lesions and that increased circulation would reduce the ischemia in these areas. The R.E.P. involves two to three rest periods of 10 to 20 minutes each during the day, with stressful exercises carried out before, or sometimes after, the period of rest. Exercises are often done on a mat and involve the upper extremities, which encourages increased circulation in the upper spinal cord and brain stem. Push-ups are considered to be a good exercise unless there is lumbar pain or considerable weakness. Weight lifting in a supine position is also used. The effort of the exercise, according to this theory, should produce dyspnea, an increased heart rate, and flushing of the skin on the face, head, and neck as evidence of increased circulation. Patients who are to be placed on the program are admitted to the hospital for 1 week. The first 24 hours are spent resting, and on the 2nd day the program is started and graded during the rest of the week to the level which is to be continued at home. The program is adapted to the degree of disability and may include running, cycling, sports, or gardening. Sixty-nine new cases of multiple sclerosis who had not received other kinds of treatment and who graded above grade 5 on the McAlpine and Compston grading scale were placed on a R.E.P. and followed for 2 to 8 years. With initiation of the program, a majority of the patients improved quickly to a significant degree. One of the most encouraging results of the study, however, related to the long-term effects. The condition of patients who had had many relapses before starting the program became static or benign as soon as the R.E.P. began. Although patients gradually declined in grade as charted each year over a period of years, the rapid decline to grades 4, 5, and 6 that usually occurs in 2 years with a malignant form of multiple sclerosis did not occur. It appears that the R.E.P. has a possible beneficial effect on the occurrence of relapses which cease, occur less frequently, or leave less residual disability when the program is persistently followed. Getting patients to readjust their daily schedules and faithfully follow the program has met with some difficulties. Those who make rapid improvements may think that they are well again and stop the exercises, and others with severe disabilities show little interest in treatment concerned only with prevention of further deterioration. Some patients with multiple sclerosis lack the self-discipline necessary to conscientiously follow the R.E.P., but for those who follow it, it appears to offer the potential that their disease will become benign with a less rapid course of decline of function.

The hypothesis of the R.E.P. program is interesting, and although successes have been reported by the group that originated the theory, reports of further studies of effectiveness are needed. Other beneficial treatments have been found. Some physicians have reported improvement of symptoms with spinal stimulation of the dorsal column. The use of cold to lower body temperature to 0.2°F to 1.3°F (−17.6°C to −17.05°C) has been found to improve symptoms.[16] Some success has been noted with the use of electrical stimulation for muscle reeducation.[16]

In any degenerative disease of unknown etiology, delay of the degenerative effects of the disease remains the primary treatment objective while efforts continue to discover the cause and/or more effective treatment methods.

The National Multiple Sclerosis Society has helpful literature, and local chapters offer many services to assist patients and their families in direct care, education, and referral to community resources.

PARKINSON'S DISEASE

Parkinson's disease is caused by degeneration of neurons in the substantia nigra. Pathways run from the substantia nigra to the globus pallidus, and degeneration of the substantia nigra reduces its neuronal influence on the globus pallidus resulting in the symptoms of parkinsonism. Infections or toxic agents may also cause this disorder.[1] Onset usually occurs between 40 and 70 years of age with no preferences for sex, race, or climate.[2] The symptoms of parkinsonism include a nonintention tremor, rigidity, bradykinesia (difficulty initiating movement), impairment of the righting reflexes, a gait with short steps and lack of arm swing, and autonomic disorders such as drooling, excessive sweating, greasy skin, bladder dysfunction, and flushing of the skin.[19, 20] The gait characteristics of stooped posture, short steps, lack of arm swing, slowness of movement, and a shuffling gait result from rigidity.[21] The stooped posture results from the fact that rigidity is more prominent in the flexor muscles of the trunk and extremities.[2] Muscles of the face are also involved with resultant lack of facial expression and reduced eye movements. There may be difficulty swallowing.[4] Speech is characteristically monotone with low volume.[22] Speech problems parallel motor problems with lack of emotional expression, tremulousness, and blocking.[21] A propulsive or festinating gait may develop in which the patient walks faster and faster as though to keep up with the center of gravity.[2, 21] Some patients have rapid explosive speech similar to the festination of gait.[21] Rigidity, bradykinesia, and tremors are the major symptoms,[4, 19] but in some patients, rigidity and bradykinesia may be more prominent than tremor.[1] Although the course of untreated Parkinson's disease involves progressive deterioration

to complete immobility and death, the rate of deterioration varies from 2 years to up to 20 years.[1, 20] Hoehn and Yahr[22] have found that patients with tremor as the major symptom have a better prognosis than patients with rigidity and slowness of movement.

Evaluation

The selection of evaluation procedures to be completed is based on knowledge of typical symptoms. Evaluation data is then gathered to enable the therapist to list the problems of a given patient. The purpose of evaluation is to identify the symptoms present and the extent to which they interfere with function. In Parkinson's disease, standard evaluations include range of motion, muscle tone, righting reactions, coordination, mobility and self care. The presence and severity of tremor, rigidity, and bradykinesia should be noted.

Wroe and Greer[20] devised a functional evaluation for Parkinson's disease which involves recording the time involved and manner of performance of selected activities of bed mobility, transfer, ambulation, repeated opposition, writing, and vital capacity. Voice taping of speech production and movies of gait patterns were also part of the evaluation to measure progress or regression.

Hoehn and Yayr[22] used the following scale as a means of recording degree of disability and rate of progression.

Stage I. Unilateral involvement only, usually with minimal or no functional impairment.

Stage II. Bilateral or midline involvement, without impairment of balance.

Stage III. First sign of impaired righting reflexes. This is evidenced by unsteadiness as the patient turns or is demonstrated when he is pushed from standing equilibrium with the feet together and eyes closed. Functionally, the patient is somewhat restricted in his activities but may have some work potential, depending upon the type of employment. Patients are physically capable of leading independent lives, and their disability is mild to moderate.

Stage IV. Fully developed, severely disabling disease; the patient is still able to walk and stand unassisted but is markedly incapacitated.

Stage V. Confinement to bed or wheelchair unless aided.

Because this rating scale is not operationally defined, it is a subjective rating.

Webster[21] devised a more detailed rating scale for the purpose of summarizing results of evaluation in 10 areas of impairment. Items in each area are sequenced in the typical progression of disability, and an overall quantitative score can be determined. The scale is as follows.

Parkinson's Disease Rating Scale

Apply a gross clinical rating to each of the 10 listed items, assigning value ratings of 0–3 for each item, wherein 0 is equated to no involvement, and 1, 2, and 3 are equated to early, moderate, and severe disease, respectively. Refer to the article for details of the examination and operational definitions of the ratings. (Note: Some of these examination procedures are summarized here at the end of the form).

Bradykinesia of Hands (Including Handwriting). 0, no involvement; 1, detectable slowing of the supination-pronation rate evidenced by beginning difficulty in handling tools, buttoning clothes, and with handwriting; 2, moderate slowing of supination-pronation rate, one or both sides, evidenced by moderate impairment of hand function. Handwriting is greatly impaired, and micrographia is present; 3, severe slowing of supination-pronation rate. Unable to write or button clothes. Marked difficulty in handling utensils.

Rigidity. 0, nondetectable; 1, detectable rigidity in neck and shoulders. Activation phenomenon is present. One or both arms show mild, negative, resting rigidity; 2, moderate rigidity in neck and shoulders. Resting rigidity is positive when patient is not on medication; 3, severe rigidity in neck and shoulders. Resting rigidity cannot be reversed by medication.

Posture. 0, normal posture. Head flexed forward less than 4 inches; 2, beginning arm flexion. Head flexed forward up to 6 inches. One or both arms raised but still below waist. 3, onset of simian posture. Head flexed forward more than 6 inches. One or both hands elevated above the waist. Sharp flexion of hand, beginning interphalangeal extension. Beginning flexion of knees.

Upper Extremity Swing. 0, swings both arms well; 1, one arm definitely decreased in amount of swing; 2, one arm fails to swing; 3, both arms fail to swing.

Gait. 0, steps out well with 18- to 30-inch stride. Turns about effortlessly. 1, gait shortened to 12- to 18-inch stride. Beginning to strike one heel. Turn around time slowing. Requires several steps; 2, stride moderately shortened (now 6 to 12 inches). Both heels beginning to strike floor forcefully; 3, onset of shuffling gait, steps less than 3 inches. Occasional stuttering-type of blocking gait. Walks on toes (turns around very slowly).

Tremor. 0, no detectable tremor found; 1, less than 1 inch of peak-to-peak tremor movement observed in limbs or head at rest or in either hand while walking or during finger-to-nose testing; 2, maximum tremor envelope fails to exceed 4 inches. Tremor is severe but not constant, and patient retains some control of hands; 3, tremor envelope exceeds 4 inches. Tremor is constant and severe. Patient cannot get free of tremor while awake unless it is a pure cerebellar type. Writing and feeding himself are impossible.

Facies. 0, normal. Full animation. No stare; 1, detectable immobility. Mouth remains closed. Beginning features of anxiety or depression; 2, moderate immobility. Emotion breaks through at markedly increased threshold. Lips parted some of the time. Moderate appearance of anxiety or depression. Drooling may be present. 3, frozen facies. Mouth open ¼ inch or more. Drooling may be severe.

Seborrhea. 0, none; 1, increased perspiration, secretion remaining thin; 2, obvious oiliness present. Secretion much thicker; and 3, marked seborrhea, entire face and head covered by thick secretion.

Speech. 0, clear, loud, resonant, easily understood; 1, beginning of hoarseness with loss of inflection and resonance. Good volume and still easily understood; 2, moderate hoarseness and weakness. Constant monotone, unvaried pitch. Beginning of dysarthria, hesitancy, stuttering, difficult to understand; 3, marked harshness and weakness. Very difficult to hear and to understand.

Self-Care. 0, no impairment; 1, still provides full self-care but rate of dressing is definitely impeded. Able to live alone and often still employable; 2, requires help in certain critical areas, such as turning in bed, rising from chairs, etc. Very slow in performing most activities but manages by taking much time. 3, continuously disabled. Unable to dress, feed himself, or walk alone.

The total score is then determined and interpreted.[21]

1–10: Early illness
11–20: Moderate disability
21–30: Severe disability

Examination procedures necessary for completion of the form are summarized from Webster's[21] article as follows.

Bradykinesia and Handwriting. Rapid alternating supination-pronation, as in testing dysdiadochokinesia, is used. Handwriting may also become slow with progressively smaller letters.

Rigidity. Rigidity in the neck is tested by passive flexion, extension, and rotation. Activation phenomenon is the presence of rigidity in one arm when the other arm is in active use, for example, wrist rotation (rigidity may be present with this test but not otherwise). Negative rigidity is smooth movement. In positive resting rigidity, there is definite resistance to passive movement.

Posture. Head position is the number of inches the occiput is in front of the most posterior body part. Stiffening of the trunk and gradually progressive elbow flexion are noted.

Upper Extremity Swing. Observed when patient is walking.

Gait. The patient is asked to walk approximately 15 feet, turn around, and return.

Tremor. Maximum distance of tremor excursion in both directions combined is observed and estimated.

Facies. Observations are made during conversation and at rest.

Seborrhea. Inquiry concerning frequency of shampooing may reveal the presence of oiliness.

Speech. Evaluate during normal conversation.

Self-Care. Asking the patient is the suggested means of evaluation.

Ackmann et al.[23] studied parkinsonian tremor by means of telemetry with a transducer attached to the patient's wrist or metacarpophalangeal (MP) joint for measurement of motion. They found that tremor is increased by stress, decreased by fatigue, and eliminated during sleep. The telemetry system together with computerized summaries of the recordings provides an objective measurement of tremor and is suggested for use in assessing treatment effectiveness.

Burke et al.[24] studied parkinsonian rigidity by means of EMG. They state that they found no basic difference in spindle activity between a normal subject during voluntary muscle contraction and a parkinsonian patient, although there was a difference when the normal subject was relaxed. This indicates that rigidity represents an inability to relax, controlled by higher motor centers rather than a deficit of the reflex mechanism.

Treatment

It has been found that dopamine (a catecholamine) is deficient in patients with parkinsonism,[1, 20] upsetting the chemical balance between the catecholamines and acetylcholine, an excitatory neurotransmitter. The administration of levodopa (L-dopa) to restore this balance has been found to be an effective drug in the treatment of parkinsonism. It is particularly effective in decreasing bradykinesia and rigidity,[1, 19, 20] but ameliorates all symptoms to some degree.[25-27] L-dopa does, however, have side effects which include gastrointestinal symptoms such as nausea, vomiting, and anorexia; cardiovascular changes such as dizziness, orthostatic hypotension, and irregularities of heart beat; and central nervous system symptoms such as involuntary dyskinetic movements, mental confusion, agitation, depression, and drowsiness.[20, 25, 28] Therapists who work with these patients daily must be alert to the possible side effects, observe behavior carefully, and report changes which might otherwise be missed.[25]

In a study of 50 patients with parkinsonism, Wroe and Greer[20] described a program of therapeutic exercises administered in conjunction with the use of L-dopa in treatment. The goal of treatment was to improve speed, mobility, and coordination. Lack of muscle strength was not found to be a problem. Active exercises following proprioceptive neuromuscular facilitation (PNF) patterns and the use of specific PNF techniques of rhythmic initiation and slow reversal were found to be effective in improving the ability to initiate movement, control movement direction, and decrease the cocontraction seen in rigidity. Neck and trunk rotation exercises were done to increase mobility and improve balance. Grasping an object while exercising was found to be effective in reducing tremor. Maintained stretch of upper extremity flexors by hanging from an overhead bar and active exercise involving prone extension, particularly horizontal abduction, were done to help correct the typically flexed posture of these patients. Breathing exercises and gait training were also included in the program. A graded program which stressed mobility was found to be effective, whereas heavy resistance was found to decrease mobility.[20] Additionally, group activities increased socialization and improved motivation toward independence.[20, 29]

It is important for both the patient and the family to understand the patient's problems and treatment program. The lack of facial expression and slowness of movement can be misinterpreted as lack of interest or stubbornness without the kind of understanding that counseling the family can provide.

Stefaniwsky and Bilowit[28-30] studied the influence of sensory stimuli on the speed of initiation of motion. Ten patients with Parkinson's disease and five normal subjects participated in the study. The time which elapsed between application of the stimulus and initiation of motion and the time elapsed between the stimulus and completion of 90° of elbow flexion and of elbow extension of the dominant arm were measured. Electromyographic readings were also taken to record action potentials. Stimuli used included a light, a click, a shout, and a touch on the shoulder. All subjects completed the eight tests to establish a base line. The patients were then placed on an exercise program in which the same stimuli were used for initiation of movement for 3 weeks. Then posttest scores were determined. There was a significant difference between the means of pretest and posttest scores of the patients on seven of the eight tests. When compared to normal subjects on the pretest, the patients scored significantly below the normal subjects, but there was no significant difference on the posttest. This study supports the use of sensory stimuli to increase speed of initiation of movement. Improvement was noted in other areas of performance with improved speech and ambulation in all patients. It was suggested that the interest and attention that the patients received in the course of the experiment were important factors in promoting improvement.

Although sensory stimuli were found effective in the above study, Hagbarth and Eklund[31] found that the use of vibration in patients with parkinsonism increases tremor and may also decrease performance of alternating movements.

Knott[32] reports that a technique called "pumping up" or "rhythm" exercise enabled a patient with parkinsonism to initiate activity and complete movement with greater speed. In this technique, the part to be used is moved passively through the range of the pattern to be used in the activity several times; then the patient assists in the rhythmical movement and after several more repetitions, resistance to the pattern is applied. When used before self-care activities which were difficult for the patient, "pumping up" enabled successful performance, and after several days the "pumping up" would be omitted. Rhythm of performance of other activities was emphasized as well as speed in the initiation and completion of movements. The application of cold compresses to promote relaxation is also recommended by the PNF approach to treatment.

Stockmeyer[33] describes application of the Rood approach to the treatment of parkinsonism to encourage protective responses of the face, to increase proximal mobility, and to decrease distal tremor. Mobility of the neck and trunk must be developed to permit the head to lead in body movements and to permit the quick position changes in equilibrium reactions. Vinegar or ammonia are used to activate facial muscles. Acceleration, deceleration, and rotation are used to stimulate the semicircular canals for mobilization of the neck and trunk. Rocking may be used, but horizontal movement is more facilitatory to rotation. Grasp of an object is used to facilitate distal stability for reduction of tremor.

Activities in occupational therapy involving active motion stressing mobility and rapid rhythmic movements rather than resistance would seem to be most appropriate. Music may be used to help establish and maintain a rhythm. Neck and trunk rotation with mobility of the proximal upper extremities could be incorporated in activities where reach on a horizontal plane is required by the activity. Many activities, such as leather punching and hammering, involve resisted grasp and could be selected for reduction of distal tremors. Resistance to proximal muscles, however, must be avoided to prevent an increase in rigidity. Tactile, visual, or auditory stimuli and "pumping up" as described could be used to see if they contributed to increased speed in self-care and other activities. Not to be overlooked is the beneficial effort of interest and attention which active participation in a well-planned and well-supervised program provides.

Although no studies have been reported, it would be interesting to try biofeedback and/or meditation to see if relaxation of the mind has any effect on relaxation of rigidity since higher centers are involved.

As more research is being done to determine the nature of the neurological deficit in parkinsonism and the mechanisms of motor control, therapeutic procedures can be based on these new findings, and their application can be tested clinically.

AMYOTROPHIC LATERAL SCLEROSIS

Amyotrophic lateral sclerosis (ALS), or motor neuron disease, is a progressive degenerative disease that involves upper and lower motor neurons and may include brain stem involvement.[34] Nerve cells are lost in the anterior horn, brain stem, and motor cortex, and there is degeneration of the corticospinal tracts.[2] Onset is usually between ages 40 and 60, and it affects men twice as frequently as women.[4] The course of the disease is rapidly progressive, and in the majority of cases, death occurs in 2 to 6 years.[2] Mulder and Howard[35] noted that 20% of their cases lived 5 years or more, and they describe a rare case in which remission occurred. The prognosis depends on the location of paralysis. Persons with bulbar involvement, atrophic or spastic, have the poorest prognosis, followed by those with spinal atrophic paralysis and then those with spastic involvement without bulbar signs.[36] Onset at an older age with early bulbar involvement and rapid progression of symptoms indicates a poor prognosis.[37] The will to live and family support are other significant factors affecting longevity.[35] The etiology is unknown but possibilities include a virus, autoimmune disease, and toxicity from lead or mercury.[4]

Early symptoms include muscle weakness with atrophy, cramping, and fasciculations.[4] Initial involvement may be in the hands, in the lower extremities, or in the shoulders. In the hands, the thenar and hypothenar eminences, as well as the interossei, atrophy.[4] Finger extensors become weakened before the flexors.[2] In the lower extremities, foot drop progresses to weakness of the gastrocnemius and quadriceps muscles. If initial weakness is in the shoulders, involvement gradually spreads distally.[4] Early weakness of neck musculature may accompany shoulder weakness.[34] In some patients, the upper extremities may become almost useless while the patient is still ambulatory.[2] No matter where it begins, weakness spreads quickly to other muscle groups, and corticospinal tract signs develop: spasticity and hyperactive tendon reflexes[4] with presence of clonus.[38] The triad of upper extremity weakness, lower extremity spasticity and hyperreflexia throughout, and the absense of sensory loss lead to certainty regarding this diagnosis.[2] In some patients, bulbar signs occur initially, and rapid progression occurs.[4] Bulbar signs result from weakness of cranial nerve-innervated musculature[34] with symptoms of difficulty speaking, coughing, swallowing, and breathing.[4, 34] These problems are the eventual cause of death from respiratory insufficiency or aspiration of secretions or food.[4, 34] Pseudobulbar palsy from brain stem upper motor neuron involvement may occur and results in symptoms of a positive sucking reflex, hyperactive gag reflex,[34] and emotional lability with mood swings and outbursts of crying.[34, 38]

Evaluation

Evaluation includes assessment of degree of disability in all areas of potential involvement. In ALS, these evaluations include range of motion, muscle strength, muscle tone, mobility and transfers, self-care, and communication. Feeding is carefully assessed to include ability to chew and swallow as well as other problems associated with dysphagia. Equipment the person already uses should be noted, and needs for additional adapted devices and equipment should also be noted.

Sinaki and Mulder[39] describe stages they have found helpful in assessment of the overall level of disability as follows.

Stage I—The patient is ambulatory and he is able to care for himself and accomplish the activities of daily living. There is mild weakness or clumsiness of the musculature.
Stage II—The patient has moderate weakness in selected muscle groups. For example, such a patient may have mild foot drop on one or both sides. He often has difficulty climbing stairs, elevating his arms, or using his hands—especially for fine activities such as buttoning garments.
Stage III—The patient is ambulatory but has severe weakness in selected muscle groups. Such a patient often has severe foot drop and pronounced weakness and atro-

phy of the intrinsic muscles of the hand. He is often unable to rise from a chair without help.

Stage IV—The patient's illness has progressed sufficiently that he is confined to a wheelchair, but he remains almost independent. These patients have severe weakness of the lower extremities, with mild involvement of the upper extremities.

Stage V—The patient is in a wheelchair and is dependent. There is pronounced weakness of the lower extremities and moderate or pronounced weakness of some of the muscle groups of the upper extremities.

Stage VI—The patient is bedridden. He is unable to perform any of the useful activities of daily living or of self-care and needs maximal assistance.

These stages do not include bulbar signs which may be present in any stage.[39] The otolaryngologist and speech therapist often evaluate bulbar and pseudobulbar signs. Tongue weakness results in difficulty moving the tongue from side to side and out or in.[34] There may also be atrophy and fasciculations in the tongue.[4] There can be weakness of the facial musculature of the lips and cheeks as well as of the muscles of mastication. The palate and pharynx may be weakened, and pseudobulbar signs of a gag reflex, sucking reflex, and jaw jerk may be elicited.[34] Speaking, swallowing, and, eventually, airway obstruction which contributes to difficulty in respiration all result from bulbar involvement.[39]

Speech is dysarthric,[40] and there are articulation errors due to weakness of the lips, tongue, and jaw.[34] Difficulty in phonation or sound production[2] resulting from laryngeal involvement[2,34] and nasality of speech resulting from palatopharyngeal weakness[2] occur.

Dysphagia is also associated with bulbar and pseudobulbar palsy.

Treatment

Treatment planning depends on recognition of existing symptoms and anticipation of the effects of rapid degeneration. Treatment is individualized because the initial symptoms and the degenerative process are highly variable, but potential needs should be anticipated, especially when purchasing expensive equipment.[39] Goals include maintaining full range of motion and preventing contractures, maintaining muscle strength, avoiding fatigue, and promoting independence in all areas of functional performance.

Active and/or passive range of motion is always necessary when there is muscle weakness. Active and active assistive exercises can be combined with passive range of motion to provide strengthening exercises as well as range of motion, depending on the amount of weakness or limitation in a given motion. For problems of muscle weakness, Sinaki and Mulder[39] recommend against strenuous exercises for involved muscles to avoid fatigue which could increase the amount of weakness, but Norris et al.[38] have found resistive exercises of involved muscles to be beneficial. Orthotic devices are useful for upper and lower extremity weakness. Hand splints for wrist support and/or thumb opposition improve hand function, and foot drop

splints of lightweight plastic have been found to be helpful in ambulation.[39] Arm splints or sling supports can relieve painful stretch on weak shoulders.[39] Mobile arm supports can be attached to the wheelchair to compensate for proximal weakness in the upper extremities.

Assistive devices for self-care and independence in other areas of function can incorporate the use of biomechanical principles. Levers to reduce the force required may be helpful, for example, a lever-type water faucet, a wooden extension on a key, or a clothespin on the knob of a lamp. Other aids appropriate to problems of muscle weakness can be found in the chapter on self-care. Aids for transfers and mobility include adjustable height chairs for ease in getting up from a sitting position, a standard wheelchair for long distance and, eventually, an electrically powered wheelchair.[39] Environmental controls can be used for lights, television, and other electronic devices.

For problems of verbal communication, speech therapy can be of assistance initially.[39] Compensatory methods may become necessary when speech is severely involved. An electrolarynx may be helpful for voice amplification,[39,40] or aids which substitute for speech may be needed such as a magic slate for writing,[39] a communication board with useful phrases,[39,40] or even a signal system using eye blinks[40] or electronic communication aids.

Patients with swallowing deficits may be unable to swallow saliva, and suctioning may be needed.[39] Medications intended to dry up secretions have been reported to alleviate the problem in the majority of cases seen by Norris et al.[38] while Sinaki and Mulder[39] report an increase in secretions in their experience. Methods to compensate for swallowing deficits have been useful when treatment is ineffectual in changing functional ability. A long-stemmed spoon permits food to be placed far back in the pharynx to increase ease of swallowing.[39] Blended, finely chopped foods[38] or formula diets[39] have been recommended. Tube feeding may eventually become necessary by means of a gastrostomy[39] or a cervical esophagostomy.[38]

Psychological support is recognized as an important part of any treatment program and is essential for patients with degenerative diseases.

CONCLUSION

For any other degenerative diseases, the process involved in treatment planning follows the same sequence. First, the disease process is studied to determine the possible cause and symptoms. Then, evaluations selected on the basis of potential symptomatology are done, and a treatment program is planned which will help to correct problems noted. Reevaluations are done periodically to measure the effectiveness of treatment and to record changes. Finally, it is important to keep up with advances in research on causes and beneficial treatment programs and to report any treatment found to be effective.

References

1. Bannister, R. *Brain's Clinical Neurology*, 4th ed. London: Oxford University Press, 1973, pp. 390–395, 248–253.
2. Adams, R. D., and Victor, M. *Principles of Neurology.* New York: McGraw-Hill, 1977.
3. Dean, G. The multiple sclerosis problem. *Sci. Am., 223*(1): 40–46, 1970.
4. Gilray, J., and Meyer, J. S. *Medical Neurology*, 3rd ed. New York: Macmillan, 1979.
5. Kahana, E., Leibowitz, U., and Alter, M. Cerebral multiple sclerosis. *Neurology, 21*(12): 1179–1185, 1971.
6. Fink, S. L., and Houser, H. B. An investigation of physical and intellectual changes in multiple sclerosis. *Arch. Phys. Med. Rehabil., 47*(2): 56–61, 1966.
7. Weinstein, E. A. Behavioral aspects of multiple sclerosis. *Mod. Treatment, 7*(5): 961–968, 1970.
8. Russell, W. R., and Palfrey, G. Disseminated sclerosis: Rest-exercise therapy—A program report. *Physiotherapy, 55:* 306–310, 1969.
9. Abrams, H. M. A comprehensive physical therapy program for the treatment of multiple sclerosis patients. *Phys. Ther., 48*(4): 337–341, 1968.
10. Kurtzke, J. F. On the evaluation of disability in multiple sclerosis. *Neurology, 11*(8): 686–694, 1961.
11. Kurtzke, J. F. Further note on disability evaluation in multiple sclerosis, with scale modifications. *Neurology, 15*(7): 654–661, 1965.
12. Kurtzke, J. F., Beebe, G. W., Nagler, B., Kurland, L. T., and Auth, T. J. Studies on the natural history of multiple sclerosis. 8. Early prognostic features of the later course of the illness. *J. Chron. Dis., 30*(12): 819–830, 1977.
13. Pedersen, E. A rating system for neurological impairment in multiple sclerosis. *Acta Neurol. Scand. 41*(Suppl 13, Part II): 557–558, 1965.
14. Fog, T. A scoring system for neurological impairment in multiple sclerosis. *Acta Neurol. Scand. 41*(Suppl 13, Part II): 551–555, 1965.
15. Block, J. M., and Kester, N. C. Role of rehabilitation in the management of multiple sclerosis. *Mod. Treatment, 7*(5): 930–940, 1970.
16. Schneitzer, L. Rehabilitation of patients with multiple sclerosis. *Arch. Phys. Med. Rehabil., 59:* 430–437, 1978.
17. Hewer, R. L., Cooper, R., and Morgan, M. H. An investigation into the Value of Treating Intention Tremor by Weighting the Affected Limb. *Brain, 95:* 579–590, 1972.
18. Chase, R. A., Cullen, J. K., and Sullivan, S. A. Modification of intention tremor in man. *Nature, 206:* 485–487, 1965.
19. Herbison, G. J. H-reflex in patients with parkinsonism: Effect of levodopa. *Arch. Phys. Med. Rehabil., 54:* 291–295, 301, 1973.
20. Wroe, M., and Greer, M. Parkinson's disease and physical management. *Phys. Ther., 53*(8): 849–854, 1973.
21. Webster, D. D. Critical analysis of the disability in Parkinson's disease. *Mod. Treatment, 5*(2): 257–282, 1968.
22. Hoehn, M. M., and Yahr, M. D. Parkinsonism: Onset, progression, and mortality. *Neurology, 17*(5): 427–442, 1967.
23. Ackmann, J. J., Sances, A., Jr., Larson, S. J., and Baker, J. B. Quantitative evaluation of long-term Parkinson tremor. *IEEE Trans. Biomed. Eng., 24*(1): 49–56, 1977.
24. Burke, D., Hagbarth, K-E, and Wallin, B. G. Reflex mechanisms in parkinsonian rigidity. *Scand. J. Rehabil. Med., 9:* 15–23, 1977.
25. Blonsky, E. R. The changing picture of parkinsonism. Part 1. Neurological modifications resulting from administration of L-dopa. *Rehabil. Lit., 32*(2): 34–37, 1971.
26. Gersten, J. W., et al. External work of walking and functional capacity in parkinsonian patients treated with L-dopa. *Arch. Phys. Med. Rehabil., 53*(12): 547–553, 1972.
27. Peterson, C. R., et al. Quantitative analysis of the effects of L-dopa on gait in 26 patients with parkinsonism. *Phys. Med., 51*(4): 171–181, 1972.
28. Meunter, M. D., and Tyce, G. M. L-dopa therapy of Parkinson's disease: Plasma L-dopa concentration, therapeutic response, and side effects. *Mayo Clin. Proc., 46*(4): 231–239, 1971.
29. Minnigh, E. C. Changing picture of Parkinsonism. Part II. The Northwestern University concept of rehabilitation through group physical therapy. *Rehabil. Lit., 32*(2): 38–39, 50, 1971.
30. Stefaniwsky, L., and Bilowit, D. Parkinsonism: Facilitation of motion by sensory stimulation. *Arch. Phys. Med. Rehabil., 54:* 75–77, 1973.
31. Hagbarth, K-E., and Eklund, B. The effects of muscle vibration in spasticity, rigidity, and cerebellar disorders. *J. Neurol. Neurosurg. Psychiatry, 31:* 207–213, 1968.
32. Knott, M. Report of a case of parkinsonism treated with proprioceptive facilitation technics. *Phys. Ther. Rev., 37*(4): 229, 1957.
33. Stockmeyer, S. A. An interpretation of the approach of Rood to the treatment of neuromuscular dysfunction. *Am. J. Phys. Med., 46*(1): 953–954, 1967.
34. Carpenter, R. J., McDonald, T. J., and Howard, F. M. The otolaryngologic presentation of amyotrophic lateral sclerosis. *Otolaryngology, 86*(3; Part 1): 479–484, 1978.
35. Mulder, D. W., and Howard, F. M. Patient resistance and prognosis in amyotrophic lateral sclerosis. *Mayo Clin. Proc., 51:* 537–541, 1976.
36. MacKay, R. P. Course and prognosis in amyotrophic lateral sclerosis. *Arch. Neurol., 8:* 117–127, 1963.
37. Boman, K., and Meurman, T. Factors influencing the prognosis of amyotrophic lateral sclerosis. *Acta Neurol. Scand., 43*(Suppl. 31): 176–177, 1967.
38. Norris, F. H., Sang, K., Denys, E. H., Archibald, K. C., and Lebo, C. Letter: Amyotrophic lateral sclerosis. *Mayo Clin. Proc., 53*(8): 544–545, 1978.
39. Sinaki, M., and Mulder, D. W. Rehabilitation techniques for patients with amyotrophic lateral sclerosis. *Mayo Clin. Proc., 53*(3): 173–178, 1978.
40. Adams, M. R. Communication aids for patients with amyotrophic lateral sclerosis. *J. Speech Hearing Dis., 31*(3): 274–275, 1966.

chapter

17

Closed Head Injuries

Patricia L. Weber, M.S., OTR

A head injury is usually caused by a dynamic loading or impact to the head from direct blows or from sudden movements produced by impacts to other body parts. This loading can result in any combination of compression, expansion, acceleration, deceleration, or rotation of the brain inside the skull.[1, 2] Pressure waves in the cerebral spinal fluid, produced by the movement of the cranial contents upon impact, can cause cavitation of the brain. Actual stretching or tearing of neural structures, brain white matter, or vascular structures may occur.[1, 3] A rotational component is believed essential for diffuse brain injury, whereas translation of the head leads to focal lesions at the site of impact (coup) or on the opposite side of the brain (contrecoup).[1, 2, 4, 5]

The brain may also suffer contusions or lacerations as it is moved by the impact across or into the bony prominences of the skull, i.e., the sphenoid wings, the petrous bones, or the orbital bones. Such contusions commonly involve the poles of the temporal and frontal lobes, the undersurfaces of the temporal lobes,[1, 2, 6] and the orbital cortex.[5] The occipital and parietal lobes, covered by smooth skull surfaces, are less likely to incur damage. The edges of the dural membranes can also cause damage to the brainstem or the superior surface of the cerebellum.[7]

The skull may fracture from the force of the impact. The type of fracture depends upon the force of the blow and ranges from a simple linear fracture to a stellate fracture and, lastly, to a depressed skull fracture which is frequently seen and is the result of the most forceful blow.[1, 2, 6] A basilar skull fracture, occuring 25% of the time,[6] frequently involves the petrous portion of the temporal bone and thus can result in cranial nerve damage. Cranial nerves I, V, VII, and VIII are frequently damaged in head injuries, because of their position and course within the skull.[7]

Secondary effects of the head injury can occur immediately or develop within hours or days.[2, 5] Trauma can abolish or disrupt autoregulation of cerebral blood flow, the blood-brain barrier, and vasomotor functions resulting in intracranial hypertension, arterial spasm, and increases in intracranial pressure (ICP) and in cerebral edema.[1, 8] Other secondary effects of head trauma include intracranial hemorrhage, uncal herniation resulting in brainstem compression, general systemic reactions to the neural impairment, electrolyte abnormalities, altered respiratory regulation, or abnormal autonomic nervous system responses.[2, 9, 10]

The patient with a head injury from a motor vehicle accident or a fall may have other systemic trauma, such as fractures of the limbs or clavicles, cervical fractures with possible spinal cord injury, abdominal trauma, or pneumothorax or other chest cavity trauma. He might also have had a craniotomy for evacuation of an epidural or subdural hematoma.

Head injury can produce a number of states of altered consciousness. The least ominous, concussion, entails a brief period of unconsciousness lasting from minutes to hours, with only transient abnormal neurological signs at most[11] and transient posttraumatic amnesia (PTA). PTA refers to the time after the accident before the return of continuous memory.[12] Contusion, actual bruising of the brain, occurs with most head injuries and can involve a loss of consciousness which varies in length. Severity of head injury has been classified according to length of coma,[13] motor picture,[14] or length of PTA. Mild to moderate head injury has been defined as entailing a PTA of under 24 hours; severe head injury, a PTA of over 24 hours but under 1 month; and prolonged unconsciousness, a PTA of longer than 1 month.[15-17]

Consciousness, unconsciousness, and coma are best viewed on a continuum from complete consciousness to death or complete absence of consciousness. Complete consciousness is defined as an awareness, a cognition of self and the surrounding environment; consciousness implies perception, interpretation of this perception, and an appropriate response.[18] A lesser level of consciousness, "arousal," is a state of wakefulness and attention to the environment on primarily a survival and basic function level. The third level, clouding of consciousness, is a state of reduced wakefulness, reduced clarity of thought with possible confusion, decreased attention span, and memory lapses. The next stage, stupor, involves unresponsiveness from which the person is aroused only by vigorous stimulation. In the unconsciousness stage, the person cannot be aroused by sensory stimulation, has eyes closed, and demonstrates an absence of observable interaction with the environment. If unconsciousness lasts more than a certain period of time, it becomes "coma."[11, 16, 19] However, it is important to realize that coma is not a stable state. A person in a coma can fluctuate spontaneously or from stimulation along the continuum towards, and indeed into, varying levels of consciousness.[18]

Neurological evaluation of a comatose patient to determine the depth of coma usually includes evaluation of motor and sensory responses to noxious stimulation, verbal responses, eye movements, and presence or absence of specific reflexes. Superficial reflexes such as the gag, corneal, and certain skin reflexes are tested, as are other brainstem reflexes such as pupillary reactions and dilatation, and oculovestibular reflexes.[13, 14] Deep tendon reflexes, such as the jaw jerk and knee jerk, are examined. Deep reflexes, normally under partial inhibition by the cerebral cortex, become exaggerated when this inhibition is interrupted.[20] The presence of various pathological reflexes, such as the Babinski, Hoffman's, snouting, ankle clonus, crossed extension, and extensor thrust, is also assessed.[13, 14] These pathological reflexes are primitive defense responses which are normally inhibited by the cerebral cortex and are not normally seen in humans after the age of 5 to 7 months.[20] The presence of such pathological reflexes, especially when seen with absent superficial reflexes and exaggerated deep reflexes, indicates release of lower centers from higher level influence.

Various scales have been proposed to standardize such assessment of depth of coma and the inferred severity of the head injury.[14, 21, 22] The most popular scale currently is the Glasgow Coma Scale (Table 17.1),[13] which assesses the following parameters: eye opening in response to a variety of stimuli, best motor response to pressure on the nail bed, and best verbal response. A modification of this scale, the Maryland Coma Scale (Table 17.2),[23] assesses eye opening, brainstem reflexes, motor performance, orientation, verbal response, and intensity of stimulation necessary to elicit motor and verbal responses. The authors stated that this scale, which excludes untestable responses, may provide a more sensitive assessment of patients with multiple injuries than would the Glasgow Coma Scale. The reader is referred to the original source for detailed testing instructions.

SYMPTOMS

The presenting picture of each patient will be slightly different, as each combination of forces producing a head injury is unique. Also, secondary effects of the damage vary from patient to patient. Possible results of a head injury include paralysis or paresis, spasticity, ataxia, sensory deficits, dysarthria, aphasia, visual field defects, and cognitive and/or perceptual deficits.[24, 25] The length of time which has passed since the injury will influence the symptoms seen by the therapist. Some of the results of a head injury will be obvious in the earlier stages of recovery, while others will not be evident until the latter stages of recovery.

Recovery from a severe traumatic head injury generally follows a recognizable pattern. The patient in a coma first evidences return of awareness of sensory stimuli (first to that of deep pain, then auditory input, cutaneous and kinesthetic stimuli and, lastly, to that of visual input),[26] followed by motor and sensory recovery to varying degrees dependent on the extent of damage and, lastly, the return of cognitive functioning and memory.[5] Najenson et al.[9] investigated the return of communicative functions after traumatic coma and discovered that comprehension precedes the recovery of the motor aspects of speech. Verbal skills usually return before nonverbal or performance skills; the patient may be able to understand more than he can demonstrate. He may be able to correctly identify left and right before he is able to put his shoe on the correct foot.[27, 28] In the process of recovery, not all patients will experience all the levels of coma described here, as some may show initial responses of a higher neurological level. Still other patients may stop at one level and plateau there indefinitely. A patient may also be at a higher level in the morning and regress with fatigue, or he may evidence brief responses of higher level scattered throughout predominantly

Table 17.1
GLASGOW COMA SCALE[a]

Eye opening	Spontaneous	4
	To sound	3
	To pain	2
	Never	1
Motor response	Obeys commands	6
	Localizes stimulus	5
	Flexion normal	4
	Flexion abnormal	3
	Extension	2
	No movement	1
Verbal response	Oriented	5
	Confused	4
	Inappropriate	3
	Incomprehensible	2
	None	1
Responsiveness or coma sum = 3–15 points		

[a] Reprinted with permission from G. Teasdale and B. Jennett.[13]

Table 17.2
NEUROLOGICAL ASSESSMENT: MARYLAND COMA SCALE[a]

Eye Opening		Pupil, Corneal, and Caloric Reflexes and Grimace		Arm Motor Response	
Spontaneously	3	Normal	2	Dextrous and strong	5
To sound	2	Decreased or abnormal	1	Paretic	4
To pain	1	Absent	0	Localizes	3
None	0	Untestable	U	Abnormal flexion	2
Untestable	U			Extension	1
Orientation		Verbal Response		None	0
				Untestable	U
Time, place, person	3	Oriented	4	Leg Motor Response	
2 of the 3	2	Confused	3		
1 of the 3	1	Inappropriate	2	Normal	2
None	0	Incomprehensible	1	Abnormal or extensor	1
Untestable	U	None	0	None	0
Stimulus		Untestable	U	Untestable	U
Voice	3				
Shake or shout	2				
Pain	1				
Central pain	0				

Date																	
Time																	
Sedation meds																	
Paralytic agents																	
Seizures																	
BP																	
HR																	
Resp.																	
Temp.																	
Eye opening																	
Orientation																	
Pupils (R/L)																	
Corneals (R/L)																	
Facial Grimace (R/L)																	
Calorics (R/L)																	
Stimulus																	
Verbal response																	
Arm motor (R/L)																	
Leg motor (R/L)																	

[a] Reprinted with permission from M. Salcman, et al.[23]

lower level neurological responses. The occupational therapy evaluation and treatment differs for each stage of coma.

EVALUATION OF THE COMATOSE PATIENT

The comatose patient may look asleep with his eyes closed, or he may open his eyes spontaneously. Most head injury patients open their eyes spontaneously or to stimulation within the 2nd to 4th week postinjury.[24, 29] Nonpurposeful eye movements or dysconjugate gaze may be present.[25, 30] Primitive automatic responses of facial grimacing, teeth clenching and grinding, and/or rhythmic chewing may occur spontaneously or in response to stimulation.[11] The patient may be breathing on his own or, more likely with prolonged coma, will have a tracheostomy or endotracheal tube and will be assisted by a respirator.

Evaluation of a comatose patient includes assessment of his passive range of motion (PROM), muscle tone, reflex level, coordination, and sensation of the upper extremities, face, jaw, and neck. Through sensory stimulation and observation of the patient's response, his motor and sensory abilities and level of consciousness can be evaluated. Stimulation is applied to muscles on both the right and left sides of the patient's body and his response, if any, is noted. Any spontaneous movements seen are described. Presence of clonus, spasticity, or contractures is also noted. The patient's brain damage may be diffuse, and he may not exhibit a clear "hemiplegic" picture of muscle weakness or tone changes.

A prefeeding evaluation is done if the patient shows some response to stimulation. Cranial nerve VII may have been injured, with resulting paresis or paralysis of facial muscles, lips, some tongue movements, and/or some soft palate movements.[7] This evaluation includes assessment of tone of individual facial muscles, facial sensation, tongue movements in response to stimulation by temperature or touch, external observation of the swallowing process and actions of muscles of the throat, jaw mobility, the gag and bite reflexes, sucking, and chewing ability.[31] Continued presence of an endotracheal tube or nasogastric tube will usually decrease the gag reflex.

Specific evaluations of the patient's self-care skills, sensory deficits, or cognitive/perceptual status must wait until he is responding to stimulation consistently, i.e., the patient must at least be localizing stimuli with one side of his body. However, throughout the stages of recovery, the therapist relies upon observation to infer specific motor, sensory, perceptual, or cognitive deficits.

Motor Responses to Stimulation

Evaluation of muscle tone and reflex levels begins with assessment of the patient's response to stimulation, which in turn indicates the depth of his coma. Patients in the very deepest level of coma will show no observable change in behavior to painful, auditory, temperature, tactile, or proprioceptive stimulation. The motor response will be flaccid. Reflexes are absent. The damage producing this lack of response is thought to be below the vestibular nuclei in the brainstem.[32]

In the next higher level of coma, the patient can respond with a generalized startle to a loud noise, with increased or decreased motor activity to auditory stimulation, or with a generalized motor reflex.[25] This motor reflex, seen in response to internal or noxious external stimulation, is known as decerebrate rigidity or extensor posturing. The patient's legs and arms extend, adduct, and internally rotate; the forearm hyperpronates, the wrist and fingers flex, and the feet plantar flex.[33] This motor picture is thought to be caused by bilateral damage in the midbrain below the red nucleus, sparing the vestibular nuclei; in effect,

removing the midbrain-pontine structures from more rostral neural influences.[11] Spinal level reflexes and lower brainstem reflexes may be seen in their entirety, or might simply be influencing the patient's muscle tone. The vestibular reflexes and postural righting reflexes are usually operable and assist in the production of increased tone in antigravity (extensor) muscles. The tonic neck reflex, grasp reflex, and sucking reflex may also be elicited at this stage of coma.[7]

The third higher level of coma entails a response to stimulation known as decorticate rigidity or flexor posturing. This sterotyped pattern of movement consists of adduction and slight flexion of the shoulder, elbow flexion, forearm pronation, and wrist and finger flexion.[33] The patient's lower extremities extend as in decerebrate rigidity.[30] Flexion of the hip and knee elicited by painful stimulation, known as "triple flexion," is a spinal reflex and indicates damage to the descending motor tracts.[34] This decorticate response is thought to indicate damage in the internal capsule or cerebral hemispheres, causing an interruption in the corticospinal pathways.[11] Midbrain reflexes and automatic movement reactions may be elicited at this stage of coma; the tonic neck reflexes can usually be readily seen also.[7]

The fourth possible motor response to stimulation is withdrawal, which is a more rapid movement than decorticate posturing and includes shoulder abduction.[30] For example, the patient withdraws the entire limb when his hand is stimulated. The patient may also show spontaneous, nonpurposeful movement of his limbs.

The fifth level motor response to stimulation is localization. At this stage, the patient may be said to be "lighter", that is, he is still comatose, but not as deeply. His responses to stimulation are quicker and becoming more appropriate. The patient may reach over and brush the painful stimulation away, move just the part being stimulated, blink to strong light or visual threat, turn toward or away from auditory stimulation, and/or visually track a moving object.[26] Cortical equilibrium reactions or protective extension reactions may be elicited at this stage. According to Finkelstein and Ropper,[34] limb abduction, or movement away from the body midline, is the only movement which is always purposeful and which indicates an intact connection from the cortex to that limb.

The highest level motor response of the patient to stimulation is an appropriate response, i.e., not withdrawing from all touch and stimuli, but only from that which is noxious or irritating, and following simple requests or initiating purposeful activity.

The patient could demonstrate any combination of the above-described responses, depending upon which areas of brain were damaged. For example, he may exhibit decerebrate rigidity with his right limbs and localizing response with his left side. He could exhibit bilateral decerebrate posturing. He may initially evidence decorticate posturing on one side and then sink to decerebrate rigidity or flaccidity on that side, which indicates a deterioration in his condition. He may exhibit hemiplegia on one side and normal muscle tone on the other. Infrequently, cerebellar dysfunction, such as intention tremor or ataxia, is seen.[35]

TREATMENT

Stage I: Absent or Generalized Response to Stimulation

The goal of occupational therapy with the deeply comatose patient, who is flaccid or posturing, is to provide the patient with organized and enhanced stimulation which requests an increasingly higher level motor response from the patient. This patient exhibits little spontaneous response to the environment, so the therapist attempts to organize and heighten the stimuli to increase the chance of a response being elicited.[26] As the patient responds more consistently, the therapist attempts to channel those responses.

Auditory, tactile, olfactory, visual, vestibular, and proprioceptive stimuli are utilized. Organized stimulation periods are done frequently throughout the day for 15 to 20 minutes each, or until a deterioration in the quality of the patient's responses occurs. Stimulation consists of two to three modalities presented in a consistent and meaningful manner, i.e., the patient is told what the therapist is doing and what is expected of him.[26, 36, 37] Verbal feedback is given on every response elicited: "Good, you are pushing your arm forward", or "I feel you pushing, but I want you to push harder." The patient's response to stimulation may be quite prolonged, as CNS processing is slowed by damage sustained, if not prevented altogether. The therapist should wait for a response to the stimulation and, if necessary, repeat the stimulus.

Auditory stimulation consists of tapes of favorite music or familiar voices, bells, loud alerting noises, direct conversation to the patient, and verbal praise and feedback. A normal but firm voice is used with this patient; a comatose patient does not need to be soothed. During therapy sessions, radios, TVs, or other noises should be eliminated as much as possible so that voice commands for motor responses or the selected auditory stimuli are the most prevalent auditory input to the patient.

Tactile stimulation includes rubbing the patient's skin with various textures or temperatures, use of vibration and firm touch to the patient's limbs.[37] The daily bath and other self-care tasks are excellent sources of cutaneous input, especially if verbal orientation to body parts being washed or handled is included.

Olfactory stimulation can be attempted with noxious or pleasant odors such as sulfur, ammonia, vanilla, peppermint, lemon, perfumes, or coffee. However, this cranial nerve is commonly injured in head trauma, and thus olfactory stimulation might not be effective.[7]

Visual stimulation, i.e., brightly colored objects, mobiles over the bed, pictures of family, friends, and the patient or members of the family itself is provided. These objects or people are used to elicit focus and visual tracking by the patient. Environmental changes from the bed to therapy room and appropriate changes in lighting are important sources of visual stimulation.

Vestibular and proprioceptive stimuli are provided by muscle facilitation techniques, body position changes, head movements, tilting the bed to sitting. The various reflexes and reactions seen normally in development can also be used to elicit muscle responses, increase tone, or decrease tone.[9, 37] The neck and cervical area receives special emphasis in treatment, as this area is important in head control and perceptual processes.[37] Vestibular stimulation begins gently, and the patient's response is monitored closely for increased ICP (see Precautions) or blood pressure changes.[38] The comatose patient is told in advance of any body position changes performed passively to decrease the possibility of posturing and other stereotypic reactions. If the stimulation causes an increase of posturing, it is stopped temporarily and resumed after the patient has rested.

Specific facilitation techniques useful with the deeply comatose patient include proprioceptive neuromuscular facilitation (PNF) techniques and patterns, Brunnstrom's flexion-extension synergy patterns of motions, and attempts to elicit any individual muscle action. Such techniques combined with quick stretch, tapping over the muscle belly, joint approximation and the request for an appropriate motor response provide proprioceptive, tactile and, auditory stimulation to the patient. Quick ice to the muscle belly is used to facilitate that muscle (see Chapter 6) or can be used for directionality of motion ("I am going to put ice on your hand. Pull away from the ice") Quick ice is perceived as a distinct noxious stimulus when applied to the face, soles of the feet, or palms.[39] Normal precautions with use of ice are observed (see Chapter 6). If the patient has a weaker side or one which responds to stimulation at a lower neurological level, the other side is worked with first. The patient may only be able to respond in one part of a muscle's range, so the shortened or slightly lengthened positions must each be tried. Verbal instructions to the patient must be consistent and simple. The movement is described as the therapist moves the patient's body through the motion. For example, "Push your arm from here to here (the therapist demonstrates by taking the patient's arm to the points indicated and pausing at each one), from here to here (therapist again demonstrates the spatial location) ready, push!" Since individualized movements will not generally be visible in this stage of coma, the therapist must feel the muscle tone changes which signify the beginnings of a voluntary effort. Such minute changes are best felt if the therapist has maximum cutaneous contact with the patient's arm. For example, to work on an extension synergy pattern or a PNF pattern, the patient's right arm is cradled in the therapist's right arm, his elbow in the crook of the therapist's elbow, his hand in the therapist's palm. Quick stretch can be provided by the therapist's right arm; the therapist's left hand is free to provide the tapping or quick ice to the patient's shoulder or arm muscle. Any increase of pressure due to the patient's attempt to move voluntarily will be felt along the therapist's entire forearm and hand. When giving a quick stretch to initiate a motion, it is difficult to separate that component from a voluntary component occurring also. As the therapist handles the comatose patient and becomes more familiar with his pattern of muscle tone, changes occurring in that muscle tone will be more obvious. Movement or pressure in a range where there was no movement before might represent the beginnings of voluntary movement. A sustained push felt near the end of the range is not likely to be the result of the quick stretch, which elicits a phasic response (see Chapter 5).

These same techniques of quick stretch, icing, and tactile stimulation are used on the facial and oral musculature to provide range of motion (ROM), decrease any hypersensitivity or abnormal reflexes, and promote resumption of normal feeding. Pressure to the tongue and oral stimulation to the gums is done. If the patient has a bite reflex, such stimulation is given on the outside of the mouth and/or teeth. If the patient does not have a hyperactive bite reflex and if he can swallow without aspiration, various tastes of sweet, sour, salty, and bitter can be used as a sensory modality.

PROM, splinting, and/or positioning to prevent or reduce upper extremity contractures or lower extremity foot drop may be necessary.[40] The family of these patients usually indicates its need to be involved in the patient's care, to feel they can do something to promote his recovery.[6] Oddy et al.[41] documented the stress on the patient's family as greatest during the first month postinjury. Family members can be shown simple ROM exercises to do with the patient. The importance of periods of organized sensory stimulation followed by rest is explained to the family. Auditory and tactile stimulation can be provided by the family, as their voices and touch will be more familiar to the patient at first, and may elicit more response than unfamiliar voices.

Precautions

If the patient is within a month of his injury, the therapist must be alert to drastic systemic changes in response to stimulation.[10] A major concern with acute head trauma is control of ICP. Increased ICP above a certain level can be fatal.[10] The patient with an ICP monitor can be readily checked during stimulation sessions; a patient not on a monitor must be closely observed for decreased neurological responses, abnormal brainstem reflexes, flaccidity, pupil changes, behavioral changes, vomiting, or changes in pulse rate, blood pressure, or respiration rate.[5, 10, 38] Fluids may be restricted or the patient's head may be positioned in neutral at 30° elevation in an attempt to regulate his ICP.[10] Turning the patient's head to one side may obstruct the internal jugular vein and result in a sudden increase of ICP. The neck should not be flexed when the patient is positioned on his side.[6, 10] Changes in the patient's blood pressure must also be monitored

and kept within the ranges designated by the physician.

Posttraumatic epilepsy occurs in 5% of patients with head injuries.[2] To reduce the chance of a seizure occurring during treatment, tactile and vestibular stimulation and icing are begun slowly and distally to assess the patient's physiological response. His heart rate, blood pressure, and facial color are monitored, as well as any autonomic changes such as sudden perspiration or increased restlessness. As the therapist becomes more familiar with the patient's responses, intensity of stimulation is gradually increased. A padded tongue blade is kept at the patient's bedside. If a seizure does occur, the therapist should position the patient supinely, insert the padded tongue blade or a rolled towel between his teeth if possible, and summon medical assistance. The patient's limbs should not be restrained during a seizure.

If the patient has had a craniotomy for evacuation of a hematoma, the bone flap may be left off, and the brain may be covered only by scalp to allow the brain room to expand. Direct pressure to this site must be avoided.

The patient may have a tear in the dura with subsequent CSF leak. In this case, the patient is usually treated by observation, precautions against nose blowing, head elevation, and antibiotics.[2]

If the patient has other systemic trauma, such as fractures or chest cavity trauma, appropriate precautions must be taken when stimulating or moving him.

Stage II: Localized Response to Stimulation

The occupational therapy goal is to refine and direct the patient's response to stimulation once the patient begins to respond to stimulation with a more localized response. Such localization is seen when the patient pulls at his nasogastric tube or catheter, or turns his head away when his cheek is stimulated. The therapist attempts to obtain greater consistency in localizing responses and avoiding stereotypic movements, more variety in the response, and a decreased interval between stimulation and response.[26] The therapist also attempts to increase the patient's ability to follow commands, to attend to an activity, and to use common objects such as a spoon, comb, or washcloth.

At this stage of coma, the therapist may be able to more precisely identify motor or sensory deficits by observing the patient's spontaneous repositioning in bed; his periods of restlessness; his motor response to stimuli of light touch, temperature, pain, and proprioception; his facial movements in response to family, friends, or stimuli; or his spontaneous response to, or manipulation of, utensils.

Treatment of motor problems continues using facilitation techniques, resistive exercises, if possible, and sensory stimulation. Mat activities for the developmental stages of head and neck control, rolling, and sitting may be appropriate, if the patient has been able to tolerate these activities in bed. Splinting to control or prevent contractures is continued if necessary.

Rudimentary self-care skills of feeding, face-washing, and light grooming are now begun. Basic self-care tasks are overlearned and may draw automatic responses from the patient. Such tasks are normally relegated to subcortical direction,[37] which may not have been impaired.[5] The attention of the patient is focused on the end result, rather than the process, to tap this subcortical direction.[37] These tasks are done at appropriate times of the day to reduce the patient's temporal confusion and to orient him. Rest periods are essential, as the patient fatigues rapidly. The patient is treated in a quiet environment. Instructions are minimal and consistent, and the variables in the task are reduced because of the patient's distractibility. For example, one dish and one spoon are used in feeding, and the rest of the tray is put out of sight. The complexity, rate of presentation and response, and the duration of the task are decreased until the patient is successful.[26] When he is consistently successful, one of these factors at a time is gradually increased.

Feeding is begun only when the patient has been assessed to have an adequate swallow and strong gag and cough reflexes. If the patient still has a tracheostomy tube, it must be closed before feeding is begun. The patient's nurse should be present at first to check closure of the tube and to assist with any necessary suctioning. During each feeding session, the therapist positions the patient appropriately, decreases the distractions, increases the patient's awareness of chewing and swallowing each bite, and monitors closely for signs of aspiration.[31, 42] The patient is begun on ice chips or popsicles to assess his ability to suck and swallow. If he manages these foods without aspiration, he is progressed to thick cold foods such as ice cream, sherbert, malts, applesauce, and then to pureed or baby foods. Before progressing to foods requiring chewing, the patient's tongue movements are assessed. He must be able to keep food in between his teeth for chewing and then move it to the back of his mouth for swallowing. Head trauma patients may show impulsivity and lack of thorough chewing and thus may be inappropriate for advancement to foods requiring chewing. If the patient is able to bring the spoon up to his mouth with minimum or moderate physical assistance, a more automatic oral response may be elicited.

Cognitive and perceptual functioning cannot be formally evaluated at this point in the recovery process; such functioning must be inferred from the patient's performance of self-care tasks. Observation will indicate if the patient notices visitors or objects on both sides of him or if he exhibits signs of homonymous hemianopsia; if he seems to use objects appropriately or needs to be shown; if he watches the therapist demonstrating usage of objects; if he is able to sustain attention to a specific task; and if his spatial and depth perception appears impaired when reaching for objects.

The patient may still have his eyes closed most of the time. If his eyes are open and tracking, he is usually highly distractible and demonstrates a very short attention span and no memory. The patient will not show carry-over of new learning from treatment session to session. Memory entails encoding an experience, storing it, and then retrieving it. Any or all of these processes can be disrupted by a head injury. The temporal lobes, hippocampus, thalamus, and anterior portions of the limbic area appear to be primarily involved in the encoding of memory,[5, 36] and these are the areas most frequently damaged.[5] The patient with a head injury will usually not remember day-to-day activities consistently until he is able to fairly consistently produce appropriate responses to external stimulation. Until then, he exists in a fugue-like state.

Once the patient begins localizing stimuli, he may become quite agitated and restless as he becomes acutely aware of internal discomfort, pain, and external restraints. The patient will usually tear at tubes and restraints, show decreased ability to cooperate with treatment, and may become aggressive.[43] Not all head trauma patients pass through this phase; those who do may experience this phase for a few days or a few weeks.[43] An appropriately restless or agitated patient has been found to be more likely to show greater improvement than an immobile or sluggishly moving patient.[9, 43]

The goal of occupational therapy during this phase is to decrease the patient's agitation as much as possible, continue focusing his attention on the external environment through engaging his participation in self-care and other "automatic" tasks, and attempt to have the patient follow simple commands. Removal of noxious stimulation, whenever possible, assists in decreasing agitation. Limb restraints are removed during therapy sessions. Inhibitory techniques of repetitive or sustained touch, warmth, rocking, slow rolling, slow vestibular stimulation, and use of the therapist's voice and presence to soothe the patient are helpful.[37, 40] A change of environment to a quieter place with less stimulation; explanation to the patient that this is a stage of recovery which will pass; and continual orientation of the patient to where he is, why, and what the therapist is doing with him can also assist in decreasing his agitation. Acknowledgment of the discomfort and gentle redirection of the patient's attention to tasks is useful.

Treatment continues as in the previous stage with simple self-care tasks, muscle reeducation, and facilitation. The patient will most likely need maximum assistance with self-care tasks, although his agitation may increase his independence in bed mobility. He may also begin transfers now, depending upon his level of muscular involvement.

The patient's orientation may be assessed if he is verbally responsive. However, such assessment should not be pursued if it further agitates the patient. Patients can be aware of their situation early in the recovery process. This awareness may be simply a knowledge that something is wrong even if it cannot be defined, that they should remember something but that they don't. These patients have undergone a total loss of control of their body and actions. Each action is isolated because the patient cannot remember what came before, yet he struggles to make cognitive sense out of each moment. At this point, the patient needs the therapist to provide consistency and predictability, feedback on reality, calmness, acceptance, and consideration of his communications, however nonsensical, inappropriate, or nonverbal. The therapist can gather information on the patient's cognitive status by observing the patient functioning in tasks or by watching his social interactions.

Stage III: Confused and Inappropriate, or Appropriate, Response to Stimulation

As the patient's agitation decreases, he will respond more to the external environment. His responses will be confused and inappropriate at first.[23] This state of confusion may or may not be accompanied by delirium. Later, his response to a given situation may be appropriate, but may still not be completely correct due to poor memory, persistent confusion, dyspraxia, and/or inconsistent orientation.[44]

Assessment of the patient's neuropsychological recovery and the duration of his PTA can begin if the patient can respond verbally in a comprehensible fashion. Most tests are given daily and include questions on basic biographical data, orientation in time and space, last memory before and first memory since the accident, naming of familiar objects, and being asked specifically to remember them the next day.[45, 46] Eson et al.[28] designed a neuropsychological recovery assessment based on development. The first segment covers 0 to 4 years of age and consists of items from infant scales. The second covers 4 to 8 years of age and tests for the ability to note differences and similarities, follow instructions, and organize perceptual arrays. The third section, 8 to 12 years, tests for basic information processing skills, serial organization, right-left discrimination, orientation in space, and selective attention to one perceptual characteristic and inhibition of another. The final segment, mature adaptive function, covers activities necessary for functioning in the community such as following road signs and reading a want ad section.

Occupational therapy goals in this phase are to increase attention span to more specific tasks, increase the process of sequential organization, increase immediate and recent memory, and increase independence in self-care tasks. The therapist continues to structure the patient's environment for him. Variables are reduced to the patient's level of ability, distractions are reduced, and his immediate environment is kept as unchanged as possible.[44, 47]

Treatment consists of continued specific muscle facilitation and/or strengthening exercises, developmental activities for upper extremity stability and mobility phases, and continued self-care tasks of feeding, hygiene, and transfer training. The patient usually continues to require moderate assistance, even if he has only minimal physical deficit, because of cognitive impairment. The therapist is prepared to repeat the task steps over and over, or to rephrase instructions if the patient appears confused.

Cognitively, the patient usually displays severe short-term and long-term memory impairment; he is unlikely to demonstrate carry-over of new learning from day to day but may begin to show carry-over of familiar tasks of self-care.[26] He appears alert but is highly distractible; he does not initiate functional tasks. Jargon, word-finding difficulty, or confabulation may be present.

In treating the cognitive impairment, specific tasks such as discrimination of differences and similarities, matching, copying, sorting, or memory drills of letters or numbers may be utilized.[26, 44, 48] The patient may be asked to verbalize all the steps involved in a specific activities of daily living (ADL) such as making a sandwich, brushing his teeth, or getting ready to go home on a weekend pass. He should be on a reliable schedule of therapy without long periods of inactivity. A written schedule is given to the patient for reference to reduce confusion.

Stage IV: Consistently Appropriate Response to Stimulation

When the patient demonstrates fairly consistent appropriate responses to the external environment, the occupational therapy goals are to gradually decrease the external structuring of the patient's environment, increase his initiation of self-care and other occupational performance tasks, and increase his responsibility for doing those tasks.[26, 28] Participation in the decision-making process of his therapy program is effective.[26] The patient can be made responsible for coming to therapy sessions, following his own exercise program, planning more advanced kitchen activities, etc.

More formal cognitive and perceptual testing and retraining can be done now, as the patient can follow simple directions. His ability to integrate, analyze, or sequence material is assessed.[28] Immediate recall, short- and long-term memory, verbal memory, and visual memory should be evaluated.[15] The results of tests administered by a psychologist, such as the Wechsler Memory Scale, the WAIS, and the Raven's Progressive Matrices, can be helpful in treatment planning.

In this stage of recovery, the patient may demonstrate specific deficits in short- and long-term memory, reasoning, concept formation, abstract thinking, organization of information, simplification of problems, judgment, or problem-solving.[36] He may also demonstrate specific visual perception deficits, apraxia, or other deficits secondary to focal areas of brain damage.

Cognitive retraining emphasizes increasing the patient's ability to concentrate on specific tasks, organize and utilize information, and remember increasing amounts of information. More complex reading and mathematical tasks are given, as well as tasks involving increasing analysis or categorization of information, or increasing abstraction, i.e., proverb interpretation, meaning of stories or poems. Other examples of tasks are sequencing cards depicting an activity such as a picnic or getting ready for school, or sequencing numbers or letters; recognizing items or objects; or the patient's keeping a daily log of events which increases in detail as his memory increases.[26, 44]

The patient may now begin evidencing feelings of denial of his injury, withdrawal, anger, or depression. The therapist can help by letting the patient express his feelings, acknowledging the validity of his feelings, showing empathy, supporting the patient within reason, encouraging him to continue to strive for recovery, remaining accessible to the patient, and avoiding judgmental responses to the patient's expressions of anger or depression.

When self-care tasks and lower level ADLs are being done consistently, the patient must be reintroduced to the community and necessary survival skills. The patient needs to learn how to manage money, write checks, go shopping, do laundry, go to restaurants, and prepare meals; he needs to be able to utilize public transportation, the telephone, and the phone book; he should know the use and care of his equipment or splints; he needs to use crosswalks and obey traffic lights. He also needs to be reintroduced to avocational interests and how to plan his day's activities. Prevocational and/or vocational skills and driver training are taught, if appropriate. The patient can participate in anticipating problems he will face upon returning home and in organizing solutions. Social skills must also be considered and treated, as the postrehabilitation progress of the patient with a head injury depends greatly on his family and other social contacts.[49] Cognitive training concentrates on improving the patient's ability to concentrate on a task to the exclusion of other events or occurrences, improving his memory and cognitive flexibility, and improving his judgment.

As the patient becomes ready to go home, he may still be evidencing a decreased level of response when fatigued, difficulty operating safely in unfamiliar situations, little flexibility in cognitive processing, a shortened attention span, and difficulty in learning new information or tasks.[5, 10] The patient may need continued cognitive rehabilitation after discharge, as recovery in this area has been shown to continue for 2 or more years postinjury.[15, 35, 40, 50] Personality or behavioral changes may also remain, for example, disinhibition, low frustration or stress tolerance, reduced insight or judgment, labile affect, irritability, and impulsivity. These are likely to lead to reduced social activity.[12, 30, 49] The patient may experience paranoia, phobias, confusion, anxiety, or delusional ideation.[15, 25, 51] Mental and emotional deficits have been found to be more difficult to adjust to than are physical deficits[12, 27] and interfere with successful rehabilitation outcomes.[15, 35, 52]

STUDIES OF THE EFFECTIVENESS OF THERAPY

There is very little agreement or evidence concerning when to initiate rehabilitation for comatose patients or for a patient with a closed head injury, or what rehabilitation measures would be included at

various stages of recovery.[47, 53, 54] The available literature on head injury concentrates on the proposed medical treatments and assessment of their efficacy[1, 30] and upon factors predictive of outcome from severe head injury.[24, 30, 35, 43, 52] The studies found which focus on the rehabilitation of such a patient primarily contain statistics on the outcome of patients with this diagnosis correlated to duration of coma or other factors and measured by return to work, social interaction, or degrees of independence in ADLs.[12, 29, 40, 55] These articles contain only the authors' opinions on the usefulness and necessity of rehabilitative measures, and little experimental documentation.

Lewin et al.[35] studied 479 patients who had had a head injury between 10 and 24 years earlier to discover predictive factors of long-term outcome. These authors did not detail the therapeutic procedures utilized, but stated that the rehabilitation units had been "clearly" helpful; however, specific effects of such procedures were not clear. Stover and Zeiger[29] concurred that there was no evidence that rehabilitation initiated in the period of coma decreased the duration of that coma, but still concluded that it was important to begin then to prevent contractures and pulmonary, gastrointestinal, and urinary complications. Rusk et al.[56] found that 46% of the patients studied returned to some form of gainful employment after rehabilitation. These authors decided that severe disability can usually be helped by an intensive rehabilitation program, but did not describe such a program or offer statistics on a control group. Forer and Miller[57] studied progress made by patients with varying diagnoses after discharge from a rehabilitation hospital. It was discovered that head trauma patients did not make significant gains in ADLs after leaving the hospital, but did make significant gains in cognition, speech, and language comprehension.

There are a few authors who have described the rehabilitation programs used with patients and presented statistics on the outcome of that group of patients. Most of these studies had no control groups or other aspects of an experimental design. Najenson et al.[40] studied the outcome of 169 patients with severe head injury who underwent a program utilizing postural reflexes, self-care tasks, locomotor tasks, and communicative training. The statistics presented showed that 84% of the patients were independent in ADLs upon discharge. A follow-up study[52] of 38 of these patients defined the subsequent improvement in locomotor disorders, cognitive performance, communication disorders, behavioral disturbances, and vocational rehabilitation. This study offered statistics supporting the need for continued follow-up of these patients after discharge from a rehabilitation hospital. Rosenbaum et al.[58] described an intensive therapeutic community setting and offered preliminary conclusions. Gerstenbrand[47] described a rehabilitation program beginning in the acute stage after trauma which included use of reflexes to influence muscle tone and more active mobilization and socialization techniques later. He briefly stated his results with 170 patients in terms of being back at work and concluded that rehabilitation at full intensity was essential. Gjone et al.[55] presented statistics comparing the pre- and postrehabilitation neurological signs of 92 patients with severe head injury and concluded that the vast majority had been "cured" or "improved," especially in the areas of paralysis or paresis (92%), spasms or contractures (71%), dysphasia (83%), dysarthria (83%), and ataxia (78%). However, the authors did not describe the exact nature of the rehabilitation program. Brink et al.[25] studied 344 children with severe closed head injury, comatose over 24 hours, who had begun rehabilitation within 3 to 6 weeks postinjury. These authors found that 73% became independent in ambulation and self-care, 10% were partially dependent, and 17% were totally dependent. The nature of the rehabilitation techniques was not described in this article, but presumably has been described in literature from Rancho Los Amigos Hospital Workshops given during the period of time covered by this study.[26] This study also was not based on an experimental design.

One study, using an experimental design, compared patients receiving a rehabilitation program with patients receiving unstructured attention.[28] This study found that the rehabilitation group was back at work much sooner than the other group of patients.

Postlesion experience in a mildly stressful, active environment has been found to be more facilitatory to behavioral and motor recovery than a more neutral, passive environment.[59-61] Other authors have emphasized the increased effectiveness of such experience when begun as soon postinjury as possible.[62, 63] Zinn,[50] in studying the rehabilitation of brain-damaged patients, found a rough correlation between the results of rehabilitation and the intensity of the stimulation and training, as well as the individual patient's ability to absorb and utilize the training. However, he concluded that comparisons between groups of patients requiring rehabilitation could not be made because of the lack of standardized assessment or criteria.

There are experimental studies utilizing control groups which document some of the subtle cognitive deficits caused by a head injury.[4, 15] However, again, there is a paucity of studies investigating efficacy of cognitive retraining with such patients. A few case studies of specific cognitive retraining strategies for patients with head injury are available in the literature.[48, 64]

Even fewer studies have been done exploring the effects of sensory stimulation or therapeutic techniques on comatose patients. McGraw and Tindall[38] found changes in heart rate, respiratory rate, and ICP in 50% of their comatose patient population in response to tactile, auditory, and painful stimulation. No gross movements were noted with these changes, but increased electrical activity was recorded in some patients' cervical muscles. In another study of three comatose patients,[65] significant differences were found in the patients' cortical activity after therapy periods compared to periods of unstructured stimulation and/or activity. The therapy in this study consisted of selected PNF patterns, quick icing, joint approximation, and verbal requests for a motor output.

As is evident, very few controlled studies on patients with head injury or brain damage are available which investigate the time of initiation of rehabilitation, the extent and intensity of rehabilitation necessary, specific procedures utilized, or if these techniques have affected the outcome of the injury.[15, 50] Bach-y-Rita[66, 67] suggested several factors contributing to such a lack of research, including difficulty in finding and matching large numbers of patients by lesion and symptoms, the long-term period of possible recovery from brain damage, the possibility that some recovery occurs because of motivation and a "mind-body" interaction which is difficult to measure and assess, and the difficulty in quantifying and defining the nature of recovery itself. In addition, researchers face the philosophical dilemma of withholding therapy from a control group of patients. However, these difficulties need to be surmounted, and research needs to be conducted on the efficacy of the therapeutic procedures utilized with head-injured patients and their effect upon the long-term outcome of the injury.

Acknowledgment. I wish to acknowledge the contribution of the staff at Rancho Los Amigos Hospital whose workshop gave me a framework by which I could organize my current treatment of the head-injured patient and from which I could expand my thinking for future treatment.

References

1. Bakay, L., and Glasauer, R. E. *Head Injuries.* Boston: Little, Brown, 1980.
2. Feiring, E. H. Management of head injuries. *Compr. Ther.*, 5(1): 53–58, 1979.
3. Walker, A. E. Mechanisms of cerebral trauma and the impairment of consciousness. In *Neurological Surgery*, edited by J. E. Youmans. Vol. 2, Philadelphia: W. B. Saunders, 1973.
4. Richardson, J. T. E. Mental imagery, human memory, and the effects of closed head injury. *Br. J. Soc. Clin. Psychol.*, 18(3): 319–327, 1979.
5. Ommaya, A. K., and Gennarelli, T. A. A physiopathologic basis for noninvasive diagnosis and prognosis of head injury severity. In *Head Injuries, Proceedings of the Second Chicago Symposium on Neural Trauma*, edited by R. L. McLaurin. New York: Grune & Stratton, 1976.
6. Walleck, C. Head trauma in children. *Nurs. Clin. North Am.*, 15(1): 115–127, 1980.
7. Gilroy, J., and Meyer, J. S. *Medical Neurology.* London: MacMillan, 1969.
8. Symon, L. Distribution of pressure within the cranial cavity and its significance. In *Head Injuries, Proceedings of the Second Chicago Symposium on Neural Trauma*, edited by R. L. McLaurin. New York: Grune & Stratton, 1976.
9. Najenson, T., Sazbon, L., Fiselzon, J., Becker, E., and Schechter, I. Recovery of communicative functions after prolonged traumatic coma. *Scand. J. Rehabil. Med.*, 10(1): 15–21, 1978.
10. Raphaely, R. C., Swedlow, D. B., Downes, J. J., and Bruce, D. A. Management of severe pediatric head trauma. *Pediatr. Clin. North Am.*, 27(3): 715–727, 1980.
11. Plum, F., and Posner, J. *The Diagnosis of Stupor and Coma*, 2nd ed. Philadelphia: F. A. Davis, 1972.
12. Oddy, M., Humphrey, M., and Uttley, D. Subjective impairment and social recovery after closed head injury. *J. Neurol. Neurosurg. Psychiatry*, 41(7): 611–616, 1978.

13. Teasdale, G., and Jennett, B. Assessment of coma and impaired consciousness: A practical scale. *Lancet, 2:* 81–84, 1974.

14. Braakman, R., Gelpke, G. J., Habbema, J. D. F., Maas, A. I. R., and Minderhoud, J. M. Systematic selection of prognostic features in patients with severe head injury. *Neurosurgery, 6*(4): 362–370, 1980.

15. Benton, A. Behavioral consequences of closed head injury. In *Central Nervous System Trauma Research Status Report*, edited by G. L. Odom. Bethesda, Md.: National Institutes of Health, 1979.

16. Lewin, W., and Roberts, A. H. Long-term prognosis after severe head injury. *Acta Neurochir. Suppl., 28:* 128–133, 1979.

17. Ommaya, A. K. Indices of neural trauma: An overview of the present status. In *Neural Trauma*, edited by A. Popp, R. S. Bourke, L. R. Nelson, and H. K. Kimelbert. New York: Raven Press, 1979.

18. Arfel, G. Introduction to clinical and EEG studies in coma. In *Handbook of EEG and Clinical Neurophysiology*, edited by R. Harner and R. Naquet. Vol. 12. Amsterdam: Elsevier, 1975.

19. Frowein, R. A. Prognostic assessment of coma in relation to age. *Acta Neurochir. Suppl., 28:* 3–12, 1979.

20. Chusid, J. G. *Correlative Neuroanatomy and Functional Neurology*, 15th ed. Los Altos, Calif., Lange, 1973.

21. Dimov, V., and Anghel, M. The clinical criteria in gravity assessment of acute head injuries associated with coma. *Acta Neurochir. Suppl., 28:* 29–34, 1979.

22. Yen, J. K., Bourke, R. S., Nelson, L. R., and Popp, A. J. Numerical grading of clinical neurological status after serious head injury. *J. Neurol. Neurosurg. Psychiatry, 41*(12): 1125–1130, 1978.

23. Salcman, M., Schepp, R. S., and Ducker, T. B. Calculated recovery rates in severe head trauma. *Neurosurgery, 8*(3): 301–308, 1981.

24. Bricolo, A., Turazzi, S., and Feriotti, G. Prolonged posttraumatic unconsciousness: Therapeutic assets and liabilities. *J. Neurosurg., 52*(5): 625–634, 1980.

25. Brink, J. D., Imbus, C., and Woo-Sam, J. Physical recovery after severe closed head trauma in children and adolescents. *J. Pediatr., 97*(5): 721–727, 1980.

26. Rancho Los Amigos. *Head Trauma Rehabilitation.* Los Angeles: Rancho Los Amigos, 1977.

27. Bond, M. R., and Brooks, D. N. Understanding the process of recovery as a basis for the investigation of rehabilitation for the brain injured. *Scand. J. Rehabil. Med., 8:* 127–133, 1976.

28. Eson, M. E., Yen, J. K., and Bourke, R. S. Assessment of recovery from serious head injury. *J. Neurol. Neurosurg. Psychiatry, 41*(11): 1036–1042, 1978.

29. Stover, S. L., and Zeiger, H. E. Head injury in children and teenagers: Functional recovery correlated with the duration of coma. *Arch. Phys. Med. Rehabil., 57*(5): 201–205, 1976.

30. Heiden, J. S., Small, R., Caton, W., Weiss, M. H. and Kurze, T. Severe head injury and outcome: A prospective study. In *Neural Trauma*, edited by A. J. Popp, R. S. Bourke, L. R. Nelson, and H. K. Kimelberg. New York: Raven Press, 1979.

31. Hargrove, R. Feeding the severely dysphagic patient. *J. Neurosurg. Nurs., 12*(2): 102–107, 1980.

32. Hooper, R. *Patterns of Acute Head Injury.* London: Edward Arnold, 1969.

33. Allen, N. Prognostic indicators in coma. *Heart Lung, 8*(6): 1075–1083, 1979.

34. Finkelstein, S., and Ropper, A. The diagnosis of coma: Its pitfalls and limitations. *Heart Lung, 8*(6): 1059–1064, 1979.

35. Lewin, W., Marshall, T. F. de C., and Roberts, A. H. Long-term outcome after severe head injury. *Br. Med. J., 2*(6204): 1533–1538, 1979.

36. Mahoney, E. K. Alterations in cognitive functioning in the brain-damaged patient. *Nurs. Clin. North Am., 15*(2): 283–292, 1980.

37. Moore, J. C. Neuroanatomical considerations relating to recovery of function following brain lesions. In *Recovery of Function: Theoretical Considerations for Brain Injury Rehabilitation*, edited by P. Bach-y-Rita. Baltimore: University Park Press, 1980.

38. McGraw, C. P., and Tindall, G. T. Cardio-respiratory alterations in head injury: Patients' response to stimulation. *Surg. Neurol., 2:* 263–266, 1974.

39. Stockmeyer, S. An interpretation of the approach of Rood to the treatment of neuromuscular dysfunction. *Am. J. Phys. Med., 46*(1): 900–956, 1967.

40. Najenson, T., Mendelson, L., Schechter, I., David, C., Mintz, N., and Grosswasser, Z. Rehabilitation after severe head injury. *Scand. J. Rehabil. Med., 6:* 5–14, 1974.

41. Oddy, M., Humphrey, M., and Uttley, D. Stresses upon the relatives of head-injured patients. *Br. J. Psychiatry, 133:* 507–513, 1978.

42. De Jersey, M. C. An approach to the problems of orofacial dysfunction in the adult. *Austr. J. Physiother., 21*(1): 5–10, 1975.

43. Reyes, R. L., Bhattacharyya, A. K., and Heller, D. Traumatic head injury: Restlessness and agitation as prognosticators of physical and psychologic improvement in patients. *Arch. Phys. Med. Rehabil., 62*(1): 20–23, 1981.

44. Stichbury, J. C., Davenport, M. J., and Middleton, F. R. I. Head-injured patients—A combined therapeutic approach. *Physiotherapy, 66*(9): 288–292, 1980.

45. Fortuny, L. A., Briggs, M., Newcombe, F., Ratcliffe, G., and Thomas, C. Measuring the duration of post traumatic amnesia. *J. Neurol. Neurosurg. Psychiatry, 43*(5): 377–379, 1980.

46. Levin, H. S., O'Donnell, V. M., and Grossman, R. G. The Galveston orientation and amnesia test: A practical scale to assess cognition after head injury. *J. Nerv. Ment. Dis., 167*(11): 675–684, 1979.

47. Gerstenbrand, F. The course of restitution of brain injury in the early and late stages and the rehabilitative measures. *Scand. J. Rehabil. Med., 4:* 85–89, 1972.

48. Gianutsos, R. What is cognitive rehabilitation? *J. Rehabil., 46*(3): 36–40, 1980.

49. Oddy, M., and Humphrey, M. Social recovery during the year following severe head injury. *J. Neurol. Neurosurg. Psychiatry, 43*(9): 798–802, 1980.

50. Zinn, W. M. Assessment, treatment and rehabilitation of adult patients with brain damage. *Int. Rehabil. Med., 1*(1): 3–9, 1978.

51. Dikmen, S., and Reitan, R. M. Emotional sequelae of head injury. *Ann. Neurol., 2*(6): 492–494, 1977.

52. Groswasser, Z., Mendelson, L., Stern, M. J., Schechter, I., and Najenson, T. Re-evaluation of prognostic factors in rehabilitation after severe head injury. *Scand. J. Rehabil. Med., 9*(4): 147–149, 1977.

53. Evans, C. D. Aspects of recovery from physical disability after head injuries. *Scott. Med. J., 23*(1): 105–106, 1978.

54. Jerva, M. J., and Flanigan, M. M. Early neurosurgical management of the head injured child. *Proc. Inst. Med. Chic., 31*(2): 30, 1976.

55. Gjone, R., Kristiansen, K., and Sponheim, N. Rehabilitation in severe head injuries. *Scand. J. Rehabil. Med., 4:* 2–4, 1972.

56. Rusk, H. A., Block, J. M., and Lowman, E. W. Rehabilitation following traumatic brain damage. *Med. Clin. North Am., 53*(3): 677–684, 1969.

57. Forer, S. K., and Miller, L. S. Rehabilitation outcome: Comparative analysis of different patient types. *Arch. Phys. Med. Rehabil., 61*(8): 359–365, 1980.

58. Rosenbaum, M., Lipsitz, N., Abraham, J., and Najenson, T. A description of an intensive treatment project for the rehabilitation of severely brain-injured soldiers. *Scand. J. Rehabil. Med., 10*(1): 1–6, 1978.

59. Sadka, M. Discussion. In *CIBA Symposium 34, Outcome of Severe Damage to the Central Nervous System.* Amsterdam: Elsevier, 1975.

60. Hewer, R. L. Comments. In *CIBA Symposium 34, Outcome of Severe Damage to the Central Nervous System.* Amsterdam: Elsevier, 1975.

61. Wall, P. D. Discussion. In *CIBA Symposium 34, Outcome of Severe Damage to the Central Nervous System.* Amsterdam: Elsevier, 1975.

62. Walsh, R. N., and Cummins, R. A. Neural responses to therapeutic sensory environments. In *Environments as Therapy for Brain Dysfunction*, edited by R. N. Walsh and W. T. Greenough. New York: Plenum Press, 1976.

63. Teuber, H-L. Recovery of function after brain injury in man. In

CIBA Symposium 34, Outcome of Severe Damage to the Central Nervous System. Amsterdam: Elsevier, 1975.

64. Glasgow, R. E., Zeiss, R. A., Barrera, M., Jr., and Lewinsohn, P. M. Case studies on remediating memory deficits in brain-damaged individuals. *J. Clin. Psychol., 33*(4): 1049–1054, 1977.

65. Weber, P. L. *The Effects of Therapeutic Sensorimotor Intervention on the Cortical Activity of Comatose Patients.* Unpublished Master's Thesis, Boston University, 1980.

66. Bach-y-Rita, P. Brain plasticity as a basis for therapeutic procedures. In *Recovery of Function: Theoretical Considerations for Brain Injury Rehabilitation,* edited by P. Bach-y-Rita. Baltimore: University Park Press, 1980.

67. Bach-y-Rita, P. *Brain Plasticity as a Basis of the Development of Rehabilitation Procedures for Hemiplegia.* Martinez, Calif., VA Medical Center, 1981.

PART EIGHT

Application of Biomechanical Approach

Treatment for commonly seen diagnoses for which the biomechanical approach is appropriate is the topic of this part. This section is intended to assist the reader in the application of the principles of the biomechanical approach to the treatment of orthopedic, cardiac, and lower motor neuron problems. The reader will note that in addition to the application of these principles, each diagnosis has specialized treatment based on the particular signs, symptoms, course, prognosis, and precautions. Only the characteristics of each diagnosis which influence occupational therapy are included.

chapter
18

Hand Therapy

Cynthia A. Philips, M.A., OTR

The recent advances in hand surgery, including microvascular surgery, joint implants, and staged tendon repair, require a specialized approach to patient care. The therapist and the physician must work closely together with the patient in a well-organized therapeutic program. The therapist must have an intimate knowledge of normal hand anatomy and must adhere to the basic principles of wound healing and the choice and timing of basic therapeutic modalities. Careful thought must be given to the biomechanical principles of splinting to ensure that the intended purpose of the splint is fulfilled.

Exercises must be done gently and always within the patient's tolerance. Forced passive motion or painful therapy sets up a vicious cycle of further injury, which increases edema, which leads to further scarring and fibrosis, which leads to greater stiffness. Psychologically, the patient becomes fearful and will not exercise. All this leads to poor results.

Hand therapy should be directed by an experienced therapist who has had specialized hand therapy training. A therapist interested in hand therapy should become proficient in general rehabilitation skills and then should seek out specialized hand therapy training. This chapter is meant only as a guideline to the treatment of some of the more common hand diagnoses. Of course, treatment procedures may vary depending upon the particular patient's circumstances.

EVALUATION

Before treatment can begin, a base line evaluation is necessary to determine your plan of treatment, monitor your patient's progress, and judge the effectiveness of your treatment procedures.

An evaluation can be divided into subjective and objective information.

Subjective Information

Subjective information, as described below, is obtained through speaking with and listening to your patient, observation, and palpation of the hand. This type of information is important from a treatment and diagnostic standpoint but cannot be used to make valid statements for research or in accurately assessing your therapeutic management.

A. History of injury or illness
B. Posture of the Hand: Normally, the wrist is in slight dorsiflexion. The digits lie with increasing flexion toward the ulnar side of the hand. The index and midfingers are slightly supinated. The fingernails lie in the direction of the scaphoid bone. Tendon injuries or certain fractures will disrupt this posture
C. Condition of the skin
D. Color of the skin
E. Edema
F. Sensibility: The patient would be asked to describe the way the hand feels. This would include any pain, numbness, tingling, etc
G. Any deformity
H. Palpation of the Hand
　1. Any masses or nodules
　2. Temperature of the skin
　3. Texture of the skin (i.e., dry, wet, soft, rough, scarred)
I. Patient's hand dominance
J. Patient's family, work, and avocational history

Objective Information

When recording objective measurements, tests which have been analyzed for validity and reliability should be used. These testing instruments must be easy to administer and produce objective, measurable, and reproducible data. This gives one a basis to evaluate the patient's progress and the treatment procedures. This type of data also lay the foundation for important research and more accurate communication among professionals.

A. Joint Range of Motion: Both active and passive motions should be recorded with a goniometer. If a discrepancy between active and passive range of motion exists, it can indicate that the problem is with tendon excursion rather than the joint itself. The Clinical Assessment Committee of the American Society for Surgery of the Hand also recommends the recording of total active range of motion and passive range of motion. Total active range of motion is the sum of the angles of the metacarpophalangeal, proximal interphalangeal, and distal interphalangeal joints when the hand is in maximum active flexion, minus any deviation from full extension. Total passive range of motion is the sum of the angles formed by the metacarpophalangeal, proximal interphalangeal, and distal interphalangeal joints when the hand is in full passive flexion, minus any passive extension deficit

B. Grip Strength: When grip strength is recorded, notations of the spacing of the handle should be recorded on the evaluation form.

C. Pinch Strength

D. Sensory Evaluation: To be discussed later in this chapter and in Chapter 3

E. Muscle testing

F. Functional Assessment Tests:
1. Activities of daily living skills
2. Endurance tests
3. Dexterity Tests: Examples of these would be the Purdue Pegboard or the Jebsen Hand Function Test. These are standardized tests.
4. Work assessment tests.

G. Edema Assessment: Edema assessment can be done with circumference measurements or volumeter measurements

In most busy clinics, it is not possible to perform a number of objective tests. Therefore, one must choose which ones are most appropriate and will be most helpful in gaining the type of data you require for a particular patient.

Reevaluation should be done on an ongoing basis throughout your patient's treatment program. The frequency of reevaluation would depend upon your patient's individual circumstances.

JOINT INJURIES

Injuries to the joints and their supporting soft tissue structures are among the most common hand injuries. Unfortunately, the full implication of these injuries is not always appreciated. This can often lead to needless disability.

These injuries will be divided into ligamentous injuries, volar plate injuries, and dislocations.

Incomplete proximal interphalangeal joint injuries probably occur with the most frequency. An incomplete tear of the ligament implies that the injured joint has enought capsular support remaining to prevent displacement of the joint, when adequately stressed.[1]

Of course, our goal is to maintain joint mobility. However, before one can begin motion, a period of rest is required in the most advantageous position for proper ligamentous healing. The joint is immobilized for 10 to 14 days in approximately 30 to 35° of flexion using a dorsal aluminum splint[2-5] (Fig. 18.1). The dorsal splint allows the palmar surface to be free and does not block the metacarpophalangeal joint or the distal interphalangeal joint. The dorsal splint also provides better support and is less likely to be worked loose.[6] In some cases, it may be wise to put the whole hand at rest for a few days, until the initial pain and

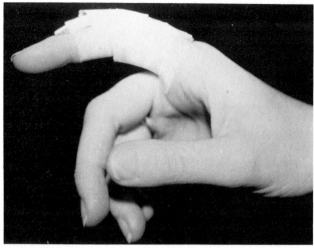

Figure 18.1 Dorsal aluminum splint to support injured proximal interphalangeal (PIP) joint in the proper position.

swelling have subsided. Then immobilize only the involved joint. The exact length of time for immobilization depends upon the amount of pain and swelling and the joint's response to the period of rest.[3, 4]

If the joint shows instability to stress, immobilization for 3 weeks is required, since this may indicate more extensive damage.[3] Following this period of immobilization, the injured finger may be taped to an adjacent digit to provide support for another 1 to 2 weeks.

Metacarpophalangeal joint ligamentous injuries of the digits occur with much less frequency than the proximal interphalangeal joint ligament injury.[3, 4, 7] It is most often the radial collateral ligament that is injured.[3-5, 7] More often, it is the metacarpophalangeal joint hyperextension injury that occurs.[3] These injuries often cause a large amount of edema and ecchymosis over both the dorsum of the hand and volar into the palm. The treatment initially is immobilization of the hand. The hand is immobilized from the proximal interphalangeal joint to the mid forearm. The metacarpophalangeal joints are placed in about 45 to 50° of flexion.[3, 7] Immobilization is continued for approximately 2 to 3 weeks before exercises are started. The exact period depends upon the degree of pain and swelling.

Collateral ligament injuries to the metacarpophalangeal joint of the thumb most often occur to the ulnar side and are handled differently than those of the digits.[2, 4] It is more often necessary to surgically repair ligamentous injuries of the thumb metacarpophalangeal joint, since soft tissue often becomes interposed between the bone and the ends of the ligaments.[2-4] This, then, would prevent healing of the ligaments without surgical intervention. Following repair, the thumb is immobilized for 5 to 6 weeks.[4] The goal is to provide a good stable joint for pinch. Active and active assistive exercises are started following the immobilization period and are generally increased, as tolerated by the patient. Ligamentous injuries may not be considered stable for as long as 10 to 12 weeks. However, the patient may experience some discomfort and weakness for as long as 6 to 12 months following the injury. Therefore, the level of activity allowed is determined on an individual basis.[3, 4] Any exercise program must be designed with this in mind and must progress accordingly.

Volar plate injuries are caused by hyperextension forces against the extended finger.[2–5] A poorly treated volar plate injury can result in a symptomatic swan-neck deformity (hyperextension of the proximal interphalangeal joint and flexion of the distal interphalangeal joint). Initially, the finger is splinted with the proximal interphalangeal joint in about 30° of flexion for 2 weeks. When motion is started, an extension block splint (fig. 18.2) is used for an additional 1 to 2 weeks to further protect the volar plate. In old volar plate injuries that have developed symptomatic swan-neck deformities, surgery may be carried out. These cases would require immobilization for 3 weeks. Extension block splinting is again used for 1 to 2 more weeks.[4, 5]

Dislocations of the proximal interphalangeal joints often occur in contact sports. The joint can become dislocated in a dorsal direction, a lateral direction, or a volar direction.[2–5] One must keep in mind that when a dislocation occurs there is always associated soft tissue damage. The structures injured depend upon the mechanism of the injury. When a dorsal dislocation occurs, the major damage is to the volar plate.[2–4] There may also be an avulsion of a small bone fragment along with the volar plate. In these cases, the joint is splinted in 20 to 30° of flexion for about 3 weeks.[2] An active exercise program is then started. An extension block splint may be used for an additional

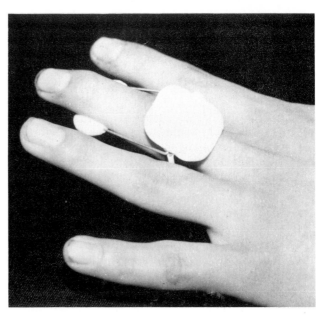

Figure 18.3   A dynamic splint used to aid in achieving or maintaining finger extension.

week or two. It is important that proper splinting be done, since the sequela of a poorly treated dorsal dislocation can be a swan-neck deformity.

Another possible complication may be a proximal interphalangeal joint flexion contracture. This may occur if the joint is left in flexion for too long a period of time. Proximal interphalangeal joint flexion deformities are difficult problems. It takes a long period of time to correct them through either a series of cylinder splints or dynamic splints or a combination of both. Some may ultimately require corrective surgery. In those that come to surgery, we have found that continued monitoring may be necessary for at least 6 months postoperatively to prevent recurrence of the deformity. It is also necessary to maintain a program of extension splinting (Figs. 18.3 and 12.24) during this period of time. The patient is progressed from extension splinting, except for exercises, to intermittent splinting for specified periods of time. A night splint is recommended for an extended period of time, since it is a person's natural tendency to sleep with the fingers in a flexed position.

Lateral dislocations occur when torsion, angular, or shearing forces are placed on the finger. This type of injury results in rupture of one of the collateral ligaments and a portion of the insertion of the volar plate.[3] The finger is splinted with the proximal interphalangeal joint in about 20° of flexion for about 2 weeks. Following this period of immobilization, the finger is protected for another 1 to 2 weeks with taping to the adjacent finger next to the side of the ruptured ligament.[3] It may also be necessary to use an extension block splint to protect the volar plate.[4] Joints that are stable to active motion, but show instability to lateral stress need to be immobilized for 3 weeks.[3]

When a volar dislocation occurs, there is either incomplete or complete protrusion of the head of the

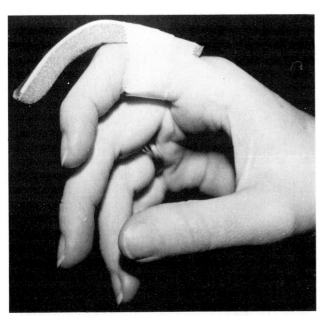

Figure 18.2   Dorsal block splinting to prevent full extension while permitting flexion.

proximal phalanx to the dorsal apparatus.[2-4] This injury is splinted in extension 4 to 6 weeks to allow the dorsal apparatus to heal.[2] A night splint and/or splinting in between exercises may be continued for another 1 to 2 weeks after the therapy program of active exercises has been started. It is again important that proper splinting be done, since the resulting complication of this injury could be a boutonniere deformity (flexion of the proximal interphalangeal joint and hyperextension of the distal interphalangeal joint). Therefore, when exercising the injured joint, extension is emphasized with gentle flexion exercises. It should be carefully observed that the patient can extend the finger well with each repetition of the exercise. If the patient has difficulty with extension, further splinting is necessary.

When a fracture-dislocation occurs, the treatment varies, depending upon the size of the fragment.[3, 4] Surgery is required to repair the joint and soft tissue damage, if the fragment is large causing the joint to be unstable. Postoperatively, then, the joint is held in plaster with the proximal interphalangeal joint in about 35° of flexion for approximately 3 weeks before beginning a therapy program. When exercises are begun, an extension block splint is used for another week. On about the 5th week, gentle controlled extension exercises are allowed. If, after 8 weeks, the patient has not gained full extension, a dynamic splint may be used to aid in achieving full extension.[3] If, when reduced closed, joint alignment and stability are satisfactory, the joint is immobilized for 10 days to 2 weeks, at which time a dorsal block splint is used for another week before extension is allowed.[3, 4]

Dislocations of the metacarpophalangeal joints are rare. When they do occur, it is usually to the index or fifth fingers. The dislocation is often dorsal and more frequently requires open reduction, since soft tissue may become caught between the joint spaces.[3-5] Following repair, the joint is immobilized for 3 weeks. Active flexion is started, but extension is not allowed for 4 weeks.[3] Dislocations of the thumb metacarpal result in a major disruption of the soft tissue structures.[2-5] These are generally reduced closed and are held for 3 to 4 weeks before initiating a therapy program. A dislocation of the carpometacarpal of the thumb usually occurs with such force that the metacarpal shaft is fractured, producing the Bennett's fracture-dislocation.[2-5] The fracture may be reduced closed, and a Kirschner wire may be placed percutaneously to maintain the reduction. The joint is immobilized for 4 weeks. Gentle exercises are begun at this time and are progressed gradually over the next few weeks.

The mallet deformity deserves mention at this time. It is a common injury to the distal interphalangeal joint. The mallet deformity results from elongation, laceration, or rupture of the terminal tendon of the dorsal apparatus.[8] The distal joint drops into flexion. Generally, the treatment is splinting of the distal joint in extension for 8 weeks.[6, 8] The patient is instructed in changing the splint and caring for the skin to prevent skin breakdown (Fig. 18.4). When the splint is changed, the patient is instructed to be very careful to maintain the joint in extension.[6] If the joint drops into flexion, the splinting must be started all over again. During the immobilization period, exercises to the proximal interphalangeal joint are done. The result of the untreated mallet deformity can be a swan-neck deformity brought about by muscle and tendon imbalance. Therefore, following the immobilization period, careful monitoring is required to be sure that extension is maintained. If an extension lag is noted, further splinting is indicated.

When one is attempting to mobilize joint injuries, there are other aspects of the rehabilitation program that are common to all the injuries discussed. All exercises must be done gently and within the patient's tolerance. Exercises should not, under any circumstances, increase pain or swelling. In some cases where swelling of the joint persists, an ice pack or an ice massage may be a useful tool in controlling edema, even after the acute period. Proximal interphalangeal joint injuries tend to remain swollen for long periods of time.[4] Therefore, edema control needs to be a part of the general hand therapy program for these and other joint injuries. These injuries often cause a great deal of swelling and pain within the whole hand as well. Therefore, exercises to maintain mobility of the rest of the hand should be done. If the rest of the hand is not exercised, stiffness and fibrosis can be the result.

One should also pay particular attention to the intrinsic muscles of the hand.[6] Because of the intimate relationship between the injured structures and the intrinsic muscles, exercises to these muscles should be started as soon as it is safe to do so. These exercises can be done in such a way as to prevent undue stress on the injured structures.

When exercising the proximal interphalangeal joint, it may be helpful to splint the distal joint temporarily,

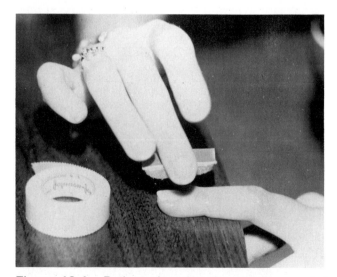

Figure 18.4 Patient changing the aluminum splint used to maintain extension of the distal interphalangeal (DIP) joint when a mallet deformity occurs.

as well as to block the metacarpophalangeal joint. This helps to concentrate the flexion and extension power at the proximal interphalangeal joint. Following proximal interphalangeal joint exercises, the distal joint splint is removed, and the distal joint is exercised. It is important that, with proximal interphalangeal joint injuries, the distal joint is also exercised. The oblique retinacular ligament can become tight, causing decreased distal joint motion. It must be remembered that, although at first glance these injuries may look benign, they are serious injuries. Recovery from these injuries is often prolonged and requires the cooperation and active participation of the patient. The therapist and physician must educate the patient to maximize this cooperation. Above all, patience and encouragement are necessary throughout treatment.

JOINT IMPLANT ARTHROPLASTIES

When a joint has been irreparably damaged through either trauma or arthritis, it is possible to reconstruct the joint using various implants now available. The ones most commonly used are the Swanson flexible hinge implants. These implants are made of silicone rubber and act as joint spacers while the new capsuloligamentous system forms during the healing process.[9-12] Dr. Swanson refers to this as the process of encapsulation.[11, 12] The following is a general rule to the postoperative management of these implants.

Metacarpophalangeal Joint Interpositional Arthroplasty

Metacarpophalangeal joint arthroplasty is most often done in patients with rheumatoid arthritis. Preoperatively, certain types of deformities are seen. Millender and Nalebuff[10] have described a classification for these deformities. Postoperatively, the hand is initially held in a bulky dressing with a plaster splint that supports the metacarpophalangeal joints in extension and some radial deviation to maintain desired joint alignment. If preoperatively the patient has very limited flexion and minimal or no ulnar deviation, the fingers may be held in some flexion.[13] On days 1 and 2 following the surgery, the exercises consist of gentle finger pumping (gentle range of motion) to help reduce edema and provide gentle active metacarpophalangeal joint motion. On days 3 to 5, exercises consist of active and active assistive range of motion to the metacarpophalangeal joints. Metacarpophalangeal joint flexion is stressed by teaching the patient to bring the metacarpophalangeal joints into a shelf-like position and then curl the interphalangeal joints into the palm. When the patient has good proximal interphalangeal joint motion, he may attempt to substitute this motion for metacarpophalangeal joint flexion. If this is allowed to continue, the patient's final range of flexion could be severely compromised. If this is a problem, the proximal interphalangeal joints can be immobilized during exercise sessions to concentrate the flexion and extension at the metacarpophalangeal joint level.[11-13] The proximal interphalangeal joints can be immobi-

lized with either alumofoam splints (Fig. 18.5) or pieces of splinting material. Usually, on about the 5th to 7th postoperative day, depending upon the amount of pain and swelling the patient has, a dynamic splint is fabricated[9-13] (Fig. 18.6). This splint is made generally as an ulnar gutter splint to provide good wrist support as well as carpometacarpal support to the fourth and fifth digits. The outrigger is placed in a radial direction to give the metacarpophalangeal joints a gentle continuous radial pull.[13] The elastics must be of appropriate tension to provide adequate extension and radial deviation but not so tight as to restrict flexion. Hyperextension of the metacarpophalangeal joints must be avoided. To be sure that the patient gets full flexion, he may be instructed to remove the cuffs for short periods of time each time he exercises.[13] If the patient is not achieving what we would consider a good range

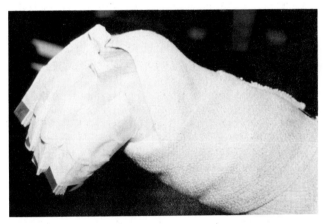

Figure 18.5 Aluminum splint immobilizing proximal interphalangeal (PIP) joints to aid in achieving better metacarpophalangeal (MCP) motion following MCP arthroplasty.

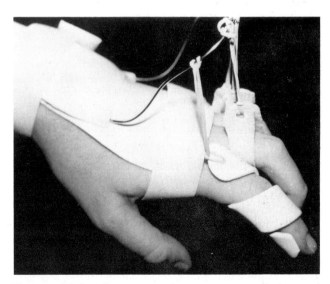

Figure 18.6 Postoperative metacarpophalangeal (MCP) arthroplasty splint with serpentine-type splint attached to help supinate the index finger.

of motion (approximately 70°), a volar outrigger may be attached to the splint to provide a flexion pull at the metacarpophalangeal joints.[13] The dynamic splint is worn all day for approximately 6 to 8 weeks. The elastics are adjusted, and the splint is modified, whenever necessary, to maintain proper functioning. At night, the patient wears a plaster resting shell to maintain the positioning of the hand. This splint is also modified, as necessary, during the postoperative program. The night splint is often worn for about 2 weeks, after the dynamic splint has been discontinued.

The exercises are done about 4 times a day for a brief period of time at each session, approximately 5 minutes. Several brief sessions of exercises spread out over the entire day are less likely to cause tissue reaction than one long session.[13] There are other considerations when treating patients with metacarpophalangeal joint arthroplasties. In some patients, the fifth finger is more difficult to mobilize than the others. One must be sure that the elastic for that finger is not too tight. In some cases, it may not be necessary to use an elastic on that finger. This, of course, has to be decided on an individual basis. Another consideration is the proper alignment of the digits. In the normal hand, there is some supination with the digits heading in the direction of the scaphoid. In some patients, the fingers, especially the index finger, may tend to assume a more pronated position.[11, 12] For this situation, a serpentine-type finger splint made of orthoplast or polyform may be wrapped around the finger to maintain the digit in some supination.[11, 12] This is attached to the outrigger with an elastic and is used in place of the usual finger cuff. After 2 to 3 weeks, the patient is allowed to begin using the hand for very light activities, such as eating, with the dynamic splint on the hand. At 6 to 8 weeks, mild resistance may be added to the exercise program for strengthening.[13] Functional use of the hand is also increased at this time. It must be kept in mind that the patient with rheumatoid disease is weakened to begin with. Therefore, one cannot expect that the implants will provide normal strength, although strength in many cases is improved. At 3 months, the patient is generally allowed to use the hand for all daily activities. This is a gradual active process and is progressed according to the patient's tolerance.

Proximal Interphalangeal Joint Implant Arthroplasty

Much of the postoperative hand therapy management of the patient who has undergone proximal interphalangeal joint implant arthroplasty depends upon the soft tissue surgery that is done at the time of the arthroplasty.[14] Therefore, the time when motion is begun has to be determined on an individual basis. Proximal interphalangeal joint arthroplasty may be done for the following indications:

A. To reconstruct a stiff, painful proximal interphalangeal joint, damaged by trauma, rheumatoid disease, or degenerative joint disease.

B. To reconstruct a boutonniere deformity.
C. To reconstruct a swan-neck deformity.

Stiff Proximal Interphalangeal Joint. When the proximal interphalangeal joint arthroplasty is done for this reason, gentle proximal interphalangeal joint motion may be started as soon as 2 to 3 days postoperatively, depending upon the amount of pain and swelling. The patient is held in a plaster splint that holds the proximal interphalangeal joint in extension between exercise periods. In some cases where postoperative stiffness appears to be a problem, the proximal interphalangeal joint may be taped down into flexion for at least part of the time between exercise sessions.[14]

Boutonniere Repair. When an arthroplasty is done for this situation, the extensor mechanism is repaired as part of the procedure. Therefore, the extensor mechanism must be protected in extension, usually with an alumofoam splint. Gentle active motion is started at about 10 to 14 days.[11, 12, 14] Between exercise sessions, the finger is placed back in the extension splint. The splint is worn for 4 to 6 weeks or until the position of the finger has stabilized. It may be necessary in some cases to delay exercises for as long as 4 weeks.

Swan-neck Repair. When this procedure has been done in conjunction with tendon reconstruction, the finger is held in approximately 20 to 30° of flexion to prevent a recurrent hyperextension deformity.[11, 12, 14] In this situation, a slight proximal interphalangeal flexion contracture may be desirable. Gentle motion allowing flexion and extension may be started at about 3 to 5 days postoperatively. The finger is then splinted, until the position of the joint has stabilized.

General Exercise Considerations

Active and active assistive exercises are done to begin with and then increased to gentle passive motion. Care must be taken to always support the metacarpophalangeal joint in extension. This can be done by the patient, with the other hand, or a piece of splinting material, padded with moleskin, can be used as a block to support the metacarpophalangeal joint while exercising the proximal interphalangeal joint. Splinting material works well, since it is rigid but thin enough not to block any proximal interphalangeal joint motion. The hand can also be positioned over a book or the edge of a table. When this method is used, care must be taken to be sure that proximal interphalangeal joint motion is not being blocked. Usually, after 6 to 8 weeks, resistance can be added to the program to improve strength. Functional use of the hand should gradually be increased over this period of time.

Silastic Wrist Implant Arthroplasty

The postoperative therapy for wrist arthroplasty begins the first day following surgery, when the drain is removed, the dressing is changed, and both volar and dorsal plaster splints are made. At this time, finger range of motion is begun to maintain digital motion.

The pumping action of the fingers aids in reducing postoperative edema. The volar and dorsal wrist splints are kept in place for 4 to 6 weeks.[11, 15] During this time, no wrist motion is done. If any laxity of the wrist is noted, the wrist will be held longer. Often, a distal ulnar excision is done in conjunction with the wrist arthroplasty. An ulnar head implant may or may not be used in these cases. When a distal ulnar excision is done, the forearm is held in some supination for 2 to 3 weeks with either a sugar tong splint or another form of plaster splinting to ensure good capsular healing.[15] Generally, wrist exercises are begun at about 4 weeks. For the first week following initiation of the exercise program, the exercises are gentle and protected active assistive motion. Exercises are then progressed to active and gentle passive range of motion. Gradually, after approximately 6 to 8 weeks postoperatively, resistance can be added to the exercise program for strengthening. Generally, at this point, splinting is discontinued, and the patient can begin using his hand unprotected for light activities of daily living. Activities of daily living are gradually increased as strength returns. In special cases, when any laxity or tendency toward drifting of the wrist is observed, a wrist splint is fabricated[14] (Fig. 18.7). The patient would wear this splint during the day to provide protected motion. At night the patient would go back into the plaster splint.

Thumb Carpometacarpal Joint Implant Arthroplasty

Arthroplasty of the carpometacarpal joint of the thumb is most often done in patients with osteoarthritis. When evaluating these patients for surgery, it is important that the other joints of the thumb be evaluated as well that maximum results from the arthroplasty be ensured. For example, an adduction deformity of the metacarpophalangeal joint of the thumb may be an associated problem with carpometacarpal joint arthritis.[11] If this is severe, the adductor pollicis may have to be released to ensure proper balance and seating of the implant. Hyperex-

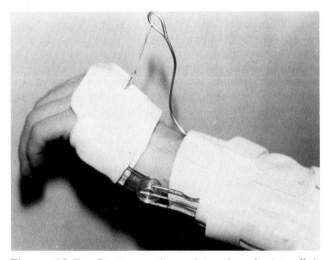

Figure 18.7 Postoperative wrist arthroplasty splint.

tension deformity of the metacarpal joint of the thumb can also contribute to the adduction deformity.[11] If the metacarpophalangeal joint of the thumb is hyperextended, it may be necessary to surgically correct this problem to prevent dislocation or subluxation of the implant. Postoperatively, the thumb is held in a plaster splint in palmar abduction for 4 to 6 weeks to ensure good capsular healing.[11, 14] During this time, range of motion of the fingers is encouraged. When the splint is removed, the patient begins opposition, abduction, and circumduction exercises. Hyperextension of the thumb should be avoided. Dexterity activities are then added to the program and are increased, as strength begins to return. Unrestricted use of the thumb is generally allowed in about 12 weeks. Strength takes considerably longer to return. It may, in fact, take up to a year before the patient feels that he has adequate strength.

NERVE INJURIES

Sensibility of the hand is a very complex subject. Obviously, without functioning nerves, one would have an essentially useless appendage. Sensibility of the hand encompasses the very essence of human experience. We require sensibility of the hand for self-expression, prehension, identification and evaluation of objects, to protect us from harmful stimuli, and to enable us to manipulate our environment. Therefore, every effort must be made to help people with nerve injuries regain as much useful function as possible.

Evaluation

The first step in the rehabilitation process is evaluation. Evaluating sensibility can be very difficult, since one is evaluating a number of things. There are many types of tests available to evaluate sensibility. However, except for the electrodiagnostic studies, there are no standardized tests currently available for this purpose. Therefore, data obtained is subjective. There is, though, certain information that one needs to obtain in order to evaluate sensory function. This information needs to be measured and recorded in such a way as to reproduce it for comparison. The evaluation should be done in a quiet, relaxed atmosphere. The evaluation should not cause pain and should not be done on a hypersensitive, painful hand. It is often helpful to first make a drawing of the patient's hand on a piece of paper, noting the level of the laceration, any callouses, or any injuries (such as burns) that would indicate lack of protective sensation. The patient is then asked to give a description of how the hand feels.[16] This includes having the patient identify where on the hand the sensation changes. As well as giving the therapist information about the level of sensibility, this information may give insight into the patient's ability to adapt to the altered sensation. It may also indicate the patient's motivation for sensory reeducation.

The patient's active and passive ranges of motion are recorded, and a muscle test is administered. Grip strength and pinch strength should be recorded on both hands, as a comparison. A Jamar dynamometer is used, and measurements are recorded with the handle in Level 2, Level 3, and, in the case of a large hand, in Level 4. A standard pinch meter is used to measure pinch. Pulp pinch (palmar pinch), lateral pinch, and 3-jaw chuck pinch (palmar pinch using index and middle fingers and thumb) are all recorded.

Weinstein-Semmes Monofilaments

Weinstein-Semmes pressure aesthesiometer tests light touch perception (Fig. 18.8). This evaluation tool consists of 20 nylon monofilaments mounted in plastic rods.[16-19] Each probe is of varying thickness and stiffness. The scale goes from 1.65 to 6.65, with the normal range between 2.44 and 2.83[18, 19] The monofilaments bend when pressed against the skin. They bend according to their length and thickness and not according to the pressure exerted by the examiner.[19] Testing is begun distal to proximal but is varied periodically to avoid patient anticipation.[16] The rod is held perpendicular to the finger.[18, 19] When testing in the area of 2.44 to 4.08, it is recommended that the monofilaments be bounced off the skin.[18, 19] Three trials are given. For the heavier monofilaments, one motion is used, and only one trial is given.[18, 19] During the application of the monofilaments, the patient should have his eyes closed. The patient is then asked to open his eyes and point to the spot on the skin touched with the monofilaments to determine point localization.[18, 19] This should then be recorded on the evaluation sheet. It is important to first do an assessment of the uninvolved hand to determine what is the normal range for that patient.[16, 18, 19]

Two-Point Discrimination

The purpose of the two-point discrimination test is to determine if the patient can distinguish being touched by one point or two points and at what distance this can be appreciated. One can use a Boley gauge, a caliper, or a paper clip to measure. The gauge is generally recommended, since a scale in millimeters is on the instrument. There is also often a barb on the edge of the paper clip which could, if allowed to stroke the patient's finger, alter results of the test. The patient's other hand is tested again to determine a base line and to help the patient become familiar with the testing procedure. Once this is done, the gauge is set at 10 mm and is held with the points in the longitudinal axis.[18, 19] Testing proceeds in a random fashion across the hand and distal to proximal alternating one and two points. One should pause about 5 seconds between point application.[18] An answer is considered correct, if 5 of 7 responses are accurate. If the examiner is satisfied with the results, the gauge is then adjusted down 1 mm. If the response is not acceptable, the gauge is then adjusted up to 1 mm. The pressure of the instrument should not produce blanching of the skin. The normal range of two-point discrimination varies depending upon the location on the hand[16, 18, 19] (see Chapter 3). The results of two-point discrimination and the Weinstein-Semmes aesthesiometer do not necessarily correlate. It is, for example, possible to have two-point discrimination recorded within a normal range but still show diminished protective sensation when tested with the Weinstein-Semmes monofilaments.[16]

Moberg Pickup Test

In 1958, Moberg[20] introduced a pickup test to help determine the patient's functional level of sensibility. A group of small objects is placed on the table. The patient is then asked to pick these objects up as quickly as possible and drop them into a small container.[18, 20] The activity is timed using a stop watch. Both hands are tested. Following this procedure, the patient is blindfolded and asked to repeat the test. While blindfolded, the patient is also asked to identify

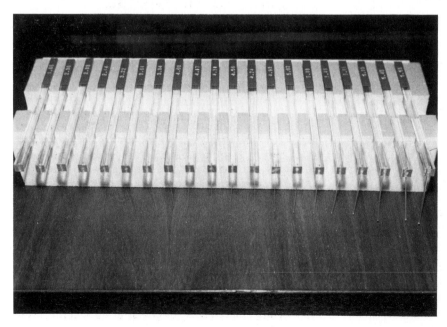

Figure 18.8 Weinstein-Semmes monofilaments used to test light touch perception.

the object.[18, 20] The time of both procedures is recorded. With vision occluded, the time is generally increased, if there is decreased sensibility.[20] The number of objects remains constant, but the objects themselves are varied to help prevent a learning factor from altering the results. It must be remembered that this is not a standardized test and is presented only as a useful tool in evaluating sensibility in median nerve or combined median and ulnar nerve lesions.[20]

Proprioception

The patient's finger is supported by the examiner and then passively moved from ½ to 1 cm in different directions. The patient is then asked to identify in what direction the finger is moved. Omer[18] states that an interphalangeal joint requires 5 to 10° of passive motion before recognition of the position is possible.

Finger and Point Identification

Using the point of a pencil, the finger is touched just enough to indent the skin but not enough to cause blanching. The patient is then asked to identify both the finger touched and the point on the finger that was touched. Results of this are recorded on the evaluation form. Nerve regeneration is generally thought to take place at approximately 1 inch per month.[21, 22] Therefore, reevaluation following nerve injury should be done approximately every 4 to 6 weeks.[21]

Sensory Reeducation

Dellon et al.[23-26] have shown that the quality of functional sensibility can be improved through a program of sensory reeducation. Not only does this reeducation process appear to improve the level of sensibility but it also seems to aid in helping the patient integrate altered sensibility, thus improving the patient's functional capacity.[21-24, 26, 27]

Sensory reeducation is begun as soon as possible following the injury. One begins training when light touch is returned to the palm and proximal phalanx.[23-26] At this stage, we begin with stimulating the area with either a finger of the other hand or an eraser on a pencil.[23-26] We introduce large objects of various shapes that can be grasped or placed in the palm.[22] The patient is also instructed to immerse his hand in substances such as sand or rice. These activities are also done with the normal hand to help the patient in the educational process.[22] As the return of sensibility progresses distally, smaller objects are introduced. These are manipulated with both the normal and the injured hands. These include things such as nuts and bolts, coins, keys, and other everyday objects.[22-25] Activities of daily living such as buttoning clothing and tying shoes are also encouraged.[22-25] If the injured hand is the dominant hand, writing skills and manipulation of eating utensils are also practiced. As the level of sensibility improves, common objects may be buried in the rice or sand.[22] The patient must then try to find these objects and identify them. When possible, the tools the patient may use at work are also introduced into the treatment program.[22-24]

Motor Reeducation

After nerve repair, the wrist and fingers are positioned in such a way as to prevent tension on the repair.[21, 28] The exact position would depend upon the available length of the nerve and is determined by the surgeon at the time of the operation. The nerve repair is immobilized from 3 to 5 weeks, before motion is allowed.[21, 28] During this period of immobilization, it may be possible to gradually bring the wrist and hand into a more natural position, while being protected in the splint. The nerve is adversely affected by tension. Rapid stretch will cause the nerve to exceed its elastic limit and may lead to interneural fibrosis.[29] Therefore, it is recommended that the joint not be extended more than 10° per week.[28, 29]

Following immobilization, gentle active exercises should be started along with gentle passive motion to the paralyzed joints, in order to maintain full joint mobility. Exercises to the rest of the extremity are important as well to maintain strength of the uninvolved muscles and to aid in circulation and nutrition of the extremity.[22] Light massage is also beneficial for circulation and is relaxing and pleasurable for the patient. Stretching exercises are generally delayed until about 8 weeks following the repair.[22] Splinting is often necessary to prevent deformity that may be caused by the muscle imbalance brought about by the nerve injury. The type of splint used is dependent upon the nerve injured and the muscles affected by the loss of nerve function. Great caution must be taken to be sure that the splint used is correct. A poorly designed or ill-conceived splint can lead to irreversible deformity. Static or dynamic splints may be used to maintain position, as the joints are gradually brought into their normal position.

Muscle atrophy of denervated muscle will take place regardless of good therapy or intermittent electrical stimulation.[22, 30] The only way, at present, to prevent atrophy is to reinnervate the muscles.[30]

TENDON TRANSFERS

When irreparable nerve and/or muscle damage occurs, it is possible to restore muscle balance and improve function through tendon transfers. Tendon transfers are used to redistribute the remaining muscle power and to utilize this in the most effective functional combination. The types of transfers used would, of course, depend upon the muscles available for transfer. Certain conditions, however, must exist before tendons can be transferred successfully.[22, 28, 31-33] First, joints in the area of the transfer must have adequate passive mobility. In the preoperative stage, it is the responsibility of the therapist to maintain joint mobility through exercise and splinting. Second, the soft tissue must also be well-healed and in good condition. The therapist can help here by using massage and active exercise to uninvolved muscles and joints. This helps to improve circulation and nutrition to the extremity and maintain strength of the normal musculature. In some cases, restoration of soft tissue through various plastic procedures may be necessary before tendon transfers can be done. Third, the proposed transfer muscle must have adequate strength to perform the desired function. Although it is generally agreed that it is easier to train a transfer when synergistic muscles are used, it is no longer thought to be a major consideration.[22, 32, 33] It is believed that the direction of the pull of the transfer is far more important in the success of the training.[31-34]

Following transfer, the hand is immobilized for 3 to 4 weeks. Extensor tendons are generally held at least 4 to 6 weeks, because of the force that is placed on them by the much stronger flexors.[31] A protective splint is then used for an additional 2 to 3 weeks between exercise sessions.[31] The exact period of immobilization depends upon the stress to be placed on the transfer. Exercises begin with controlled active motion. Any forced manipulation must be avoided. Active range of motion to the rest of the extremity is encouraged. The therapy program should then progress to gradually increasing resistance for strengthening. PNF techniques are quite helpful in the training of certain transfers.[22] Functional activities are introduced as early as possible into the program to encourage the use of the extremity and to improve strength (Fig. 18.9). In patients who are having difficulty with the retraining process, biofeedback can be a very useful adjunct to the treatment program. The exact timing for the introduction of various modalities is determined by the surgeon. Generally, relearning progresses quickly with very little difficulty.

TENDON REPAIR

Tendon lacerations are among the more common types of hand injuries. Rehabilitation of these patients offers a special challenge to the therapist. New advances in research to understand tendon healing and in microsurgical techniques are exciting and make the

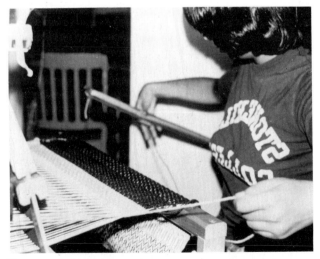

Figure 18.9 Patient performing functional activities to aid in transfer training.

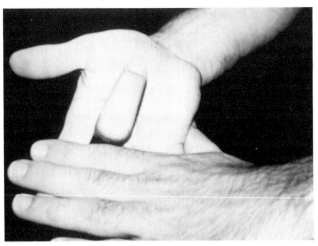

Figure 18.10 Testing for superficialis function.

area of tendon rehabilitation very dynamic for both the surgeon and the therapist.

Flexor Tendons

When discussing flexor tendon injuries, it is best done by dividing the injuries into 5 zones.[35, 36] Zone 1 is the area distal to where the superficialis divides. Zone 2 is the area that begins at the proximal part of the flexor tendon sheath proximal to the metacarpophalangeal joint and extends to the middle portion of the middle phalanx. This area is an especially difficult area in which to restore smooth tendon gliding. Both flexor tendons pass through a tight fibro-osseous canal. This leaves very little room for any scarring. Even a small amount of adhesion formation can disrupt the gliding mechanism and cause decreased range of motion. Zone 3 is the area from the origin of the lumbricals to, but not including, the carpal tunnel. Zone 4 includes the carpal tunnel. Repairs in this area may necessitate placing the wrist in neutral or slight dorsiflexion, because of the repair of the transverse carpal ligament. This would require that the metacarpophalangeal joints be blocked about 45 to 60° to ensure that there is no tension placed on the repair.[36] In other zones, the wrist is generally placed in about 40° of palmarflexion with the metacarpophalangeal joints and the proximal interphalangeal joints in about 20° of flexion. Zone 5 extends from the distal forearm to the wrist, proximal to the transverse carpal ligament.

Another consideration to be kept in mind is the position of the hand when it was injured. If the finger was flexed, the actual laceration of the tendon will be distal to the skin laceration. If the finger was in extension at the time of the injury, then the skin laceration would correspond to the tendon laceration.[35]

One should also know how to test individual tendon function (Figs. 18.10 and 18.11). To test for superficialis function, support all the fingers in extension, except the one being tested. If the superficialis is intact, the proximal interphalangeal joint should be able to flex.[35] The exception to this may be the fifth finger. In a study done by Baker *et al.*,[37] they concluded in a large portion of the population that the fifth finger superficialis is functionally deficient. To test for profundus function, put the finger in extension and ask the patient to flex the distal joint. If the profundus is intact, he will be able to do so.[35]

Postoperative Management

The use of dynamic traction for early controlled mobilization adds another dimension to the management of tendon repair in Zones 2 and 3. Duran and Hauser[1, 38] have shown that 3 to 5 mm of extension motion of the tendon repair done in a "controlled passive exercise program" is generally enough to prevent the formation of firm adhesions in Zone 2 repairs. Postoperatively, the wrist is held in about 20 to 45° of flexion, and the metacarpophalangeal joints and the proximal interphalangeal joints in about 20° of flexion using a dorsal block splint[1, 35, 38–40] (Fig. 18.12). An elastic is attached to the fingernail of the involved finger using a dress hook and is attached proximally to the wrist with a safety pin that is fastened to the ace bandage. When the finger is flexed, there should not be any tension on the elastic. The exercise program begins on days 2 to 5. At this time, the patient is instructed to extend the finger within the limits of the splint. He then allows the elastic to bring the digit into flexion. Active finger flexion or passive extension is not permitted.[35, 36, 39, 40] With the Duran[1, 38] method, only passive motion within the splint is allowed. At 3½ to 4 weeks, the dorsal splint is removed, and the traction is attached to a wrist cuff or ace wrap. At this time, active exercises are started, but the patient is not allowed to use the hand for any strong grasping or any passive extension. At about 6 weeks, dynamic traction is generally discontinued. Very mild resistance may be added at 6 to 8 weeks. If a flexion contracture appears to be developing, assistive extension and dynamic and static splinting may be started at 8 to 10 weeks.[36, 39, 40] Generally, the patient is allowed to resume normal activities at about 12 weeks following repair. It must be noted that, because early motion

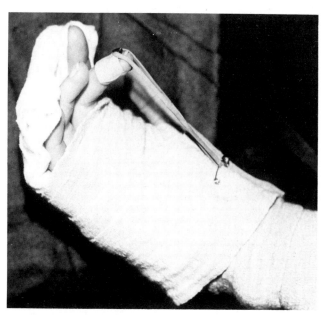

Figure 18.12 Elastic traction used for early flexor tendon mobilization.

inhibits the formation of firm scar, one complication of early motion is tendon rupture. Therefore, if the patient early on has good smooth motion, the progression of the program should be delayed.[41] This smooth motion indicates that the scarring has been light. Therefore, the tendon juncture is vulnerable to rupture at this point.

In cases of flexor tendon grafts, the hand is immobilized for 3 weeks. At this point, gentle, controlled, active exercises are begun to provide tendon pull-through. Protection in the splint is continued for another 1 to 2 weeks in between exercises. At 4 weeks, the wrist can be brought into neutral. Dorsiflexion of the wrist is achieved gradually, so as not to place stress on the graft. If there is a proximal interphalangeal joint flexion contracture, an extension assist splint can be used intermittently at about 6 weeks. The extension assist splint also can provide mild resistance against flexion. Light massage is used at this time to help soften and maintain the skin in good condition. It is important to note that, when training the patient, the proximal joint must be blocked to place the flexor power at the joint being exercised. For example, when exercising the proximal interphalangeal joint, the metacarpophalangeal joint should be blocked. When exercising the distal interphalangeal joint, the metacarpophalangeal and the proximal interphalangeal joints should be blocked. This can be achieved by using a Bunnell block or by having the patient block with the other hand. Blocking exercises are usually started at 4 to 5 weeks.[42–47] For part of the exercise program, the proximal interphalangeal joint should also be exercised with the metacarpophalangeal joint supported in flexion to provide tendon glide in this range.

Staged Tendon Reconstruction. In cases of a severely damaged tendon system, the reconstructive ten-

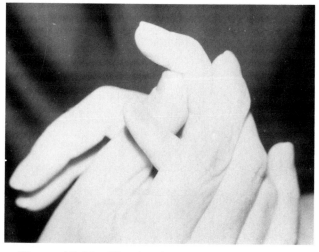

Figure 18.11 Testing for profundus function.

don procedure may be done in two stages. This technique of staged tendon surgery has improved the results of flexor tendon graft. Dr. James Hunter developed a method of implanting a flexible silicone rod around which a pseudosheath grows.[42-45] Later, the rod is removed, and a tendon graft is placed within this sheath providing a reconstructed tendon system. A necessary part of the pseudosheath formation is an organized program of passive gliding of the prosthesis. The implant is generally left in place for approximately 3 months before grafting is undertaken. This technique may also be used in some cases for damaged extensor tendons.

Stage I. Evelyn Mackin, L.P.T., and Dr. Hunter have given us careful guidelines to follow in the care of these patients.[42, 47] The silicone prosthesis is implanted in the finger and sutured at the distal end to the distal stump of the profundus. Following the surgery, the wrist is placed in about 30 to 40° of flexion with the metacarpophalangeal joints in about 40 to 60° of flexion and the interphalangeal joints in 20 to 30° of flexion.[42-45] The hand is maintained in this position for about 3 weeks. During the first week, controlled passive motion of the finger is started.[46, 47] The therapist must be careful to note any signs of synovitis in the finger. Exercises that are done too vigorously will result in swelling and pain. If this does occur, the finger must be rested, and infection or failure of the implant must be ruled out.[42-47] Therefore, close communication is essential between the surgeon and the therapist. Stretching exercises may be allowed under the supervision of the therapist during the 5th week.[42-44] Finger trapping using the adjacent finger to aid in gaining further passive motion may also be started at this time. If no sign of synovitis is present at 6 weeks, the patient is allowed to return to his normal activities.

Stage II. The Stage II procedure is the introduction of the tendon graft. Following surgery, the patient is protected in a dorsal splint with the hand in the same position as for Stage I. At about 5 to 7 days, with the hand still carefully protected in the dorsal splint, gentle passive flexion of the finger is done. Ten repetitions are done about 4 times per day. The patient may be allowed a limited amount of active wiggling of the finger.[42-44, 47] Again, this is done only within the confines of the splint. At about 4 weeks, finger blocking to encourage tendon pull-through may be allowed. This would be determined by the surgeon who would base his decision upon the condition of the tendon and how much tension he feels can be safely placed upon the tendon juncture.[42-47] At about 4 to 5 weeks, the pull-out wire is removed, and the active exercise program is increased.[47] It may be possible, at this time, to discontinue wearing the dorsal splint.[47] In some patients, however, it may be necessary to protect the hand a bit longer in the dorsal splint between exercises. This is decided on an individual basis depending upon the patient's circumstances. A block is then introduced to exercise each joint.[42-47] At about 6 to 8 weeks, the patient may be allowed to begin a program of graded activities to improve strength.[47]

Prior to a staged flexor tendon reconstruction, it is important that the therapist see the patient to improve the general condition of the hand by improving passive mobility of the injured finger and active and passive mobility of the uninvolved digits. Every effort must be made to improve as much as possible the condition of the soft tissue prior to surgery.

Extensor Tendon Repairs

The laceration of the extensor tendons is also a significant injury and can have a serious affect on hand function. Not only could one lose full extension but, because of scarring and a decrease of tendon excursion, one could also lose flexion.

The extensor tendons, in contrast to the flexor tendons, do not glide in a synovial sheath, except at the wrist.[8, 48] At the wrist, the synovial sheath extends about 1 inch above and 1 inch below the extensor retinaculum. The blood supply to the extensors comes from the soft tissue and paratenon rather than the vincula, as it does for the flexor tendons.[48]

Laceration of the extensor tendons at the distal joint level results in a mallet deformity. The management of this injury has been previously discussed.

Extensor tendon injuries that occur at the proximal interphalangeal joint level can result in a boutonniere deformity, since the central slip is often lacerated at that level.[48, 49] The treatment for this injury is immobilization of the proximal interphalangeal joint in full extension for about 5 to 6 weeks.[48] Active motion of the metacarpophalangeal joint and the distal interphalangeal joint is allowed during this time. When active proximal interphalangeal joint motion is started, it is necessary to monitor extension of the proximal interphalangeal joint carefully to be sure that no extensor lag develops. Further splinting would be necessary if a lag occurs.

Extensor tendon injuries to the rest of the hand are immobilized for approximately 4 weeks.[48] The hand is immobilized in a volar splint that extends from the proximal interphalangeal joint to two-thirds up the forearm. The wrist is held in about 20° of dorsiflexion with the metacarpophalangeal joints in extension.[48] The proximal interphalangeal joints are free to move. Following this period of immobilization, active and active assistive extension are started. At 5 weeks, gentle active flexion is allowed but must be done carefully. Remember, the flexors are much stronger than the extensors. Strong flexion could disrupt the repair. If the wrist extensors only are lacerated, the digits may be left free, and just the wrist may be immobilized. Immobilization is continued for 4 weeks.[48] An exercise we have found helpful in gaining extension following extensor tendon repair is to tape the proximal interphalangeal joints into flexion. The patient then flexes and extends the metacarpophalangeal joints in this manner[13] (Figs. 18.13 and 18.14). This position helps to isolate the long extensors and

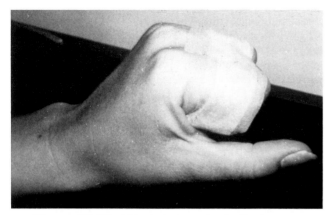

Figure 18.13 Taping exercise in flexion.

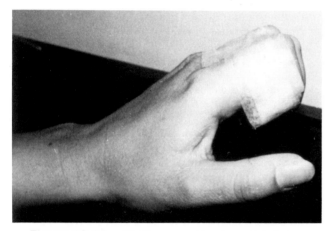

Figure 18.14 Taping exercise in extension.

places the extensor power at the metacarpophalangeal joint level. One must remember that the excursion of the extensor tendons can be decreased due to the adherence of the extensor tendons to the surrounding tissues. Therefore, when safe to do so, gentle stretching exercises to the extensors should be done. In some cases, a dynamic splint to aid in stretching may be necessary.[8] In cases where an extensor lag persists, a dynamic splint is fabricated to support the fingers in extension.[13] These injuries often progress slowly, and recovery may require several months. Biofeedback can be a useful tool in the treatment of these injuries. Generally, however, good results can be achieved.

Extensor Tendon Ruptures in Rheumatoid Arthritis

Extensor tendon rupture is a serious complication of rheumatoid arthritis. It requires a prolonged rehabilitation program. The patient needs to be told that it may take 3 to 4 months or longer to reach an end result. There are thought to be several causes of spontaneous tendon rupture in rheumatoid arthritis.[50-53] First, attrition rupture, when a tendon ruptures on a piece of bone, usually the distal ulna; second,

tenosynovitis that infiltrates the tendon; third, pressure from a hypertrophied synovial membrane beneath the tight dorsal retinaculum; and fourth, multiple steroid injections.

Single tendon ruptures cause a minimal extension lag because of the junctura tendonae which connect the tendons over the metacarpophalangeal joints.[52, 53] The patients will often have very little disability and may not even see a physician.[52-54] However, when two tendons rupture, the disability becomes more obvious. Any acute extensor tendon rupture is treated with urgency, as a single tendon rupture is followed by a second or a third.[52, 53] In patients with rheumatoid arthritis, either tendon transfer, usually the extensor indicis proprius, or adjacent tendon suture, is most often used to restore tendon function.[50-53] For more complicated ruptures, wrist extensors or the flexor digitorum superficialis tendons may be used. Generally, the poor condition of the soft tissue and the time elapsed between the actual rupture and the surgical repair prevents end-to-end suture. The final results of the repair are, of course, influenced by the number of tendons ruptured and the status of the surrounding joints and soft tissue.[52, 53] Following the transfer, the hand is immobilized for about 3½ weeks with the wrist in slight extension and the metacarpophalangeal joints in extension. The proximal interphalangeal joints are free to move. At 3½ weeks, the patient is started on gentle assisted active and passive extension and controlled active flexion.[13] Exercises are increased gradually over the next few weeks. We also utilize the taping exercise, as described previously. In some cases, it may also be necessary to fabricate a dynamic splint to support the tendons in extension.[13] The splint would be worn during the day. At night, the patient would return to the resting splint.[13]

Tenolysis

In some patients in whom therapy has failed to restore the tendon gliding, it may be necessary to perform a tenolysis following a tendon graft or repair. As we have previously mentioned, sometimes scar binds down the tendon and prevents it from gliding. The tenolysis frees the tendon from the scar.[55, 56] Generally, the surgeon waits about 3 to 6 months before performing tenolysis to see if the patient is able to get tendon pull-through without further surgery.[55]

Hand therapy, following a tenolysis, begins on the day following the surgery.[55, 56] Motion is done briefly 3 times per day. Care must be taken to teach the patient to exercise gently, so as not to increase swelling. The patient is carefully monitored over the next several weeks. During tenolysis, there is an interruption of the blood supply to the tendon. This makes the tendon more vulnerable to rupture. Therefore, no resistive activities are generally allowed before 6 to 8 weeks.[55] The exact time frame is determined by the surgeon and depends upon the condition of the tendon at surgery.

PAIN PROBLEMS

Problems of pain are among the most challenging and, without a doubt, often the most frustrating for all concerned. This is primarily due to the fact that we, as professionals, still do not understand about the mechanisms of pain and how to adequately control it.

Reflex Sympathetic Dystrophy

Reflex sympathetic dystrophy appears to result from an abnormal response of the autonomic nervous system to trauma. This, then, sets up a cycle of pain, immobility, swelling, and vasospasm which eventually leads to a stiff, nonfunctioning hand.[41, 57-60] This entity has been called by a number of names. These include minor causalgia, minor traumatic dystrophy, shoulder/hand syndrome, major traumatic dystrophy, and major causalgia. These, however, can all be considered classifications under the heading of reflex sympathetic dystrophy.[41, 57-60] This entity was described in 1864 by Silas Weir Mitchell.[41, 57-60] He reported this condition during the Civil War in soldiers who sustained gunshot wounds involving injuries to nerves. He termed this "burning pain" as causalgia. We know now that this syndrome does not necessarily result from nerve injury. It can result from carpal tunnel compression, release of Dupuytren's contracture, a crush injury, or fractures. It can be a devastating complication of Colles' fracture.[57, 59, 60] It may also be a sequela of a very minor injury. The predominant symptoms of reflex sympathetic dystrophy are pain and swelling which are out of all proportion to the injury. The patient often describes this pain as burning or stinging.[41, 57-60] The patient may also describe this as a constricting or pressure-type pain. This pain often may be aggravated by motion. As the dystrophy progresses, the hand becomes stiff from lack of motion. There is usually a change in skin color which often progresses from redness to a wax-like appearance. One often sees either excessive sweating or dryness of the skin. The hand may at first feel warm but in later stages will feel cool. There will also be progressive atrophy of the skin and muscles. One may also note changes in hair growth and nail growth. X-rays of the hand in the late stages may show demineralization of bone and narrowing of joint spaces.[57, 59] The pain may become so intense that even a breeze across the arm will cause unbearable pain, and the pain may progress to previously uninvolved areas.

These patients often manifest psychosocial problems. They are often angry and fearful.[57, 59, 60] These people have often been pushed from doctor to doctor and may be suspicious and, therefore, not always able to cooperate in their treatment. They expect the medical team to "make it better." These patients need to be shown that someone cares about them. They need a lot of emotional support. All treatment must be well coordinated with no discrepancies among the professionals involved in their treatment. These patients tend to be very suggestible. Therefore, consistent,

positive reinforcement is very beneficial. Various treatment procedures are used in an effort to relieve these unfortunate patients of their pain. Sympathetic blocks are frequently used by the physician to try to break the sympathetic arc. In some cases, it may be necessary to permanently interrupt the sympathetic arc by performing a surgical sympathectomy.

Hand Therapy Procedures

The main goal of treatment of these patients is to, first, help decrease pain and, second, to help increase their range of motion. However, before these goals can be accomplished, a trusting relationship between the therapist and the patient must be established.

The program of hand therapy should begin with modalities that will decrease pain. Hot packs or paraffin may be helpful in providing relief and can be used prior to exercises or activities.[41, 57-60] A trial of transcutaneous nerve stimulation (TENS) is given.[61-64] The electrode placement of the TENS depends upon the area of pain, the cause of the pain, and the nature of the pain. The electrodes may be placed over trigger points, the location of the greatest pain, distant or contralateral locations, specific dermatones or spinal segmental levels, points along the peripheral nerves, and linear pathways.[65] In some cases, alternative placements may be necessary in order to produce relief. If pain relief is obtained with the TENS, the patient may rent a unit which can be used at home. Naturally, once pain is decreased, a program to improve motion is much easier. Active exercises and activities are done by the patient and are done within the patient's tolerance. Therapy that increases pain is counterproductive and only adds to the patient's anxiety. Splinting to help correct deformity and improve mobility is used as soon as can be tolerated by the patient. Edema control, through elevation and massage in conjunction with active exercise, is also an important aspect of treatment. Massage is always done by the patient. In conjunction with massage, the patient is put on a program of systemic desensitization. This program involves the use of materials of varying textures. The patient begins stroking the hand and arm with the texture that can best be tolerated, doing this until it begins to become uncomfortable and repeating this procedure several times a day. The patient progresses, as tolerated, through the various textures, each one with increasing roughness. When this can be tolerated, the patient progresses to immersion therapy in which the hand is immersed in substances such as rice, beans, macaroni, etc.

Functional activities are also an important part of the treatment and are introduced as soon as possible. Since these patients often withdraw from social contacts, group activities are very helpful in getting these people back into the mainstream of life.

In cases of painful neuromas, the use of percussion and vibration of the neuroma, in conjunction with the previously outlined therapeutic measures, is often successful in relieving pain in selected patients.[41]

PSYCHOLOGICAL IMPLICATIONS

It must be kept in mind that people who sustain hand injuries or develop hand problems have to make a number of psychological adjustments to their disability. Their daily lives are interrupted, and their function is altered. In many cases, the disability is temporary and, in a period of time, they will return to their regular routine. However, in more serious problems, the person's life can be permanently changed. It can mean loss of the ability to perform his usual work or to pursue his various avocational interests. A person may lose self-esteem and become depressed, when unable to do regular work. Often, a patient who appears to lack motivation is really depressed or may be fearful of returning to the machine on which the injury occurred. The therapist can help the patient set realistic goals and act as a resource for needed information or referrals to outside agencies.

Some patients may require professional psychiatric help to deal with these issues. However, the supportive hand therapy environment and encouragement (not false hope) can help in making the adjustment period much smoother and less traumatic.

Acknowledgment. The author would like to give special acknowledgment to Mrs. Elaine Ames for her help in the preparation of this chapter.

References

1. Duran, R. J., Hauser, R. G., and Staver, M. G. Management of flexor tendon lacerations in Zone 2 using controlled passive motion post-operatively. In *Rehabilitation of the Hand*, edited by J. M. Hunter, L. H. Schneider, E. J. Mackin, and J. A. Bell. St. Louis: C. V. Mosby, 1978.
2. Burton, R. I. Acute Hand Joint Injuries. In *Acute Hand Injuries, A Multispecialty Approach*, edited by F. G. Walfort. Boston: Little, Brown, 1980.
3. Eaton, R. G. *Joint Injuries of the Hand*. Springfield, Ill.: Charles C Thomas, 1971.
4. Millender, L. H. Joint injuries. In *The Practice of Hand Surgery*, edited by D. W. Lamb and K. Kuczynski. Boston: Blackwell Scientific Publications, 1981.
5. Nalebuff, E. A., and Millender, L. H. Skeletal and ligamentous injuries of the hand. In *Trauma Management*, edited by E. Cave and R. Boyd. Chicago: Year Book Medical Publishers, 1974.
6. Burton, R. I., Beasley, R. W., Newmeyer, W. L., and Eaton, R. G. The jammed finger or thumb. *Contemp. Orthop.* 56–81, April 1979.
7. Dray, G., Millender, L. H., and Nalebuff, E. A. Rupture of the radial collateral ligament of the metacarpophalangeal joint to one of the ulnar three fingers. *J. Hand Surg.*, 4 (4): 346–350, 1979.
8. Rosenthal, E. A. The extensor tendons. In *Rehabilitation of the Hand*, edited by J. M. Hunter, L. H. Schneider, E. J. Mackin, and J. A. Bell. St. Louis: C. V. Mosby, 1978.
9. Madden, J. W., DeVore, G., and Arem, A. J. A rational postoperative management program for metacarpophalangeal joint implant arthroplasty. *J. Hand Surg.*, 2 (5): 358–366, 1977.
10. Millender, L. H., and Nalebuff, E. A. Metacarpophalangeal joint arthroplasty utilizing the silicone rubber prosthesis. *Orthop. Clin. North Am.*, 4 (2): 349–371, 1973.
11. Swanson, A. B. *Flexible Implant Resection Arthroplasty in the Hand and Extremities*. St. Louis: C. V. Mosby, 1973.
12. Swanson, A. B., Swanson, G., and Leonard, J. Post-operative rehabilitation program in flexible implant arthroplasty of the digits. In *Rehabilitation of the Hand*, edited by J. M. Hunter, L. H. Schneider, E. J. Mackin, and J. A. Bell. St. Louis: C. V. Mosby, 1978.
13. Philips, C. A., McCann, V. H., and Quigley, T. R. Preoperative and Post-operative Management: The Role of the Allied Health Professionals. *Orthop. Clin. North Am.*, 6 (3): 881–906, 1975.
14. Nalebuff, E. A., and Millender, L. H. Personal communication, 1981.
15. Goodman, M. J., Millender, L. H., Nalebuff, E. A., and Philips, C. A. Arthroplasty of the rheumatoid wrist with silicone rubber: An early evaluation. *J. Hand Surg.*, 2: 114–121, 1980.
16. Bell, J. A. Sensibility evaluation. In *Rehabilitation of the Hand*, edited by J. M. Hunter, L. H. Schneider, E. J. Mackin, and J. A. Bell. St. Louis: C. V. Mosby, 1978.
17. Levin, S., Pearsall, G., and Ruderman, R. J. Von Frey's method of measuring pressure sensibility in the hand: An engineering analysis of the Weinstein-Semmes pressure aesthesiometer. *J. Hand Surg.*, 3 (3): 211–216, 1978.
18. Omer, G. E. Sensibility testing. In *Management of Peripheral Nerve Problems*, edited by G. E. Omer and M. Spinner. Philadelphia: W. B. Saunders, 1980.
19. Werner, J. L., and Omer, G. E. Evaluating cutaneous pressure sensation of the hand. *Am. J. Occup. Ther.*, 24 (5): 347–376, 1970.
20. Moberg, E. Objective methods for determining the functional value of sensibility in the hand. *J. Bone Joint Surg.*, 40B (3): 454–459, 1958.
21. Parry, R. G. Nerve injuries. In *Acute Hand Injuries, A Multispecialty Approach*, edited by F. G. Walfort. Boston, Little, Brown, 1980.
22. Wynn Parry, C. B. *Rehabilitation of the Hand*. 3rd ed. London: Butterworth, 1973.
23. Curtis, R. M., and Dellon, A. L. Sensory re-education after peripheral nerve injury. In *Management of Peripheral Nerve Problems*, edited by G. E. Omer and M. Spinner. Philadelphia: W. B. Saunders, 1980.
24. Dellon, A. L., Curtis, R. M., and Edgerton, M. T. Re-education of sensation in the hand after nerve injury and repair. *Plast. Reconstr. Surg.*, 53: 297–305, 1974.
25. Maynard, C. J. Sensory re-education following peripheral nerve injury. In *Rehabilitation of the Hand*, edited by J. M. Hunter, L. H. Schneider, E. J. Mackin, and J. A. Bell. St. Louis: C. V. Mosby, 1978.
26. Dellon, A. L., Curtis, R. M., and Edgerton, M. T. Evaluating recovery of sensation in the hand following nerve injury. *Johns Hopkins Med. J.*, 130: 235–243, 1972.
27. Almquist, E. E. The effect of training on sensory function. In *Traumatic Nerve Lesions of the Upper Extremity*, edited by J. Mechon, and Moberg, E. New York: Churchill Livingstone, 1975.
28. Braun, R. M. Epineural nerve repair. In *Management of Peripheral Problems*, edited by G. E. Omer and M. Spinner. Philadelphia: W. B. Saunders, 1980.
29. Schultz, R. J. Management of nerve gaps. In *Management of Peripheral Nerve Problems*, edited by G. E. Omer and M. Spinner. Philadelphia: W. B. Saunders, 1980.
30. Ducker, T. B. Pathophysiology of peripheral nerve trauma. In *Management of Peripheral Nerve Problems*, edited by G. E. Omer and M. Spinner. Philadelphia: W. B. Saunders, 1980.
31. Omer, G. E. Tendon transfers for reconstruction of the forearm and hand following peripheral nerve injuries. In *Management of Peripheral Nerve Problems*, edited by G. E. Omer and M. Spinner. Philadelphia: W. B. Saunders, 1980.
32. Schneider, L. H. Tendon transfers in the upper extremity. In *Rehabilitation of the Hand*, edited by J. M. Hunter, L. H. Schneider, E. J. Mackin, and J. A. Bell. St. Louis: C. V. Mosby, 1978.
33. Verdan, C. The general principles of tendon transfer in the hand and forearm. In *Tendon Surgery of the Hand, G. E. M. Monograph 4*, edited by C. Verdan. New York: Churchill Livingstone, 1979.
34. Beasley, R. W. Basic considerations for tendon transfer operations in the upper extremity. In *American Academy of Orthopedic Surgeons Symposium on Tendon Surgery in the Hand*. St. Louis: C. V. Mosby, 1975.

35. McKay, D. Flexor tendon injuries. In *Acute Hand Injuries, a Multispecialty Approach*, edited by F. G. Walfort. Boston: Little, Brown, 1980.

36. Nissenbaum, M. Early care of flexor tendon injuries: Application of principles of tendon healing and early motion. In *Rehabilitation of the Hand*, edited by J. M. Hunter, L. H. Schneider, E. J. Mackin and J. A. Bell. St. Louis: C. V. Mosby, 1978.

37. Baker, D. S., Gaul, J. S., Williams, V. K., and Graves, M. The little finger superficialis—a clinical investigation of its anatomic and functional shortcomings. *J. Hand Surg.*, 6 (4): 374–378, 1981.

38. Duran, R. J., and Hauser, R. G. Controlled passive motion following flexor tendon repair in Zones 2 and 3. In *American Academy of Orthopaedic Surgeons Symposium on Tendon Surgery in the Hand*. St. Louis: C. V. Mosby, 1975.

39. Kleinert, H. E., Kutz, J. E., and Cohen, M. J. Primary repair of Zone 2 flexor tendon lacerations. In *American Academy of Orthopaedic Surgeons Symposium on Tendon Surgery in the Hand*. St. Louis: C. V. Mosby, 1975.

40. Kleinert, H. E., and Weiland, H. E. Primary repair of flexor tendon lacerations in Zone II. In *Tendon Surgery of the Hand, G. E. M. Monograph 4*, edited by C. Verdan. New York: Churchill Livingstone, 1979.

41. Omer, G. E., Jr. Management of pain syndromes in the upper extremity. In *Rehabilitation of the Hand*, edited by J. M. Hunter, L. H. Schneider, E. J. Mackin, and J. A. Bell. St. Louis: C. V. Mosby, 1978.

42. Hunter, J. M. Staged flexor tendon reconstruction. In *Rehabilitation of the Hand*, edited by J. M. Hunter, L. H. Schneider, E. J. Mackin, and J. A. Bell. St. Louis: C. V. Mosby, 1978.

43. Hunter, J. M. Two stage flexor tendon reconstruction: A technique using a tendon prosthesis prior to tendon grafting. In *Tendon Surgery of the Hand, G. E. M. Monograph 4*, edited by C. Verdan. New York: Churchill Livingstone, 1979.

44. Hunter, J. M., and Salisbury, R. E. Flexor-tendon reconstruction in severely damaged hands. *J. Bone Joint Surg.*, 53A (5): 829–857, 1971.

45. Hunter, J. M., and Schneider, L. H. Staged flexor tendon reconstruction current status. In *American Academy of Orthopaedic Surgeons Symposium on Tendon Surgery in the Hand*. St. Louis: C. V. Mosby, 1975.

46. Mackin, E. J. Physical therapy and the staged tendon graft: Pre-operative and post-operative management. In *American Academy of Orthopaedic Surgeons Symposium on Tendon Surgery in the Hand*. St. Louis: C. V. Mosby, 1975.

47. Mackin, E. J., and Mainano, L. Post-operative therapy following staged flexor tendon reconstruction. In *Rehabilitation of the Hand*, edited by J. M. Hunter, L. H. Schneider, E. J. Mackin, and J. A. Bell. St. Louis: C. V. Mosby, 1978.

48. Jabaley, M. E., and Heckler, F. R. Extensor tendon injuries. In *Acute Hand Injuries, a Multispecialty Approach*, edited by F. G. Walfort. Boston: Little, Brown, 1980.

49. Tubiana, R. Injuries to the extensor apparatus on the dorsum of the fingers. In *Tendon Surgery of the Hand, G. E. M. Monograph 4*, edited by C. Verdan. New York: Churchill Livingstone, 1979.

50. Egloff, D., and Verdan, C. Spontaneous tendon ruptures at the wrist in rheumatoid arthritis. In *Tendon Surgery of the Hand, G. E. M. Monograph 4*, edited by C. Verdan. New York: Churchill Livingstone, 1979.

51. Gschwend, N. Tendon involvement in rheumatoid arthritis. In *Tendon Surgery of the Hand, G. E. M. Monograph 4*, edited by C. Verdan. New York: Churchill Livingstone, 1979.

52. Nalebuff, E. A. The recognition and treatment of tendon ruptures of the rheumatoid hand. In *American Academy of Orthopaedic Surgeons Symposium of Tendon Surgery in the Hand*. St. Louis: C. V. Mosby, 1975.

53. Nalebuff, E. A. Surgical treatment of tendon rupture in the rheumatoid hand. *Surg. Clin. North Am.*, 49 (4): 811–822, 1969.

54. Cantero, J., and Chamay, A. Extensor tendon lesions on the dorsum of the hand and wrist. In *Tendon Surgery of the Hand, G. E. M. Monograph 4*, edited by C. Verdan. New York: Churchill Livingstone, 1979.

55. Schneider, L. H., and Hunter, J. M. Flexor tenolysis. In *American Academy of Orthopaedic Surgeons Symposium on Tendon Surgery in the Hand*. St. Louis: C. V. Mosby, 1975.

56. Verdan, C. Tenolysis. In *Tendon Surgery of the Hand, G. E. M. Monograph 4*, edited by C. Verdan. New York: Churchill Livingstone, 1979.

57. Clark, G. L. Causalgia: A discussion of chronic pain syndromes in the upper limb. In *Rehabilitation of the Hand*, edited by J. M. Hunter, L. H. Schneider, E. J. Mackin, and J. A. Bell. St. Louis: C. V. Mosby, 1978.

58. Erickson, J. C., III. Evaluation and management of autonomic dystrophies of the upper extremity. In *Rehabilitation of the Hand*, edited by J. M. Hunter, L.H. Schneider, E. J. Mackin, and J. A. Bell. St. Louis: C. V. Mosby, 1978.

59. Lankford, L. L. Reflex sympathetic dystrophy. In *Management of Peripheral Nerve Problems*, edited by G. E. Omer and M. Spinner. Philadelphia: W. B. Saunders, 1980.

60. Morgan, J. E. Sympathetic dystrophy. In *Acute Hand Injuries, a Multispecialty Approach*, edited by F. G. Walfort. Boston: Little, Brown, 1980.

61. Lampe, G. N. Introduction to the use of transcutaneous electrical nerve stimulation devices. *Phys. Ther.*, 58 (12): 1450–1454, 1978.

62. Wolf, S. L., Gersh, M. R., and Kutner, M. Relationship of selected clinical variables to current delivered during transcutaneous electrical nerve stimulation. *Phys. Ther.*, 58 (12): 1478–1485, 1978.

63. Wolf, S. L. Perspective on central nervous system responsiveness to transcutaneous electrical nerve stimulation. *Phys. Ther.*, 58 (12): 1443–1447, 1978.

64. Kleinert, H. E., Norberg, H., and McDonough, J. J. Surgical sympathectomy of the upper and lower extremity. In *Management of Peripheral Nerve Problems*, edited by G. E. Omer and M. Spinner. Philadelphia: W. B. Saunders, 1980.

65. Mannheimer, J. S. Electrode placements for transcutaneous electrical nerve stimulation. *Phys. Ther.*, 58 (12): 1455–1462, 1978.

Supplementary Reading

Fess, E. Evaluation of the hand by objective measurement. In *Rehabilitation of the Hand*, edited by J. M. Hunter, L. H. Schneider, E. J. Mackin, and J. A. Bell. St. Louis: C. V. Mosby, 1978.

Fess, E. E., Gettle, K. S., and Strickland, J. W. *Hand Splinting: Principles and Methods*. St. Louis: C. V. Mosby, 1981.

Flatt, A. *Care of Rheumatoid Hand*. 3rd Edition. St. Louis: C. V. Mosby, 1974.

Jebsen, R. H., Taylor, N., Triegchmann, R. B., Trotter, M. J., and Howard, L. A. An objective and standardized test of hand function. *Arch. Phys. Med. Rehabil.*, 50: 311, 1969.

Lamb, D. W., and Kuczynski, K. (eds.). *The Practice of Hand Surgery*. Boston: Blackwell Scientific Publications, 1981.

The Hand: Examination and Diagnosis. Aurora, Colo. The American Society for Surgery of the Hand, 1978.

chapter

19

Fractures

Lillian Hoyle Parent, M.A., OTR

Improvements in orthopedic surgical and immobilization techniques have resulted in methods that lead to earlier motion of the fractured extremity, and enhanced healing of the fracture. Patients can resume normal activity sooner. Once a fracture has stable reduction from a plaster cast or internal fixation, active motion is begun in muscles and uninjured joints in the extremity. The kind and amount of movement depends on the site of the fracture and the patient's general condition.[1]

A fracture is an interruption of the continuity of bone or an epiphyseal plate, usually caused by trauma. A direct blow to the extremity often causes a transverse fracture, whereas a twisting force causes a spiral fracture. A crushing injury often results in a comminuted fracture, one with multiple bone fragments. Symptoms of a fracture are pain and loss of function. The presence of a fracture is confirmed by x-ray.[2]

An open fracture has skin and soft tissue wounds, whereas a closed fracture does not interrupt the skin. A comminuted fracture may be an open or closed fracture. The goals of fracture treatment are to reduce, that is, to place the bone fragments in as close to anatomical position as possible, and to create an environment for the bone cells to proliferate to form a union between or among the bone parts and eventually to consolidate so there is adequate strength to support neuromuscular activity without pain.[2]

A pathological fracture is one that occurs spontaneously from some abnormal condition such as osteoporosis or metastatic disease that causes bone to weaken. These fractures can be stabilized by open reduction and internal fixation; the patient's overall condition and function determine the procedure to be used.[3] Closed reduction is done by an orthopedic surgeon and confirmed by x-ray. If a more accurate reduction can be achieved for earlier mobilization of the patient, surgery will be done to place an internal fixation device such as an orthopedic nail, pin, screw, rod, or compression plate to promote faster healing.

The goal of fracture treatment is to prevent malunion. There are also various prosthetic devices for implantation to restore joint motion.[2]

Fracture healing has a general timetable which is observed by repeated x-rays during the course of treatment. Union of a fracture, characterized by proliferation of calcified callus, is an incomplete repair. The fracture site is still tender, and although when tested the bone moves in one piece, the healing is incomplete, and the bone is not yet strong enough for stress without the protection of some type of immobilization. Consolidation, or complete repair, has occurred when the calcified callus has ossified; the fracture site is no longer tender and painful, and there is no movement when the fractured bone is manipulated. Further protection is not necessary. A general estimate of healing time for an uncomplicated fracture is[2]:

	Union	Consolidation
Upper extremity spiral fracture	3 weeks	6 to 8 weeks
Upper extremity transverse fracture	6 weeks	12 weeks
Lower extremity spiral fracture	6 weeks	12 to 16 weeks
Lower extremity transverse fracture	12 to 15 weeks	24 to 30 weeks

The goal of fracture rehabilitation is to return the patient to the previous level of function, and this begins as soon as the fracture is reduced and immobilized. Although the fractured bone is immobilized, the supporting structures such as soft tissue, muscle, nerve, and skin should be active from the start of fracture immobilization, which occurs when the plaster cast is dry, after about 48 to 60 hours,[3] and within a day or two after surgery for open reduction. The amount and kind of activity depend on the place of the fracture, the treatment procedure selected by the orthopedist and, in some instances, the age of the patient.[2]

Fractures are treated as an emergency, reduced and immobilized. The patient may not be referred to occupational therapy. Newer approaches to treatment indicate that early but specific use of the immobilized extremities may foster bone healing and reduce disuse atrophy and stiffness that are the residuals of immobilization of joints and tissues. It is important to obtain early referral to occupational therapy with the goal of teaching these patients activities to be done during the fracture immobilization.

Evaluation is done for active range of motion of any joint available for testing. Also, if fingers are not included in the cast, pinch evaluation can be done. The program is planned to prevent disuse and stiffness rather than to treat the conditions that exist when the cast is removed. A program based on activities of daily living and work modalities will cause the patient to use the muscles and joints repeatedly. The OT's goal is to teach the patient that movement and use of the involved extremity is more desirable than inactivity.

STAGES OF FRACTURE CARE

Fracture care is divided into two stages. Stage one is the period from reduction and immobilization through the period of consolidation. The final functional result after a fracture depends not only on the treatment for the injured bone, but also the treatment of associated soft tissue injuries.[4] Adequate treatment while the fracture is healing decreases the amount of postimmobilization treatment.[5] This includes upper extremity movement, as well as movement of lower extremities which require longer periods of nonweight bearing or immobilization because fractures here take longer to consolidate. Stage 2 follows immobilization and extends through return of optimum range of motion and strength in the extremity. This second stage may be minimized through active treatment programs during the first stage of treatment.[4]

First Stage

Because many upper extremity fractures are seen in an emergency room where reduction and immobilization are done immediately, at any hour, patients may not be referred to occupational therapy and may not be taught a treatment program designed for their specific needs. If occupational therapists are to receive referrals for these patients, it is necessary to set up treatment protocols and to establish a working referral system with the orthopedic surgeons and emergency room physicians. Patients with fractures treated in outpatient clinics may not otherwise know the benefits from muscular exercise while the fracture heals. Written instructions for therapeutic activities can be issued, and routine visits to change the program can be scheduled as necessary. Current research indicates that an adequate program for the use of all muscles and joints that are not immobilized leads to quicker

functional return and diminishes, or in some instances eliminates, the need for treatment after immobilization and prevents the occurrence of some side effects of immobilization, such as stiff joints and weakness.[5]

Also, after initial immobilization, the patient needs a program of definitive movement to prevent or eliminate edema and disuse atrophy of bone and muscles that occur with inactivity and are common following immobilization.[6] Contraction of muscles that cross the fracture site actually cause the bone ends to impinge on each other, which encourages bone healing.[2] During immobilization in a cast or a fracture brace for the upper extremity, patients are encouraged to use the muscles and joints through functional use of the extremity.[5, 6] However, older patients may be fearful that early mobilization of fractures, as currently practiced, will do more damage.[7] The therapist needs to emphasize the benefits from doing activities and teach the patients how to do them.[4] Patients with upper extremity fractures may need information on self-care (see Chapter 26) and perhaps how to use assistive devices. Also, occupational therapists can design a therapeutic program incorporating work, leisure, and self-care activities into the program.

Precautions

Plaster casts are commonly used for immobilization of fractures. Patients wearing casts must be observed for signs of edema forming within the extremity inside the cast. Soft tissue damage associated with a fracture results in extracellular edema. Unless this condition is treated quickly, the extracellular fluid will gel and bind down all the tissue with adhesions, a condition that retards restoration of movement and function. The best treatment for this condition is muscular contraction to pump away the edema fluid and to keep torn muscle fibers from adhering to other structures.[2] The upper extremity can be elevated with an arm sling, or an overhead sling, or other equipment to support or to suspend the extremity with the hand held above the heart level, while avoiding acute elbow flexion.[8]

Excessive edema, or damage to arterial circulation, can result in compression of nerve and muscle. Nerve will regenerate, but muscle can survive ischemia for only 6 to 8 hours and cannot regenerate. Arterial occlusion, if complete, leads to Volkmann's ischemia, which can be caused by edema or acute elbow flexion that compresses an artery against bone. If occlusion is complete, gangrene can result. Signs of ischemia are pale bluish color of skin, absence of forearm radial pulse, or decreased hand sensation accompanied by severe pain. Any of these signs indicate that arterial circulation may be compromised. The patient's physician must be notified immediately. If not treated, either by reduction of edema, change of position, removal of cast, or exploration of the vascular system, the condition can lead to Volkmann's contracture, a sequelae of ischemia of the forearm. If not treated quickly, muscles become fibrosed and contracted, leaving deformity, stiffness, and perhaps sensory loss to the hand. This typically results in a claw hand (proximal interphalangeal (PIP) and distal interphalangeal (DIP) flexion) in which tenodesis action can provide some grip, but this hand is a needlessly weak and severely impaired hand from a preventable condition.[2,3]

Ischemia of the hand can follow forearm injuries and involve the intrinsic muscles leaving a deformity of metacarpophalangeal (MP) flexion and interphalangeal (IP) extension with the thumb held in adduction. Lower extremities can be subject to ischemia with similar residuals in the foreleg and foot.[2]

Other complications of a fracture may include venous thrombosis and pulmonary embolism. Tetanus may be a problem in an open fracture. Muscles, tendons, and nerves may be damaged by an open fracture of the humerus, particularly in the supracondylar area because the radial, median, and ulnar nerves are in close proximity to the humerus before spreading into the forearm.[2] Nerve and tendon injuries that accompany a fracture will be treated according to methods described in Chapter 18.

If a patient in a cast complains of burning pain under the cast, the physician should be notified because the pain may be a signal that a pressure sore is developing and the cast needs revision to prevent further problems. A well-made properly fitted cast should provide comfort, never pain.[2]

Second Stage

The second stage of fracture treatment follows consolidation of bone. When the patient's immobilization is ended, evaluation of active range of motion can be done and, if it is deficient, a program of activity can be started. No passive motion such as stretching should be done once the patient is out of the cast. This is particularly true of the elbow. It is considered that passive movement is involved in myositis ossificans in which calcium is deposited outside of the bone.[2] If the patient has not used muscles consistently during the immobilization, early movement may be painful because all structures will be tight, shortened, and weak, and the joints will probably be stiff. The patient should have a treatment program of gentle active motion to gain strength and range of motion to correct any deficits noted. Strengthening can begin with active motion, and as this becomes comfortable, gentle, progressively resistive activities may be started. Elderly patients may not gain full anatomical range of motion following a fracture.[2,4,9] Evaluate the other extremity to determine the patient's usual range of motion before a vigorous program is started. If it is not complete, perhaps the patient has been independent with less than anatomical range. The goal is to obtain enough range of motion in the immobilized extremity, and the other one, sufficient for the patient's needs for activities of daily living. If not, adapted techniques can be taught and, if necessary, adaptive equipment can be provided to restore independence.

UPPER EXTREMITY FRACTURES

As soon as pain diminishes in a fracture, any upper extremity immobilized or placed in a sling must have all uninvolved joints used daily. This is especially important in the elderly. Special attention is given to mobilization of the shoulder and fingers because they are easily subject to loss of range of motion. The goal is to decrease atrophy and maintain muscle function and range of motion in any joint not immobilized.[2] Following removal of the plaster cast or other forms of immobilization, only active motion should be done. Codman's exercises are a gentle active motion that is used to reestablish function following upper extremity fractures. Codman's pendulum exercises are done by having the patient bend over at the waist, either standing or sitting, so that the trunk is parallel to the floor. The arm is allowed to assume a position away from the body, either with or without a sling, as much as pain and stiffness permit. In this position the patient can move the arm forward in flexion or back in extension. In this position the motions are performed with gravity minimized, compared with trying to do the movements in the upright position.[9] If a patient is seated, an activity to encourage this motion might be movement of pieces on a game board that has been placed on a low stool or the floor. Codman's exercises should not be used with an edematous upper extremity. An overhead sling would permit gravity minimized shoulder movement while the edematous upper extremity is being elevated.

Clavicle

Fractures of the middle or distal third of the clavicle are treated with the arm in a sling, and no physical activity of the shoulder until the pain and tenderness diminish. Then gentle active movements of the shoulder, elbow, wrist and fingers are started to avoid stiffness, a common residual of these fractures.[3]

Fractures of the middle third of the clavicle are treated with a figure of eight bandage. The elbow and hand are exercised from the beginning, and active shoulder motions should be started when it is comfortable for the patient. The shoulder movement may be done in gravity-minimized positions (as in muscle testing) to maintain shoulder mobility or Codman's movements may be used. The patient should be advised not to do heavy activity on the side of the fracture for 3 months postinjury.[3]

A fracture of the coracoid process is treated in an arm sling for a week and athletic activities are restricted for about 2 months.[3]

Shoulder

A fracture dislocation of the shoulder, after reduction, is immobilized in a sling for a few days. Because this injury quickly results in stiffness, a minimal period of immobilization is used. Passive movement is used sparingly in the shoulder and should be avoided in the elderly.[4] All other joints should do active movement.

External rotation is emphasized during recovery because full abduction is not possible without external rotation which may become limited, especially in the elderly because of loss of elasticity in the joint capsule. Recurrent dislocations require surgical correction and are immobilized 3 weeks postoperatively in athletic individuals and 1 week in the elderly.[3] Graded range of motion exercises are initiated gradually with Codman's movements in which flexion is followed by abduction. Strengthening can be started when active shoulder range of motion is achieved. No forced range of motion should be attempted.[2, 3]

Humerus

A fracture of the neck of the humerus is treated in a sling with the elbow free. The weight of the arm provides traction on the fracture for the first week. The wrist is supported by a sling from around the neck. The patient should bend over from the waist, with the arm still in the sling, to do simple movements with the shoulder to try to increase shoulder motion each day.[3] Motions should be started early to prevent soft tissue scarring in the glenohumeral joint. Shoulder flexion movement is strengthened by voluntary movement forward until 90° is achieved. When the fracture is consolidated, voluntary abduction activities can begin. When these are comfortable, all shoulder motions can be resumed. The fracture usually heals in 6 to 8 weeks, and strengthening activities can begin when full range of motion is achieved.[4]

Although fractures of the humerus unite quickly, treatment in a sling keeps the arm in adduction and internal rotation, which leads to joint stiffness in the extremity, especially in the shoulder. This is a great problem for the elderly because of pain and fear of moving. Active motion must be initiated early and regularly.[2, 7]

Humeral shaft fractures may be treated in a splint of thermoplastic material that circles the humerus over the fracture site. The arm may be supported in a sling for the first week. This allows for shoulder, elbow, and hand movements, although strenuous exercise is discouraged. The patient is relatively comfortable and can do activities of daily living. The sling is discontinued when pain is no longer present. The thermoplastic splint is used until the fracture has consolidated.[10]

Elbow

Supracondylar fractures of the humerus may be treated in plaster or with open reduction. The elbow is placed in 90 to 100° of flexion with a plaster slab or splint, and the arm is supported in a collar and cuff sling. This sling is a circle of material that is placed around the neck. The forearm is placed in the circle and supported only at the wrist. The length of the sling should place the radial side of the wrist just below the nipple line.[2] After the first week the plaster slab is removed daily for gentle active motion and then reapplied between activity sessions.[3] Active motions for fractures around the elbow emphasize flexion rather than extension and may be done in a gravity-minimized position.

Treatment following dislocation of the elbow, trauma, or fracture to the humerus, radius, or ulna in the immediate vicinity of the elbow joint emphasizes active movement. Passive motion should not be attempted because of the possibility of myositis ossificans occurring with further limitation. An injury in this area may result in some permanent limitation in elbow extension. However, many patients with injuries in this area achieve close to full range of motion in from 6 months to a year without specific treatment.[2, 3, 4, 9] A complication of supracondylar fractures may be Volkmann's ischemia or peripheral nerve injury.[6]

Complex fractures of the elbow may require open reduction with well-secured fixation. Active motion can begin within 5 days. Fractures of the elbow are usually splinted in flexion rather than extension because in flexion the hand can be placed to the face and head for activities of daily living.[1, 3, 4] In the elderly, elbow fractures may be treated in a collar and cuff sling, described above, and mobilized early. Otherwise, they become stiff, painful joints. A useful arc of motion for daily activities can be regained, although the elderly may never achieve full range of motion.[7]

Forearm

A fracture of the radial head is treated with a sling or plaster slab for comfort. The arm is out of the sling for active movement of the elbow 15 to 20 minutes daily. If function does not return, then the radial head may be excised.[3]

A Monteggia fracture is a fracture of the ulna and dislocation of the radial head. The fracture is treated with open reduction and internal fixation for adult patients.[6] When there is a fracture of both bones of the forearm, closed reduction and immobilization with plaster is used. If the reduction cannot be maintained in plaster, or cannot be obtained, then open reduction and internal fixation are done. This requires 6 to 8 weeks to heal.[3]

A Colles' fracture involves the distal end of the radius with avulsion of the ulnar styloid. This is usually reduced and held in plaster. Use of the hand and whole extremity should be encouraged during immobilization because finger stiffness is a severe sequelae.[3] If movement is maintained, little treatment is needed after immobilization.[5]

For fractures of the hand, see Chapter 18.

LOWER EXTREMITY FRACTURES

There are an estimated 200,000 hip fractures that occur annually in the United States, and the majority of them occur in elderly women, more often in the left hip. Moderate trauma is a common cause of hip fracture in women and may occur while walking, in a fall from a chair or bed, often when getting up at night to void,[11, 12] from a change in posture,[13] and perhaps from changes of visual functions in the elderly,[14] particularly

ticularly those related to poor lighting.[12] Hip fracture in middle-aged or elderly men usually results from severe trauma.[11] If patients are treated in the recumbent position, this increases calcium loss and, therefore, bone strength diminishes in extended immobilization in the elderly. These patients need to be mobilized early, and this is a consideration for the choice of the type of surgery to repair fractures of the hip.[6, 11, 15] The cost of caring for these patients exceeds $750,000,000 per year.[11] The long-term care of these patients will increase that cost because many of these patients were independent prior to the hip fracture, but require nursing home care following the fracture.[16] About 19% of these patients die as a result of complications secondary to the fracture.[11]

Elderly women are a population at risk for falls, commonly on level ground, often without apparent cause. There seems to be a deterioration of sensorimotor abilities, and the elderly are slow to react in an emergency such as tripping, or missing the last step in descending stairs. If a planned movement must be changed quickly, an older person may not be able to do so rapidly enough. An apparently trivial accident may prove severe in terms of physical and social abilities.[12] The elderly who fall tend to show changes in gait to gain stability at the expense of efficiency. Speed and length of step decrease, and there is marked variability in the frequency of step length. It is suggested that there may be some loss of central control over automatic stepping.[13] Hasselkus[17] reports that in some elderly patients the more primitive protective response patterns tend to reappear, which may interfere with refined equilibrium responses of the normal adult. Patients who are to be ambulatory or non- or partially weight bearing after hip surgery, should be evaluated for righting and equilibrium reactions and, if decreased in these reactions, some training or modified techniques could be attempted.

Prognostic indicators for elderly patients to return home after a hip fracture, in addition to age and general medical condition, include whether they lived with someone and had a preinjury pattern of social contacts outside of their home. Also those patients who were ambulated early in the hospital and could manage dressing, personal hygiene, and toileting during the first 2 postoperative weeks were statistically more likely to return home. Physical therapists' ratings on weight bearing and strength of the uninvolved lower extremity, endurance, balance, mental clarity, and evidence of motivation were also indicators of individual rehabilitation potential.[18]

Patients with hip fractures, hip arthroplasties, and other lower extremity fractures are referred routinely to physical therapy for gait training, transfer, and other mobility activities. Once the patient has learned the basic techniques, often cognitively and consciously, occupational therapy programs can be used to apply mobility skills to other activities of daily living concurrently so that mobility is automatic while the patient concentrates on activities of daily living, homemaking responsibilities, or return to work. Oc-

cupational therapy programs can concentrate on ADL using a walker with partial weight bearing and to help these patients regain confidence in their overall abilities.[19]

Fractures of the Hip

Orthopedic surgical procedures for the hip are divided into two categories, emergency surgery for hip fractures and elective surgery for relief of pain and restoration of range of motion and function. Hip fractures have various classifications, but the following terms are commonly used.[3] The method of treatment for a fracture will depend on the history of the patient's activities immediately prior to the injury, the type of fracture, and the anticipated level of activity after recovery.[20]

Intracapsular Fractures

Subcapital fractures occur at the base of the head of the femur or the high portion of the femoral neck.[3] If this fracture is impacted and undisplaced, with bone fragments in good position, closed treatment may be used.[21] However, because there is about 100% success for healing with reduction and internal fixation, this is the usual treatment to promote immediate weight bearing.[3] In some instances a prosthetic replacement of the femoral head may be used.[21]

Transcervical or midcervical fractures occur in the midportion of the femoral neck. These are treated with reduction and internal fixation with a nail, multiple pins, or a nail and plate.[3]

Basilar neck (basicervical) fractures are located at the lower portion of the femoral neck and are treated with reduction and internal fixation.[3]

Postoperative Treatment. Patients with intracapsular fractures treated with internal fixation are mobilized by transferring to a chair the second or third postoperative day assisted by the physical therapist, and the following day should begin ambulation training with a walker. The physical therapist teaches the patient to place no more than 40 to 50 lbs. of weight on the operated leg during ambulation for the first 2 to 3 weeks.[22] High femoral neck fractures (subcapital, midcervical) should not do full weight bearing until the fracture is healed. However, patients with low femoral neck fractures can progress to weight bearing rapidly. The average length of hospital stay for patients with intracapsular fractures is 2 weeks, and they should be mobilized quickly, whether weight bearing or nonweight bearing.[3]

A method for teaching patients to do gradual or partial weight bearing and to learn how a certain amount of pressure feels is to have the patient in a standing table, foot of the uninvolved leg placed on a wooden block the height of a bathroom scale. The scale is placed parallel to the block, and the patient touches down on the scale with the foot of the involved leg. The therapist reads the amount of weight registered. The patient can touch down a bit more until the desired weight is reached. The patient then practices doing a specific amount to get the feel for partial weight bearing.[21]

Extracapsular Fractures

These fractures tend to occur in women in their 70s who have osteoporosis. Trochanteric fractures tend to heal better than femoral neck fractures. In general they are treated with reduction and internal fixation to promote early mobilization.[3]

Intertrochanteric fractures occur along the trochanteric line without involving the trochanters. The fractures are reduced and held with internal fixation. Some treatment protocols suggest that the patient should be nonweight-bearing until there is x-ray evidence of clinical union, which may take up to 11 weeks.[23] If the treatment is closed intramedullary nailing, the patient is transferred from bed to chair the first or second postoperative day, and the next day is progressed to ambulation in parallel bars or a walker with no weight bearing on the operated leg. Depending upon the internal fixation device used by the surgeon, such as a sliding compression screw, the patient can progress to full weight bearing with the walker.[24] Although some patients with adequate balance can progress to crutchwalking, if there is any doubt about balance and mental competence, or there is concurrent neurological, musculoskeletal, or cardiac involvement, these patients should use a walker.[21]

Pertrochanteric fractures involve the greater trochanter, or both trochanters. Treatment of a comminuted fracture may restrict the patient to partial weight bearing for the first 6 months following fixation. Full weight bearing may not be allowed until there is x-ray evidence of union.[3]

Subtrochanteric fractures are difficult to classify because there is no precise anatomical definition of the area. Young patients who have these fractures, as a result of severe direct trauma, are usually treated in traction which requires three months. Eighteen weeks is required for clinical union, and the patient must be nonweight-bearing for 6 months after injury. A young patient who may be unreliable about weight bearing can be treated in a hip spica cast. The postoperative plan depends on the amount of stability achieved with internal fixation.[3] For this reason, close collaboration between the orthopedic surgeon and the therapists is important in the management of these patients.

Subtrochanteric fractures occur frequently in the elderly, and the goal is early ambulation to avoid secondary medical complications. They are treated with internal fixation and may begin ambulation within the first week after surgery and by 3 weeks may achieve full weight bearing.[2] With oblique and badly comminuted fractures, even with internal fixation, these patients may be treated as bed to chair patients with therapists making sure that all joints maintain range of motion and that strength is preserved in the upper extremities.[3] These patients may be mobilized in a rocking chair to promote contraction of lower extremity muscles without weight bearing.[23]

Other aspects of successful rehabilitation include a consistent program to give information about hip fractures and recovery to patients and their families. Emphasis is placed on convincing the patient of the importance of doing optimum self-care[18] and giving reassurance to the family that interruption of independence is temporary and that they can help the patient return to independence. This must be tempered with the awareness that because of other medical problems, debility, and age, many of these patients may not survive a hip fracture. In such cases, heroic measures may not be humane.[7]

Fractures of the Shaft of the Femur

Treatment for femoral shaft fracture can be closed reduction and skeletal traction for 6 weeks or until union is achieved.[2] Muscle function in the thigh and range of motion of the knee and ankle are encouraged while in traction.[4] After fracture union, a cast brace may be applied to allow partial weight bearing, as tolerated, progressing to full weight bearing because this facilitates healing. Although the cast brace may be used for another 3 months, the patient can resume social and work routines.[3]

In the elderly a femoral shaft fracture may be treated with intramedullary nailing because it allows early mobilization.[1] The patient may sit in a chair the day following surgery and should be taught transfers and activities of daily living within the restraints of limited weight bearing until the fracture heals.[9] For elderly patients, partial or nonweight bearing may not be a viable goal. They should be encouraged to bear as much weight on the leg as is comfortable. Nonweight bearing may protect the fracture from excessive load, but active muscular contraction is important for fracture healing.[3]

Supracondylar Fracture

Supracondylar fractures of the femur and fractures of the tibial plateau are treated with internal fixation to prevent delayed union and to permit knee motion. If the supracondylar fracture reduction is well aligned and stable, early weight bearing may be permitted. However, for fractures of the tibial plateau, weight bearing is delayed 3 months, although nonweight bearing knee movement is encouraged.[3]

Tibial Fractures

Fracture of the tibia may be treated in a long leg cast for early weight bearing. After there is fracture union, about 4 weeks, a functional below-knee cast can be applied, and weight bearing, which facilitates healing, is begun.[1, 3]

Ankle Fractures

Fractures of the ankle may be treated with open or closed reduction and a below-knee cast. Nonweight bearing may last for up to 3 months for these fractures.[3]

LOWER EXTREMITY ELECTIVE SURGERY

A hip fracture is considered an emergency and is an acute problem requiring immediate and definitive care. Other conditions of the hip joint may have an insidious progressive onset. The surgical correction for relief of pain is an elective procedure. Some hip joint problems, for which surgery is an elective procedure, are congenital hip disease, rheumatoid arthritis, and osteoarthritis or degenerative joint disease. Osteoarthritis is a common form of arthritis of unknown etiology, and it results in the inability of the joint cartilages to repair themselves as quickly as they degenerate. Osteophytes form on the joint surface, leaving an uneven surface, which results in painful joint movement. The onset is gradual and may involve one or a few joints. The hip joint is a common site where osteoarthritis occurs and leads to a painful limp which can result in great restriction of a person's activities over time. In severe cases canes, crutches, or a walker may help to protect weight-bearing joints.[25] Body mechanics are an important consideration. Displacement of weight from painful joints to other joints can produce overload or stress on otherwise satisfactory joints.

Conservative treatment of this condition results in reduction of activities, use of a cane, crutches, or a wheelchair, weight control, and use of analgesics.[21] Energy conservation techniques are taught to reduce the kind and amount of homemaking and activities of daily living to conserve energy for vocational and leisure activities. Disabling pain is usually the reason for the patient's final decision to seek surgical relief.[26]

There are a number of surgical procedures for reduction of hip disability and pain. They include osteotomy, arthrodesis or hip fusion, THARIES (total hip replacement with internal eccentric shells), and total hip arthroplasty (THA). In selecting the procedure, the orthopedic surgeon will consider the degree of deformity and the amount of bone stock available, compared with knowledge of the patient's age, occupation, life-style, and potential for cooperation in the postoperative rehabilitation. Also, the patient's weight and activity levels must be balanced with what is known of the selected procedure's capability of providing a predictably good result with decreasing possibility of failure.[27] Any orthopedic procedure being considered must take into consideration the patient's level of self-care and activities of daily living, including occupation and leisure. In younger patients, work activities are considered carefully. For the older patient, who may not be employed, it is important to find out the living arrangements and social support network the patient will have available following a given procedure.[7] Also, the surgeon may select the least radical procedure in order to make possible some later procedure, if this should become necessary.

Osteotomy

An intertrochanteric osteotomy, a procedure to change the alignment of the femur to relieve weight bearing on the hip joint, can be used. This may be the surgery of choice if it is done in the early stages of the osteoarthritic process. When the procedure is done, compression plates are used to stabilize the bone, and the patient can begin early postoperative mobilization with passive movement. However, no active, resisted exercise is permitted for the first postoperative weeks. The knee should be mobilized. No weight bearing can be done for 6 months because this increases pressure on the hip joint. A successful outcome of a hip osteotomy depends on this long period of nonweight bearing.[28]

Arthrodesis

An arthrodesis of the hip fuses the hip joint at about 30° of flexion and neutral abduction and rotation, and it results in a stable, pain-free joint. This procedure is considered for patients under age 60 who are in good physical condition and have one painful osteoarthritic hip. Preoperative assessment for an arthrodesis will consider the patient's physical needs for work, the physical requirements of the occupation, life-style, and the kind of disability caused by the pain. The patient must have full range of motion of the knee on the side to be operated and full hip and knee range of motion on the opposite side.[2, 29]

The patient with a hip arthrodesis, fixed by a metal plate, is mobilized about a week after surgery and is allowed gradual weight bearing up to full weight bearing in 2 months. Some patients may use a cane for ambulation for a long time after surgery.[29]

The patient with an arthrodesis of the hip sits with a curved lumbar spine. In the early postoperative stages, these patients require assistive devices for lower extremity dressing and bathing. The patients may ultimately be able to put on a sock and shoe by bending the knee and reaching behind to guide them onto the foot by touch without visual guidance. Although it may seem that this procedure leaves the patient with residual disability, it does give the patient a strong, stable, pain-free hip that is adequate for endurance needed for standing at work. Follow-up studies indicate that many of these patients participate in active sports such as walking, hiking, sailing, and horseback riding.[29]

Hip Arthroplasty

A procedure used with younger patients with painful stiff hips is the Smith-Petersen cup arthroplasty. A metal cup is placed over the head of the femur, and the acetabulum is shaped to fit the cup. Postoperative training must be done carefully, and no weight is allowed on the operated leg for more than 6 months because it requires that long for a fibrous cartilage to regenerate on both sides of the metal cup. All movements of the hip are done without pressure to enhance the development of the cartilage for better function. Because of the long period of nonweight bearing, the patient and his life-style must be evaluated carefully before a decision is made to do this surgery. Once done, the occupational therapist can teach the patient activities of daily living without weight bearing on the operated side.[2, 30]

For some fractures of the neck and head of the femur, a partial joint replacement is done. An Austin-Moore prosthesis can be used, particularly in the older patient, to ensure quick postsurgical mobilization. After excision of the head of the femur, the metal prosthesis is inserted into the femur, and it articulates with the normal acetabulum. This procedure has tended to be replaced by the total hip arthroplasty, and the postoperative procedures are similar because there is no bone to heal.[2, 9, 21]

THARIES

This procedure is total hip articular replacement by internal eccentric shells. This procedure saves more of the femur by placing a shell over the prepared head of the femur that articulates with an acetabular component. It is considered a useful procedure for younger active patients to buy time while waiting for development of improvements in the technology of hip surgery. Because bone is retained, further revision can be done later. The hip must be protected, and the bone interface must not be stressed early in the postoperative period.[31]

Postoperative care includes immediate muscle setting of quadriceps, gluteus maximus, and hamstrings. On the second or third day, active flexion, rotation, and extension of the hip begins, progressing to a walker for touchdown weight bearing on the 4th day. However, only partial weight bearing is allowed for 2 months. Hip flexion contracture occurs more easily in the THARIES procedure and must be prevented. Also, these patients should not do any heavy lifting. The rehabilitation procedures and precautions are similar to those for total hip arthroplasty (THA).[32]

Total Hip Arthroplasty

Total hip arthroplasty (THA), or total hip replacement, is a recent development in orthopedic surgery. The procedure, developed by John Charnley in England, became available in the United States in 1971 when the Food and Drug Administration approved the use of methyl methacrylate, a self-curing acrylic resin, to cement a plastic acetabular cup to the pelvis and a metal prosthetic femoral head in a hollowed out femur.[33] Because the head and neck of the femur are removed to place the Charnley prosthesis, and the behavior of the components over time is not fully known, this procedure is usually reserved for older patients. Before the procedure is selected for younger patients all medical and social aspects are considered, and the patient must know that there are specific restrictions on activity once this surgery is performed.[34] However, it can be used at any age if the hip disease is severe enough.[26]

Success of the THA depends on a special operating room environment to decrease the incidence of infection, the greatest cause of failure in this procedure, exacting surgical technique, and very careful postoperative mobilization of the patient. To date the success rate is about 90% for patients receiving the Charnley procedure for relief of pain and to increase functional ability.[26]

If a patient has other disabilities, such as arthritis involving numerous joints, a careful plan of sequential surgeries and preparation of the patient must be made. It is important that there be a careful evaluation and planning among surgeons and occupational and physical therapists to select the sequence of surgeries and rehabilitation procedures for severely involved patients.[35] The patient with THA needs ability in the upper extremities for postoperative crutchwalking, an important part of THA rehabilitation. Arthritic patients with multiple joint involvement may require four to six procedures to become ambulatory and independent.[36] Therefore, patients being considered for multiple joint replacement, such as hips and knees, must be evaluated for all joint function because patients with multiple involvement of the upper extremities have more problems in rehabilitation. Without hip and knee flexion, adequate to climb stairs or rise from a chair, the patients are less able to compensate for diminished abilities.[35]

Postoperative Treatment for Total Hip Arthroplasty

A specific treatment program follows total hip arthroplasty, and the first 2 months of activity are critical for protection and function of the new joint. During the Charnley procedure for THA, the greater trochanter is removed with muscle attachments intact and is reflected back for a surgical approach to the hip joint. At the end of the prosthetic placement, the trochanter is wired back into place.[26] The postsurgical program is designed to allow for healing of the trochanter and soft tissues, and to develop a capsule around the joint for future stability. It is a time for muscle re-education to gain strength and stability for walking.[9, 37] When supine, the patient must keep hips abducted, and a splint is used for this postoperatively.[37] Some centers may also use balanced sling suspension postoperatively.[32] Hip flexion beyond 70 to 80° is avoided for the first 2 months postsurgery, until soft tissue healing is secure. Passive motion is never used with THA. The artificial hip joint design permits only 90° of hip flexion and combined with abduction may equal 120°, which is adequate for most functional activities. Patients who are candidates for this surgery usually have had a limited range of hip flexion prior to surgery. About two-thirds of that motion is regained through walking the first 3 weeks postsurgery.[37]

An occupational therapy evaluation can be done prior to surgery to estimate the abilities and other disabilities the patient may have. A patient with a painful hip comes to surgery after an insidious onset of pain and reduction of activities. Find out what the patient has not been able to do. It may be possible to rehearse some of the activities for remediation prior to surgery. At the least, the OT can describe the occupational therapy program for the postsurgical period. The patient should be evaluated for ADL, home environment, home responsibilities, and the social network available for posthospital events. What are the requirements for the patient to do homemaking, drive a car, etc.? It will be necessary to teach the patient safe methods of performance that will encourage independence while protecting the operated hip.

Following surgery, the physical therapist mobilizes the patient quickly to promote walking. The patient learns to transfer from supine to standing without flexing the operated hip, keeping the knees apart and the hips abducted, sliding out of a raised bed to take weight on the unoperated leg. The patient is then encouraged to bear full weight on the operated leg from the beginning of ambulation training, which may start with a walker. There is quick progression to crutches, which are used for about 6 weeks, and then a cane is recommended until the Trendelenburg gait disappears. Older patients may use a walker or a cane for extended periods for safety or reassurance.[37]

During the early postoperative period the patient should avoid sitting on low chairs or stools because this flexes the hip acutely and has resulted in dislocation of the prosthesis. He should not lean over to pull on socks and shoes. The patient is urged not to gain hip flexion motion too quickly after surgery.[37] Patients who sit upright in the hospital bed too soon after surgery are at risk for dislocating the prosthesis. If dislocation occurs, the hip is realigned, and the patient is placed in a hip spica cast for 3 weeks, thus delaying rehabilitation.[26]

When the patient gains about 55° of hip flexion, usually about the 2nd week after surgery, the patient may sit in a chair with a seat that has been elevated by use of a cushion or extended legs. Armrests are useful to help the patient get out of the chair. The raised chair is to avoid passive hip flexion caused by sitting in an upright position. The patient should sit with the hip extended, and the knee should be kept in extension,[37] thus breaking up the hip-knee flexion pattern. Sitting on a firm wedge cushion promotes hip extension and comfort for the patient.

A wedge cushion of firm foam can be cut easily with an electric carving knife. The dimensions are approximately 20 inches (50 cm) across for the chair width, by 10 inches (25 cm) for chair depth, and 6 inches (15 cm) deep. The cushion should taper from the 6-inch thickness on the long side to nothing on its opposite edge to make the wedge. The thick edge is placed at the back of the chair.[38] It can also be used as a backrest that keeps the patient from sitting back in the chair at 90° if the 6-inch side is placed flat on the chair seat. If this cushion is covered and a handle attached, the patient can carry it easily to a car, or any place that he will be sitting to remind him to keep the hip extended. This is particularly important during the first 2 months postsurgery.

When the patient can sit, modified dressing techniques can be taught for lower extremity dressing and hygiene, such as showering or bathing using a tub seat. For any activity, the patient must be reminded that the hip is not to be passively flexed or the leg adducted.[37] To get into a bathtub to take a standing shower, the patient stands with feet parallel to the tub with the operated leg next to tub, and stabilizes the body by holding onto a grab bar or wall or counter, with weight on the unoperated leg. With the operated leg in hip extension, he flexes the knee on the same side and abducts it over the edge of the tub, extends the knee and places the foot on a nonskid applique. When balance is secure and weight is transferred to the operated leg, he lifts the unoperated leg over the edge of the tub and places the foot in the tub. To get out, the patient needs to turn around carefully to face the opposite direction and to repeat the procedure to avoid unnecessary adduction of the operated hip.

The operated hip should not be adducted, that is, the operated leg should not be crossed over the other leg in either sitting or standing position. Passive hip flexion is to be avoided, such as when sitting in a straight chair. The patient should not lean forward to get closer to a table or desk because this is equivalent to hip flexion. Teach the patient to place the chair closer to the table to allow leaning back, or use the wedge cushion which helps to maintain the proper reclining position.

Equipment used by THA patients are a raised toilet seat, with a cut out for the surgical side, a sock donner, a long-handled shoe horn, and a reacher, plus a long-handled bath brush for feet and legs. Ideally, their use should be taught prior to discharge from the hospital.[37]

The patient with THA needs to be upright, walking more than sitting, since sitting tends to flex the hip, while walking improves the hip range of motion and strength.[37] The patient can work at the kitchen sink, bathroom counter, or home workbench. Practice in side stepping in abduction for getting around when working at counter heights is a good activity for the hip. However, adduction of the operated side should not be carried across the midline.

Usually, patients do not receive outpatient therapy following THA. After receiving the appropriate training in ambulation and ADL in the hospital, the patient is discharged with a written list of what he can do or should not do. During the hospital stay, the patient should have been taught the skills he will need, such as stairclimbing, using reachers, and using adapted equipment for lower extremity dressing and bathing. The preoperative evaluation of the patient's home environment and responsibilities should have indicated skills the patient will need most. Simple walking is the most important activity at home because it improves hip motion and strength.

The therapist may want to advise that the patient arrange for someone to reorganize household storage so that things to be used for the next 6 months are placed in the midrange of not too high overhead and not too close to the floor so that the patient can get to them for use. This is especially true for kitchen, bathroom, and closets.

Patients can be taught to reach something on the floor in an emergency. First, the patient should use a stable piece of furniture to hold onto for balance, then extend the operated leg posteriorly in hip extension while bending the other hip and knee to get closer to the floor with the hand. However, a reacher is a better solution.

If a patient must sit in a regular height chair, he should be taught to stand up without overflexing the operated hip, which can lead to dislocation of the hip prosthesis. In a regular chair with armrests, the patient can scoot to the edge of the chair, keeping hip extended, and then use the armrests to push up without bending forward at the hip. In a chair without armrests, the patient can move to the side of the chair so that the operated thigh is over the edge with the foot placed back to the midline of the chair. This places the foot closer to the center of gravity and enables standing up without excessive hip flexion to gain momentum. The same technique can be used for a regular height toilet seat.[9] In public facilities a patient should use the wheelchair accommodation because it often has a raised toilet.

When sleeping in supine position, the patient should keep a pillow between the legs to prevent adduction. The patient should not sleep on the operated side, but can sleep on the unoperated side, if a pillow is placed between the knees to prevent adduction.[37] To facilitate getting out of bed at home the first few months, the height of the bed can be raised using leg extenders or even by putting another mattress on the patient's bed to avoid acute hip flexion when entering or leaving the bed.

Patients are advised not to use a car with bucket seats for the first few months. To enter an automobile the patient can stand with his back to the front seat, sit down, and then scoot toward the middle of the car seat. Then the patient can swing legs around to face the front of the car without too much hip flexion.[39] Resumption of driving will depend on the surgeon's approval and the side of the operation. For example, a patient with an automatic transmission car and a THA on the left will be able to resume driving sooner than a patient with a right side THA.

Social dancing can be done if the precautions are observed and the dance is moderate, such as a slow waltz. However, very vigorous dance activity should not be done.[40]

Physical problems related to sexual expression presurgically have related to pain, stiffness, and limited hip motion, rather than to loss of libido, and this can be the source of marital problems. THA is a more enabling procedure for sexual activity than other hip procedures, whereas the hip arthrodesis greatly limits function for women in coition.[41] Following THA, sexual activity, which may begin 2 to 3 months postsurgically, is no problem for the patient in the supine position. Pillows can be used to position the operated leg to prevent excessive hip internal rotation and adduction. Kneeling should be avoided for any activity for 3 to 4 months after surgery.[37, 39] Patients surveyed thought that written information about the hip procedures related to sexual activity would be helpful if supplied to a patient and his sexual partner.[42]

Between the second and third month postsurgically, all routine daily activities can be resumed with restrictions related to too much hip flexion and no adduction or internal rotation still applicable. Strenuous sports such as tennis, skiing, or jogging should not be encouraged.[37] The Charnley prosthesis is designed for walking, not running or other athletic activities. One problem that has occurred is the loosening of the femoral components of the prosthesis. Patients who put too much stress, through work or recreation activities, on the prosthetic-cement-bone components tend to have a higher incidence of loosening. Even with x-ray evidence of loosening, the signs may not progress if the patient reduces his activity level and reduces body weight. Failures of THA reported in the literature followed walking on uneven ground daily at work, climbing ladders, and long distance running. Probably the procedure should not be considered for the patient who is highly motivated to perform activities of daily stress to the hip replacement. No failures have been reported for moderate levels of swimming, hiking, or horseback riding.[43-46]

Four year follow-up studies of THA patients showed that most patients have dramatic relief of pain and improved functional performance by 6 months after surgery. At the end of 2 years, most functional activities showed improvement which was maintained through the 4-year period of the study. Some patients reported slight pain when beginning motion, but the pain decreased as they continued the activity. Patients who developed ossification around the prosthetic head had reduction of hip flexion and internal rotation which made lower extremity dressing a bit more difficult but not impossible.[47]

For some patients lower extremity dressing is a problem for quite a while after surgery but is solved through the use of equipment. Postsurgically, mobility for the THA patient can be measured by the ability to put on stockings and tie shoes. Stability can be measured by the ability to do cleaning and shopping.[48]

References

1. Parker, H. G., and Reitman, H. K. Changing patterns in fracture management emphasizing early motion and function. *Surg. Clin. North Am., 56* (3): 667-672, 1976.
2. Apley, A. G. *System of Orthopaedics and Fractures,* 5th ed. London: Butterworth, 1977.
3. Heppenstall, R. B. (Ed.) *Fracture Treatment and Healing.* Philadelphia: W.B. Saunders, 1980.
4. Nichols, P. J. R. *Rehabilitation Medicine, The Management of Physical Disabilities.* London: Butterworth, 1976, pp. 161-180.
5. Sarmiento, A., Latta, L., and Sinclair, W. F. Functional bracing of fractures. In *American Academy of Orthopaedic Surgeons Instructional Course Lectures,* Vol. 25, 1976. St. Louis: C.V. Mosby, 1976, 184-237.
6. Mercier, L. R., and Pettid, F. J. *Practical Orthopaedics.* Chicago: Year Book Medical Publishers, 1980.
7. Devas, M. (ed.). *Geriatric Orthopaedics.* London: Academic Press, 1977.
8. Vasudevan, S. V., and Melvin, J. L. Upper extremity edema control: Rationale of the techniques. *Am. J. Occup. Ther., 33* (8): 520-523, 1979.
9. Glazer, R. M. Rehabilitation. in *Fracture Treatment and Healing,* edited by R. B. Heppenstall. Philadelphia: W.B. Saunders Co., 1980, pp. 1041-1069.

10. Bell, C. H., Jr. Construction of orthoplast splints for humeral shaft fractures. *Am. J. Occup. Ther.*, *33* (2): 114–115, 1979.

11. Lewinnek, G. E., *et al.* The significance and a comparative analysis of the epidemiology of hip fractures. *Clin. Orthop., 152:* 35–43, 1980.

12. Boucher, C. A. Accidents among old persons. *Geriatrics, 14* (5): 293–300, 1959.

13. Guimaraes, R. M., and Isaacs, B. Characteristics of the gait in old people who fall. *Int. Rehabil. Med., 2* (4): 177–180, 1980.

14. Cristarella, M. C. Visual functions of the elderly. *Am. J. Occup. Ther., 31* (7): 432–440, 1977.

15. Jowsey, J. Osteoporosis and its relationship to femoral neck fractures. In *The Hip*, Proceedings of the Fifth Open Scientific Meeting of the Hip Society, 1977. St. Louis: C.V. Mosby, pp. 3–11, 1977.

16. Owen, R. A., *et al.* The national cost of acute care of hip fractures associated with osteoporosis. *Clin. Orthop., 150:* 172–176, 1980.

17. Hasselkus, B. R. Aging and the human nervous system. *Am. J. Occup. Ther., 28* (1): 16–21, 1974.

18. Ceder, L., Thorngren, K-G., and Wallden, B. Prognostic indicators and early home rehabilitation in elderly patients with hip fractures. *Clin. Orthop., 152:* 173–184, 1980.

19. Schaefer, R. Occupational therapy for lower extremity problems. *Am. J. Occup. Ther., 27* (3): 132–137, 1973.

20. Simm, F. H., and Stauffer, R. N. Fractures of the neck of the femur. In *American Academy of Orthopaedic Surgeons Instructional Course Lectures, 29.* St. Louis: C.V. Mosby, 1980, pp. 14–15.

21. Hirschberg, G. G., Lewis, L., and Vaughan, P. *Rehabilitation: A Manual for the Care of the Disabled and Elderly*, 2nd Ed. Philadelphia: J. B. Lippincott, 1976.

22. Arnold, W. D. Percutaneous Knowles pinnings: Primary treatment for femoral neck fractures. In *The Hip*. Proceedings of the Fifth Open Scientific Meeting of the Hip Society, 1977. St. Louis: C.V. Mosby, 1977, pp. 21–34.

23. Laskin, R. S., Gruber, M. A., and Zimmerman, A. J. Intertrochanteric fractures of the hip in the elderly, a retrospective analysis of 236 cases. *Clin. Orthop., 141:* 188–195, 1979.

24. Harris, L. J. Closed intramedullary nailing of intertrochanteric and subtrochanteric fractures of the femur. *American Academy of Orthopaedic Surgeons Instructional Course Lectures, 29.* St. Louis: C.V. Mosby, 1980, pp. 17–29.

25. Berkow, R. (Ed.). *The Merck Manual of Diagnosis and Therapy*, 13th ed. Rahway, N.J.: Merck Sharp & Dohme Research Laboratories, 1977.

26. Eftekhar, N. S. *Principles of Total Hip Arthroplasty.* St. Louis: C.V. Mosby, 1978.

27. Coventry, M. B. Total hip replacement. In *The Hip*, edited by L. H. Riley, Jr. The Hip Society Eighth Scientific Meeting, 1980. St. Louis: C.V. Mosby, 1980, pp. 68–81.

28. Morscher, E. W. Intertrochanteric osteotomy in osteoarthritis of the hip. In *The Hip*, edited by L. H. Riley, Jr., The Hip Society Eighth Scientific Meeting, 1980. St. Louis: C.V. Mosby, 1980, pp. 24–46.

29. Liechti, R. *Hip Arthrodesis and Associated Problems.* Berlin: Springer-Verlag, 1978.

30. Friedebold, G. The Smith-Peterson cup arthroplasty: An analysis of failures. In *Arthroplasty of the Hip*, edited by G. Chapchal. Stuttgart: Georg Thieme, 1973, pp. 68–70.

31. Amstutz, H. C. Surface replacement of the hip. In *The Hip*, edited by L. H. Riley, Jr., Proceedings of the Hip Society, 1980, St. Louis: C.V. Mosby, 1980, pp. 47–66.

32. Amstutz, H. C., *et al.* Total hip articular replacement by internal eccentric shells. *Clin. Orthop., 128:* 261–284, 1977.

33. Muller, M. E. Late complications of total hip replacement. In *The Hip*, edited by W. H. Harris, The Hip Society Proceedings, 1974. St. Louis: C.V. Mosby, 1974, p. 319.

34. Manzoni, A. Prophylactic indication for total replacement of the hip. In *Arthroplasty of the Hip*, edited by G. Chapchal. Stuttgart: Georg Thieme, 1973, pp. 81–83.

35. Jergesen, H. E., Poss, R., and Sledge, C. B. Bilateral total hip and knee replacement in adults with rheumatoid arthritis: An evaluation of function. *Clin. Orthop., 137:* 120–128, 1978.

36. Poss, R. Total hip replacement in the patient with rheumatoid arthritis. In *American Academy of Orthopaedic Surgeons, Instructional Course Lectures, 28*, 1979, 298–302.

37. Aufranc, O. E. Postoperative management. In *Principles of Total Hip Arthroplasty*, edited by N. S. Eftekhar, St. Louis: C.V. Mosby, 1978, pp. 313–326.

38. McKee, J. I. Foam wedges aid sitting posture of patients with total hip replacement. *Phys. Ther., 55* (7): 767, 1975.

39. Yoslow, W., Simeone, J., and Huestis, D. Hip replacement rehabilitation. *Arch. Phys. Med. Rehabil., 57* (6): 275–278, 1976.

40. Carpenter, E. S., *et al. Information for Our Patients: Total Hip Joint Replacement.* Downey, Calif.: Professional Staff Association, Rancho Los Amigos Hospital, revised 1979.

41. Harris, J., and Currey, H. L. F. Sexual problems due to disease of the hip joint: Its relevance to hip surgery. In *Total Hip Replacement*, edited by M. Jayson. Philadelphia: J. B. Lippincott, 1971, pp. 144–148.

42. Todd, R. C., Lightowler, C. D. R., and Harris, J. Low friction arthroplasty of the hip joint and sexual activity. *Acta Orthop. Scand., 44* (6): 690–693, 1973.

43. Stinchfeld, F. E., guest editor, Symposium—Statistics in total hip replacement. *Clin. Orthop., 95:* 9–223, 1973.

44. Ling, R. S. M. Prevention of loosening of total hip components. In *The Hip*, edited by L. H. Riley, Jr., The Hip Society Proceedings, 1980. St. Louis: C.V. Mosby, 1980, pp. 292–307.

45. Moreland, J. R., *et al.* Aseptic loosening of total hip replacement: incidence and significance. In *The Hip*, edited by L. H. Riley, Jr., The Hip Society Proceedings, 1980. St. Louis: C.V. Mosby, 1980, pp. 281–291.

46. Weaver, J. K. Activity expectations and limitations following total joint replacement. *Clin. Orthop., 137:* 55–61, 1978.

47. Murray, M. P., *et al.* Joint function after total hip arthroplasty: A four-year follow-up of 72 cases with Charnley and Müller replacements. *Clin. Orthop., 157:* 119–124, 1981.

48. Visuri, T., and Honkanen, R. The influence of total hip replacement on selected activities of daily living and on the use of domestic aid. *Scand. J. Rehabil. Med., 10* (4): 221–225, 1978.

Supplementary Readings

Brown, D. M., and Clark, S. Elevation crutch in the treatment of the edematous hand. *Am. J. Occup. Ther., 32* (5): 320–321, 1978.

DeVore, G., and Hamilton, G. Volume measuring of the severely injured hand. *Am. J. Occup. Ther., 22* (1): 16–18, 1968.

Feinberg, M. A. Dynamic foot splint for the Hoffman apparatus. *Am. J. Occup. Ther., 34* (1): 45, 1980.

McKee, P. R. and Brintnell, E. S. Trends in lower limb splinting by Canadian occupational and physical therapists. *Can. J. Occup. Ther., 48* (2): 65–71, 1981.

Pincus, A. New findings on learning in old age: Implications for occupational therapy. *Am. J. Occup. Ther., 22* (4): 300–303, 1968.

Seeger, M. S., and Fisher, L. A. Occupational therapy in total hip replacement/total surface replacement. *Arthr. Newsletter, 14* (1): 1–9, 1980.

Steinberg, F. U. *The Immobilized Patient: Functional Pathology and Management.* New York: Plenum, 1980.

chapter

20

Arthritis

Catherine A. Trombly, M.A., OTR

Two of the many types of arthritic diseases are discussed in this chapter: rheumatoid arthritis and degenerative joint disease, also known as osteoarthritis.

RHEUMATOID ARTHRITIS

Rheumatoid arthritis is a systemic disease characterized by remissions and exacerbations which vary in severity and time among people.[1,2] Two to three times more women are stricken than men.[1,2] Onset is usually between the 25th and 50th year of age. Etiology is unknown. Two theories, not mutually exclusive, are being studied: the infection and the autoimmunity theories. The infection theory hypothesizes that a virus may be the cause. The autoimmune theory holds that there is a disruption of the immune process that allows abnormal antibodies to be produced which attack the body's own tissues.[2] Stress is not a causative factor, but may precipitate the onset of symptoms and aggravate the disease, once established.[2] There is no cure at this time.[2]

The chronic nature and often degenerative course causes those treating patients with rheumatoid arthritis to follow the philosophy utilized in the care of patients with any degenerative disease: maintain the patient's physical, psychological, and functional abilities for as long as possible through an ongoing, carefully planned treatment program and patient education. Team treatment is essential.[3,4]

Symptoms include malaise, tiredness, anemia, wasting of the muscles around a joint, stiffness, and limited movement.[3] The disease begins within the joints as inflammation of the synovium.[1,3] Rheumatoid arthritis affects many joints, most commonly, the small joints of the hands.[2] The joints become swollen, hot, red, and tender. Once the active disease process burns out, the patient is left with residual joint deformities[1,3] and resultant limitation of function. The primary objective of treatment is to prevent joint destruction, which is nonreversible.[2]

Goals of Occupational Therapy

Specific goals of occupational therapy in the treatment of patients with reheumatoid arthritis depend on the problems and needs of the particular person and the stage of the disease. However, in general, the goals to be considered are:

1. Maintenance or increase of joint mobility.
2. Prevention of deformities.
3. Maintenance or increase of strength.
4. Maintenance or increase of endurance.
5. Maintenance or increase of skill in functional tasks.
6. Education of the patient regarding recognition of the continued need for activity balanced with rest, energy conservation, and use of techniques to protect the joints and prevent pain during occupational performance tasks.

Evaluation

The occupational therapist assesses and grades functional impairment[3] as well as joint stability and mobility, muscle strength, endurance, and the presence of deformities or the precursors to deformity. Hand function, and the function of the upper extremity in so far as it serves hand function, are of particular interest. Maintenance of hand function is important since the disabling nature of this disease may limit employment to the sedentary type, for which good hand function is a necessity.[5] Sensory evaluation should be done if systemic involvement includes polyneuropathies or nerve compression.[1]

Joint Mobility

Changes in joint mobility occur due to excess joint play due to loosened ligaments and joint capsules and due to contractures of muscles and other connective tissue. Range of motion is measured as described in Chapter 7. One researcher has reported an attempt to standardize the technique by applying 0.45 kg of force to the movable arm of the goniometer 10 cm from the axis of rotation. The goniometer is held dorsal or volar to the joint, not laterally, for better reliability.[6]

Deformities or Their Precursors

These deformities and their precursors are evaluated by determining whether the ligaments and capsule are slack, resulting in excess joint play, whether the muscles are too tight, whether swelling or nodules are present, and whether the integrity of the tendons and joints has been preserved.

Ligamentous stability of the fingers is evaluated by placing the proximal interphalangeal (PIP) and distal interphalangeal (DIP) joints in full passive extension (0°), stabilizing the proximal bone, and moving the distal one from side to side.[7] The amount of joint play should be little; however, normality is determined by comparing to a normal joint, since the amount of normal joint play differs among people.[7] Abnormal laxity of the radial collateral ligament at the metacarpophalangeal (MP) joint is evaluated by placing the patient's MP joints in 90° of flexion; the therapist then pushes the digit ulnarly. The ligament is stretched if the finger can be pushed easily.

To test for shortened ulnar intrinsic muscles, the patient flexes the PIP joint while the MP joint is held in 0° of deviation. The amount of PIP flexion is measured with a goniometer. The patient then ulnarly deviates the MP joint and flexes the PIP joint again. The amount of PIP flexion is measured and compared to the previous measurement. If the ulnar intrinsics are tight, there will be more PIP flexion with the MP joint in ulnar deviation than with the MP joint in 0° of deviation.[8]

Nodules are sometimes found on the extrinsic tendons of the finger muscles. Although extensor tendon nodules can be easily detected visually, flexor tendon nodules are less obvious. Nodules are more likely to form on the flexor digitorum sublimis (superficialis) than on the flexor digitorum profundus.[5] Flexor tendon nodules can be detected using the following method. If active finger flexion motion is less than normal, but passive motion is normal, then flexor tendon nodules can be suspected. To test, have the patient flex each finger; if active range of motion is limited, check passive range of motion. It will be normal, but the finger will meet a stopping point (the nodule) and have to be moved slowly to full range.[8]

Tendon rupture is uncommon,[5] but due to the disease process, may occur. If the tendon has ruptured, the full passive range of motion will be achieved without resistance. The most common tendons to rupture are those of the extensor digitorum due to rubbing of the tendons on the distal ulna. A single rupture stands out because the finger droops. Multiple ruptures become evident when the patient is asked to flex and extend the metacarpophalangeal joints. Flexor tendon rupture can follow development of nodules on the flexor tendons and is usually preceded by the "trigger" or "locking" phenomenon of the finger with a nodule. An isolated rupture of any of the flexor tendons causes little functional loss. These can be found, however, using standard muscle testing procedures: there will be a loss of flexor motion of either the distal interphalangeal joint or the proximal interphalangeal joint of one finger while motion is preserved in the fingers unaffected by the rupture.[8]

The location of pain, hot and inflamed joints, swelling, tendon rupture, nodules, crepitus, and subluxations or dislocations are noted in such a way as to allow comparison from evaluation to evaluation. Some clinics use xerography, and others use photography to supplement written descriptions.

The severity of pain can be graded based on its occurrence during activity; it is graded mild if it occurs only with stressful activity, moderate if it occurs with active motion, and severe if it occurs even at rest.[9]

The typical deformities of the wrist and hand and the underlying mechanisms thought to produce these deformities are being described in detail not only so that they may be evaluated, but also because it will be seen that normal use of the hands produces forces which promote the deformities. Therapy must be guided by this information. The exact cause of deformity is not yet fully understood, but it appears that hypertrophy of the synovium due to the inflammation process pushes against the joint structures from within. The ligaments become stretched, and when the swelling of the synovium subsides, the ligaments are left lax. The force moments of the tendons are changed because of the ligamentous abnormality, and their pull becomes deforming.[5]

Deformities of the Wrist. Volar subluxation of the hand in relation to the ulna is caused by erosion of the intercarpal ligaments and volar displacement of the extensor carpi ulnaris[10] which, in effect, causes this muscle to act as a flexor force.

The wrist commonly radially deviates due to a loss of support of the radial and ulnar ligaments.[7] Loss of this support allows the carpal bones to ulnarly sublux, which results in the radial deviation.[7, 11] The fingers, especially the index, then ulnarly deviate in an effort to realign the index with the radius, its normal position.[7, 11] This completes the zig-zag deformity: wrist radial deviation with MP ulnar deviation.

Deformities of the Metacarpophalangeal Joints. Volar subluxation of the fingers appears to develop in the following way.[5] Synovitis of the MP joint stretches the extensor mechanism. The extensor hood is thinner radially, and the hypertrophied synovium tends to herniate on the radial side of the extensor tendons. The hood is pushed distally, which causes the extensor tendons to slip ulnarly off the tops of the joints to the "valleys" between. This places them below the joint axes; therefore, their force becomes a flexor force.[5, 8] In addition, the large volar forces generated at the mouth of the flexor tunnels during pinch or grasp cause mechanical damage to the metacarpoglenoidal ligaments supporting them. The tunnel mouths are displaced volarly.[12] A new equilibrium of forces is established between the pull of the flexors and the supporting structure: the rim of the phalanx and the metacarpophalangeal (collateral) ligaments. If the rim wears down, or the ligaments are stretched, the deformity of volar subluxation results.[12]

One theory is that ulnar deviation deformity develops when the tissues surrounding the joint, especially the radial collateral ligaments,[10] become permanently stretched due to the push of the synovium. Normally, the ulnar interossei exert a stronger pull than the radial ones do.[5, 7, 12] This, combined with the pull of the flexor tendons on the mouths of the tendon sheaths in an ulnar direction, contributes to the force which causes the dynamic ulnar deviation.[12] In time, the ulnar intrinsics become shortened, creating a constant pull toward ulnar deviation. Although it is hypothesized that a protective MP flexor response is induced in the interossei muscles as a pain avoidance mechanism which eventually results in fibrous, fixed shortening of the intrinsics,[13] electromyographical evidence has failed to validate spasm as a possible source of this deformity and supports the findings that muscle action normally present in the hand is the cause of deformity.[12, 14] Another theory is that ulnar deviation deformity results as a compensation for wrist radial deviation deformity.[15] Pahle and Raunio[11] conclude from their study that the two theories supplement one another in that the ulnarly deviating forces of the extrinsic flexor muscles at the base of the fingers can be seen to decrease as the wrist is ulnarly deviated because this tends to align the metacarpal part of the flexor tendons with the wrist part.

The Interphalangeal Joint Deformities. The deformities of the interphalangeal joints caused by rheumatoid arthritis, degenerative joint disease, and traumatic arthritis are swan neck deformity, boutonniere deformity, and fixed flexor or extensor deformities.[6]

A swan neck deformity (intrinsic plus hand) is a combination of PIP hyperextension and DIP flexion caused by tight interossei which pull abnormally on the extensor tendons and cause hyperextension of the hypermobile PIP joints.[8, 10] This deformity may be flexible or fixed. To test for flexibility, support the metacarpophalangeal joints in extension and have the patient flex the PIP joint.[8] If full flexion of the PIP joint occurs, the deformity is flexible, and the volar plate which prevents hyperextension is only slightly stretched. If PIP flexion is impossible with the metacarpophalangeal joint extended but can be accomplished with the metacarpophalangeal joint flexed, a fixed deformity due to tight intrinsics is present.

The intrinsic muscles are on stretch when the MP joints are extended and the interphalangeal joints are flexed. Early detection of tightness of the intrinsics is important so treatment can be instituted. Tightness can be detected by noting if a difference exists in the amount of flexion of the PIP joints when the MP joints are flexed or extended.[7]

A fixed swan neck deformity may also be caused by

sticking lateral bands. In this case, PIP flexion is impossible, regardless of the position of the metacarpophalangeal joint.[8]

A boutonniere deformity is a combination of PIP flexion and DIP hyperextension caused by the PIP joint slipping up between the lateral bands of the extensor digitorum,[8, 10] which then act to flex the PIP joint. The relationship between the flexor digitorum profundus and the extensor digitorum is changed, and the extensor acts unopposed at the DIP joint.[10] To test for shortening of the lateral bands, hold the PIP extended and passively try to flex the DIP; if this is difficult, there is shortening.[10]

Deformities of the Thumb. Interphalangeal hyperextension is caused by intrinsic-plus pull on the extensor mechanism of the hypermobile interphalangeal joint when metacarpophalangeal extension is lost due to volar displacement of the long extensor secondary to capsular and extensor apparatus stretch caused by inflammation of the MP joint.[10]

Metacarpophalangeal hyperextension occurs in response to the pull of a tight adductor pollicis on weakened joint structures.[10]

Strength

The systemic nature of rheumatoid arthritis, along with atrophy of disuse, produces muscle weakness.[16] Use of manual muscle testing involving resistance is controversial. On the one hand, it is necessary to know the patient's strength, expecially the comparative strength of muscles around a joint; on the other hand, resistance causes harm to the diseased tissue, which causes pain. Pain causes the patient to protect the part and results in an unreliable test. Some rheumatologists prohibit any resistance beyond that which is necessary for self-care due to the deforming forces of muscle contraction when joint structures are stretched and weakened.[14] The dynamometer and pinchmeter would therefore also be prohibited by physicians holding that philosophy. Others feel that knowledge of level of muscle strength and the effectiveness of strengthening exercises is important.[16] The muscle test should be done isometrically, not isotonically; isotonic movement against resistance tends to increase inflammation and pain in arthritic joints.[16]

Endurance

Endurance is evaluated as outlined in Chapter 7 or by noticing the patient's limits of endurance during daily activity. The patient must learn to evaluate this for himself, since he must learn to rest before fatigue becomes a factor in the performance of activities.

Activities of Daily Living

Activities of daily living (ADL) are evaluated as described in Chapter 25. It may be useful to add two categories to the scoring criteria for "independent," one category for activity which is possible to complete independently but not entirely without pain and one category for those activities which are very difficult or painful.[17] These would clue the therapist to help the patient find alternative methods of doing these tasks since pain is to be avoided. Melvin[1] suggests that it is good, when evaluating functional impairment, to end the evaluation with a task the patient can do in order to focus the patient on ability rather than disability. It is also suggested, in order to contain the feelings of total disablement and to help clarify the limits of dysfunction, that the patient be asked to be very specific when he reports the inability to do something.[7]

A factor analytical study of ADL/homemaking activities was done to determine if certain factors could be identified with the hope of developing a "screening approach to ADL," i.e., activities representative of different types of function could be selected and only if difficulties were encountered with the screening task would there be a need to assess the whole group of tasks.[17] It was determined that tasks seemed to relate to what areas of the body were involved. However, the analysis requires further validation before it is ready for clinical use.[17]

Assessment of Hand Function

Both the prehensile and nonprehensile functions of the hand should be evaluated.[7] Prehensile functions are pinch and grasp; nonprehensile functions are those that use the hand statically held either flexed (hook grasp) or extended (e.g., tucking in clothing, smoothing sheets, sorting coins on a surface).[7] In rheumatoid arthritis, the prehensile functions are potentially deforming; therefore, if nonprehensile functions can be substituted, the joints may be protected from deformity.

A number of hand function tests exist. Two of the more common ones are the Jebsen "Objective and Standardized Test of Hand Function"[18] and the "Functional Assessment of the Rheumatoid Hand."[19] These tests focus on the prehensile functions. The reader is referred to the original articles for directions for administration of these tests.

Treatment

Treatment corresponds to the progress of the disease in the particular joint. Two programs have been published which illustrate this principle, one for the shoulder[20] and one for the hands.[5]

The three stages of development of joint damage in the rheumatoid shoulder are: (1) simple synovitis—there is pain and a loss of movement, but the joint structures are normal. (2) There is more advanced involvement of the joint. Movement is painful, range of motion is decreased, the joint space is narrowed, and erosions are visible on X-ray. The synovium has become proliferative. Rupture of the rotator cuff may occur. There is rarely full functional recovery from this state. (3) There is advanced joint damage with advanced narrowing of the joint space; the humeral head may be distorted or disappear.[20]

The motions that are affected are hand to back of the head, hand to buttocks, and hand to opposite shoulder.

Treatment during the early stage consists of steroid drugs and gentle mobilizing exercise directed toward recovery of function. Isometric contractions of the shoulder muscles are done 3 to 6 times each treatment. The scapula is mobilized with the humerus held immobile as soon as the inflammation diminishes. The shoulder is positioned into abduction to avoid the typical pattern of deformity (adduction and internal rotation) which is adopted because it is comfortable. Movement is done in functional patterns to the limit of pain and without resistance. Mobility exercises and activities to encourage gentle abduction and elevation of the upper limb are used. The shoulder is supported in a sling if painful. Treatment is offered in short periods of increasing frequency to avoid fatigue. Adaptive devices, organization of the work area, support for the shoulder, elimination of tasks, and energy conservation comprise treatment in the later stages. In the final stage, the joint may be surgically replaced if deterioration severely interferes with function.

The progress of disease in the rheumatoid hand proceeds through three stages also: (1) early proliferative stage; (2) a period of regression of synovitis; and (3) stage of fixed deformity.[5] Therapy in the active proliferative stage is aimed at limiting damage caused by the synovitis. Drugs are used to reduce the bulk of the synovium, and the actively involved joints are rested in splints that hold the part in functional position, especially flexion of the metacarpophalangeal joints. During the second stage, which is the most important stage in the management of the rheumatoid hand, the goal is to prevent progression of the deformities to a fixed status. As the swelling decreases, stretched capsule and other joint tissues result in joint laxity; in this condition, the joint is vulnerable to abnormal forces. In this stage, therapy includes exercises to encourage strength of the radial interossei, joint protection techniques by which the hands are used in the least damaging way, and extensor exercises to counteract the flexion/extension imbalance caused by stretched extensor tendons whose mechanical effectiveness has decreased. In the third stage, the stage of fixed deformity, treatment is surgical replacement of the joint(s).

Treatment for specific goals will now be considered. The implementation of treatment depends upon the stage of the disease process.[21] During the acute stage (synovial inflammation) or in severe generalized rheumatoid arthritis, gentle exercise to maintain mobility interrupts the rest that the joint otherwise receives. During the subacute or chronic stages, or in cases of mild to moderate disease, the goals are to maintain or increase mobility and strength.[21] Throughout treatment, the joints are positioned for comfort and to decrease stress. Fatigue is avoided. In the case of severe joint destruction, surgical replacement of the joint may be done. See Chapter 18 for a discussion of therapy following joint replacement procedures.

Maintenance or Increase of Mobility of Joints

In acute disease, passive or very gentle active-assistive motion is done for each joint daily to maintain the mobility. As the disease subsides, the therapist assists less. The patient should be treated in three or four short periods per day, treating different joints at each session.[22]

Exercise is best done when pain has been decreased by drugs or heat and when morning stiffness has subsided.[23] Neutral warmth may be sufficient to reduce pain, and since it avoids the possibility of a rebound effect that occurs with other methods of warming, it may be preferred.

In the postinflammatory stage, passive range of motion to just beyond the point of pain to provide gentle prolonged stretch may be necessary if the patient lacks full active range.[21, 23] The stretching is done to prevent the muscles and connective tissue from shortening into fixed deformities. Warming before the passive exercises is also beneficial. Abrupt application of stretch may rupture the tissue.[21]

If the occupational therapist is to take responsibility for passive ranging, then it should be done directly after the patient receives heat treatments in physical therapy. If the physical therapist does the ranging, that is enough. If pain persists several hours after therapy, the amount of exercise should be cut in half.[22, 23] If pain persists, the joint must be rested.

Nonresistive activities which require the patient to move to full range in nondeforming motion patterns are desirable media. However, repetitive use of the joints or overexercise may aggravate the disease by causing inflammation.[21, 23] Therefore, the patient's pain and joint swelling must be monitored carefully. Pain should not last more than 2 hours on therapy day and on the next day should be no worse than before therapy.[23]

Prevention of Deformity

Exercise is used to maintain muscle power to help maintain joint alignment, but consideration of minimizing stress on joints is also necessary.[3]

Static deforming positions, or motions in the direction of potential deformity, should be strictly avoided. In fact, in all cases, motions in the direction opposite to the deformity or potential deformity are desirable. Knitting, hammering, and leather lacing are examples of activities to be avoided because they involve static resisted grasp or pinch with some force toward ulnar deviation.

Activities should avoid strong grasp or pinch which are deforming forces in the rheumatoid hand.[8, 12, 14, 24] Looper potholder weaving from right to left using the right hand is an example of an acceptable choice of activity because it involves minimal resistance and movement in a radial direction.

Actively inflamed joints need local rest by splinting in functional positions.[3] The full hand splint is usually worn at night,[25] and the hand is left free for light activity in the day. Based on the biomechanical analysis of deformity at the MP joint, it is suggested by one author that the hand be splinted with the MPs in extension with no deviation, which would protect the flexor tunnel mouths from damaging forces.[12] In this position, the joint capsule would be in the slack position (off stretch),[26] and if maintained there might tighten to its normal tautness. Others suggest MP flexion[5, 25] and slight radial deviation.[11] One guideline for a resting hand splint is 30 to 40° wrist dorsiflexion, 70 to 80° MP flexion, and 10 to 20° PIP and DIP flexion.[25]

Some advocate removing the resting splint several times a day for ranging,[3] and others say that splints can be left on up to 4 weeks without range of motion exercises with no loss of mobility.[21, 23]

In a study of 50 rheumatoid arthritic patients splinted in full-hand resting splints, it was found at follow-up that no significant differences occurred in the range of motion between the compliant (splints worn more than 50% of the time) and the noncompliant group (splints worn less than 50% of the time).[9] The noncompliant group actually improved slightly more than the compliant group in range of motion, which leads one to wonder if splints need closer monitoring and should be discarded at the moment inflammation is no longer active to allow free use of the joints to maintain the range.

During the day, if a splint is used, a design which is less confining is chosen. A wrist cock-up splint (Fig. 12.4) frees the hand for use while supporting the wrist.[25] It should be lightweight and constructed to put the wrist in about 5° of ulnar deviation.[11] If the MP joints need support, the splint can be extended to support them in extension with no deviation; finger IP flexion would still be possible[12] (Fig. 20.1).

In addition to using splints to rest the joint, prevent deformity, and to stabilize the joint during movement to increase function, splints are also used for correcting contractures (serial casting or splinting) and to assist in the postsurgical rehabilitation of the hand (dynamic splints).[23]

The Principles of Joint Protection. The principles of joint protection are as follows: (1) maintenance of muscle strength and joint range of motion; (2) avoidance of positions of deformity and avoidance of external and internal pressures and stresses to the joint in positions of deformity; (3) use of the strongest joints available for the job; (4) use of each joint in its most stable anatomical and functional plane; (5) use of correct patterns of motion; (6) avoidance of holding joints or using muscles in one position for any undue length of time; (7) avoidance of starting an activity which cannot be stopped part way if it proves beyond the patient's power to complete; and (8) respect for pain.

The patient has to learn the application of these principles through supervised practice of specific joint protection techniques, some of which follow.

Avoidance of Strong Grasp and Pinch. Avoidance of positions of deformity is a particularly applicable principle to be aware of when the hands are used functionally since the forces generated during grasp and pinch become increasingly deforming as resistance increases. To avoid this, the hand is used in nonprehensile functional ways if possible, or the joints are supported to counteract the deforming pull of the

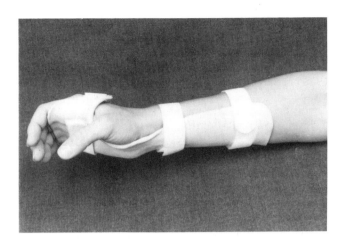

Figure 20.1 Splint to support wrist and metacarpophalangeal joints in extension.

muscles or the motion is done in a way opposite to the deformity. Some suggestions are as follows.

When opening jars, one correct way is to stabilize the jar on a wet towel, place the palm of the hand on the jar lid, press down and turn in a radial direction. A better solution is to use the Zim jar opener (Fig. 20.2).

Press water from a cloth or sponge rather than wring it.

Hold a knife with the blade protruding from the ulnar side of the hand, which pushes the hand toward radial deviation (Fig. 20.3). The knife should be sharp to offer less resistance.

Hold stirring spoons so that the bowl of the spoon is on the ulnar side of the hand.

Avoidance of Pressure that Pushes the Metacarpophalangeal or Wrist Joints in an Ulnar Direction. (a). Smooth ironing, bedsheets, etc. by moving the hand in a radial direction. (b). Turn handles or lids in a radial direction; this may mean using the nondominant hand. (c). In using the hands to assist standing up, avoid putting pressure anywhere except on the heel of the hand and especially not on the radial side of the index finger. (d). Using an adapted knife which is specially constructed to keep the blade surface in contact with the material being cut while keeping the handle parallel to the MP joints[29] prevents ulnar deviation during the cutting process.

If Shapiro's thesis[15] that radial wrist deviation is an important factor in the development of MP ulnar deviation, then it may be necessary to avoid the combination of wrist radial deviation and MP ulnar deviation. Further testing, both in the laboratory and the clinic, needs to be done to establish the effectiveness of these measures in preventing deformities.

Use of the Proximal Body Parts in Lieu of the More Distal Ones. Use of the proximal body parts in lieu of the more distal ones utilizes the stronger body parts and protects the weaker ones. (a) Slip a pocketbook or shopping bag over the forearm. (b) Pots can be carried by putting one hand flat underneath and by steadying with the other. (c) Forearm platform

crutches are an application of the principle applied to ambulation.

Use of Each Joint in Its Most Stable and Func-

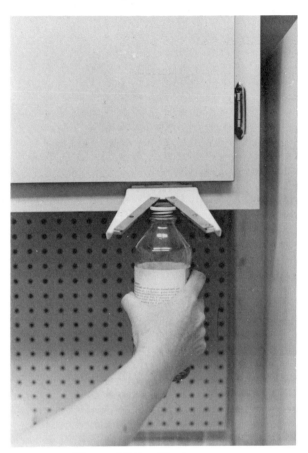

Figure 20.2 Zim jar opener.

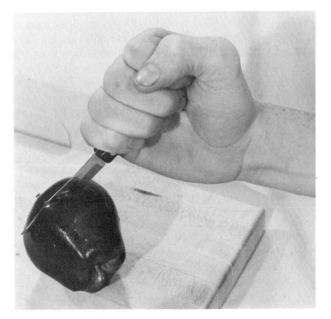

Figure 20.3 Cutting an apple using a dagger-grip on the knife to force the fingers in a radial direction during cutting.

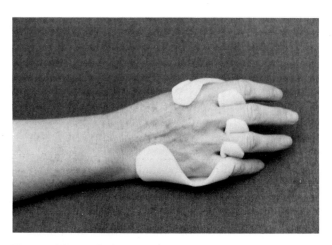

Figure 20.4 Splint to prevent ulnar deviation during hand use.

tional Plane. Avoid twisting the knees when standing up by standing up first and then turning. A splint can be used to hold the fingers in good alignment and to prevent ulnar deviation during hand usage (Fig. 20.4).

Maintenance or Increase of Strength

Exercise for strengthening is avoided during the acute systemic illness[7] and during the stage of inflammation of the joints.[21] During the subacute stage, isometric exercise is used.[7, 23] One maximum contraction per muscle group is enough.[21] Others recommend repetition of the isometric exercise three times per muscle group, once per day.[7, 23] The goal is to maintain the static holding ability of muscle so that proper positioning can be maintained during functional activities.[21] Strengthening exercises follow a period of warm-up and are done when pain and stiffness are at a minimum.[21]

Activities to maintain and increase strength should be gently resistive, done for short periods of time within the limits of pain, and balanced with rest of the part. Activities which require reaching to pick up objects are good choices for the upper extremities, trunk, and neck; the joints exercised and the extent of the exercise are controlled by the location of the pieces to be picked up. An example is to place pieces for a project in various locations in relation to the patient. He reaches for them and then into another plane to work each piece of material into the project.

It is important that the patient be kept interested in moving actively throughout the day but within limits of pain and fatigue. Care should be exercised that repetitive exercise/activity is not exacerbating the joint disease.

Resistance for patients having rheumatoid arthritis is controversial; because resistive forces cause deformity, some authorities advocate avoidance of resistance. Flatt[24] believes that resistive exercise is deforming because of the alteration of relationships of tendons to the axes of movement. Resistive exercise cannot improve weakened joint structures nor reposition the tendons. Swezey[21] states that there is not enough

research to support whether resistive exercises are helpful or harmful in cases of myositis, and he therefore defers resistive exercises until serum enzymes are normal to avoid exacerbating the myositis. Both Flatt[24] and Swezey[21] advocate graduated exercise programs and protection of supporting joint structures during exercise. The graduation of resistance is *very* gradual, and in estimating the initial amount of resistance, as well as the graduated increments, it is better to err on the side of too little rather than too much.

Maintenance or Increase of Endurance

Endurance is increased by involving the patient in interesting activities. This provides the opportunity for the patient to learn to gauge his own endurance and to rest before fatigue ensues. Fatigue not only may cause careless use of joints, but also requires a longer rest period, which means longer immobilization. The total day of the patient with rheumatoid arthritis must be examined to coordinate rest with activity. This balance of rest and activity is carried over to home planning also.

Recreational activities to overcome the depression associated with chronic disability and pain, yet which are nonstressful to joints, should be promoted. Swimming is one especially good activity for most persons.[21]

Maintenance or Increase of Skill in Functional Tasks

Principles and methods of self-care and homemaking activities for a patient with limited range of motion are described in the section on the rehabilitative approach. Essentially, the methods involve the use of long handles to extend the reach and enlarged handles to decrease the grasp force required. A warm morning bath or shower helps the patient overcome morning stiffness and "get moving."

It is important to instruct the patient how to reduce joint strain during activities of daily living.[3] All functional activities that involve MP flexion (especially grasp and pinch) increase ulnar forces across the MP joints because the flexor profundus tendon can bowstring if the flexor sheath is damaged or weakened by synovitis. Also, the ulnar interossei are more powerful than the radial during functional use.[7, 12] Any means of substituting for grasp or reducing the force required are sought.

Additionally, the rheumatoid arthritic person needs to learn energy conservation principles and techniques outlined in the chapter on homemaking.

Patients with advanced inflammatory polyarthritis may develop such deformities and muscle weakness that a powered wheelchair becomes a necessity.[30]

Patient Education

The topics that are included in patient education for the rheumatoid arthritic included the importance of rest, positioning, and protection of joint function, energy conservation principles and work simplification techniques, and home program.

When instructing the patient, attention should be paid to the instructional process as well as the patient's specific needs and methods of coping with his disability.[7] Instructional sessions should have specific goals and should clearly present the material through discussion and audiovisual means. After assessing what the patient has learned, the information may have to be repeated because it is not retained all at once.[3] The therapist should assess the psychological readiness of the patient to learn the new techniques or suggestions.[7] Pain, concern with the disease, and the effects of medication may interfere with the learning process; written information is therefore helpful for future reference.[3, 7]

Patients with generalized synovitis who are systemically unwell need increased rest periods, but not complete bedrest which can result in weakness, stiffening, and loss of mobility.[3] Exercise increases as the disease activity decreases.[23] The patient is taught not to push beyond capacity, but that inactivity is to be avoided since it starts a cycle of discouragement, depression, and further inactivity.[31] Fulfilling work is creative and involves problem-solving. One registered nurse, herself a victim of rheumatoid arthritis for 30 years, teaches that too much rest is more disabling than a life of activity in terms of weakness and loss of function.[31]

Methods of energy conservation must become part of the patient's new habit repertoire: he must learn to use lightweight, energy-saving equipment, delete some jobs, plan ahead to balance rest with exertion, gather all necessary equipment ahead of time, make storage convenient, and sit to work when possible.

The topic of sex should receive some attention during patient education. Some of this may be the occupational therapist's duty since it is related to protected use of the joints and avoidance of pain. Sex is difficult to do or enjoy for the rheumatoid arthritic because of pain and joint limitations.[32] The difficulty is not only related to the mechanics, but also has to do with fear about the effect sex will have on the condition; guilt feelings connected to the idea that the disease is punishment for some previous wrong; role anxieties related to change in role due to the disease; and feelings of anger, depression, and poor self-image. There is also a concern with the inability to physically obtain or use certain types of contraceptive methods. There may be worry that the disease is hereditary. Sexual counseling beyond the information concerning joint protection should be available.[32]

Regarding the mechanics of sex, it is recommended that the patient take pain medication beforehand, use cushions to support painful limbs, use positions that are found to be most comfortable,[33] and make other methods of sexual satisfaction an important part of intimacy.[32] It is recommended that the patient identify comfortable reclining positions for himself and then adapt them for sexual intercourse; the positions should minimize stress on the joints.[34] Sexual intercourse should be avoided during periods of fatigue and during flare-ups of the disease.[35]

An essential part of the treatment program of a rheumatoid arthritic is a written and rehearsed home program of activity to maintain gains. The therapist carefully explains to the patient and family the rationale for all stages of the treatment program, including the home program. The patient's acceptance of responsibility for his own program is sought. The patient must be educated to the importance of mobility and joint protection throughout life and must learn the techniques prior to discharge.

Group therapy to deal with issues of disturbance of self-image, body image, job status, family relationships, and coping mechanisms would be useful.[35]

An "Arthritis Club" run by and for persons with arthritis and their families would improve the person's chances of coping successfully with the disease on a long-term day-to-day basis. One such club is described which educates in lay terms, organizes recreational programs, and provides peer counseling and many other services.[36]

DEGENERATIVE JOINT DISEASE

Degenerative joint disease, or osteoarthritis, is more common than rheumatoid arthritis, but less damaging.[2] It results from a combination of aging, irritation of the joints, and normal wear and tear caused by obesity, poor body mechanics, and poor posture.[1, 2] It is localized to the traumatized joint(s). The weight-bearing joints are the most often affected. The knees are most commonly affected, but more disability results from involvement of the hip. The DIP joints of the fingers are also often affected.

The disease process is one of wearing away or deterioration of the articular cartilage and formation of new bone in subchondral areas and margins.[1] Heberden's nodes, which form on the sides of the distal interphalangeal joints, are examples of the formation of excess spurs of bone.

Treatment is directed toward relief of pain, restoration of joint function, prevention of avoidable deformity or progression of the joint deterioration.[2] There are no specific treatments.[1] The joint is rested for some time daily. Support to the joint may be needed, unnecessary use or stress to the joint is avoided, and exercises to correct any muscle imbalance or atrophy so as to prevent joint instability are done[1] using progressive resistance.

Occupational therapy treatment is concerned with increasing the strength of muscles surrounding the joint so that they may more effectively support the joint. Relief of pain by resting the joint and relieving stress to the joint, maintenance of joint mobility balanced with rest to the part, and avoidance of deforming positions of immobilization are also important. Movement increases the nutrition to the avascular articular cartilage, the component damaged in osteoarthritis, in a way not yet clearly understood.[1] Therefore, movement in therapy is important for this reason as well as for the usual reasons of strengthening and mobility. It is also important to teach the patient to be functionally independent using the least stress to the joint. This may require use of adapted devices, joint protection techniques, and/or use of energy-conserving methods such as sitting while working to relieve stress to the affected hip or knee.

Surgical correction of deformed weight-bearing joints, especially the hip, is very successful and is being done more routinely for the relief of pain. See Chapter 19 on fractures for treatment following hip replacement surgery.

References

1. Rodnon, G. P. (ed.) *Primer on the Rheumatic Diseases*, 7th ed. Reprinted from JAMA 224, (Suppl. 5), 1973. Distributed by The Arthritis Foundation, 1212 Avenue of the Americas, New York, N.Y. 10036.
2. National Institute of Arthritis, Metabolism, and Digestive Diseases. *How to Cope with Arthritis*, DHEW Publication No. (NIH) 78-1092 Washington, D.C. U.S. Government Printing Office, 1978.
3. Edmonds, J. The management of rheumatoid arthritis. *Aust. Fam. Phys.*, 7 (8): 925–935, 1978.
4. Barrows, D. M., Berezny, L. M., and Reynolds, M. D. Physical and occupational therapy for arthritic patients: A cooperative effort among hospital departments. *Arch. Phys. Med. Rehabil.*, 59 (2): 64–67, 1978.
5. Kay, A. G. L. Management of the rheumatoid hand. *Rheumat. Rehabil.*, 18 (Suppl. 1): 76–81, 1979.
6. Swanson, A. B. Flexible implant arthroplasty for arthritic finger joints. *J. Bone Joint Surg.*, 54A (3): 435–455, 1972.
7. Melvin, J. L. *Rheumatic Disease: Occupational Therapy and Rehabilitation*. Philadelphia: F. A. Davis, 1977.
8. English, C. B., and Nalebuff, E. A. Understanding the arthritic hand. *Am. J. Occup. Ther.*, 25 (7): 353–358, 1971.
9. Feinberg, J., and Brandt, K. D. Use of resting splints by patients with rheumatoid arthritis. *Am. J. Occup. Ther.*, 35 (3): 173–178, 1981.
10. Swezey, R. L. Dynamic factors in deformity of the rheumatoid arthritic hand. *Bull. Rheumat. Dis.*, 22 (1 and 2): 651–654, 1971–72. The Arthritis Foundation, 1212 Avenue of the Americas, New York, N.Y. 10036.
11. Pahle, J. A., and Raunio, P. The influence of wrist position on finger deviation in the rheumatoid hand. *J. Bone Joint Surg.*, 5 (4): 664–676, 1969.
12. Smith, E. M., Juvinall, R. C., Bender, L. F., and Pearson, J. R. Role of the finger flexors in rheumatoid deformities of the metacarpophalangeal joints. *Arthritis Rheumat.*, 7 (5): 467–480, 1964.
13. Swezey, R. L., and Fiegenberg, D. S. Inappropriate intrinsic muscle action in the rheumatoid hand. *Ann. Rheum. Dis.*, 30: 619–625, 1971.
14. Wozny, W., and Long, C. Electromyographic kinesiology of the rheumatoid hand. *Arch. Phys. Med. Rehabil.*, 47 (11): 702–703, 1966.
15. Shapiro, J. S. The etiology of ulnar drift: A new factor. *J. Bone Joint Surg.*, 50A: 634, 1968.
16. Vignos, P. J. Editorial: Physiotherapy in rheumatoid arthritis. *J. Rheumatol.*, 7 (3): 269–271, 1980.
17. Badley, E. M., Lee, J., and Wood, P. H. N. Patterns of disability related to joint involvement in rheumatoid arthritis. *Rheumatol. Rehabil.*, 18 (2): 105–109, 1979.
18. Jebsen, R. H., *et al.* An objective and standardized test of hand function. *Arch. Phys. Med. Rehabil.*, 50 (6): 311–319, 1969.
19. Carthum, C. J., Clawson, D. K., and Decker, J. L. Functional assessment of the rheumatoid hand. *Am. J. Occup. Ther.*, 23 (2): 122–125, 1969.
20. Simon, L. Rehabilitation of the rheumatoid shoulder. *Rheumatol. Rehabil.*, 18 (Suppl. 1): 81–85, 1979.
21. Swezey, R. L. Rehabilitation aspects in arthritis. In *Arthritis and Allied Conditions*, 9th ed., edited by D. J. McCarty. Philadelphia: Lea & Febiger, 1979.
22. Long, C. Lecture. Highland View Hospital, Cleveland, Ohio. June 1962.
23. Glass, J. Physical medicine in rheumatology. *Aust. N.Z. J Med.*, 8 (Suppl. 1): 168–171, 1978.
24. Flatt, A. E. *The Care of the Rheumatoid Hand*, 3rd ed. St. Louis: C. V. Mosby, 1974.
25. Davis, J., and Janecki, C. J. Rehabilitation of the rheumatoid upper limb. *Orthop. Clin. North Am.*, 9 (2): 559–568, 1978.
26. Kaplan, E. B. *Functional and Surgical Anatomy of the Hand*. Philadelphia: J. B. Lippincott, 1965.
27. Long, C. Upper Limb Orthotics. In *Orthotics Etcetera*, 2nd ed., edited by J. B. Redford. Baltimore: Williams & Wilkins, 1980.
28. Cordery, J. Joint protection: A responsiblity of the occupational therapist. *Am. J. Occup. Ther.*, 19 (5): 285–294, 1965.
29. Moore, J. W. Adapted knife for rheumatoid arthritics. *Am. J. Occup. Ther.*, 32 (2): 112–113, 1978.
30. Bossingham, D. H., and Russell, P. The usefulness of powered wheelchairs in advanced inflammatory polyarthritis. *Rheumatol. Rehabil.*, 19 (2): 131–135, 1980.
31. Schwaid, M. C. Advice to arthritics: Keep moving. *Am. J. Nurs.*: 1708–1709, 1978.
32. Greengross, W. Sex and arthritis. *Rheumatol. Rehabil.*, 18 (Suppl. 1): 68–70, 1979.
33. Frederick, B. B., *et al. Body Mechanics Instruction Manual: A Guide for Therapists*. Redmond, Wash.: Express Publications, 1979.
34. Onder, J., Lachniet, D., and Becker, M. C. Sexual counselling, arthritis, and women. *Allied Health Professions Section Newsletter*, 7 (3 and 4): 1–6, 1973. Distributed by the Arthritis Foundation, 1212 The Avenue of the Americas, New York, N.Y. 10036.
35. Krawitz, M., and Wolman, T. Group therapy in rheumatoid arthritis. *Pennsylvania Med.*, 82 (12): 35–37, 1979.
36. Gatter, R. A., Richmond, J. D., and Andrews, R. P. Arthritis community outreach program. *N. Engl. J. Med.*, 301 (1): 52, 1979.

Supplementary Reading

Amis, A. A., *et al.* Elbow joint forces in patients with rheumatoid arthritis. *Rheumatol. Rehabil.*, 18 (4): 230–234, 1979.

Brattström, M. Gelenkschutz bei Progredient-Chronischer Polyarthritis. Sweden: Student-litteratur. ISBN 91-44-09551-1. (Useful photographs for patient education.)

Chamberlain, M. A. Aids and equipment for the arthritic. *Practitioner*, 224 (1339): 65–71, 1980.

Dworecka, F. F., *et al.* A practical approach to the evaluation of rheumatoid hand deformity. *Am. J. Orthop. Surg.*: 1968.

Home Care Programs in Arthritis: A Manual for Patients. The Arthritis Foundation, 1212 The Avenue of the Americas, New York, NY 10036.

Johnson, B. M., Flynn, M. J. G., and Beckenbaugh, R. D. A dynamic splint for use after total wrist arthroplasty. *Am. J. Occup. Ther.*, 35 (3): 179–184, 1981.

Klinger, J. L., Gruen, H., Navarro, A. H., Reilly, M. M., and McLean, M. A. *Self Help Manual for Patients with Arthritis*. Atlanta: the Arthritis Foundation, 1980.

Meenan, R. F., Gertmen, P. M., and Mason, J. H. Measuring health status in arthritis: The arthritis impact measurement scales. *Arth. Rheumat.*, 23 (2): 146–152, 1980.

Melvin, J. L. *Rheumatic Disease: Occupational Therapy and Rehabilitation*, ed. 2. Philadelphia: F. A. Davis, 1982.

Paradis, D. K., and Ferlic, D. C. Shoulder arthroplasty in rheumatoid arthritis. *Phys. Ther.*, 55 (2): 157–159, 1975.

Swezey, R. L. *Arthritis: Rational Therapy and Rehabilitation*. Philadelphia: W. B. Saunders, 1978.

University of Michigan Pilot Geriatric Arthritis Program, *Joint Protection for Osteoarthritis*.

University of Michigan Pilot Geriatric Arthritis Program, *Osteoarthritis*.

chapter

21

Spinal Cord Injury

Catherine A. Trombly, M.A., OTR

The spinal cord contains the neural connecting tracts which transmit sensory and motor impulses to and from the brain. Internuncial cells and the anterior horn cells are also located in the spinal cord. Disease or injury to the spinal cord will affect the sensory motor function of the person in that lower motor neuron signs will be seen at the site of the lesion due to destruction of the anterior horn cells or peripheral nerves (cauda equina), and upper motor neuron signs will be visible below the level of the lesion if the sensory and motor tracts are interrupted. Spinal cord-injured patients do not have brain damage; therefore, cognition and perception are intact. Spinal cord function can be disrupted by disease, such as multiple sclerosis (MS) or amyotrophic lateral sclerosis (ALS); by tumors; by congenital deformities, such as spina bifida; or by trauma, such as automobile accidents, gunshot wounds, knife wounds, or diving accidents. This chapter will concentrate on therapy devised for the traumatic spinal cord-injured (SCI) patient; however, the ideas are selectively appropriate for patients with other types of spinal cord dysfunction.

It is estimated that 10,000 spinal cord injuries occur annually[1] (35 per 1,000,000 persons in the U.S.A.[2]) and that there is a population of 200,000 spinal cord-injured (SCI) persons in the United States at this time.[1]

Unless the cord is physically cut as in knife or gunshot wounds, the usual injury is a compression fracture in which the cord is squeezed by the damaged or displaced vertebrae. A major cord compression injury results in profound ischemia of the cord, not only at the injury site but also for a considerable distance proximal and distal to the site.[3] Traumatic spinal cord injury can be complete (no function below the level of the lesion) or incomplete (sparing of sensory and/or motor function below the lesion level). Innervation of muscles is arranged in an orderly progression so that the lower the location of the lesion, the more upper extremity (proximal to distal), trunk, and finally lower extremity musculature is preserved. Spinal cord injury is designated by the last segmental level of the cord that is preserved. For example, C_6 quadriplegia (complete) designates that all motor, sensory, and autonomic functions mediated by the nervous system at the sixth cervical level of the cord and above are preserved. Injuries to the cord may be diagonal which results in greater preservation of function on one side of the body than on the other. In this case, both levels are noted. For example, $C_{5,6}$ means that the functions of the fifth cervical segment are preserved on one side and those of the sixth on the other. There are no shorthand methods of labeling for incomplete lesions with distal sparing.

In one type of incomplete lesion, the functions of the central cord are preserved, while the peripheral functions are lost below the lesion level. This results in sparing of the lower extremity function because of the location of the tracts serving these limbs within the cord. Sacral sparing is confirmed by evidence of perianal sensation and active toe flexion.[4]

Effective emergency and immediate care of spinal cord-injured patients have increased the number of patients coming for rehabilitation and their functional potential. The preservation of one additional spinal cord segment can contribute significantly to the functional capabilities of the patient (see Table 21.1). For that reason, improved handling at the accident scene and transportation techniques are now in common usage for persons suspected of having spinal injury. One immediate care technique that has some effect in preserving function is hypothermic irrigation, or cord cooling, which, if done within hours of the compression injury, may prevent the secondary neurological deficits due to cord swelling and compression within the unyielding vertebral column. However, after more careful recent study, this method cannot be considered a panacea since it has been found only variably effective and only for injuries of limited severity.[3]

CLINICAL PICTURE

The immediate consequence of spinal cord injury is spinal shock which may last several days to weeks. It is characterized by areflexia of the limbs, bowel, and bladder.[1] As soon as spinal shock subsides, reflex spasticity develops, and return of some motor function begins, which continues for approximately 1 year.

Spinal cord injury is a physically and psychologically devastating disability. In addition to the spasticity and loss of voluntary motor control below the level of the lesion, there are many other sequelae. There is a loss of sensory discrimination and awareness below lesion level. Bowel, bladder, and sexual functions are no longer under voluntary control. In high level lesions, the autonomic nervous system fails to regulate body temperature and blood pressure as it normally would. The injury usually precipitates an abrupt change from vigorous activity to infantile dependency which plummets the patient and his family into depression and denial.

Many complications can arise from these sequelae and must be carefully attended to in order to ensure that the patient does not lose potential functional ability because of their effects. Some of the complications which directly affect therapy are listed here.

In time, spasticity may develop into spasms, either clonic or tonic. Spasms are usually triggered by a certain sensory stimulus, such as infection, sudden touch, or other irritation. Mild spasms can be controlled by ensuring that the patient is free of the triggering stimuli. Clonus, spasmodic alternation of contraction of agonist and antagonist, can be stopped by holding the part steady for a few moments, which dampens the oscillations. Some patients use their spasms to accomplish certain functions, and they learn to trigger them in a controlled way. Severe spasms may interfere with the achievement of independence, and medical or surgical relief may be required.

Contractures tend to develop in patterns of spasticity and in each joint which is not kept mobile by either active or passive range of motion exercises. On the other hand, periarticular ossification may occur at joints innervated below the level of lesion due to too much (or too little) exercise, although these causative factors are as yet unproven.[5] This complication limits use of the extremity and decreases functional independence. Surgical removal provides at least temporary relief; however, there is a tendency for recurrence.

High level lesions (C_{1-4}) damage the phrenic nerve, and paralysis of the diaphragm is the result. Few survive the acute state.[5-6] Those who do must be artificially respirated at all times. Although chest respirators are the most common method of doing this, phrenic nerve stimulators have been developed by rehabilitation engineers and are currently finding acceptance, since they allow elimination of the bulky respirator during part of the day.[7] They can only be used if the anterior horn cells of the phrenic nerve are intact.[4] The stimulator paces the diaphragm with an electrical impulse to the phrenic nerve.[7] These patients and others with lesions at T_6 and above require therapy for hygiene of their lungs.[1] They are unable to cough to rid themselves of the waste in their lungs as persons with normally innervated respiratory muscles are able to do.

High level spinal cord-injured patients (above T_7)[5] suffer from severely disturbed autonomic function. An emergency associated with this is called sympathetic hyperreflexia[6] or autonomic dysreflexia in which the blood pressure of the patient rises dangerously or even fatally. The stimulus may be visceral distension or bladder distension, the latter being more common. The patient has some or all of these symptoms: he is flushed, restless, perspiring, nauseous,[6] chilled, has increased spasticity, and headache.[8] Immediately check to see if the patient's catheter is unclamped and free flowing, then call the nurse or physician. Do not recline the patient because that will increase the already high blood pressure in the cerebral arteries. Eventually patients learn to recognize the onset of symptoms early, what the triggering stimulus is, and how to guide the person who assists them.

High level quadriplegic patients also cannot regulate their temperature automatically and need to be artificially kept warm in winter and cool in summer. The latter is especially important because hyperthermia may ensue. Therapy should be discontinued if air conditioning is unavailable and the patient is experiencing a rise in body temperature.

The lack of sensory awareness coupled with the reduced blood flow to tissue results in a propensity to develop decubiti from prolonged pressure.[1, 6] At all times, *and for the rest of his life*, the patient must be constantly vigilant against this. At first the personnel take responsibility for instructing, turning, and positioning the patient. Gradually the responsibility is shifted to the patient even if he can only direct someone else to move him. Patients at lesion levels of C_6 and below can learn to relieve pressure themselves, and achieving this becomes a major goal of therapy.

Bowel and bladder regulation can be achieved through special training and use of adaptive techniques and equipment. The rehabilitation nurse usually assumes responsibility for this aspect of the patient's rehabilitation, although others become involved as their expertise warrants. Rehabilitation engineers are working on electrical stimulation methods for micturition.[7] The occupational therapist may get involved by developing special aids to enable the patients to assume independent self-care.

The bowel is regulated via diet and regular use of suppositories. Upper motor neuron lesion may result in neurogenic bladder[6] or detrusor-external urethral sphincter dyssynergia in which the urethral sphincter fails to relax as in normal voiding.[9] This results in spasmodic and incomplete voiding, potential sources of infection and embarrassment. It has been found that one way this problem can be overcome is by anal sphincter stretch during voiding which causes a reflex relaxation of the urethral sphincter.[9] An orthotic finger appliance has been devised to assist selected C_7, C_8

quadriplegics to maintain a sustained stretch on the anal sphincter.[9] Patients with lower level lesions do not require the appliance and those with higher lesions lack the trunk balance and/or upper extremity requirements to do the procedure. Intermittent catheterization is another method of controlling the bladder problem and is beginning to replace the use of indwelling catheters in some patients. Intermittent catheterization can be done by patients with lesions as high as C_6 with adaptations and practice.[10]

Sexual functions are less disturbed in female than male patients. The female usually resumes menstruation within 6 months postinjury and must consider birth control if a child is not wanted.[1] There may be a reduction in reflex vaginal lubrication during intercourse[1] which can be rectified by use of recommended lubricants. In male patients who suffer lesions to $S_{2,3}$ or $_4$, there is a loss of erection (flaccidity).[1] In all other male patients, reflex, though not psychogenic, erection is preserved.[1] In high level lesions, erections occur frequently in response to various stimuli[5] which is a potential source of embarrassment to the patient and needs to be dealt with as part of sexual counseling. Ejaculation occurs less often than erections; patients with levels T_{11} to L_2 preserved are more likely to have this function.[5] It is rare for SCI patients to father children both because of inability to ejaculate and because of decreased and altered motility of the sperm.[1]

Sexual counseling needs to be done with these patients by a knowledgeable team member. Four aspects of sexuality need to be addressed: satisfaction, including information about attitudes and methods that can be used as alternatives to genital sexual satisfaction[1]; function[1, 11]; fertility; and desirability which becomes a true concern given the values of society.[1]

The psychological complications must be addressed in therapy from the beginning. Rehabilitation can only occur in the patient whose motivation is not blocked by depression and denial.

The typical patient is the young, athletic male of 15 to 25 years. This fact presents several problems to rehabilitation. One is that the patient is in a period of his life when physical prowess, independence, developing sexuality, and preparation for life's work are important issues. Immediately the accident renders him dependent on others for basic self-care needs, unable to move, doubtful about his masculinity and future abilities. Another problem is that if he were a person who used physical activity to dissipate feelings of frustration and anger, that avenue may be closed to him if paralysis is extensive. Young adults often consider physical appearance of prime importance in the valuing of self or others, and patients may reject their new appearance, the use of special techniques or necessary mechanical devices, such as wheelchairs, splints, etc., on this basis.

It has been found by a physical therapist that a program of progressively vigorous handling of quadriplegics with stable fracture sites seemed to be psychologically beneficial in that there was less fear of falling, more body control developed, less feelings of fragility, and greater feelings of being "touchable."[12] Also, the use of recreational and sports activities may engage the patient's interest and participation in therapy aimed at increasing strength and endurance, while allowing some friendly competition and socialization which are normal life tasks of this age group.

OCCUPATIONAL THERAPY GOALS AND TREATMENT PLANNING

Rehabilitation of the spinal cord-injured patient is lengthy, requiring 100 to 160 days for a paraplegic[5] and 180 to 300 days for a quadriplegic.[5, 13] The rehabilitation process must be comprehensive and involve not only the restoration and compensation for lost function but also therapy to help the patient accept and value his changed self. The patient is helped to take the responsibility for directing and carrying out his rehabilitative process. Rehabilitation of a spinal cord-injured patient is complex and is effective only if a true team effort is put forth by the patient as well as the SCI unit personnel.

The primary goal of the occupational therapist in the rehabilitation of spinal cord-injured patients is to teach the person to be as independent as he is able to become in all aspects of occupational performance tasks. Adjunctive to increased independence is maintenance of range of motion, increase of strength and endurance, prevention of decubiti, acceptance of body image, and containment of depression and denial to within workable limits. To become independent, the person needs to learn techniques that compensate for weakness and lack of function, especially lack of hand function in quadriplegics. The person needs to learn to use gravity and leverage to handle his own body and objects. In early treatment, goal setting may not involve active decision-making on the part of the patient if he is emotionally overwhelmed. However, at the earliest point that the patient can participate in goal setting, he should. An informative study by Taylor[14] indicates a need for closer collaboration between the occupational therapist and the quadriplegic patient in establishing goals and priorities. Therapy goals considered by OTR's to be important for C_5, C_6 quadriplegics were different from those considered important by the patients themselves. The patients of the particular sample valued development of work tolerance first, then muscle strengthening, and then bowel and bladder control. They placed least value on bathing and dressing. The therapists ranked development of adapted equipment and devices first, followed by eating, socialization, and wheelchair mobility. Low value was given by the therapists to driver education and to bowel and bladder control. There was greater compatibility between the paraplegic's values and those of the OTR, probably because the goals are more circumscribed and there was less chance of variability.[14]

Neurologic functions, as measured by manual muscle testing and sensation of pinprick, were found to correlate positively, at the time of discharge and at 1 year follow-up, with function as measured by movement of the limbs, ability to do essential self-care, walk 50 meters on level ground, and transfers.[15] These types of observations over the years have led therapists and physicians to develop guidelines for certain expected levels of achievement in performance of daily life tasks by SCI patients. These expectations are outlined in Table 21.1. Use of such guidelines helps the therapist to know what levels of accomplishment to expect and to keep goal setting realistic. The guidelines suppose that the patient is a healthy, athletic male who is free from secondarily limiting factors, such as spasm, decubiti, contractures, an unstable fracture site, etc. They also presume that the patient has been active in therapy to develop sufficient strength and endurance equal to each task. These guidelines ought not to be considered limiting; some patients of unusual drive, strength, and resourcefulness are able to become more independent than one would expect, based on the experience of the accomplishments of other spinal cord-injured patients of similar level. However, it is psychologically crucial that the patient not be asked to try to do tasks that will cause him to experience failure.

In developing priorities for daily therapy, the therapist uses as a guide the fact that the patient needs to have prerequisite psychological attitudes and physical abilities to do daily living tasks. Therapy is aimed at establishing these prerequisites and then introducing the functional task with expectations for success. A good sequence of training is to start with light activities, such as feeding and hygiene, and progress to bed mobility, wheelchair mobility, transfers, toileting, bathing, dressing, and finally driving.

OCCUPATIONAL THERAPY EVALUATION AND TREATMENT

Occupational therapy evaluation includes measurements, as appropriate to the patient's lesion level, of passive range of motion, muscle strength, endurance for sustained activity, sensory awareness and discrimination, level of independence in occupational performance tasks, and stage of recovery of psychological equilibrium. Therapy to restore or maintain range of motion, strength, and endurance is biomechanical in nature (see Chapter 8). All muscles with any remaining supraspinal innervation are strengthened by exercise to recruit motor units and then to hypertrophy the motor fibers of the units through repetitive resistive exercise. If the lesion is complete, no hope of regaining control of the muscles innervated below the level of lesion is held. Sometimes neurodevelopmental inhibition techniques are helpful in reducing the spasticity of the muscles below the lesion, but this is reflexive in nature and never develops beyond this. In patients with incomplete lesions, there may be a combination of spasticity and weak voluntary power in some muscles. The neurodevelopmental techniques may prove beneficial in these cases. Therapy for sensory loss and

functional loss is compensatory (see Chapter 3 and Part 9). Orthoses may also be needed, especially for quadriplegics, and are suggested in Table 21.1 and described in Chapter 12. The information in Chapter 2 will assist the occupational therapist to devise an appropriate psychosocial therapeutic program that must be inherently interwoven with the therapy program directed toward increased physical functioning.

The occupational therapy program must interdigitate with the rest of the rehabilitation program, all of which is dictated by the recovery process.

Early Treatment Program for SCI Patients

To maintain normal alignment of the spine, patients are immobilized in bed or on turning frames until the vertebral fracture site is healed. Patients with cervical injuries may be further immobilized in correct alignment by use of skeletal traction attached by cranial tongs or head halter.[1] Halo braces are also used to provide traction and alignment.[1] Thoracolumbar injuries may be immobilized in a plaster jacket or brace.[1] The immobilization places limits on the types of therapy possible. Precautions are exercised by all hospital personnel when handling the patient to prevent movement of the fracture site which could jeopardize the neurological functioning of the patient, and, in high cervical lesions, even his life. No upright, rotary, or flexion/extension movement of the spine is allowed until the orthopedist clears the patient for such movement.[1] Turning frames not only enable nursing staff to safely and easily turn the immobilized patient over every 2 hours, thus preventing the development of decubiti over bony prominences, but also put the patient in positions which facilitate exercise and practice of functional tasks. Stryker or Foster turning frames have sectional mattresses to eliminate pressure over bony prominences. The frame pivots around its longitudinal axis and turns the patient as if he were on a rotisserie. Circoelectric beds pivot around a horizontal axis so the patient is turned from back lying, to standing, to prone-lying. Their use is controversial. Some believe that use of circoelectric beds is contraindicated in treatment of the recently injured spine due to the axial loading during turning,[1] and others cite the frequency of calcaneous decubiti developed during the standing position as a reason for not using them. Those who prefer it, cite the opportunity to be upright for a period of time as the positive factor.

Maintenance of range of motion requires a concerted effort of therapists and nurses. The occupational therapist is particularly responsible for seeing that all joints of the upper extremities maintain adequate range of motion so that future independence in daily life tasks is not precluded or limited. Attention to the upper extremity is critical from the earliest point because functional achievement depends on the upper extremities.[6] It is extremely important, however, that the finger flexors of the C_6 quadriplegic be allowed to tighten into a partially flexed position so that he will have a more effective tenodesis grasp. During range of motion exercise, when the fingers are flexed,

Table 21.1
EXPECTED LEVELS OF ACHIEVEMENT AND SUGGESTED METHODS FOR SPINAL CORD-INJURED PATIENTS

Last Fully Innervated Level and Key Muscles Added	Movements the Patient Can Do	Achievement	Technique and/or Equipment

C_1, C_2, C_3
 	
 Facial and neck muscles innervated by cranial nerves
	Chew
	 Swallow
	 Talk
	 Blow
		Self-care
		 None
		
		 Mobility
		  1. W/c locomotion
		
		  2. Recline
		
		 Communication
		  1. Typing
		
		  2. Control appliances
			a. Needs respirator. Phrenic nerve stimulator may be used in daytime.[4]
			
			 a. Electronically controlled electric w/c with gradual acceleration feature[12] and safety belt; can use sip and puff or microswitch controls.
			 b. May need corset; cushion needed.
			 a. Electronically controlled reclining electric w/c.[1]
			
			 a. Electric typewriter and mouthstick or sip and puff controls. (POSSUM)[34]
			 b. Paper on a roll.[35]
			 a. Environmental Control Unit[18,36] to control TV on/off and channel selection, lamp, electric bed, nurse call, tape recorder, page turner, automatic telephone dialer.[18, 35]
			 b. Speaker phone.[36]

C_4
 Diaphragm
 Trapezius
	Respiration
	 Scapular elevation
		Self-care
		  1. Some feeding
		
		 Mobility
		  Locomotion and weight shift
			a. Mobile Arm supports which may need to have a powered elbow.
			 b. Externally powered flexor hinge hand splint for the stronger extremity.[34–40] Long opponens with double "T" bars for other, assistive extremity. A ratchet splint can be used in lieu of external power.[32,41]
			 c. Lapboard. A plexiglass lapboard is preferred for patients who use an electric w/c so they can see where their feet are and avoid bumping them while traveling.
			 d. Plate guard or scoop dish so the food can be "captured."
			 e. Long straw with a strawholder because the patient cannot pick up the glass.
			 f. Swivel "spork" with built-up, friction handle.[35]
			 g. The dish may need to be elevated off the lapboard until the patient gains skills. The dish must be stabilized by a nonskid pad or wet towel.
			
			 a. Electronically controlled w/c with reclining back; controls can be sip and puff,[1] chin switches,[42] or switches mounted on the lapboard or in a shoulder harness. A gradual acceleration accessory on the w/c to prevent sudden starts and a seat belt are good safety measures.

Table 21.1—*Continued*

Last Fully Innervated Level and Key Muscles Added	Movements the Patient Can Do	Achievement	Technique and/or Equipment
			b. Cushion.
			c. Trunk support if necessary.[43]
		Communication	
		1. Typing	a. Electric ball-type typewriter with automatic pushbutton return; can be used with a mouthstick or sip and puff controls.
			b. Self-correcting ribbon.[35]
			c. Paper in roll[35] or use a modified mouthstick to put the paper in.[35,44]
			d. Some patients use a rubber-tipped stick held in the splint to type.
			e. A good bookstand is a commercially available industrial catalogue rack.[44]
		2. Telephoning	a. Automatic telephone dialer.[18,35]
			b. Speaker phone.[35]
		3. Notetaking in school or business	a. Adapted tape recorder which must have electronic switching to allow adaptation to remote push button control unit.
		4. Control appliances	a. Environmental control units.[18,35,36,45] An ultrasound remote control unit that can take 16 appliances and can summon aid from nearby house has been developed.[44]
		Recreation	
		1. Table games	a. The same orthotic equipment used for feeding can be used to move playing pieces which may need to be adapted as to size, shape, or texture.[46]
		2. Painting or drawing.	a. Mouthstick with brush or pencil attached. A battery-operated oral telescoping orthosis with a mouthpiece that covers the complete dentition has been developed; it has interchangeable terminal pieces.[47]
C$_5$ Biceps Brachialis[6] Brachioradialis[6] Supinator[6] Infraspinatus[6] Deltoid	Elbow flexion and supination Shoulder external rotation Shoulder abduction to 80–90° Gravity provides: shoulder adduction pronation internal rotation	All of the above tasks are done more easily.	The patient may not need some adaptations and may be able to use others. He will not need a powered elbow on the mobile arm support (MAS); some patients get strong enough to discard the MAS altogether in time. The controls of the electric bed can be lever type adaptations to the regular controls which the patient operates by elbow flexion.[48]
C$_6$ Pectoralis major	Shoulder flexion and extension	Self-care	
Serratus anterior Latissimus dorsi	Reach forward Shoulder internal rotation Shoulder adduction More respiratory reserve (accessory breathing muscles)	1. Feeding	a. May use a universal cuff, thread the utensil through his fingers ("interlacing grip"[21]), or use a wrist-driven flexor hinge hand splint; does not use MAS, but may need to initially.

Table 21.1—*Continued*

Last Fully Innervated Level and Key Muscles Added	Movements the Patient Can Do	Achievement	Technique and/or Equipment
C$_6$ (con't) Pronator teres Radial wrist extensors	Pronation Wrist extension (tenodesis grasp)		b. Rocker knife or very sharp paring knife for cutting. c. Does not need long straw; may use cup or mug with a large handle. d. Does not need plate guard.
		2. Dressing	a. Uses flexor hinge hand splint when pinch is necessary. If wrist extension only rates P to F a SAFRA (Sequential Advancing Flexion Retention Attachment) locking mechanism can be added to a standard flexor hinge splint.[49] b. Dresses lower extremities in bed as described in Chapter 26. Uses momentum and substitute movements to turn over, sit up, pull up clothing.[50] c. Uses button hook and zipper pull. d. Cannot tie shoes. e. Clothes should be of correct size or one size larger.
		3. Bathing and grooming	a. Uses bath mitt with a pocket to hold the soap. b. In a tub bath or shower, the patient sits on a padded shower bench. Faucets must be within reach. c. In tub or shower, uses a hand-held spray attachment to rinse and to shampoo. d. Toothbrushing, shaving, makeup can all be done using the pinch of the flexor hinge splint.
		4. Bowel and bladder care	a. Uses bowel routine, inserts suppositories with adapted device.[35] b. May be independent in transfer to toilet or commode chair. A transfer commode seat may be necessary.[51] c. Self-catherization may be an option for the patient[1,10] d. If external drainage for urine is used, the patient learns to apply the drainage system which usually consists of a condom, tubing, and storage bag. e. May need adapted means to clamp and unclamp the tubing and to empty the drainage bag.
		Mobility 1. Locomotion	a. Pushes standard wheelchair with friction material on the rims or by using push mitt.[52] He may need projection knobs on the rims in the beginning.[6] An electric wheelchair would be required if the person had to wheel long distances.[52]
		2. Transfer	a. Uses a transfer board and partial depression or swivel transfer. Assistance may be needed.
		3. Bed mobility	a. Independent in rolling over[52] and sit-

Table 21.1—*Continued*

Last Fully Innervated Level and Key Muscles Added	Movements the Patient Can Do	Achievement	Technique and/or Equipment
C₆ (con't)			ting up using the method described in Chapter 26.
			b. Loops attached to the overhead bed frame may be needed initially to come to sitting position.[52]
		4. Automobile	a. May be able to drive a car adapted with hand controls, and "U" shaped cuff attached to steering wheel.
			b. Will need assistance (human or mechanical) to put the wheelchair into the car.
		Communication 1. Writing	a. Can hold the pencil using the wrist-driven flexor hinge hand splint or a special writing splint which abducts the thumb and holds the pencil in place.[53]
		2. Typing	a. Can put paper into the typewriter.
			b. Uses an electric typewriter with push button return.
			c. May use typing splints that fit over the index fingers only[54] in preference to holding typing sticks with the flexor splint.
		3. Notetaking	a. Can use adapted tape recorder.[55]
			b. Can write short notes as above.
		4. Telephoning	a. Can use a standard phone, dialing with a pencil held in a universal cuff or threaded through the fingers.
		Recreation	a. Can turn radio, TV, etc. on and off.
			b. Can play table games with some adaptation.[56]
			c. Can participate in some w/c sports.
		Vocation	a. Homebound work is most practical.
			b. Cannot use hand tools that require strength.
			c. Electronic office mechines are very well suited to these patients.
			d. Is able to independently relieve pressure while in the wheelchair; therefore is able to work out of the home.
			e. Homemaking: at best can be an assistive homemaker. Can only do some cooking and light cleaning with great expenditure of energy and time. Needs w/c accessible kitchen.
C₇ Triceps Extrinsic finger extensors Flexor carpi radialis	Elbow extension Active finger extension (tenodesis grasp) Wrist flexion	Self-care 1. Feeding 2. Dressing 3. Bathing and grooming 4. Bowel and bladder	Independent Independent with aid of buttonhook. Same as for C₆ but easier. Same as for C₆ but easier.
		Mobility 1. Locomotion 2. Bed mobility 3. Transfers	Wheels standard chair easily. Independent. Independent using depression transfer; does push-ups to relieve ischial pressure.

Table 21.1—*Continued*

Last Fully Innervated Level and Key Muscles Added	Movements the Patient Can Do	Achievement	Technique and/or Equipment
C_7 (con't)		4. Driving	Uses adapted car; may need help getting the wheelchair into the car.
		Communication	Independent without adapted equipment.
		Recreation	Games without adaptation; w/c sports.
		Vocation	Same as for C_6, but easier.
C_8 T_1 Intrinsics including thumb Ulnar wrist flexors and extensors Extrinsic finger and thumb flexors Extrinsic thumb extensor	Full upper extremity control including fine coordination and strong grasp	1. Independent in feeding, dressing, bathing, bowel and bladder care, skin inspection, locomotion	Uses minimal adapted equipment.
		2. Work	Homebound work or work in a building free of architectural barriers. Travel by private car, Handi-Cabs,[35] or accessible public transportation.
		3. Housekeeping	Can do light housekeeping independently, but this is time-consuming. Needs a wheelchair-accessible house.
T_6 Top half of intercostals Long muscles of the back	Increased endurance due to larger respiratory reserve Pectoral girdle stabilized for heavy lifting	1. Independent in all self-care	Will use full braces (including trunk and pelvic bracing) and a standing aid for physiological standing only. Can ambulate with *great* difficulty, on level surface, but is not practical for locomotion.
		2. Work	Can work with tools and do fairly heavy lifting from a sedentary position.
	Better trunk control	3. Sports	Active wheelchair sports (basketball, archery, hunting, etc.).
		4. Housekeeping	Independent but needs help with seasonal cleaning. Needs a wheelchair-accessible house.
T_{12} Full innervations of intercostals Abdominal musculature	Better endurance Better trunk control	1. Independent in self-care, work, sports, housekeeping when architectural barriers do not prevent independence.	
		2. Locomotion	Chooses wheelchair for energy conservation. Ambulates with difficulty using long-leg braces and crutches. Can use ride-on snow plow, grass cutter, etc. if adapted with hand controls.
L_4 Low back muscles Hip flexors Quadriceps	Hip flexion Knee extension	1. Independent in all activities plus ambulation.	Uses canes to prevent deforming effects of gait (recurvatum of knee and lumbar lordosis) which could cause, in time, degenerative arthritis. Uses short-leg braces with dorsiflexion stop. Wheelchair may still be a convenience at work and at home. Bowel and bladder control is not voluntary.

the wrist must be extended, and when the fingers are extended, the wrist must be flexed.[13] In this case, range is done to keep the joint capsules free,[13] not to stretch the extrinsic muscles. If the intrinsic muscles need to be stretched, that is done by flexing the interphalangeal joints with the MP extended. Positioning is important between sessions of range of motion exercise. Any hand splint used should protect the alignment of the fingers, thumb, and wrist for future function or dynamic splinting. If the web space tightens, for example, a flexor hinge hand splint for prehension will not fit properly for a secure palmar pinch. For C_6 patients, who will depend on their tenodesis grasp, some SCI units utilize a hand roll,[6] or a thermoplastic splint, which has a roll to support the fingers in a flexed position. The splint also preserves the width of the webspace and extends over the volar wrist to protect the weak wrist extensors from being stretched (Fig. 21.1).

The patient is taught to compensate visually for lost sensation as a protective measure. Burns, abrasions, and pressure are all potentially dangerous to the insensitive extremities, and the patient must be alerted to avoid situations that could cause these. Some less obvious situations include dragging the body across the sheet during dressing or transfer and sitting too close to a hot radiator.

The strength of remaining musculature is increased within the limitations imposed by the patient's recumbent position and the precaution regarding avoidance of fatigue of very weak muscles. Sling suspensions with springs can be used on the patient's bed to offer active assistive exercise for proximal muscles. These are suspended from an orthopedic frame mounted on the bed. Activities or exercise to increase forearm, wrist, and hand strength should be included if these muscles are innervated. The C_4, C_5 quadriplegic patient can begin controls training for use of his externally powered

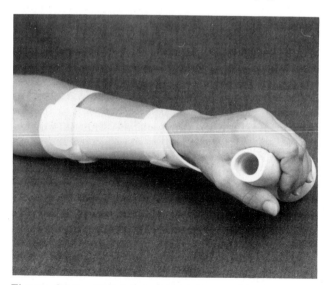

Figure 21.1 Splint to support C_6 quadriplegic's fingers in flexion, to maintain the web space, and to keep the wrist supported in neutral.

hand splint; this would be beneficial because he would then be ready to start use training when permitted to sit up. See Chapter 12 for controls and use training.

Those independent living activities which can be done within the limitations of position and weakness are initiated. For example, the C_7 quadriplegic patient can do self-feeding and some grooming while in the prone position on a turning frame. C_4, C_5 patients will be unable to do any functional activities in this position, however.

Intermediate Treatment Program for SCI Patients

Once cleared to begin sitting, the patient begins a new phase of rehabilitation. SCI patients usually begin sitting at less than 90° upright and for short periods of time. A fully reclining wheelchair is used initially for quadriplegic patients to enable them to gradually develop tolerance for upright sitting. After being recumbent for several weeks, any SCI patient may experience syncope if he is moved to a sitting position too quickly. Fainting may also occur when in a sitting position because blood pools in the lower extremities due to the loss of the muscular pumping action that helps venous return. Elastic stockings and sometimes an abdominal binder are worn to help alleviate this problem. If fainting or syncope occur during treatment, stand behind the locked wheelchair and tip it backward so that the patient's feet are higher than his head.[13] Raise the chair slowly to its upright position when the patient feels better.

Sitting tolerance is evaluated and improved until the patient can sit upright for an average day. Concurrent with development of sitting tolerance, the patient's awareness and sense of responsibility are heightened regarding ischial pressure relief. Each patient must develop the habit of using his chosen method routinely even if it means only taking the responsibility of reminding someone else to do it for him.[13] Prevention of decubiti requires that two factors are attended to. One is a proper cushion (see Chapter 14). But since no cushion provides less than capillary pressure on soft tissue, relief of pressure by change of position must also be done.[1]

Patients with lesions of C_7 and below have the muscle innervation (triceps) to do push-ups, that is, raise the buttocks off the seat by pressing down with the extended arms. A rocking platform has been developed which essentially makes a wheelchair into a rocking chair.[16] It is suggested by the developer that paraplegics can use it as a diversional device which also relieves constant pressure by alternating pressure in a more equitable distribution over the buttocks similar to a rocking bed.[16] Methods by which C_6 patients may independently relieve ischial pressure include the following. A web belt loop can be attached to the wheelchair arm.[17] This loop allows the patient to pull himself upright after laterally flexing the trunk, with the wheelchair armrest removed to relieve the pressure from one buttock. He must then bend to the other side. Alternately, two such web loops can be attached to the uprights of the wheelchair back. With the wheelchair locked, the feet on the floor, and the arms through the loops, the patient bends fully forward for 1 minute, then uses the loops to regain upright sitting.[13]

The C_5 patient will need assistance in relieving pressure. Full reclining with the legs raised to horizontal is a method used by lightweight persons. Another is, with the wheelchair locked, a person sits next to the patient, removes the armrest, and pulls the patient's trunk onto the attending person's lap. This posture is maintained for 1 minute.[13] The occupational therapist should reinforce the instructions of the physical therapist and rehabilitation nurse regarding pushups and other maneuvers that the patient has been taught to use to relieve pressure. Patients who find it difficult to remember to relieve pressure can learn by using an electronic device which gives off an audible signal if pressure is not relieved every period of a preset duration, usually beginning with 10-minute intervals.

The rehabilitation nurse teaches the patient methods of skin inspection and helps him to inspect his skin for reddened areas each night. Hand mirrors are used and are one way that the patient compensates visually for his sensory loss.

Not only ischial decubiti are of concern, but also any other source of decubiti which will result from pressure greater than capillary pressure (25 to 35 mm Hg[7]). Any equipment or splint which leaves a reddened area on the skin that lasts 20 minutes after removal needs modification. Do not pad it; this adds rather than relieves pressure. Instead, relieve the pressure by enlarging the device at that point. The corrected equipment should not be used again until the reddened area disappears.

Therapy to maintain range is continued. This will be necessary as long as the patient cannot move a joint actively through full range. Patients with lower level lesions can learn to range their own limbs daily. Evaluations are done regularly to determine if passive range of motion is being preserved.

Therapy to increase the strength and the endurance of innervated musculature continues. Regular muscle tests and measures of endurance are done to document progress. For the C_{1-4} patient, therapy to increase strength and control of facial and neck muscles is used in preparation for use of mouthstick, microswitches, or sip and puff controls.[4, 6] Mouthsticks are used to turn pages, write, draw, type, and push buttons of electronic devices. Microswitches can be mounted so they are tongue or chin-operated and control electric wheelchairs, environmental control units, and upper limb orthoses. Sip and puff controls are used on electric wheelchairs, environmental control units, and electric typewriters.[18]

As the patient gains adequate strength and endurance, activities of daily living (ADL) are taught using appropriate methods and equipment. A problem-solving approach is used in teaching ADL because the person needs to be able to independently solve new problems as they arise in his life. Results of one study showed that patients continue to improve in self-care and transfer activities between discharge and follow-up 1 year later.[15]

The rehabilitation nurse works with the patient to develop bowel and bladder hygiene and programs for independent care. Most male patients eventually change from indwelling catheters to intermittent catheterization or external drainage. The OTR will be involved in devising ways for the patient to apply the external drainage devices, to clamp the catheter between voidings, to empty the collection bag, or to insert a catheter.

Later Treatment Program for SCI Patients

As the patient progresses through the stages of rehabilitation, discharge, and community reintegration, he assumes increased responsibility for, and control over, his own care.[1] One decision that may present itself to the patient is whether to have reconstructive hand surgery. At the time of maximal return of strength, estimated to be 1 year postinjury,[5, 6, 19] hand reconstructive surgery may increase the function of a C_6, C_7, or C_8 level patient and allow him to discard his orthosis.[20] Restoration is aimed at preserving the hand as a means of human contact as well as its function as a gripping tool.[21] Surgical reconstruction is still not a routine treatment, although it is beginning to be considered more of a feasible alternative to splinting.[20] Zancolli[22] believes that "splinting cannot replace a good surgical result; therefore in the absence of surgical contraindications, the patient should be operated on."

The types of reconstructive work done currently are less complicated, and seemingly more successful, than former types of surgery which included multiple joint arthrodeses.[20] The exact type of surgery is determined by the preserved function in the upper extremity. Any procedure must be reversible because any loss of function that may occur would be a disaster to the patient and would not be acceptable.[21]

Prerequisites to reconstructive hand surgery that some surgeons look for are a realistic attitude toward the outcome; afferent input either visual or preferably two-point discrimination in the thumb, index, and long fingers of 10 to 12 mm[20, 21]; strength of transferable muscles of grades 4 to 5[20, 21] (G to N); and one moveable joint in the thumb.[21] If the only sensory input is by visual observation of the hand, only one hand can be restored successfully.[21]

The surgical procedures performed on C_5, C_6 patients with good results are as follows[20, 21]: Active wrist extension is achieved by use of the brachioradialis. Tenodesis thumb flexor grip (lateral pinch), which is estimated to be the preferred pincer function,[21] is achieved by allowing the flexor pollicis longus (FPL) to bowstring from the metacarpophalangeal joint to increase the moment arm and therefore decrease the power needed; by tenodesing the FPL to the radius; and by stabilizing the interphalangeal joint. Elbow extension is provided to some patients by attaching the posterior half of the deltoid to the triceps aponeurosis and by lengthening the deltoid with free grafts from the toe extensors.

Procedures used for C_7, C_8 patients are aimed at refining hand function, specifically finger flexion and opposition. To provide the finger flexion, the extensor carpi radialis longus, which is synergistic to finger flexion,[19] is transferred if the more centrally located brevis is strong.[19, 20] The brachioradialis is transferred to provide thumb flexion[20] or adduction/opposition of the thumb.[19] The expected average strength of grasp is 5.5 kg and pinch is 3.0 kg.[19]

The occupational therapist provides both preoperative and postoperative treatment.[23] The goals of preop treatment are to educate the patient regarding the surgery, its expected outcomes, and the problems that are to be expected during the convalescent stage.[23] The major problem during that time is the inability to independently relieve ischial pressure, since the operated hand is casted or too fragile yet to withstand the stresses patients put on their hands during push-ups or other pressure-relieving maneuvers. The patient is taught alternate pressure-relief techniques, or if that is not within the patient's capabilities, he is helped to work out a plan for assistance in this crucial function during the 3 to 6 weeks of immobilization.[19-23] Postop treatment begins when the cast is removed. A half shell is still used to protect against stretching and rupture of the healing tissue. The half shell is removed for treatment twice daily. If joint fusion has been done, e.g., carpometacarpal joint of the thumb, a splint is made to prevent movement but to allow some use of the part. Other splints may be needed, depending on the type of surgery done and healing requirements; these will be specifically ordered by the hand surgeon.

Goals of post-op therapy are to increase range of motion, strength, endurance, coordination, and ADL independence.[23] Therapy for range, strength, and endurance during the 1st month involves only active range of motion exercises. Aggressive passive range of motion and resistive exercise are avoided for fear the tendon(s) would be stretched or detached as a result. Evaluation of strength of pinch and grasp is made only after healing is complete. EMG biofeedback is beneficial in helping the patient learn to use the transferred tendon in its new function (see Chapter 11). Coordination is achieved through use of unresistive hand activities. Speed is measured as an index of improved coordination. The Physical Capacities Evaluation of Hand Skill, developed by the Occupational Therapy Department of Texas Rehabilitation Hospital, allows evaluation of hand function pre- and postsurgery as well as pre- and postorthosis.[24] It provides a graphic comparison of hand function to determine which functions are enhanced and which are decreased.[24] Activities of daily living are reevaluated with the purpose of discarding adaptive devices if possible as a result of improved function following surgery.[23] Also, the need to teach new techniques that will protect the transferred tendon is also evaluated. One such new technique is the use of the hands during transfer: normally

quadriplegics transfer with the fingers and wrist in full extension, but this would put too much stress on the newly arranged tendons; therefore, the patients are taught to transfer with the hand fisted or with the fingers extending over the surface's edge.[23]

As the patient nears his maximal strength, endurance, and self-care ability, more specific planning must be done with him and his family regarding vocational and recreational pursuits that he plans to follow postdischarge. It may be necessary to explore new avenues of vocation and recreation due to the extent of disability. The occupational therapy clinic becomes a valuable laboratory for testing skills within a secure environment (see Chapters 28 and 30).

A community reintegration program that includes trips into the community to practice skills needed as a wheelchair-bound citizen are made in the beginning with the occupational or physical therapist to help work out the problems as they arise (see Chapter 29). As the patient resumes social interactions, personal grooming may become an important issue. Clothing designed for wheelchair-bound persons is available, but the need remains only partially addressed.[25] One example of adaptive clothing is men's suits which are tailored so that the trousers do not ride up even though the person is sitting and the jacket fits neatly without bunching into the chair seat.

Shortly before the time of discharge, the home is visited by the occupational and physical therapists to evaluate the wheelchair accessibility and to help the patient and his family determine what changes need to be made to facilitate independence and to preserve the life-style of the patient as much as possible. Weekend visits by the patient to his home during the ongoing rehabilitation process are valuable in pointing out accessibility problems (see Chapter 29) prior to the home evaluation. An alternative to discharge to home or to nursing home is the Independent Living Centers which are developing in larger cities as a result of congressional concern and governmental funding. The specific services offered differ between centers and therefore may or may not offer the full services needed by a particular spinal cord-injured person. The patient can be directed to the center to negotiate his discharge plans based on his needs and the services offered. The C_{1-4} quadriplegic will require an attendant for life to take care of all dressing, bathing, grooming, transfer, toilet needs, respiratory equipment maintenance, out of the home locomotion, and possibly feeding or set up of complicated orthotic equipment. These patients will probably be best served in a protective environment, if not living with full-time attendant care.

To prevent deterioration of physical fitness gained in rehabilitation, continued involvement in activities (wheelchair ambulation uphill, crutch ambulation), sports (basketball), and fitness training has been recommended following a study of six paraplegics.[26] Using heart rate monitors to record heart rate during a 48-hour period, it was found that training in addition to normal ADL was needed to maintain circulatory and physical fitness of these rehabilitated paraplegics. The ADL activities did not tax the heart rate reserve enough for a training effect to occur.[26] Wheelchair sports and recreational opportunities are improving. It would be beneficial if the patient were introduced to these as part of his rehabilitation process since they not only add significantly to the quality of life, but also to maintenance of physical fitness.

Before discharge, the patient should be put in touch with the local chapter of the National Spinal Cord Injury Foundation. He should also be made aware of helpful publications, such as *Accent on Living*, a quarterly periodical which offers realistic and practical solutions to the problems encountered in daily life by patients with spinal cord injuries.

EFFECTIVENESS STUDIES

There is currently a study underway to collect and update data from thousands of SCI persons in the U.S.A. and abroad to answer questions related to the preinjury characteristics of the patient, the events of the injury, the type, quality, and cost of acute and rehabilitative care, the outcome in terms of quality and length of life, and the productivity of the rehabilitated person.[2] A similar study was completed in 1966.[27] Unitary focus studies have also been done to determine the continued satisfaction with certain orthoses[28-31] and whether achieved levels of independence continued postdischarge.[32-33] Whether the patient uses orthoses postdischarge seems to depend on the value of the function added relative to the energy required to do the function, the trouble in putting on the equipment, and the functions lost by use of the equipment. Reliability, cosmesis, and thorough training are also important factors in the patient's acceptance of the orthosis.

One follow-up study of 35 quadriplegic persons (20 with radial wrist extensors and 15 without), 1 to 4 years postdischarge, indicated that level of independence in self-care was generally maintained posthospitalization, especially in the areas of feeding and desk skills.[32] Regression in grooming, bathing, toileting, and lower extremity dressing seemed to be secondary to a reordering of time and energy priorities.[32] The equipment issued at the time of discharge and still in use were splints, universal cuffs, push cuffs (to propel wheelchair), and quad clamp (for catheter). Other equipment, including mobile arm supports, lapboard, button hooks, reachers, and mouthsticks had been abandoned.[32] More study is needed concerning the nature and extent of rehabilitation services that should be offered to be both fiscally responsible and to afford the person with this devastating injury all the opportunity he can benefit from to regain a quality life.

References

1. King, R. B., and Dudas, S. Rehabilitation of the patient with a spinal cord injury. *Nurs. Clin. North Am.*, 15(2): 225-243, 1980.
2. Young, J. S. The United States national spinal cord injury data research centre. *Paraplegia*, 14: 81-86, 1976.
3. Tator, C. H. Spinal cord cooling and irrigation for treatment of acute cord injury. In *Neural Trauma*, edited by A. J. Popp *et al.* New York: Raven Press, 1979.
4. Van Steen, H. Treatment of a patient with a complete C_1 quadriplegia. *Phys. Ther.*, 55(1): 35-38, 1975.
5. Panchal, P. D. Rehabilitation of the patient with spinal cord injury. *Curr. Probl. Surg.*, 17(4): 254-262, 1980.
6. Rozin, R. The upper limb in spinal cord injury. *Prog. Surg.*, 16: 207-220, 1978.
7. Reswick, M. B., and Simoes, N. Application of engineering principles in management of spinal cord injured patients. *Clin. Orthop.*, 112: 4-129, 1975.
8. Long, C. Congenital and traumatic lesions of the spinal cord. In *Handbook of Physical Medicine and Rehabilitation*, 2nd ed., edited by F. H. Krusen, F. J. Kottke, and P. M. Ellwood. Philadelphia: W. B. Saunders, 1971.
9. Donovan, W. H., Macri, D., and Clowers, D. E. A finger device for obtaining satisfactory voiding in spinal cord-injured patients. *Am. J. Occup. Ther.*, 31(2): 107-108, 1977.
10. Dailey, J., and Michael, R. Nonsterile self-intermittent catherization for male quadriplegic patients. *Am. J. Occup. Ther.*, 31(2): 86-89, 1977.
11. Mooney, T., Cole, T., and Chilgren, R. *Sexual Options for Paraplegics and Quadriplegics.* Boston: Little, Brown, 1975.
12. Gerhart, K. A. Increasing sensory and motor stimulation for the patient with quadriplegia. *Phys. Ther.*, 59(12): 1518-1520, 1979.
13. McKenzie, M. W., and Buck, G. L. Combined motor and peripheral sensory insufficiency. III. Management of spinal cord injury. *Phys. Ther.*, 58(3): 294-303, 1978.
14. Taylor, D. P. Treatment goals for quadriplegic patients. *Am. J. Occup. Ther.*, 28(1): 22-29, 1974.
15. Bracken, M. B., Hildreth, N., Freeman, D. H., and Webb, S. B. Relationship between neurological and functional status after acute spinal cord injury: An epidemiological study. *J. Chronic. Dis.*, 33: 115-125, 1980.
16. Jackson, F. E., Wojcik, V. F., and Wojcik, W. R. Rocking platform for paraplegic patients in wheelchairs. *J. Neurosurg.*, 42(3): 358-359, 1975.
17. Agrawal, B. K., Arnold, T., and Vicich, J. Web-belt loop for relief of pressure on buttocks. *Arch. Phys. Med. Rehabil.*, 59(7): 346-347, 1978.
18. Prentke-Romich Company. *Electronic Aids for the Severely Handicapped.* Shreve, Ohio, 1982.
19. House, J. H., Gwathmey, F. W., and Lundsgaard, D. K. Restoration of strong grasp and lateral pinch in tetraplegia due to cervical cord injury. *J. Hand Surg.*, 1(2): 152-159, 1976.
20. Hentz, V. R., and Keoshian, L. A. Changing perspectives in surgical hand rehabilitation in quadriplegic patients. *Plast. Reconstr. Surg.*, 64(4): 509-515, 1979.
21. Moberg, E. Surgical treatment for absent single-hand grip and elbow extension in quadriplegia. *J. Bone Joint Surg.*, 57-A(2): 196-206, 1975.
22. Zancolli, E. Surgery for the quadriplegic hand with active, strong wrist extension preserved: A study of 97 cases. *Clin. Orthop.*, 112: 101-113, 1975.
23. Mathiowetz, V., and Brambilla, M. Tendon transfers for quadriplegics: Implications for therapy. *American Occupational Therapy Association Physical Disabilities Specialty Section Newsletter*, 2(3): 3, 1979.
24. Bell, E., Jurek, K., and Wilson, T. Hand skill measurement: A gauge for treatment. *Am. J. Occup. Ther.*, 30(2): 80-86, 1976.
25. Nessley, E., and King, R. R. Textile fabric and clothing needs of paraplegic and quadriplegic persons confined to wheelchairs. *J. Rehabil.*, 46(2): 63-67, 1980.
26. Hjeltnes, N., and Vokac, Z. Circulatory strain in everyday life of paraplegics. *Scand. J. Rehabil. Med.*, 11: 67-73, 1979.
27. Kaplan, L., Pwell, B. R., Brynbaum, B. B. and Rusk, H. A. Comprehensive Follow-up Study of Spinal Cord Dysfunction and its Resultant Disabilities. Institute of Rehabilitation Medicine, New York University Medical Center, 1966.
28. Knox, C. C., Engel, W. H., and Siebens, A. A. Results of a survey on the use of a wrist-driven splint for prehension. *Am. J. Occup. Ther.*, 25(2): 109-111, 1971.
29. Allen, V. R. Follow-up study of wrist-driven flexor-hinge splint

use. *Am. J. Occup. Ther.*, *25*(8): 420–422, 1971.

30. Trombly, C. A. Myoelectric control of orthotic devices for the severely paralyzed. *Am. J. Occup. Ther.*, *22*(5): 385–389, 1968.

31. Nichols, P. J., Peach, S. L., Haworth, R. J., and Ennis, J. The value of flexor hinge hand splints. *Prosthet. Orthot. Int.*, *2*(2): 86–94, 1978.

32. Rogers, J. C., and Figone, J. J. Traumatic quadriplegia: Follow-up study of self-care skills. *Arch. Phys. Med. Rehabil.*, *61*(7): 316–321, 1980.

33. Runge, M. Follow-up study of self-care activities in traumatic spinal cord injury quadriplegics and quadriparetics. *Am. J. Occup. Ther.*, *20*(5): 241–249, 1966.

34. Possum Controls Ltd., POB 7033, Van Nuys, Calif. 95125.

35. Lowman, E., and Klinger, J. *Aids to Independent Living.* New York: McGraw Hill, Blakiston Division, 1969.

36. Parish, J. G. A study of the use of electronic environmental control systems by severely paralysed patients. *Paraplegia, 17*: 147–156, 1979–80.

37. Long, C., and Masciarelli, V. An electrophysiologic splint for the hand. *Arch. Phys. Med. Rehabil.*, *44*(9): 499–503, 1963.

38. Kelly, S., and Hartman, H. Switch control concepts in a myoelectric control system. *Am. J. Occup. Ther.*, *25*(3): 164–169, 1971.

39. Trombly, C. A. Principles of operant conditioning related to orthotic training of quadriplegic patients. *Am. J. Occup. Ther.*, *20*(5): 217–220, 1966.

40. Barber, L., and Nickel, V. Carbon dioxide-powered arm and hand devices. *Am. J. Occup. Ther.*, *23*(3): 215–225, 1969.

41. McKenzie, M. The ratchet hand-splint. *Am. J. Occup. Ther.*, *27*(8): 477–479, 1973.

42. Schmeisser, G., and Seamone, W. An assistive equipment controller for quadriplegics. *Johns Hopkins Med. J.*, *145*: 84–88, 1979.

43. McKenzie, M., and Rogers, J. Use of trunk supports for severely paralyzed people. *Am. J. Occup. Ther.*, *27*(3): 147–148, 1973.

44. Schmeisser, G., and Seamone, W. Low cost assistive device systems for a high spinal cord-injured person in the home environment—a technical note. *Bull. Prosthet. Res.*, *16*(2): 212–223, 1979.

45. Sell, G. H., Stratford, C. D., Zimmerman, M. E., Youdin, M. and Milner, D. Environmental and typewriter control systems for high-level quadriplegic patients: Evaluation and prescription. *Arch. Phys. Med. Rehabil.*, *60*(6): 246–251, 1979.

46. Berard, E., Bourret, J., Girard, R., Minaire, P., and Ratinet, G. The technical aids of tetraplegic patients. *Paraplegia, 17*: 157–160, 1979–80.

47. Cloran, A. J., Lotz, J. W., Campbell, H. D., and Wiechers, D. O. Oral telescoping orthosis: An aid to functional rehabilitation of quadriplegic patients. *J.A.D.A.*, *100*(6): 876–879, 1980.

48. Smith, B. Adapted bed controls and the quadriplegic patient. *Am. J. Occup. Ther.*, *32*(5): 322, 1978.

49. Bacon, G., and Olszewski, E. Sequential advancing flexion retention attachment. *Am. J. Occup. Ther.*, *32*(9): 577–585, 1978.

50. Ford, J. R., and Duckworth, B. *Physical Management for the Quadriplegic Patient.* Philadelphia: F. A. Davis, 1974.

51. Bortner, E. The transfer commode seat. *Am. J. Occup. Ther.*, *33*(10): 655, 1979.

52. McGee, M., and Hertling, D. Equipment and transfer techniques used by C_6 quadriplegic patients. *Phys. Ther.*, *57*(12): 1372–1375, 1977.

53. Feinberg, J. Writing device for the quadriplegic patient. *Am. J. Occup. Ther.*, *29*(2): 101, 1975.

54. Craver, P. N. Typing splints for the quadriplegic patient. *Am. J. Occup. Ther.*, *29*(9): 551, 1975.

55. Grahn, E. Tape recorder modifications for use by quadriplegics. *Am. J. Occup. Ther.*, *24*(5): 360–361, 1970.

56. Slatter, E. R., and Gibb, M. M. A table tennis glove for tetraplegics. *Paraplegia, 17*(2): 259–261, 1979.

Supplementary Reading

Billings, C. V. Emotional first aid. *Am. J. Nurs.*, *80*(11): 2006–2009, 1980.

Brereton, W. D., *et al.* Power reclined wheelchair back. *J. Med. Eng. Technol.*, *2*(6): 315–316, 1978.

Burnham, B. A., and Werner, G. The high-level tetraplegic: Psychological survival and adjustment. *Paraplegia, 16*: 184–192, 1978–79.

Carlson, C. E. Conceptual style and life satisfaction following spinal cord injury. *Arch. Phys. Med. Rehabil.*, *60*(8): 346–352, 1979.

Crewe, N. M., Athelstan, G. T., and Krumberger, J. Spinal cord injury: A comparison of preinjury and postinjury marriages. *Arch. Phys. Med. Rehabil.*, *60*(6): 252–256, 1979.

Dingemans, L. M., and Hawn, J. M. Mobility and equipment for the ventilator dependent tetraplegic. *Paraplegia, 16*(2): 175–183, 1978.

Kofkin, J., Tobing, M., and Dellon, A. L. Dynamic elbow splint following tendon transfer to restore triceps function. *Am. J. Occup. Ther.*, *34*(10): 680–681, 1980.

Osborne, P., and Carne, N. Learning from experience. *Nurs. Mirror, 146*(8): 26–29, 1978.

Rogers, J. C., and Figone, J. J. Psychosocial parameters in treating the person with quadriplegia. *Am. J. Occup. Ther.*, *33*(7): 432–439, 1979.

Rogers, J. C. and Figone, J. J. The avocational pursuits of rehabilitants with traumatic quadriplegia. *Am. J. Occup. Ther.*, *32*(8): 571–576, 1978.

Romano, M. D., and Lassiter, R. E. Sexual counseling with the spinal-cord injured. *Arch. Phys. Med. Rehabil.*, *53*(12): 568–572, 1972.

Sigman, J. M. Sexual functioning and the physically disabled adult. *Am. J. Occup. Ther.*, *31*(2): 81–85, 1977.

Sinha, A. K., and Schaffer, F. J. External urinary collecting device for the incontinent male. *Am. J. Occup. Ther.*, *32*(4): 238–239, 1978.

Williams, G. O., *et al.* Rehabilitation of a young quadriplegic: A team approach. *J. Family Pract.*, *10*(3): 517–523, 1980.

Williams, L., and Garetz, D. Independent leg bag emptying technique for cervical five quadriplegic clients. *Am. J. Occup. Ther.*, *35*(1): 40–42, 1981.

chapter
22

Burns

Lillian Hoyle Parent, M.A., OTR

An estimated 2 million Americans have serious burns annually and from 6 to 7% require hospitalization.[1] Significant advances in the care of burned patients have improved survival rates while decreasing the length of hospitalization for all types of burns.[2] These advances include improved medications to reduce or prevent burn wound infection, improvement in many life support measures, the use of biological dressings for immediate care in extensive burns, and vigorous rehabilitation measures.[3] However, Larson[4] emphasizes that one can no longer be satisfied with just survival in the treatment of burns. The goal is to help patients reach their maximum rehabilitation status.[4]

A burned patient has an acute illness of weeks to months and requires a therapeutic regimen that may extend for a year or longer beyond hospitalization.[1] Treatment for burns can occur in any emergency room, hospital, or doctor's office. However, for large, deep burns, hospitalization is essential. Some hospitals have burn programs where there is a method of consistent management for burn patients. This includes special training for some staff and an available doctor who has special skills in the treatment of burns. A burn unit within a hospital refers to beds set aside for the exclusive use of burn patients to be treated by trained personnel. A burn center, on the other hand, in addition to the previous requirements, also promotes education and research.[5]

A burn wound is a tissue response to heat. The source of heat may be thermal, chemical, or electrical. The resultant problems and their resolution depend on the depth and extent of the trauma. Flame burns, more common in the adult, cause the most severe burns because of the extent and depth of the burn. Scald burns from hot liquid, the common burn injury among the very young, may be superficial or deep in a limited area. Explosive flash burns tend to be superficial and limited to exposed body parts.[6, 7] Chemical burns are always third degree and may penetrate deeply into tissues until the substance is washed away, leaving a full thickness burn.[3] Electrical burns have special characteristics.

Electrical burns are a small proportion of all burns, but because of their nature, patients with these burns have special problems.[8] While the extent of thermal burns can be identified and are predictable, electrical burns usually have an entry and exit point, and those areas have a dessicated grayish yellow appearance outlined by acute erythema. The skin between the entry and exit points may appear normal, but the passage of current beneath the skin through muscle and nerve, between those points, may have damaged those structures and the vascular supply, and the extent of damage cannot be estimated early. The division between necrotic and surviving tissue is slow to develop and is highly susceptible to infection.[9] Edema may also compromise vascular supply, which affects muscle and nerve, resulting in peripheral nerve injury. Treatment can include fasciotomy to relieve pressure and debridement to remove necrotic tissue. The goal is to turn a base of tissue loss into clean wounds for early grafting.[10] The sequelae of electrical burns are progressive muscular fibrosis, contracture, and loss of function. Amputation is often necessary to save life by preventing the spread of infection or gangrene after an electrical burn. The patients often require intensive rehabilitation procedures.[8] Many of the procedures applied to the treatment of thermal burns can be applied to the patient with electrical burns.

SYMPTOMS

The extent of a burn is estimated by the rule of nines. In adults the percentage of total body surface area with second and third degree burns is calculated by the formula: head 7% and neck 2% equal 9%; each upper extremity is 9%, for a total of 18%; anterior trunk is 2 times 9%, which equals 18%; posterior trunk at 13% plus buttocks at 5% equals 18%; each lower extremity is 18%, equaling 36%, and the genitalia are 1%, for a total of 100%. The extent of an individual's burn is then given in a percentage figure assessment.[6] The amount of total body surface burn is a factor for predicting outcome of a burn injury. Major burns are those that involve 25 to 30% of total body surface with deep second and third degree burns. Massive burns of more than 60% of body surface have a very high mortality,[11] and very few people survive a burn of 80% or more. Patients over age 60 with large burns are at greatest risk for survival.[2]

The depth of trauma is based on the intensity of heat on the skin surface. A first degree burn involves only the superficial outer layer of the epidermis and is capable of regeneration. When this dead layer 'peels' off, as in sunburn, a new epithelial layer has regenerated from the epidermis. This is a painful burn. A second degree burn is a partial thickness burn, characterized by redness and blisters. It involves epidermis and some of the underlying dermis. The epithelial structures of sebaceous and sweat glands and hair follicles, because they are deep in the skin, survive and are a source for regeneration of new epidermis to reepithelize the wound.[6] These are painful burns.[12] Third degree burns are full thickness burns characterized by a hard dry surface. They produce trauma to the entire skin thickness and the deep epithelial structures. There is no ability for spontaneous healing or regeneration of the epithelium.[6] In third degree burns healing is slow and produces fibrosis and heavy scar. New skin, in the form of a graft, is placed on the area to promote healing. Third degree burn surfaces are inelastic and anesthetic because the sensory nerve endings are destroyed.[7]

Comprehensive care of a burn patient requires the special skills and knowledge of a multidisciplinary team effort, and the coordination of responsibilities of all personnel for optimum care. Many body systems are involved in a severe burn resulting in physical and psychosocial consequences. The burn care team includes several medical and surgical specialists, nurses, physical and occupational therapists, a nutritionist, a psychologist, and a social worker.[13] Emergency room care institutes fluid resuscitation to correct fluid, electrolyte, and protein deficits. It is an attempt to maintain fluid balance without overloading the circulation which can result in excess edema formation. Medical complications of a burn may involve the respiratory tract from inhalation injury, cardiovascular and renal function, and acute gastroduodenal ulceration from stress. The ulcers can be prevented by early prophylactic use of medication and adequate nutrition to compensate for the hypermetabolic state. The burn patient is hypermetabolic and requires a high calorie diet until skin coverage is complete.[11]

A burn injury destroys protective skin covering, leaving an open wound with the tissue becoming a medium for bacteria growth and ultimate sepsis which can cause death. Until the burn wound is closed through healing or grafting, it is essential to prevent bacterial contamination of the wound. Prevention of infection is a prime goal in burn units. There may be special arrangements for air flow out of the area or elaborate bubble reverse isolation systems.[14, 15] Reverse isolation or protective isolation is used for burn patients to prevent them from an increased risk of infection. Each institution may have its own procedures. However, general guidelines are to have the patient in a private room, or if the patient is on a ward the bed is surrounded by screens or other devices. Handwashing is done before working with a patient. Those entering the area of a burn patient may be required to put on a special gown and mask. These are removed after working with the patient and placed in an appropriate receptacle. Hands are washed again. Disposable equipment is used wherever possible, and other equipment, including splints and braces, is sterilized according to institutional standards.[16, 17]

Infection in a deep second degree burn can convert the wound to a third degree burn. Topical antibacterial creams and ointments are used as dressings to prevent infection, soften eschar (the coagulated burn slough), and permit movement before grafting. The primary substances are sulfamylon and silver sulfadiazine, the latter having patient preference because it is not as painful when applied. The antibacterial ointments require minimal or no dressings and permit the patient to move unless restricted by splints.[17] Biological dressings are used as temporary skin cover to reduce infection and pain, and to promote development of the wound site for autografting.[11] Biological dressings may be allografts or homografts, skin from the same species, or xenografts, skin from another species, or amnion, the fetal membrane. Only the patient's own skin can be used for autografting because the others do not adhere to the patient.[18]

Deep burns result in much edema that may invade adjacent tissues, leading to ischemic necrosis and contracture.[7] Edema begins to form within 6 hours post-injury in third degree burns and may result in capillary damage. The elasticity of the skin is lost, and the resultant eschar does not stretch, which may result in pressure great enough to cause venous occlusion or ischemia in the trunk or extremities.[12, 19] The pressure is relieved by escharotomy, an incision into burned skin and subcutaneous tissue which is anesthetic because the sensory nerve endings have been destroyed. Although escharotomy is not painful in such a deep burn, the procedure must be explained to the patient before it is done.[12]

THERAPY RELATED TO STAGES OF CARE

Burn care is divided into stages or time intervals. The emergent stage is from 0 to 72 hours postburn.[12] The patient is in emotional shock with emotional lability, and his adaptation in this stage may be expressed by withdrawal or protest behaviors.[15] Between 48 and 72 hours, the patient begins to recover from the physiologic shock and initial emotional shock.[12] Patients with extensive injuries of 50% or more of body surface area involved may not be able to cooperate actively with the therapist's treatment program during the early phases.[20] Severely burned patients, aggravated by the stress reaction, may exhibit a variety of emotional problems. There is pain, shock, and fear. A patient's response may be excitation, delerium, or hallucinations. Pain can be the focus of a patient's behavior. A stable well-adjusted person may accept the treatment routine better than a frightened immature person. When prolonged treatment is necessary, the continuing stress may lead to depression or hostility toward the personnel responsible for their care.[21]

A burn patient's response to personnel may create hostility and resentment among the staff. Daily contact with emotionally distraught, disfigured, and critically ill patients may provoke strong emotions and anxiety in professionals working with them.[22] During these times the therapist needs to accept the patient without attaching judgmental labels to behavior. It is situational and the patient's response to trauma.[12, 22] Often, burn team members work through their negative feelings and depression with the support of more experienced personnel.[21] The difficult patient behaviors are often reduced when physiological functions are stabilized,[23] and improvements in emotional stress are noted when most of the burn wounds have healed or have been covered with grafts.[15]

The acute phase is from 72 hours until skin coverage is complete which may be weeks or months. Treatments that cause the most pain begin during the early phases of this period. In order to prevent infection that can lead to sepsis and death and to prepare the burn wound for eventual grafting, there are dressing changes, hydrotherapy to debride the exchar, and some surgical debridement.[12] In an acute burn it takes from 1 to 2 weeks to remove eschar from a deep burn to prepare it for grafting.[7] All of these procedures are difficult for the patient, and this may be a time when the most obnoxious behavior is manifested.[15] During this phase, as his condition permits, the patient should begin to participate in activities of daily living such as eating and any daily hygiene possible using adapted methods or equipment. Early involvement of the patient is important to avoid progressive dependency and passivity and to promote self-esteem, self-reliance, and a more positive feeling for the future.[19]

Prevention of deformity is a prime consideration after the patient has become medically stable. Most alterations in the musculoskeletal system occur after the acute injury and are not the direct result of it.[24] It is important to anticipate potential impairment and to use measures to prevent and to reduce the time of hospitalization and rehabilitation.[25] Typical deformities occur in joints, and a specific positioning program is used to minimize or to prevent the deformities from occurring. All positioning, to be effective, must be enforced from the first day of the burn.[26]

Some surgeons rely on skeletal traction for positioning circumferential burns of the extremities, either early in treatment or at the time of grafting. Other methods to position include the use of splints and braces and other devices to maintain the burn patient in optimum position. Early prophylactic use of splints and braces on or around burned areas, particularly if joints are under a burn, can decrease the development of secondary deformities.[26] During the first 10 days postburn, splints and braces may require many revisions not only because of edema but also to obtain range of motion and the desired antideformity position. All splints should be checked frequently to make certain there is no pressure from the splint or straps that could compromise the vascular system.[19]

A specific positioning program is used with a burn patient to prevent deformity and contracture of joints under burns. A body segment is positioned opposite to the anticipated deformity. The prone and supine positions are similar, except that in prone positions the forehead should be supported on a foam rubber contoured piece to maintain an airway and to keep the neck in slight extension.[27]

The deforming position for a burn on the face, neck, or chest is neck flexion. The eyelids and mouth structures, as well as the neck and shoulders, can be deformed by neck flexion contractures. The antideformity position places the neck in slight extension off the edge of a short mattress,[26] or a thermoplastic neck conformer is used[23] (Fig. 22.1). A patient allowed to sit up will require a conformer for the upright as well as the supine position for 24-hour wear. The conformer is removed for meals and regular cleaning daily.[17]

The deforming position for the shoulder or axilla with burn wounds is the anatomical position with the arms at the side in adduction. The antideformity position places the shoulder in 90° of abduction with shoulder girdle retraction and neutral rotation.[28] The shoulder should be placed in slight flexion because positioning the shoulder in marked extension can result in a brachial palsy or anterior shoulder dislocation.[28, 29] If the axilla is also burned, the arm is placed in abduction to 90° with slight shoulder flexion. The

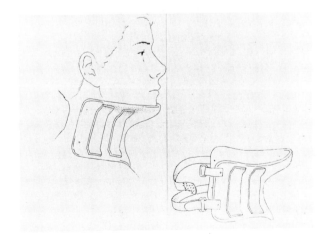

Figure 22.1 Conformer neck splint made of Orthoplast. (Reproduced with permission from Shirley Baty, illustrator, and Emergency Medicine.[41])

position can be maintained by skeletal traction, or axillary conformers (Fig. 22.2) when the patient is supine.[28–30] In the upright position, semicircular sponges are placed in the axilla and secured with an elastic figure-of-eight wrap[28] (Fig. 22.3). Edema in the upper extremity is treated by elevation, either by

skeletal traction or positioning with the elbow above the shoulder.[31]

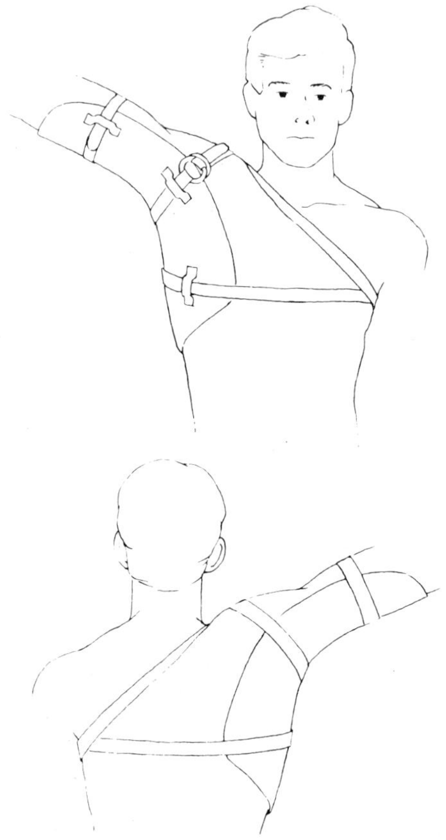

The deforming position for the elbow is elbow flexion, and the antideformity position is for the elbow to be positioned in complete extension with the forearm in midposition. Extension contractures are rare. To maintain the elbow in extension, a simple three-point extension brace[32] is used (Fig. 22.4).

The position of deformity for the burned hand is wrist flexion, MP hyperextension, and PIP flexion with the thumb adducted and the palmar arch flattened.[20, 24] This is the "intrinsic-minus hand."[33] The deformity can occur within a day or two if the burned hand is allowed to rest unsplinted on a bed.[26]

People experiencing thermal injuries tend to put their hands to the face protectively, which results in burns to the dorsum of the hand and fingers. A burn on the dorsum of the hand results in loss of elasticity of the skin and leads to the intrinsic minus hand position.[34] Positioning for deep acute burns on the dorsum of the hand places the wrist in neutral with the MPs flexed and IPs extended. Only slight flexion is used to maintain capsular ligaments in the elongated position to prevent shortening and later restriction of movement. Ninety degrees of MP flexion can stretch capsular structures as well as cause dorsal ischemia over injured tendons, fascia, and skin. As the wound is more defined, positioning can be modified.[7] Early treatment using a resting splint (Fig. 12.5) can reduce the development of anatomic deformities if the wrist and hand are placed in a position to avoid secondary contractures and to maintain tendon balance through the course of treatment.[20]

General articles on the treatment of the burned hand indicate that the hand should be splinted in the position of function. The position of function described by Bunnell[35] is the midrange of all joints. It places the wrist in dorsiflexion, with all fingers slightly flexed and the thumb in partial opposition. Certainly, this is a position from which all movements can begin. However, maintaining this as a static position has not been found functional for the ultimate recovery of the burned hand.[27, 31] Many authors describe a specific antideformity position for the burned hand. There is general agreement that the wrist should be in dorsiflexion, although the degrees range from maximum,[36] to moderate,[20] to 10°[37] or neutral.[24, 28, 31] Also, the MPs

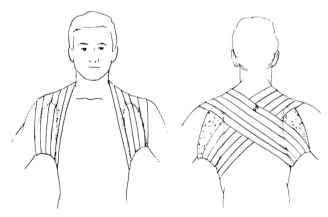

Figure 22.2 Axillary conformer splint made of Orthoplast. (Reproduced with permission from Shirley Baty, illustrator, and *Emergency Medicine*.[41])

Figure 22.3 Semicircular foam pads held in place at axilla by figure of eight Ace bandage. (Reproduced with permission from Shirley Baty, illustrator, and *Emergency Medicine*.[41])

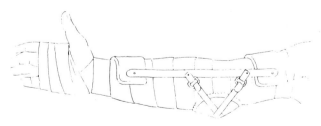

Figure 22.4 Three-point extension splint. (Reproduced with permission from Shirley Baty, illustrator, and *Emergency Medicine*.[41])

are placed in flexion and the degrees vary from 90°[24] and acute[37] to 15 to 20°.[32] It is easier to position the thumb if the MPs are not flexed to 90°.

A rationale for splinting in MP flexion and IP extension is proposed by James, who described the MP ligaments as being slack when the MP joint is extended, and if positioned in MP extension, the ligaments can become tight and unyielding. The PIP and DIP joints have slack ligaments when placed in flexion. The volar plates are also involved. To correct these deforming forces, the MP joints are placed in flexion and the IPs in extension where all lateral ligaments are taut and less likely to contract.[38]

Most authors place the fingers (PIP and DIP joints) in complete extension. The exceptions are those who allow slight flexion,[36] and McCormack,[34] who allows 30 to 60° of PIP and DIP flexion because he has noted that total immobilization in extension promotes stiffness. However, the burned hand should be in and out of splints for active motion several times per day.

There is general agreement that the thumb should be placed in abduction to preserve the thumb web space, because contracture of the thumb web space is difficult to correct. The position given is thumb abduction with MP and IP joints extended[37] or slight flexion.[28, 34]

The volar surface of the hand is not involved in burns as often as the dorsum[20] because direct contact of long duration is necessary to cause a full thickness burn in the palm.[34] Volar injuries, caused by hot metal or electricity, are often full thickness burns. Flexion deformities to all joints are most likely to occur and depend on the location of the injury. Flexion/adduction deformity of the thumb occurs from burns of the palmar thenar area. Volar surface burn deformities cannot be prevented by active motion.[20] These deformities are more easily corrected surgically than dorsal injuries because joint capsules and other structures are less likely to be involved. A dorsal splint is used to position the wrist in extension and the fingers in extension and abduction, and to maintain the thumb web space.[33] Hooks may be attached to fingernails to secure the fingers in extension with rubber bands.[39]

Lateral burns of the trunk may result in a hemithoracic scar resulting in contracture toward scoliosis. There is convexity of the curve to the contralateral side. The trunk should be positioned in a straight line to prevent incipient contracture toward a scoliosis-like position.[26]

The position of deformity for the hip is hip flexion and adduction. Once established, this deformity will require surgical correction. Hips are placed in extension, and 15 to 20° of hip abduction to prevent hip flexion contracture.[26] A severe burn over the anterior hip joint requires great vigilance to keep the hips and legs in position. A three-point extension splint on the leg will discourage hip flexion in the supine position.[28]

A burned knee, as does the elbow, tends to develop a flexion deformity, especially when the popliteal area is involved. The antideformity position is knee extension which is maintained in a 3-point extension splint.

To avoid a popliteal palsy, the knee with a popliteal burn should not be hyperextended.[24]

The deforming position for the ankle is plantar flexion. The ankle should be maintained in neutral to allow for later weight-bearing. A footboard or a posterior splint can be used to support the foot. When the patient is in the prone position, if a short mattress is used, the feet can be placed over the edge to maintain the ankle joint in a neutral position.[32, 40]

OCCUPATIONAL THERAPY EVALUATION AND TREATMENT

From the moment a burn patient enters an emergency room the occupational therapy goals for physical restoration are established for any body segment with a burn. The goals are to prevent contracture and deformity, to maintain range of motion, muscle function, and strength. The goals are accomplished by a program of positioning and splinting to prevent contractures of joints and active range of motion to maintain strength. After grafting is completed, elastic bandages or Anti/Burnscar garments, combined with splints, are used to prevent contracture and the proliferation of hypertrophic scar when the burn wounds are closed. The long-range goal is to return the patient to pretrauma functional ability.[19, 33]

The immediate care of a burn patient concentrates on the shock and physiological complications of the burn to save life.[11] Life support measures and rigid techniques that isolate the patient from infection tend to result also in social isolation, itself psychologically stressful.[15] The occupational therapist can provide some social involvement at every visit to fit and adjust splints and at that time explain to the patient what is being done and why. All of the positioning and splinting is to ensure a more functional patient when skin cover is achieved by the surgical staff. This is evidence for the patient that his recovery is anticipated. The occupational therapist can foster the patient's efforts in his own treatment from the initiation of contact. Hope for life is a powerful ally.

Knowledge of the patient's occupation and its physical requirements, his leisure activities, and age may indicate approximate extent of function prior to the injury. The usual OT evaluations, such as goniometric range of motion and manual muscle testing, may not be feasible for a patient with acute and extensive burns. Any body segments unaffected by the injury may be evaluated, and a comparison may be made with burned segments to establish an information base. If a patient's history and occupation indicate functional ability up to the time of the burn, one might assume that range of motion and strength were within normal limits. As the patient becomes able to do active motion, goniometric measures can be estimated. As skin cover is attained, the usual tests may be used. Although physicians may test sensation to determine the depth of a burn,[7] it is not considered a useful measure by others.[34] An occupational therapist probably would not want to repeat the test because the findings are not useful at this stage. It is known that second degree burns are very painful, whereas third degree burns destroy the free nerve endings and those areas do not have sensation.[7]

TREATMENT

Pregraft Treatment

As the care of the burn patient progresses through stages, the goals for preventing deformity and maintaining range of motion and strength are consistent with each stage. At times, in extensive burns, the patient will have some full thickness wounds in the pregraft stage, while other body parts are in postgraft or healed stages. Specific procedures are used for each until total skin coverage is achieved and the rehabilitation stage begins.[28]

The burn wound is cleansed daily, usually in the Hubbard tank or whirlpool, and debridement of full thickness burns continues. Antibacterial ointments are applied daily after cleansing, and this is an optimum time for the patient to do active motion while the tissues are soft and moist. All nonburned areas should be exercised daily.[19] Splints and positioning devices are removed several times daily and cleaned so that they do not become reservoirs for bacteria.[41] At that time the patient may be asked to move, or is assisted to move all joints. Active exercise should be supervised by the therapist two times per day. The patient should be taught to move every 2 hours for up to 10 repetitions of movement each time. However, an activity list can be kept at bedside to remind the patient and other personnel of the treatment program.[31] When a patient is able to participate in the treatment program, some splints are worn only during rest and sleep, and the patient is encouraged to use the extremities for self-care and other treatment procedures.[20]

It is essential, in addition to maintaining proper positioning, for the burn patient to perform active movement from the day of admission to prevent deformity and contracture, the most disabling sequelae of burns. The greatest obstacle to this goal is the patient's anticipation of pain in moving a burned extremity. One sequence for gaining patient cooperation has been described by Evans.[24] The therapist approaches the patient and describes what needs to be done and why, meanwhile surveying the patient to identify joints without burns. Then the patient is coached to do active and active-assisted motion with unburned joints. The patient is then taught to do isometric exercises, or muscle setting, in any unburned part. Next, the patient is coaxed to do isometric contraction under burned areas. As the patient learns that some muscle contraction can be done without extreme discomfort, he should be able to begin to cooperate with maintaining muscle awareness. Then the patient is asked to perform some active, or active-assisted motion with a burned part. Daily contraction of all muscles and movement of uninvolved joints is essential to maintain contact with the environment.[24] Dur-

ing periods of strict positioning, before and after grafting, it is important that the burn patient be allowed to initiate some voluntary active motion of the parts that are not being immobilized, either in or out of splints. Experiments have shown that immobilization alone can result in behavioral changes involving cognition and mood, similar to those that result from being in a sensory or perceptual deprivation environment. However, exercise or simple movements by the subjects were found to decrease the behavioral changes.[42, 43] Therefore, it is important for burn patients, immobilized after grafting, to be able to initiate some movement in some body part.

If active voluntary joint movement is too painful for the burn patient, isometric contractions within splints may be encouraged. During the acute stage, muscle awareness is the goal rather than strength building.[31] If a patient is allowed to be immobile for a few days, he will become fearful of moving and avoid any active or passive motion. If a patient, such as an uncooperative or an unconscious patient is unable to do active motion, gentle passive motion should be done at least once per day.[7, 33]

Passive motion must be done slowly and gently, and never beyond tissue resistance. Passive stretching is harmful and can result in edema and cause hemorrhage in the wound before or after skin cover is achieved. Damage can occur from stretching proliferating or immature scar.[24] Vigorous alternating rapid stretching can cause surface bacteria from the wound to enter the blood stream and can lead to sepsis. Mild sustained motions are used in passive motion to avoid additional damage to the wound or healing areas.[20, 37]

Areas of partial thickness burns should begin active motion early in treatment because surgery will not be done. Antibacterial cream, used to control sepsis, permits active movement from the time of admission. The motions should be done after tubbing or after analgesics in the early painful stages of care.[7] Because partial-thickness burns expose nerve endings, a patient with a large second degree burn can experience more pain than a patient with a deeper burn.[12] A superficial second degree burn may receive active and passive exercise to maintain range of motion.[31] Ambulation and self-care are encouraged early, depending on the extent and complications of the burn.[37] To achieve the goal of preventing deformity, it may be necessary at this time to use pressure wraps and Anti/Burnscar garments for these areas earlier than for burn sites that require grafting.[28]

The hand with deep second and third degree burns on the dorsum must be given special care. Burns on the dorsum of the fingers may threaten the integrity of the extensor mechanism. Deep second and third degree burns can distort the joints because of thermal destruction, or because of fibrosis of joint capsules and loss of continuity of the extensor tendons. Neither active nor passive motion should be allowed to place tension on the extensor mechanism, such as actively making a tight fist, or pushing the fingers passively into total flexion, which can cause the extensor mechanism to split, slip, or be damaged.[31] Acute flexion of MP and IP joints can result in disruption of the central slip, creating a boutonniere deformity which requires surgical repair.[44] Splinting the wrist in neutral with only slight MP flexion and the interphalangeal joints extended is a counteracting force.[28]

One method to achieve movement for burns on the dorsum of the hand suggests that when one joint is flexed, the other joints should remain in extension. (These are muscle testing positions for MP, PIP, and DIP flexion; see Chapter 7.) That is, MP flexion is done with the PIP and DIP joints in neutral or extension; PIP joint is flexed with the MP and DIP joints in neutral extension, and the DIP joint is flexed with MP and PIP in neutral extension.[31] A Bunnell block could be used to assist positioning for such activity.[35, 45] For thumb flexion the carpometacarpal (CM) joint is in neutral and thumb MP flexion is done with PIP in neutral. Thumb IP flexion can be done with CM and MP joints in neutral. Isometric exercises can be done in the hand splint to preserve muscle awareness.[31]

After the eschar has been removed from full-thickness burns, temporary covers of allografts are used in extensive burns to decrease fluid loss and to provide comfort. These biological dressings are not accepted by the body and are removed for placement of autografts, the patient's own skin.[7, 11] Prior to placement of this final graft, the surgeon and the occupational therapist may confer to plan the positioning devices to be used with the grafting procedure. Splints may be made prior to surgery or in the operating room.[31] The extremity can be placed in the splint and the grafts laid over the open wound without sutures or dressings, or they may be secured with tape.[46] A splint immobilizes the part while the graft takes.[31] The immobilization results in greater success and decreases the chance that the graft will be lost.[25]

After grafting, the wound is painless but the donor site is painful and requires about 3 weeks to heal.[12] To avoid the patient's disappointment in the appearance of the graft at first, he should be told that it will not have the appearance of his skin as it was before the burn.[21]

Postgraft Treatment

During immobilization after grafting, positioning continues, and during that time isometric contractions may be done under the grafted areas, but not if a graft covers a joint.[7, 24] The grafts adhere in a week to 10 days. Active or assisted motion continues for joints not grafted.

Although reinnervation of the grafted area may begin within 2 weeks after the graft is placed, when the nerve fibers may enter vacant neurilemma sheaths of the graft, the return of sensation is not complete for some time after grafting. It depends on the accessibility of neurilemma sheaths in the donor graft. Split thickness grafts have a better return of sensation. Touch, pain, temperature, and two-point discrimination return at varying rates.[18]

After the grafts take and are healed, the patient can begin a program of active motion. In the hand the patient can begin to move the finger joints carefully. A program of hourly repetitions is established to restore range of motion and hand function. All joints must be kept mobile, and the patient must be taught to avoid heat, friction, and trauma to the grafted areas.[47] Hand strength can be evaluated when skin cover is obtained, and the patient can perform pinch, grip, and goniometric measures safely.[33]

Following grafting to the lower extremities, the patient is not permitted to ambulate until venous drainage has been achieved in the grafted area, or the graft may be lost. After 10 days the patient may be allowed to walk if the legs are wrapped in elastic bandages.[37]

After the autografts take and each body area achieves skin cover, the area is wrapped in elastic bandages to prevent the formation of hypertrophic scar, and splints are used at night with the elastic bandages to prevent contracture. The early results of wound healing may be satisfactory, but in a few months smooth skin becomes contracted scar.[4] Hypertrophic scar and the contractures that follow closure of a burn wound are a frustrating sequelae of healed burns. When the deep reticular portion of the dermis is disturbed, hypertrophic scarring begins. Increased vascularity in the grafted area leaves a bright red healing wound. Collagen fibers develop to bridge the wound and begin to form a tangled mass that may take a year to mature. Continuous gentle pressure influences the arrangement of the collagen fibers so that they align in parallel rows rather than in rope-like whorls, as happens without pressure. It is thought that the pressure decreases the circulation to the area and retards scar development. As long as the scar is active it can be influenced by pressure and positioning. Once the scar becomes mature, only surgical correction is possible to remove the deforming force. If grafts cover a joint, the hypertrophic scar may be strong enough to dislocate the joint. Hypertrophic scar tends to involve flexor surfaces. These deformities can be avoided through a program of pressure dressing and conforming splinting for a long period, sometimes more than a year, after the wounds have healed.[4, 28]

Rehabilitation

After the grafted skin has securely covered the burn wound, the program of positioning and splinting continues. In addition, elastic bandages, and later Anti/Burnscar garments, are used to prevent contractures as the burn wounds heal and mature. Custom knit Anti/Burnscar garments are ordered to replace the elastic bandages after the patient's body weight stabilizes following skin cover.[28] The elastic bandages are used until the Anti/Burnscar garments are received.

The Anti/Burnscar garments are custom made for each patient by Jobst Institute in Toledo, Ohio.[48] The company provides instructions for measuring and ordering. Because the garments are worn continuously, two sets are ordered to permit laundering. The garments are removed only for bathing, or during exercise if they interfere with exercise movements. However, for the best results they should not be removed for more than an hour at a time.[41] Healing scar itches, and scratching can injure grafted skin.[7] Tolhurst[49] suggests that a thin cotton shirt can be worn under the elastic garment for this problem.

The splinting and positioning program postgraft is similar to the acute stage, but with some modifications. Anti/Burnscar garments are available for every body part and used in conjunction with thermoplastic conformers to provide pressure in specific areas.

An Anti/Burnscar mask is available to cover the head, face, and neck for burns to that area. A thermoplastic face conformer is made to provide consistent pressure to the areas of the face, particularly for scars around the nose and mouth, under the Anti/Burnscar garment.[50, 51] A transparent face mask can also be used,[52] and there are special splints for increasing the mouth opening for burns to that area.[53]

In areas such as the shoulder, neck, and axilla, where it is difficult to fit thermoplastic materials, a flexible elastomer is available to make contour molds to wear under the elastic garments.[54] The neck conformer is applied for total contact to burns of the neck. The method of preparation, described in 1970,[17] has been modified slightly.[41] The use of the neck conformer, following partial or full thickness burns, has decreased the incidence and severity of neck contractures in patients with severe burns from an expected 37 to only 9%.[55]

The shoulder area is difficult to maintain, and any scar that reduces the shoulder range of motion to less than 90° abduction will probably require a surgical release.[50] Conventional airplane splints can be used to maintain the arm in abduction.[27] Also, foam semicircles in the axilla secured with elastic bandages in a figure eight wrapping, (Fig. 22.3) or an Anti/Burnscar garment can be used to position and prevent hypertrophic scarring.[23]

To prevent flexion contracture at the elbow, a three-point extension brace, or an anterior splint of thermoplastic material, is used. It is possible to stretch out contracture until the hypertrophic scar matures by using serial splints to the forearm. The anterior splint may be worn with the elastic garment and changed as the elbow extension range of motion increases[4, 41] (Fig. 22.5).

Anti/Burnscar gloves are available and can be detached from the garment sleeves to permit hand washing. They are useful to keep the finger webs from

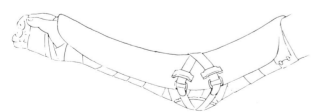

Figure 22.5 Elbow conformer splint made of Orthoplast. (Reproduced with permission from Shirley Baty, illustrator, and *Emergency Medicine.*[41])

becoming adherent and scarred. The positioning hand splint is worn at night over the Anti/Burnscar garment.[28] Elastomer molds have been used to improve the thumb web space.[54]

Hypertrophic scar to the trunk can be reduced by Anti/Burnscar garments worn over the area.[32] If the scar begins to cause a spinal curvature to develop, the scar will require surgical release and the use of an airplane splint to maintain the upright position.[37]

If hip and knee contractures are a potential problem, a three-point extension brace can be used on the leg to avoid a knee flexion, as well as a hip flexion contracture when the patient is supine. It is difficult to keep the hip flexed with the knee straight.[28] Full-thickness burns over the shoulder, anterior elbow, and hip have resulted in bridging of the joints with heterotopic bone. This has occurred in patients who were either unable, or were resistant to, participation in an active therapy program. Joints that do not yield to usual measures for range of motion should be x-rayed, because if heterotopic bone is present, surgical excision is required to restore range of motion.[24]

Burns to the dorsum of the foot are treated by the use of high tennis shoes lined with sheepskin and laced firmly to apply pressure.[28]

Von Prince and Yeakel[27] suggest that the program of splinting and positioning can be relaxed when the patient awakens from sleep and does not feel tightness when moving the joints. However, Larson[28] indicates that the program must be continued as long as there is evidence that the scar tissue has not matured.[28] Immature hypertrophic scar is firm, raised, and red. Mature hypertrophic scar tissue is pale, flat, and soft.[32]

A home program for wearing splints and antiburnscar garments requires the occupational therapist to demonstrate for the patient and to check out with the patient and caregiver how to apply the antiburnscar garments and splints accurately. The reasons for splinting, instructions for wearing garments and doing exercises, as well as the consequences of not following the program, must be explained. Also, the therapist should give the patient the name and telephone number of the person at the occupational therapy department to call to have questions answered.[28]

Although prolonged use of pressure garments and splints is necessary to achieve better function and cosmesis following a burn, the wearing program as outlined appears to be an incredible burden for an extended period of 12 to 18 months for an injured patient who has already been through the rigors of all that the care of an acute or extensive burn requires. On what basis can a therapist encourage and convince a patient or a family that this treatment must be continued for a year or more? Prior to this regimen, contractures and multiple readmissions for reconstructive surgery were common and were the accepted sequelae of a burn. A review of 625 patients at follow-up showed that the longer the pressure garments were worn, the fewer number of contractures and ultimate surgical releases of contracture were needed. In the population, 219 patients were treated prior to the introduction of the splint and pressure garment procedures. Of that group 92% required one or more follow-up surgeries after recovery from the burn. Of the 406 patients who were treated with splints and pressure, only 25% required one or more operations following recovery. An assessment was made of the length of time the garments and splints were worn, and it showed that 70% of the patients who wore them for 6 months required follow-up surgery. Only 23% of those wearing splints and garments for from 6 to 12 months required surgery. Of the patients who followed the wearing program for more than 12 months, only 15% required additional surgery. The savings in inpatient hospitalization and the trauma of surgery are impressive, but of greater interest is the information that the program is truly preventive and of great benefit for restoration of function following a burn.[56] Therefore, following discharge, patients should be rechecked regularly for a year or more, or until the grafts mature and there is no evidence of hypertrophic scar activity.

A large burn leaves physical and emotional scars. This is particularly true of the facially disfigured. The patients must call up coping and adapting mechanisms to get through repeated surgeries and uncomfortable procedures. It may take a long time to make painful adjustments, especially for the patient with a facial burn.[15]

Although the quality of burn care, measured in survival statistics improves yearly,[2, 57] the quality of life following a burn has not been investigated extentensively. Psychosocial studies of adult burn patients indicate that about 30% of burn patients have long-term psychosocial problems, commonly anxiety and depression.[58] That percentage suggests that about 70% manage to cope and adapt following a burn, although it requires about a year for patients to resolve the depression which seems unrelated to the extent of the burn injury.[57, 58] A patient's social network system, particularly the family, has been found to relate to measures of self-esteem and life satisfaction following a burn.[57, 59, 60]

Occupational therapy for burn patients is primarily prevention of the deforming sequelae of the burn. It may be difficult to realize when confronted with a severely injured burn patient that most of these patients, with current knowledge and practice, have a good prognosis for functional recovery. Occupational therapy makes a substantial contribution to that functional recovery.

References

1. Cuono, C. B. Early management of severe thermal injury. *Surg.Clin. North Am.*, 60 (5): 1021–1033, 1980.
2. Feller, I., Tholen, D., and Cornell, R. G. Improvements in burn care, 1965–1979. *J.A.M.A.*, 244 (18): 2074–2078, 1980.
3. Georgiade, N. D., Management of the burn wound. In *Symposium on the Treatment of Burns*, Vol. 5, edited by J. R. Lynch, and S. R. Lewis. St. Louis: C. V. Mosby, 1973.
4. Larson, D. L., *et al.* Mechanisms of hypertrophic scar and contracture formation in burns. *Burns*, 1 (2): 119–127, 1975.
5. Feller, I., and Crane, K. H. Classification of burn-care facilities in the United States. *J.A.M.A.*, 215 (3): 463–466, 1971.
6. Ollstein, R. Burn injury: Outpatient evaluation and treatment. *Qual. Rev. Bull.*, 5: 9–11, 1979.
7. Remensnyder, J. P., and Wray, R. C. Burn and frostbite injuries. In: *Acute Hand Injuries: A Multispecialty Approach* edited by F. G. Wolfort. Boston: Little, Brown, 1980.
8. Hunt, J. L., Sato, R. M., and Baxter, C. R. Acute electrical burns: Current diagnostic and therapeutic approaches to management. *Arch. Surg.*, 115: 434–438, 1980.
9. Masters, F. W., Robinson, D. W., and Ketchum, L. D. Management of electrical burns. In: *Symposium on the Treatment of Burns*, Vol. 5, edited by S. R. Lynch, and S. R. Lewis. St. Louis: C. V. Mosby, 1973.
10. Bingham, H. G. Electrical injuries to the upper extremity—A review. *Burns*, 7 (3): 155–157, 1981.
11. Parks, D. H., Carvajal, H. F., and Larson, D. L. Management of burns. *Surg. Clin. North Am.*, 57 (5): 875–894, 1977.
12. Wagner, M. Pain and nursing care associated with burns. In: *Pain: A Source Book for Nurses and Other Health Professionals*, edited by A. K. Jacox. Boston: Little, Brown, 1977.
13. Ward, C. G. Burn care: A multidisciplinary specialty. *Qual. Rev. Bull.*, 5: 2–3, 1979.
14. Ollstein, R. N., and McDonald, C. Topical and systemic antimicrobial agents in burns. *Ann. Plastic Surg.*, 5 (5): 386–391, 1980.
15. Bernstein, N. R. *Emotional Care of the Facially Burned and Disfigured*. Boston: Little, Brown, 1976.
16. Berkow, R. (ed). *The Merck Manual of Diagnosis and Therapy*, 13th ed. Rahway, N.J.: Merck Sharpe & Dohme Research Laboratories, 1977.
17. Willis, B. The use of orthoplast isoprene splints in the treatment of the acutely burned child. *Am. J. Occup. Ther.*, 24 (3): 187–191, 1970.
18. Šmahel, J. The healing of skin grafts. *Clin. Plast. Surg.*, 4 (3): 409–424, 1977.
19. Curreri, P. W., and Pruitt, B. A., Jr. Evaluation and treatment of the burned patient. *Am. J. Occup. Ther.*, 24 (7): 475–480, 1970.
20. Boswick, Jr., J. A. The management of fresh burns of the hand and deformities resulting from burn injuries. *Clin. Plastic Surg*, 1 (4): 621–631, 1974.
21. Knorr, N. J., and Sheehan, J. Burn unit: Patient-team interaction. In: *Symposium on the Treatment of Burns*, Vol. 5, edited by J. B. Lynch, and J. R. Lewis. St. Louis: C. V. Mosby, 1973.
22. Jones, C. A., and Feller, I. *Procedures for Nursing the Burned Patient*. Ann Arbor: National Institute of Burn Medicine, 1973.
23. Rudowski, W. *Burn Therapy and Research*. Baltimore: The Johns Hopkins University Press, 1976.
24. Evans, E. B. Orthopaedic measures in the treatment of severe burns. *J. Bone Joint Surg.*, 48-A (4): 643–669, 1966.
25. Feller, I., *et al.* Rehabilitation of the burned patient. In: *Symposium on the Treatment of Burns*, Vol. 5, edited by J. B. Lynch, and J. R. Lewis. St. Louis: C. V. Mosby, 1973.
26. Evans, E. B., *et al.* Prevention and correction of deformity after severe burns. *Surg. Clin. North Am.*, 50 (6): 1361–1375, 1970.
27. Von Prince, K. M. P., and Yeakel, M. H. *The Splinting of Burn Patients*. Springfield, Ill.: Charles C Thomas, 1974.
28. Linares, H. A., Larson, D. L., and Baur, Jr., P. S. Influence of mechanical forces on burn scar contracture and hypertrophy. In: *Symposium on Basic Science in Plastic Surgery*, Vol. 15, edited by T. J. Krizek, and J. E. Hoopes. St. Louis: C. V. Mosby, 1976.
29. Larson, D. L. *et al.* The use of skeletal suspension in grafting burned patients. In: *Symposium on the Treatment of Burns*, Vol. 5, edited by J. B. Lynch, and S. R. Lewis. St. Louis: C. V. Mosby, 1973.
30. Willis, B. Splinting the burn patient. Galveston: Shriners Burns Institute (Undated).
31. Salisbury, R. E., Reeves, S., and Wright, P. Rehabilitation of the burned hand. In: *Rehabilitation of the Hand*, edited by J. M. Hunter, *et al.* St. Louis: C. V. Mosby, 1978.
32. Parks, D. H., Evans, E. B., and Larson, D. L. Prevention and correction of deformity after severe burns. *Surg. Clin. North Am.*, 58 (6): 1279–1289, 1978.

33. Olivett, B. L. Rehabilitating the burned hand. In: *Rehabilitation of the Hand*, edited by J. M. Hunter, *et al.* St. Louis: C. V. Mosby, 1978.
34. McCormack, R. M. Problems in the treatment of burnt hands. *Clin. Plastic Surg.*, 3 (1): 77–83, 1976.
35. Bunnell, S. *Surgery of the Hand*. Philadelphia: J. B. Lippincott, 1944.
36. Swanson, A. B. Treatment of the stiff hand and flexible implant arthroplasty in the fingers. A.A.O.S. Instructional Course Lectures, Vol. 21. St. Louis: C. V. Mosby, 1972.
37. Koepke, G. H. The role of physical medicine in the treatment of burns. *Surg. Clin. North Am.*, 50 (6): 1385–1399, 1970.
38. James, J. I. P. Assessment and management of the injured hand. *The Hand*, 2 (2): 97–105, 1970.
39. Von Prince, K. M. P., Curreri, P. W., and Pruitt, B. A., Jr. Application of fingernail hooks in splinting of burned hands. *Am. J. Occup. Ther.*, 24 (8): 556–559, 1970.
40. Daniels, L. E. *Physical Therapy for the Acute Burn Patient*. Galveston: Shriners Burns Institute, 1968.
41. Making the Least of Burn Scars. *Emergency Medicine*, 4: 24–35, 1972.
42. Zubek, J. P., and MacNeill, M. Effects of immobilization: Behavioural and EEG changes. *Can. J. Psychiatry*, 20 (3): 316–336, 1966.
43. Zubek, J. P. Counteracting effects of physical exercises performed during prolonged perceptual deprivation. *Science*, 142 (3591): 504–506, 1963.
44. Larson, D. L., *et al.* Repair of the boutonniere deformity of the burned hand. *J. Trauma*, 10 (6): 481–487, 1970.
45. Becker, C. G. Adaptation of Bunnell block. *Am. J. Occup. Ther.*, 29 (2): 108, 1975.
46. Lynch, J. B. Current status of treatment of burns. *South Med. J.*, 69 (8): 1085–1089, 1976.
47. Wynn-Parry, C. B. Problems in rehabilitation of the burnt hand. *The Hand*, 2 (2): 140–144, 1970.
48. Blair, K. L. Prevention and control of hypertrophic scarring and contractures by the application of the Jobst Custom-Made Anti/Burnscar® Supports. Toledo, Ohio: Jobst Institute, 1977.
49. Tolhurst, D. E. The treatment of burns. *Ann. R. Coll. Surg. Engl.*, 62 (2): 120–124, 1980.
50. Parks, D. H., Baur, Jr., P. S., and Larson, D. L. Late problems in burns. *Clin. Plas. Surg.*, 4 (4): 547–560, 1977.
51. Peterson, P. A conformer for the reduction of facial burn con-tractures: A preliminary report. *Am. J. Occup. Ther.*, 31 (2): 101–104, 1977.
52. Rivers, E. A., Strate, R. G., and Solem, L. D. The transparent face mask. *Am. J. Occup. Ther.*, 33 (2): 108–113, 1979.
53. Gorham, J. A. A mouth splint for burn microstomia. *Am. J. Occup. Ther.*, 31 (2): 105–106, 1977.
54. Malick, M. H., and Carr, J. A. Flexible elastomer molds in burn scar control. *Am. J. Occup. Ther.*, 34 (9): 603–608, 1980.
55. Bunchman, II, H. H., *et al.* Prevention and management of contractures in patients with burns of the neck. *Am. J. Surg.*, 130: 700–703, 1975.
56. Huang, T. T., Blackwell, S. J., and Lewis, S. R. Ten years of experience in managing patients with burn contractures of axilla, elbow, wrist and knee joints. *Plastic Reconstr. Surg.*, 61 (1): 70–76, 1978.
57. Blades, B. C., Jones, C., and Munster, A. M. Quality of life after major burns. *J. Trauma*, 19 (8): 556–558, 1979.
58. Malt, U. Long-term psychosocial follow-up studies of burned adults: Review of literature. *Burns*, 6 (3): 190–197, 1980.
59. Bowden, M. L., *et al.* Self-Esteem of severely burned patients. *Arch. Phys. Med. Rehabil.*, 61 (10): 449–452, 1980.
60. Davidson, T., *et al.* Social support and post-burn adjustment. *Arch. Phys. Med. Rehabil*, 62 (6): 274–278, 1981.

Supplementary Reading

Feller, I., and Crane, K. *Planning and Designing A Burn Care Facility*. Ann Arbor: National Institute for Burn Medicine, 1971.
Feller, I., and Grabb, W. C. *Reconstruction and Rehabilitation of the Burned Patient*. Ann Arbor: National Institute for Burn Medicine, 1979.
Fishwick, G. M., and Tobin, D. G. Splinting the burned hand with primary excision and early grafting. *Am. J. Occup. Ther.*, 32 (3): 182–183, 1978.
Granite, U. Multidisciplinary discharge and rehabilitation planning for burn patients. *Qual. Rev. Bull.*, 5: 30–34, 1979.
Stamba, L. M. Early motion and splinting of hands following burns: A literature review. *Can. J. Occup. Ther.*, 48 (1): 27–32, 1981.
Sykes, W. M. Role of the child psychiatrist on the burn team and the psychiatric problems of the burned child. In: *Pediatric Burns*, edited by W. C. Bailey, Chicago: Yearbook Medical Publisher, 1979.

chapter

23

Cardiac Rehabilitation

Catherine A. Trombly, M.A., OTR

Cardiac rehabilitation is appropriate for persons who have suffered an uncomplicated myocardial infarction (MI) or "heart attack." Complications which preclude a rehabilitation program as described here include congestive heart failure, myocarditis, use of a pacemaker, or unstable angina.

The goals of cardiac rehabilitation are to increase functional capacity (ability to do work without stress or symptoms) through a graded exercise program, to alleviate depression, to change behaviors that place the patient at risk for a recurrence, and to return the person to his previous work and recreation if possible.[1]

SYMPTOMS

In coronary artery disease, the lumen of the coronary blood vessels narrows due to deposits of fat on the walls, a process called atherosclerosis.[2] Narrowed arteries reduce the flow of oxygen-carrying blood to the heart muscle.[2, 3] A greater demand for oxygen than can be supplied manifests itself by angina pectoris.[4, 5] Angina pectoris is a severe, "squeezing" pain in the chest which may radiate to the neck, left shoulder, or down the left arm.[2, 3] It is brought on by physical activity or emotional stress. It is relieved by rest, and it predictably occurs under the same demands.[4] Angina pectoris does not necessarily develop into an MI. If the person recognizes it as a warning and takes steps to reduce his risk of developing greater cardiac disease, he may avert an MI.[6]

If a coronary artery becomes obstructed, the tissue which is supplied with oxygen by that artery dies; this is a myocardial infarction. An MI is not necessarily fatal, but it always decreases the pumping efficiency of the heart.[2] Its severity depends upon the extent and location of the infarction.

Signs and symptoms of an MI include dyspnea, angina pectoris, palpitations, anxiety, diaphoresis, rapid and thready pulse, irregular heart rhythm, a low grade fever, nausea or vomiting, and/or fatigue or weakness. In one quarter of the cases, the first sign of MI is sudden death.[2]

Cardiac patients are classified according to the amount of work or kinds of activities they may safely perform. The American Heart Association's functional and therapeutic classifications of patients with disease of the heart[7] are found in Table 23.1.

VALUE OF REHABILITATION

Supervised programs of exercise are beneficial for three reasons: weight reduction (obesity requires the heart to work harder); conditioning the heart and other muscles to enable them to handle stress and strain;[2] and as a demonstration to the patient that certain levels of physical activity can be done safely. Exercise results in a training effect in which more blood is pumped during each beat (increased stroke volume) and the heart beats less times per minute (decreased heart rate) for the same amount of work, indicating improved functional capacity.

A person starts an exercise program at a level of energy expenditure which puts demands on cardiac output but is safe for that person. When the training effect from activity at the initial level is experienced, the frequency, intensity, and/or duration of activity may be increased. The training effect will occur at successive levels of cardiac output up to a maximal level for a given individual.

Covert depression which arises due to tensions and anxieties related to changes in roles in the sex act and other areas of life-style[8] can be alleviated by physical exercise programs combined with psychotherapy. Because of the myths surrounding heart function and heart disease, psychotherapy that addresses the person's need for information; his fears concerning death, recurrence, and lost abilities; and modification of behaviors to reduce certain risk factors is as necessary as exercise.

Table 23.1
THE FUNCTIONAL AND THERAPEUTIC CLASSIFICATIONS OF PATIENTS WITH DISEASES OF THE HEART

	Functional Classification	Maximal METs
Class I	Patients with cardiac disease but without resulting limitations of physical activity. Ordinary physical activity does not cause undue fatigue, palpitation, dyspnea, or anginal pain.	6.5
Class II	Patients with cardiac disease resulting in slight limitation of physical activity. They are comfortable at rest. Ordinary physical activity results in fatigue, palpitation, dyspnea, or anginal pain.	4.5
Class III	Patients with cardiac disease resulting in marked limitation of physical activity. They are comfortable at rest. Less than ordinary physical activity causes fatigue, palpitation, dyspnea, or anginal pain.	3.0
Class IV	Patinets with cardiac disease resulting in inability to carry on any physical activity without discomfort. Symptoms of cardiac insufficiency or of the anginal syndrome may be present even at rest. If any physical activity is undertaken, discomfort is increased.	1.5

Therapeutic Classification	
Class A	Patients with cardiac disease whose physical activity need not be restricted in any way.
Class B	Patients with cardiac disease whose ordinary physical activity need not be restricted, but who should be advised against severe or competitive efforts.
Class C	Patients with cardiac disease whose ordinary physical activity should be moderately restricted, and whose more strenuous efforts should be discontinued.
Class D	Patients with cardiac disease whose ordinary physical activity should be markedly restricted.
Class E	Patients with cardiac disease who should be at complete rest, confined to bed or chair.

Rehabilitation is also financially beneficial both to the individual and to society. One study of 123 post-MI patients who were divided into an experimental and two control groups concluded, after examining alternate explanations, that a cardiac rehabilitation program significantly ($p < 0.001$) reduced the length of hospitalization and improved the level of functional capacity at discharge.[9]

REHABILITATION PROGRAM

The cardiac rehabilitation program is ordered by the physician who, because of his ultimate responsibility for the patient's life, must approve the initiation and continuance of the program.

All personnel who participate in the program must be qualified. All must be certified in CPR (cardiopulmonary resuscitation).[10, 11] Failure to have these qualifications could result in legal action against the person and institution in the event of a mishap.[10]

CPR is an emergency method of substituting for cardiorespiratory function without the use of equipment. The ABCs of CPR are to clear the Airway, Breathe for the patient, and Circulate the oxygenated blood.[2] The airway is cleared by putting the patient in a supine position, hyperextending the neck, and removing anything that may be obstructing it, including dentures. Artificial breathing is accomplished by pinching the patient's nose closed, by the resuscitator completely covering the patient's mouth with his mouth, and by then blowing into the patient's mouth with enough force so that the chest expands. Initially four breaths are given followed by cardiac compression which is done by pressing over the sternum approximately 1½ inches above the end of the xyphoid process with the heels of both hands, one pressing over the other. Fifteen compressions, at a rate of 80/minute, are done. Then two quick breaths are alternated with 15 compressions until the advanced life support team arrives or the patient revives.[12, 13] Certification in CPR is available by taking courses offered by the American Heart Association or the American Red Cross. Certification must be renewed yearly.

The rehabilitation program is usually divided into phases, each placing greater demand on the patient's heart function. The best results occur when the patient participates in all phases.

Inpatient Program

The inpatient program begins early in the coronary care unit as soon as the patient is pain-free, exhibits no arrhythmias at rest, and has a resting pulse of <100.[14] The goals of the inpatient program are to prevent deconditioning; to educate regarding risk factors, physical activity, and physiologic responses to emotion and effort; to provide psychological support to the patient and his family; and to develop psychological readiness and valuing of continuation of the program as an outpatient.

The exercise program begins with light diversional and self-care activities for the purposes of increasing cardiac capacity and reducing anxiety, which in turn reduces cardiac stress. During the first few days following MI, when the patient is functionally classified in Class IV, activities requiring a maximum of 1.5 metabolic equivalents (METs) are allowed. The patient is placed in a fully supported sitting position with the proximal extremities supported so that activities or exercise are restricted to the distal parts of the extremities and utilize phasic movements[15] on a gravity-eliminated plane. An example is feeding with the elbows resting on the over-bed table which has been raised to axilla height.

The evening resting pulse rate is a guideline to rehabilitation progress. If it exceeds the morning resting rate by more than 20%, then the program may be progressing too rapidly.[14]

As a training effect becomes apparent by obtaining a low pulse rate while the patient is doing the same activity, the frequency of the activity can be increased. The Grady Memorial Hospital program serves as a model to others and is included at the end of this chapter. It should be remembered that each person should be advanced according to his particular response to exercise. As the training effect is seen for all activities within the classification, the patient is probably ready to be reclassified by the physician into Class III, in which the METs are increased to 3.0. The patient may be transferred to the Progressive Care Unit[16] to continue rehabilitation.

When the patient is classified Class III, use of full movement of the upper extremities while sitting, proximal stabilization without resistance, trunk balancing, and hand activities while standing are permitted.[15] For example, upper extremity dressing and standing at the basin to shave are acceptable activities. Frequency and duration are increased as tolerated.

In Class II, activities may require a maximum of 4.5 METs. Resistance can be graded, and more expansive movements utilizing the larger muscle groups are permitted. The patient is usually discharged home 14 to 20 days postonset and can be expected to have reached about 4.0 METs functional capacity.[14]

Intermediate or Outpatient Program

The intermediate or outpatient program begins as early as 3 to 4 weeks post-MI[11, 14] for patients with stable angina pectoris or as late as 8 weeks.[16] The goals for the outpatient phase include continued physical conditioning through supervised exercise; behavioral counseling and modification relative to risk factors; vocational counseling and evaluation; and continued psychological support.[11] Those patients who begin the outpatient program closer to the time of onset continue the supervised step-by-step progression gauged by pulse (not to exceed 100/minute) and fatigue (disappears 10 to 20 minutes after activity).[14] At 8 weeks, the level of physical activity can be guided by a graded exercise test (GXT).[16] Following this test, the person usually enters into a walk/jog program under medical supervision[16] in which the heart rate attains 70 to 85%

of maximum achieved during the stress test carried to symptomatic endpoint.[14]

Community Program

After 4 to 6 months the patient may safely participate in a community program[16] or exercise independently if he has the self-discipline. He is discharged to this program when he achieves the functional capacity that is necessary for his occupation and life-style.[11]

The components of the rehabilitation program will be described in greater detail on the following pages.

Physical Activity/Exercise

The information in this section relates not only to conditioning exercise engaged in to gain a training effect, but also to all physical activity related to occupational performance tasks. The goal is to return the person to his original life-style. If he is unable to regain his original functional capacity, or if it is desirable to reduce the energy level required of daily tasks, work simplification and energy conservation techniques are taught.

Relationship of VO_2 and Exercise. Muscle uses energy from food to do work. The energy is obtained through oxidation; therefore, oxygen is needed which the muscle receives from the arterial blood. Skeletal muscle can work for short periods at levels that exceed O_2 supply, during which anaerobic breakdown of substances produces the energy. Anaerobic work results in an oxygen debt, and the oxygen requirement is increased by this debt.

In order to function, the heart, like skeletal muscle, requires oxygen. Although the heart contains oxygenated blood in its chambers, the myocardium is not supplied with oxygen by this source. Oxygen is carried to the myocardium by the left and right coronary arteries. The oxygen supply must meet the oxygen demand of the myocardium. Unlike skeletal muscle, the cardiac muscle cannot work anaerobically nor can it tolerate an oxygen debt.[4] If the oxygen supply does not meet the oxygen demand, angina pectoris signals the discrepancy.[5]

The oxygen supply is determined by cardiac output, blood flow, and the amount of oxygen in the blood. The cardiac output is the amount of blood pumped out (stroke volume) at each beat (heart rate).[17] The blood flow depends on the patency of the coronary arteries; atherosclerosis or blockage of the arteries decrease or terminate the blood flow. The amount of oxygen depends on the blood's ability to carry oxygen in the hemoglobin; a decrease in hemoglobin would decrease the amount of oxygen available. An increased work load creates an increased demand for oxygen by the myocardium (MVO_2).

There is a maximal amount of oxygen that a person can take in and dispense to muscle during exercise; it is termed maximal oxygen uptake and abbreviated $\dot{V}O_2$ max. The $\dot{V}O_2$ max is proportional to weight, especially lean body mass.[5] It increases with physical training and decreases with bed rest and age.[5] It is a standard measure of cardiovascular fitness.[5] The $\dot{V}O_2$

max, as determined by stress testing, relates to the person's maximal MET level.[18]

One MET (metabolic equivalent) equals basal metabolic rate and is equal to 3.5 ml of oxygen per kilogram of body weight per minute.[2, 11, 19] Basal metabolic rate is the minimal amount of energy or oxygen consumption necessary to maintain metabolic processes (respiration, circulation, peristalsis, temperature, glandular function, etc.) of the body at rest.[3] The energy cost of activities or exercise can be rated using multiples of METs.[11] An exercise that is rated 4.0 METs requires 4 times the amount of oxygen per kilogram of body weight per minute than basal rate.[11, 20]

METs and calories are both used to estimate the metabolic cost of activity. Beyond the basal rate, however, METs and calories are not equivalent. The average number of calories required to sustain the basal metabolic rate of a person resting in a supine position is 1.0 Calorie/kg/hour. One Calorie equals approximately 200 ml of oxygen consumption.[21] METs are a convenient and reliable measure of energy cost because their calculation considers the oxygen requirements of activities without having to calculate the amount of oxygen consumed separately as one would have to do if calories were used. Although the MET level of an activity is equivalent for different persons, the oxygen requirement is not. For example, a 4.0 MET activity done by a 50-kg person requires 4.0×3.5 ml $O_2 \times 50$ kg/minute or 700 ml O_2/minute, whereas a 70-kg person would use 980 ml O_2/minute.

Clearly it can be seen that a person reduces the oxygen demand by reducing his weight. Beyond that, the oxygen supply must increase by increasing cardiac output.

As an immediate effect of exercise, the stroke volume and heart rate do increase.[17] Increased stroke volume is primarily due to increased venous flow into the heart during diastole.[17] The mechanical response of the ventricle is based on Starling's Law: the force of the contraction is a function of the degree of stretch of the muscle fibers during diastole.[17] Over time, a training effect is seen when the heart rate and blood pressure are less than previously required for the same amount of work.[20]

Heart rate (HR) linearly relates to $\dot{V}O_2$ max except at the upper limits (80 to 90%) of maximal capacity.[17] For example, if a person's HR is 70% of maximal HR (HR max), that means he is using approximately 70% of $\dot{V}O_2$ max.[17] HR max is age-dependent[17] and is calculated by subtracting the person's age from 220. Heart rate also correlates with coronary blood flow which increases in response to MVO_2.[17] Therefore, heart rate indicates how hard the heart is working or how well it is performing.[17] A stable heart rate during exercise indicates a steady state, that is, the right amount of O_2 is being supplied to meet the work demand.[17]

Heart rate is therefore monitored during exercise to determine the effect the exercise is having on the person's heart. In addition to rate, rhythm is also monitored in recent post-MI patients, since the tissue death often results in irritability of the remaining tissue or pacing system.

Monitoring Heart Response to Exercise. Heart rate and blood pressure change in response to exercise. In a cardiac patient heart rhythm may also change. Heart rate is monitored by taking radial or carotid pulse, by ascultation, or by counting the beats on an ECG monitor to which newly infarcted patients are often attached. Resting heart rate is taken with the patient reclined or sitting, after 5 minutes of rest.[22] The pulse is counted for a full minute for greatest accuracy, but can be taken for less time and the result multiplied to determine the number of beats per minute.[22] Radial pulse is felt at the wrist at approximately the level of the radial styloid. Light, firm pressure is applied using the index and middle fingers. Carotid pulse is felt lateral to the trachea; care must be exercised to prevent too great a pressure which could occlude the artery and trigger the carotid sinus reflex which will affect blood pressure. Or, the heart rate can be counted by using a stethoscope over the heart (ascultation).

The exercise heart rate is measured very quickly after exercise. Rate drops fast; therefore, the beats are counted for 10 seconds only and multiplied to determine the rate per minute. This method is accurate to ± 6 beats per minute.[22] Another method is to time the first 10 beats and extrapolate to determine beats per minute.[21]

Blood pressure is measured during exercise testing to see if the heart is responding as it should to exercise. Blood pressure is measured using a sphygmomanometer and stethoscope. The deflated sphygmomanometer cuff is applied firmly to the arm proximal to the elbow. The stethoscope is placed over the brachial artery under the edge of the cuff. The valve of the sphygmomanometer is closed and pumped up to a level above that expected for the patient. The valve is slowly opened to release the air from the cuff. Listening by stethoscope, the heart beat can soon be heard. The reading is noted; this is the systolic pressure. The air continues to be released. When the sound disappears, the reading is noted; this is the diastolic pressure. The results are recorded: systolic/diastolic.

The normal heart beat, as monitored by electrocardiogram (ECG) is shown in Figure 23.1. The schematic indicates the waves or deflections from baseline of one heart beat. The P wave represents the electrical activity associated with depolarization of the atria. The P-R interval represents the time that elapses from the beginning of the atrial contraction to the beginning of the ventricular contraction. The QRS complex represents the electrical activity associated with the depolarization of the ventricles. The T wave represents ventricular recovery or repolarization.[23, 24] The U wave is little understood but is thought to be the last part of ventricular recovery or the recovery wave of the Purkinje system.[24] The junction between S and T waves is called the J point.

These parts, with the possible exception of the U wave, are always present, but may appear different in orientation, depending on the lead from which the

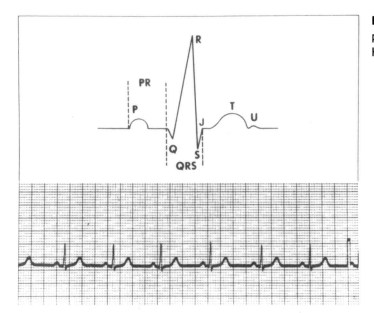

Figure 23.1   The normal ECG. (Reproduced with permission from R. H. Menard and the California Heart Association.[23])

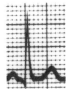

Figure 23.2   Normal EKG from V_5 lead. (Reproduced with permission from T. Winsor and the Ciba Pharmaceutical Co.[25])

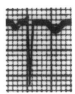

Figure 23.3   Normal EKG from AVR lead. (Reproduced with permission from T. Winsor and the Ciba Pharmaceutical Co.[25])

recording was made. The resting ECG is recorded from 12 leads in succession to look at the heart from many angles. There are three limb leads (I, II, III), three augmented limb leads (aVR, aVL, aVF), and six precordial leads (V_1 through V_6). The precordial leads extend from the 4th intercostal space on the right of the sternum to the left midlateral chest wall at the 5th intercostal space. Whether the deflection of the wave appears positive (upright) or negative depends on whether the electrode "sees" the advancing wave of depolarization (positive) or whether it "sees" a receding wave of depolarization.[25] For example, the recording from V_5 appears like the schematic (Fig. 23.2), but the normal appearance of aVR is quite different (Fig. 23.3). During exercise testing the ECG may be monitored using the CM5 placement, a modification of the V_5 placement (Fig. 23.4); however, this placement is

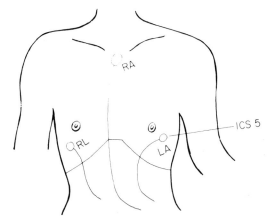

Figure 23.4   Electrode placement for exercise cardiogram. Right arm electrode (RA) is placed on the manubrium and is used as the reference. Right leg electrode (RL) is placed on the right chest and is the ground. Left arm electrode (LA) is placed on the left chest at the fifth intercostal space (ICS 5) in a line with the middle of the clavicle. This set-up optimizes the ST-segment display and minimizes noise. (Reproduced with permission from B. D. Erb and the Tennessee Heart Association.[19])

less sensitive than V_5 to detect S-T segment depression.[20]

Heart rate can be determined from ECG by counting the time elapsed between one R-R interval and dividing that into 60 seconds to determine the heart rate per minute.[24] Each five-space block (5 mm), which is marked by a heavier line on the chart paper, indicates 0.20 seconds with the paper moving at a rate of 25 mm/second. Each 1-mm block represents 0.04 seconds. Therefore, five of the large blocks or 25 of the small blocks indicates 1 second. For example, in Figure

23.1 the time elapsed between an R-R interval is 0.8 seconds which, divided into 60 seconds, equals 75 beats/minute.

Rate sticks eliminate the need for doing the mathematical calculation. The reference line of the rate stick is lined up exactly with an R peak, and three R-R intervals are counted. The heart rate is read from the value on the stick which coincides with the point of the last R peak. Another method has been described by Dubin: an R wave that falls on a dark line on the ECG paper is located; then the rate is determined by counting 300, 150, 100, 75, 60, and 50 for each successive dark line until the next R wave that falls on a line is encountered.[26] This method has the advantage of not requiring special equipment or mathematics; however, it may require a fairly long strip of ECG. For example, the rate could not be determined for the strip in Figure 23.1 because only one R wave falls on a line.

It is important for all personnel involved in the physical activity portion of the rehabilitation program to be able to recognize abnormal rates or arrhythmias on the ECG and to know which are outside of normal limits so that the activity can be appropriately discontinued and help sought if necessary. In learning to read ECGs, one should note both the rate and rhythm. In particular, ventricular rate, ventricular regularity (same R-R interval over time), presence or absence of a P wave, association of a P wave with the QRS complex, atrial rate, and QRS width are noted.[27] If the P or P-R interval are abnormal, this indicates a disruption of the electrical flow above the bundle branches. If the QRS, S-T, or T are affected, this indicates that the disruption is at the bundle branches or below.

The abnormalities that are within normal limits include S-T segment depression of 1 mm or less (the J point is compared to the PQ junction to note the amount of depression)[4, 17]; if the T-wave, which should deflect in the same direction as the QRS, flips during exercise it is not diagnostic; however, if it inverts during rest, it is abnormal[4]; steeply upsloping S-T segment so that within 0.04 to 0.06 seconds after the J point it has returned to baseline[17]; and an occasional, unifocal (same shape) premature ventricular contraction (PVC).[4] A premature ventricular contraction is an abnormal QRS complex not preceded by a P wave, but followed by a compensatory pause (Fig. 23.5). Each focus of irritability in the ventricles produces a wave form of distinctive shape.

ECG indications of intolerance to exercise include the following. (1) Ventricular tachycardia,[6, 19] defined as three or more successive PVCs[6, 26] (Fig. 23.6). The probability of developing fibrillation increases if PVCs occur in couplets, bigeminy (every other one), or are multifocal[4, 26]; therefore, exercise is terminated when any of these occur. Ventricular fibrillation (Fig. 23.7) is equivalent to cardiac standstill, and unless defibrillation and cardiopulmonary resuscitation is instituted immediately, death will ensue within minutes.[23] Cardiac arrest is indicated on the ECG by a flat line, but a disconnected or broken ECG electrode or lead may produce the same flat line in a nonemergency situation. (2) Ischemic changes (>1 mm of horizontal or downsloping S-T segment depression)[6, 19, 28] (Fig. 23.8A and B). S-T segment depression >2 mm is often accompanied by angina, a warning signal; however, in one study it was found that 72% of S-T segment depressions occurred without angina in coronary heart disease patients who were at rest or doing activity at levels below their functional capacity as determined by exercise testing.[29] This finding needs further study to determine its full implications. (3) 2 or 3° heart block.[6, 19, 28] Impairment of conduction through the A-V node is designated as a first, second, or third degree block, depending on the severity. A second degree A-V block is one in which the impairment of conduction is such that some of the impulses from the atria fail to get through to activate the ventricles, resulting in skipped beats (Fig. 23.9). In a third degree A-V block no impulses from the atria reach the ventricles. In order for the ventricles to contract, they must develop their own pacing system from nervous tissue within the heart, producing a very slow rate with abnormal QRS complexes (Fig. 23.10). Both the ST-segment depression and the A-V blocks indicate a probable impending myocardial infarction. Exercise should cease, and the physician should be notified immediately.

Neither supraventricular dysrhythmias nor bundle branch blocks (BBB) (Figs. 23.11 and 23.12) are absolute contraindications to exercise, but the patient requires close supervision. In the case of a LBBB, an MI cannot be diagnosed by ECG[4, 26] because the left ventricle fires late; therefore, the first portion of the QRS complex represents right ventricular activity. Q waves, indicating infarct, cannot be identified for the left ventricle.[26]

Monitoring activity during daily living activities can be done using telemetry or a Holter monitor. When using telemetry, the ECG is radioed from the battery-operated transmitter to the receiver where it is viewed and/or recorded. The person must stay within a certain range of the receiver and electrodes must be very well applied (see Chapter 11 for electrode application techniques). The Holter monitor is a battery-operated receiver and tape recorder which can be worn by the person for periods up to 24 hours. The tape can later be processed to print out a 24-hour heart rate record which is correlated with a detailed diary kept by the patient during that period.

Exercise Testing. Six to eight weeks after an uncomplicated MI, patients can be tested to determine their nonsymptomatic $\dot{V}O_2$ max, and from this, a fairly precise exercise prescription, in METs, can be given each patient. The occupational therapist may be a member of the testing team, the composition of which varies from center to center, but which should include a physician.[11]

Graded exercise testing (GXT) is contraindicated for those persons for whom a rehabilitation program

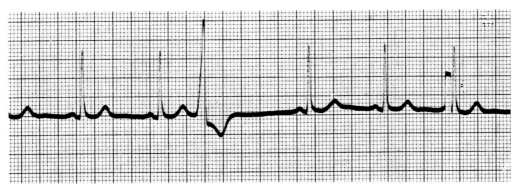

Figure 23.5 Premature ventricular contraction (PVC). There is no P wave before the abnormal PVC and there is a compensatory pause following it. (Reproduced with permission from the R. H. Menard and The California Heart Association.[23])

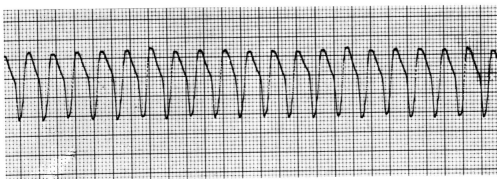

Figure 23.6 Ventricular tachycardia. (Reproduced with permission from California Heart Association.[23])

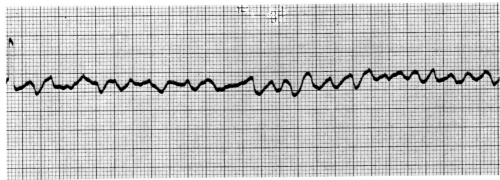

Figure 23.7 Ventricular fibrillation. (Reproduced with permission from the California Heart Association.[23])

is inappropriate, as mentioned earlier, and for the acute MI patient,[28] or patient with LBBB abnormality.[4]

An informed consent form which explains the purpose, procedure, risks, and benefits of the GXT is given the patient for signature.[10, 11, 18] The consent form does not protect the personnel from legal actions arising from negligence or malpractice, but only protects the patient's right of choice and full disclosure. The patient must also understand that he has the responsibility to report symptoms.[10]

Stress testing (exercise testing) can be done using

an automated treadmill, a bicycle ergometer, or by ascending and descending a standard size and number of steps.[6, 17-19] A study to test the reliability of treadmill *vs.* bicycle ergometer concluded that they were equally reliable in a test-retest (1 year) design, but that three out of four persons preferred the treadmill.[31]

Exercise testing is preceded by a warm-up period and followed by a cool-down period of exercise.[20] The actual testing begins with a low-intensity work load estimated from the patient's body size and current activity level. He works at this level for 4 to 6 minutes at a controlled rate to reach a steady state of oxygen uptake,[21] although some believe 3 minutes is enough to reach steady state.[6] The BP and HR by ECG are recorded at the end of each minute of exercise, and the ECG is continuously monitored for arrhythmias.[21] The patient proceeds to the next work load if HR is steady and less than target (usually 85% of HR max: 220 − age × 0.85) and he is free of symptoms. The symptoms that indicate endpoint of exercise testing are: dyspnea, weakness, changes in sensorium, angina, 2 or 3° AV blocks, S-T segment depression, decreased BP or HR for increased work load, increased ventricular arrhythmias, supraventricular tachyarrhythmias, or pallor or cyanosis.[5] The patient may signal to stop at any time. Some cardiologists believe that the endpoint of GXT should be the functional maximum or a HR of 160/minute, not a target HR which may be misleading in post-MI patients.[32] Some believe that a maximal symptom-limited exercise test should be done before the patient returns to full-time work and that the average work load should be limited to one-third to one-half of the maximal capacity.[5]

At the end of the test, the patient works at a low level for a minute or two before stopping the test and then rests. ECG monitoring continues throughout the cooldown and rest periods because ECG abnormalities may occur only during these periods.[6]

If the patient is on drugs, the particular drug may alter the interpretation of the stress test. Nitroglycerin will allow the patient to exercise longer at higher levels because it decreases the MVO_2.[17] Inderal (propranolol) may decrease S-T segment depression during the GXT. Many diuretics cause a loss of potassium (hypokalemia) which causes ventricular irritability and increased PVCs and other arrhythmias.

A method of testing and documenting the patient's cardiovascular response to activities of daily living has been devised by occupational and physical therapists at Rancho Los Amigos Hospital in California.[33, 34] It is called *Monitored Task Evaluation* and essentially stress tests the patient on daily tasks starting with supine, sitting, and standing postures. It is used with both complicated and noncomplicated cardiac cases. Five parameters are assessed: blood pressure, ECG by telemetry, heart sounds by ascultation, symptoms, and heart rate. Upper extremity activities of daily living (ADL) tasks are graded to produce a gradual increase in the cardiovascular work load. The method of grading the tasks takes such variables as arm position,

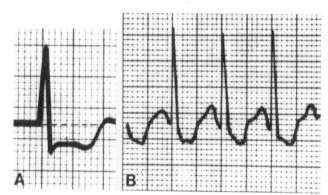

Figure 23.8 *A.* Horizontal S-T segment depression greater than 1 mm. (Reproduced with permission from D. Dubin.[26]) *B.* Downsloping S-T segment depression. (Reproduced with permission from M. H. Ellestad.[17])

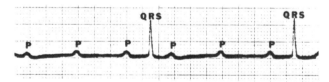

Figure 23.9 Second degree A-V block. In this case, three atrial pulses are required to stimulate the ventricular response. (Reproduced with permission from D. Dubin.[26])

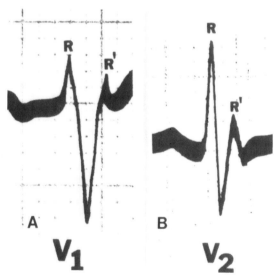

Figure 23.11 Right bundle branch block indicated by R-R′ in EKG leads V_1 and V_2. (Reproduced with permission from D. Dubin.[26])

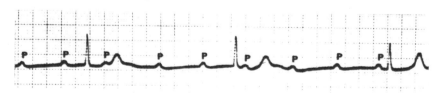

Figure 23.10 Third degree A-V block. The unstimulated ventricles set their own slow independent pace. (Reproduced with permission from D. Dubin.[26])

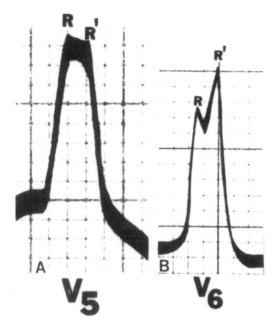

Figure 23.12 Left bundle branch block indicated by R-R' in EKG leads V_5 and V_6. (Reproduced with permission from D. Dubin.[26])

types of muscle groups used, involvement of trunk, and isometric work producing Valsalva into account.[34]

Exercise Prescription. The recommended target level of prescribed exercise in an outpatient program is 60 to 80% of maximum,[5, 22] or an average of 70%[18] and should not exceed 90%[18] as determined by GXT. A very unfit person would see a training effect at less than 60%. An example of prescribing activities or exercise is as follows:[18]

Maximal capacity as determined by GXT = 6.0 METs.
Average conditioning intensity = 0.70 × 6 = 4.2 = 4 METs.
Peak intensity = 0.90 × 6 = 5.4 = 5 METs.

Activity or exercise that averages 4 METs but less than 5 METs would be appropriate for the person. Heart rate is used to monitor response to exercise. If HR attained at maximal capacity of GXT = 170/minute, then the average conditioning HR (target HR) should not exceed 0.70 × 170 = 119/minute and peak HR should not exceed 0.90 × 170 = 153/minute.

The energy expended in different positions and while performing various activities has been measured in many studies of energy metabolism. Oxygen consumption of daily living, recreational, and vocational tasks was measured, and the METs required for each task were calculated. Many charts of the metabolic cost of activities have been published. Some of these are included at the end of this chapter. Knowledge of the energy cost of activities is valuable in determining the intensity of effort required by activities. There are slight discrepancies in the amount of energy recorded for similar activities in different charts. This is a

function of differing test situations or specific methods of performance of the activity. Because the method of performance is not described in these charts, the therapist can only consider the MET charts as a guideline for exercise prescription and should be conservative in the selection of activities.

Cardiac work or stress is influenced by many factors in addition to the energy requirements of activities. *Posture* affects cardiac output. Sitting relaxed in an easy chair with the head, back, arms, and thighs supported and with the feet on the floor is the position least demanding on the heart. Sitting on the edge of the bed, sitting in a straight chair, or even relaxed standing are less demanding than lying supine or semireclined in bed.[15] *Anxiety* increases muscular tension and blood pressure and consequently places more demand on the heart.[15] The *rate* of work influences the energy requirements of an activity, and energy expenditure increases as speed of performance increases.[15, 11] Temperature also influences cardiac stress, and a hot, humid environment increases cardiac work.[15] Other influencing factors include drugs, fatigue, emotion, hydration, and time since the last meal.[6, 35] Digestion of food results in a reflex dilation of blood vessels of the alimentary canal, thereby increasing circulation there and reducing the available circulating blood to other muscles, including the heart.[36] No exercise should be done within 1 hour of finishing a meal.[14]

Contraindications for an exercise program as stated by Nanette Kass Wenger, M.D., include[28]:

New or progressive angina pectoris
Uncontrolled congestive heart failure
Impending or very recent myocardial infarction
Uncontrolled hypertension
Arrhythmias
    Second and third degree A-V block
    Fixed rate pacemakers
    Ventricular tachycardia
    Uncontrolled atrial fibrillation
    Frequent premature ventricular contractions at rest which increase with exercise
Gross cardiac enlargement
Moderate to severe valvular disease
Outflow tract obstructive disease
Recent pulmonary embolism
Uncontrolled diabetes mellitus

For those able to participate, an individual exercise program is established taking into consideration the type, as well as the intensity, duration, and frequency of exercise.[5, 22] The person's exercise history, musculoskeletal stability, motivation, and athletic ability also must be considered.[11] Exercise prescription has to be as specific as possible, since there is a dose-effect relationship just as there is with drugs.[5] Like drugs, there is a therapeutic level, a potential for overdose, contraindications, side effects, and precautions.[5]

As with all patients, the response to therapy is carefully observed. Discontinuance or decrease of activity is indicated by one or more of the following:[5, 28]

(1) the appearance of chest pain or dyspnea; (2) an increase in the heart rate to over 120 beats/minute; (3) a decrease in systolic blood pressure of over 20 mm Hg; (4) increased ST segment displacement on the electrocardiogram; or (5) the occurrence of significant arrhythmias. The exercise prescription is reviewed and modified as often as is appropriate.[11]

Type of Exercise. Small muscle or arm exercise requires more energy than large muscle or lower extremity exercise.[5] Dynamic exercise of large muscles offers the best consistency of energy expenditure.[5] Sustained isometric contraction produces more cardiovascular stress than dynamic contractions.[2, 5] The response of increased HR and BP during isometric contraction is proportional to the percent maximal voluntary contraction of the particular muscle group involved[5, 37] and mental concentration. Ramos *et al.*[38] studied the cardiovascular effects of prolonged isometric exercise (grip) at varying intensities on six healthy subjects, aged 24 to 35 years, and found a significant elevation in blood pressure ($p < 0.01$) and heart rate ($p < 0.005$) at different predetermined levels of intensity ranging from 10 to 35% of maximum. They hypothesized that the difference in cardiac response to dynamic and static exercise occurs because dynamic exercise does not require constant cortical monitoring, whereas maintaining a predetermined level of isometric contraction does.[38] Cardiac patients should avoid exercise that is primarily isometric.[5]

Exercise used to increase muscle strength and endurance should be included in the program to enable the patient to do job tasks without stress. Stress decreases as strength increases.[18] Dynamic exercise is preferred to avoid the natural tendency to hold one's breath during activities that require exertion, known as the Valsalva effect[5]; this causes an increase in vagal stimulation which may add to cardiac stress above the level permitted. If a person can talk or count aloud while doing exercise, he is probably breathing correctly.

Flexibility and relaxation exercise, such as active range of motion (AROM) or Yoga, should also be included in the program and can be used as warm up and cool down exercises[18] that are part of each exercise period.[5, 19]

Intensity of Exercise. The MET level of an activity is a measure of its intensity. The MET load is monitored by HR response immediately following the workout.[5, 11] An indication for increasing the intensity is determination that the patient's peak exercise HR is consistently (three workouts in a row) below target HR.[5] After increasing the intensity, if the HR is more than 4 beats/minute above target HR during exercise, the intensity should be decreased.[5]

Before the patient has had a GXT, the initial MET level of activity is barely above resting and progresses as described earlier. A training effect occurs even at this low level because the patient is so debilitated. As the patient recovers, his MET level increases to the point that a regular, well-supervised dynamic exercise program can be instituted following GXT to gain a substantial training effect so that the patient's functional capacity exceeds his work and play requirements.

Activities are graded not only by the intensity (METs) but also by the duration or frequency. All of these variables are interrelated and each can be graded within a given classification, but the intensity is the most critical because it is the intensity that taxes the heart. Therefore, grading should begin with frequency and duration at low METs.[21]

Duration of Exercise. This refers to the length of time or number of repetitions of exercise done. An indication of the correct duration is that the patient experiences full recovery and feels rested within an hour after the exercise period.[18] The duration is inversely related to the intensity.[5, 18] A normal person can work almost indefinitely at 50% of VO_2 capacity, whereas he would be limited to 30 to 40 minutes of work at 70% $\dot{V}O_2$ max.[21] Not counting warm up and cool down, 20 to 30 minutes of exercise is best for most[18] on an outpatient exercise program.

Frequency of Exercise. This refers to the number of exercise sessions within a given time period. It depends on the intensity and duration.[18] In early rehabilitation, frequency is 2 to 3 times per day for 1 to 2 minutes duration each time. In late stages of rehabilitation, the frequency is reduced to 3 to 5 times per week, but the duration is increased to 20 to 45 minutes. A guideline is: for patients at 3 METs, frequency is several times a day and duration is less than 5 minutes; for those at 3 to 5 METs, the frequency is daily and duration is minimal; for those ≥8 METs, frequency is 3 times a week on alternating days.[18] Exercise frequency of 1 to 2 times/week will prevent loss in $\dot{V}O_2$max that occurs due to sedentary life-style, but 3 to 5 times/week is needed to increase $\dot{V}O_2$ max.[5]

Sex is one physical activity that both patient and spouse fear will precipitate a recurrence.[39] This fear is often not physiologically sound. It is beneficial to the couple if the energy requirement of the sex act is explained in terms of METs as is other physical activity. The MET level is 4.7 to 5.5 METs, approximately equal to climbing two flights of stairs within one minute[14] or vigorous walking.[40] Sexual activity is permitted when the person has reached a functional capacity of 6 METs. The couple who develops a loving, unhurried approach to sex, in which positions for coitus are chosen to reduce strain on the heart patient and the mate becomes the more active partner, will find sex satisfactory. Normal sex offers no particular risk to the average post-MI and may increase his self-esteem and encourage regular participation in an exercise program which in turn improves his prognosis.[8] Like other exercise, sex should be avoided after a meal, in extremes of temperature, after ingesting alcohol, when the patient is fatigued or under tension, and also if the conditions are illicit.[40]

Energy Conservation. By using the principles of work simplification and energy conservation (Chapters 20 and 27) and electrical appliances, the person can conserve his personal energy during some tasks to use it for other activities. The MET level of activity should never exceed 90% of maximal capacity[18]; the patient should work at an average level of 50 to 70%. Average implies that some activities require less than 50% and some more. The patient should be taught pacing which includes rest breaks, as frequently as every 10 to 15 minutes at first. Pacing helps to extend the function of even a severely limited patient.[33] By interspersing rest periods, the average work load can be held within very acceptable limits.

The MET values of occupational performance tasks are listed in charts such as those found at the end of this chapter. Remember that these charts are bare-bone guides and do not take into consideration a particular person's method of doing the activity in a particular environment. The actual cardiac response to the task must be determined by HR response. Adapted methods of doing activities can be tested by noting if a decrease in HR actually results. Adapted methods should be devised to allow the patient to avoid stressful positions (e.g., working with the arms overhead; working in a squatting position) or motions.[41] Methods to stabilize the thing being worked on will allow the patient to avoid isometric muscle contractions.

Psychological Support

Counseling the patient and his family are important aspects of cardiac rehabilitation.[11] The goals include relief of stress, improvement of self-esteem, and lessening of depression, as well as patient and family education regarding the cardiac condition, risk factors, and physical activity restrictions.

There are two sources of stress for the post-MI patient: (1) the threat to life during the MI and (2) the threat to life-style and livelihood that begins to develop from day 3 onward.[42] The threat to life-style produces anxiety and depression toward which the patient develops coping tactics, especially denial. Denial reduces the anxiety. The protective environment of the hospital also tends to reduce the anxiety. At the time of discharge the name and telephone number of a person to contact should be given to the patient in case he has questions.[41] This also helps to relieve anxiety. However, these do not relieve the depression, which remains "the most formidable problem in cardiac convalescence and rehabilitation."[42] Even if the depression is not noticeable, Hackett and Cassem[42] suggest that it should be assumed to be present and treated. The basis of the depression is fear of invalidism and loss of autonomy or independence; therefore, the best way to increase self-esteem and relieve depression is through activity.[42] Arts and crafts or pleasant recreational activities, chosen according to MET level permitted and the particular person's response, serve these goals. Physical activity and "physical conditioning programs are do's in a sea of don'ts and offer an affirmation of life to the patient."[42]

The educational program should inform the patient and his family about cardiovascular physiology in understandable terms. The patient should be knowl-edgeable about safe activity selection based on MET tables which are given to him in writing. He should understand the limitations of the tables as well and be able to monitor his own response to exercise (pulse). The patient should be instructed about which symptoms are significant, how to recognize them, and what to do about them beyond reporting them immediately. The patient and his family need to learn about CPR and a family member should become certified.

For patients who demonstrated noncompliance with activity restrictions, one program devised that seemed successful has been reported.[43] Information was given concerning the fact that an MI actually meant death to tissue and that rest was required to allow a scar to develop. The patients were given some control by being allowed to establish activity priorities within guidelines, by taking their own pulse to judge response to activity, and by requiring that they assume responsibility for reporting symptoms. Frequent positive reinforcement was offered. The program was task-oriented; that is, the patient was kept busy doing tasks within his capabilities which removed the emphasis from other activities which were restricted.[43]

In another study of the effectiveness of group therapy using an educational approach, it was found that a significantly higher percentage of patients receiving group therapy returned to work than the control patients. Information given was forgotten 1 year later, but the supportive aspects of the group were valued by the patients.[44]

The patient may benefit, postdischarge, from contacting the local chapter of "Mended Hearts," a club for former cardiac patients.

Modification of Risk Behavior. It is fairly well agreed that behavior and life-style may contribute to the onset, and recurrence, of cardiovascular disease.[11] To counteract this, most cardiac rehabilitation programs include identification of risk factors and modification of behavior to reduce risk factors.[11]

The goals of this aspect of the program should be expressed behaviorally and operationally to allow measurement of success. For example, instead of stating the goal as "patient will stop smoking," it is stated more specifically and in smaller increments: "patient will smoke no cigarettes before 10 AM tomorrow." Each successive short-term goal leads the person toward the long-term goal.

Some coronary risk factors cannot be changed. These include family history of cardiac disease, increasing age, or being male. Risk factors which can be changed include smoking, elevated blood pressure, high levels of blood cholesterol, glucose intolerance (diabetes), a stressful life situation, and a sedentary existence.[28] There is also an association between Type A behavior pattern and the incidence of ischemic heart disease.[45, 46] In studies of 3,400 men and 9,097 men it was found to be a highly significant predictor of heart disease and of a second MI, even when the effects of other risk factors were statistically controlled.[46] Obesity is not a direct risk factor but it intensifies other risks: BP, cholesterol, and blood sugar levels.[2]

Table 23.2
GRADY MEMORIAL HOSPITAL 14-STEP PROGRAM—INPATIENT REHABILITATION AFTER MYOCARDIAL INFARCTION[28]

	Exercise	Ward Activity	Educational & Craft Activity
Step 1	Passive ROM to all extremities (5X ea), teach pt *active* plantar and dorsiflexion of ankles to do several times per day.	Feeding self sitting with bed rolled up to 45°, trunk and arms supported by over-bed table.	Initial interview and brief orientation to program.
Step 2	Repeat exercises of Step #1.	1. Feeding self. 2. Partial AM care (washing hands & face, brushing teeth) in bed. 3. Dangle legs on side of bed (1X).	Light recreational activity, such as reading.
Step 3	Active assistive exercise in shoulder flexion and elbow flexion and extension, hip flexion, extension and rotation, knee flexion and extension, rotate feet. (4X ea).	1. Begin sitting in chair for short periods as tolerated, 2X/day. 2. Bathing whole body. 3. Use of bedside commode.	More detailed explanation of program. Continue light recreation.
Step 4	Minimal resistance, lying in bed in above ROM 5X ea. Stiffen all muscles to the count of 2, (3X).	1. Increase sitting 3X/day. 2. Change gown.	Begin explanation of what is an MI. Give pt pamphlets to read, begin craft activity: 1. Leather lacing. 2. Link belt. 3. Hand sewing, embroidery. 4. Copper tooling.

	Exercise	Ward Activity	Educational & Craft Activity
Step 5	Moderate resistance in bed at 45° above ROM exercises, hands on shoulders elbow circling (5X ea arm).	1. Sitting ad lib. 2. Sitting in chair at bedside for meals. 3. Dressing, shaving, combing hair—*sitting down.* 4. Walking in room 2X/day.	Continue education about healing of heart, reasons for early restrictions in activity.
Step 6	1. Further resistive exercises sitting on side of bed, manual resistance of knee extension & flexion, (7X ea movement). 2. Walk distance to nearest bathroom and back, (note if patient needs assistance).	1. Walk to bathroom, ad lib if pt can tolerate. 2. Stand at sink to shave.	Continue craft activity or supply pt with another one. Pt may attend group meetings in a wheelchair for no more than 1 hour.
Step 7	1. Standing warm-up exercises: a. Arms in extension and shoulder abduction, rotate arms together in circles, (circumduction) 5X ea leg. b. Stand on toes, 10X. c. May substitute abduction 5X ea leg. 2. Walk length of ward hall (50 ft) and back to room at average pace.	1. Bathe in tub. 2. Walk to telephone or sit in waiting room (1X/day).	1. May walk to group meetings on the same floor.

Table 23.2—*continued*

	Exercise	Ward Activity	Educational & Craft Activity
Step 8	1. Warm-up exercises: a. Lateral side bending, 5X ea side. b. Trunk twisting, 5X ea side. 2. Walk 1½ lengths of hall, down 1 flight of stairs, take elevator up.	1. Walk to waiting room 2X/day. 2. Stay sitting up most of the day.	Continue all previous craft and educational activities.
Step 9	1. Warm-up exercises: a. Lateral side bending, 10X ea side. b. Slight knee bends 10X with hands on hips. 2. Increase walking distance, walk down 1 flight of stairs.	Continue above activities.	Discussion of work simplification techniques and pacing of activities.
Step 10	1. Warm-up exercises: a. Lateral side bending with 1 lb weight (10X). b. Standing—leg raising leaning against wall, 5X ea. 2. Walk 2 lengths of hall and downstairs, take elevator up.	Continue all of previous ward activities.	1. Pt may walk to OT Clinic & work on craft proj. for ½ hr. a. Copper tooling; b. Woodworking; c. Ceramics; d. Small weaving proj. e. Metal hammering; f. Mosaic tile. 2. Discussion of what exercises pt will do at home.

	Exercise	Ward Activity	Educational & Craft Activity
Step 11	1. Warm-up exercises: a. Lateral side bending with 1 lb weight leaning against wall 10X ea side; b. Standing leg raising 5X ea. c. Trunk twisting with 1 lb weight 5X ea side. 2. Repeat part 2 of Step 10.	Continue all of previous ward activities.	Increase time in OT Clinic to 1 hour.
Step 12	1. Warm-up exercises: a. Lateral side bending with 2 lb weight 10X. b. Standing—leg raising leaning against wall, 10X ea. c. Trunk twisting with 2 lb weight, 10X. 2. Walk down 2 flights of stairs.	Continue all of previous ward activities.	Continue craft activity with increased resistance.
Step 13	Repeat all exercises of Step 12.	Continue all of previous ward activities.	Complete all projects.
Step 14	1. Warm-up exercises: a. Lateral side bending with 2 lb weight 10X ea side. b. Trunk twisting with 2 lb weight 10X ea side. c. Touch toes from sitting position, 10X. 2. Walk up flight of 10 stairs and down.	Continue all of previous ward activities.	Final instructions about home activities.

Table 23.3
APPROXIMATE METABOLIC COST OF ACTIVITIES[a, b]

	Occupational	Recreational
1½–2 METs[c] 4–7 ml O₂/min/kg 2–2½ kcal/min (70 kg person)	Desk work Auto driving[d] Typing Electric calculating machine operation	Standing Walking (strolling 1.6 km or 1 mile/hr) Flying,[d] motorcycling[d] Playing cards[d] Sewing, knitting
2–3 METs 7–11 ml O₂/min/kg 2½–4 kcal/min (70 kg person)	Auto repair Radio, TV repair Janitorial work Typing, manual Bartending	Level walking (3¼ km or 2 miles/hr) Level bicycling (8 km or 5 miles/hr) Riding lawn mower Billiards, bowling Skeet,[d] shuffleboard Woodworking (light) Powerboat driving[d] Golf (power cart) Canoeing (4 km or 2½ miles/hr) Horseback riding (walk) Playing piano and many musical instruments
3–4 METs 11–14 ml O₂/min/kg 4–5 kcal/min (70 kg person)	Brick laying, plastering Wheelbarrow (220-kg or 100-lb load) Machine assembly Trailer-truck in traffic Welding (moderate load) Cleaning windows	Walking (5 km or 3 miles/hr) Cycling (10 km or 6 miles/hr) Horseshoe pitching Volleyball (6-man noncompetitive) Golf (pulling bag cart) Archery Sailing (handling small boat) Fly fishing (standing with waders) Horseback (sitting to trot) Badminton (social doubles) Pushing light power mower Energetic musician
4–5 METs 14–18 ml O₂/min/kg 5–6 kcal/min (70 kg person)	Painting, masonry Paperhanging Light carpentry	Walking (5½ km or 3½ miles/hr) Cycling (13 km or 8 miles/hr) Table tennis Golf (carrying clubs) Dancing (foxtrot) Badminton (singles) Tennis (doubles) Raking leaves Hoeing Many calisthenics
5–6 METs 18–21 ml O₂/min/kg 6–7 kcal/min (70 kg person)	Digging garden Shoveling light earth	Walking (6½ km or 4 miles/hr) Cycling (16 km or 10 miles/hr) Canoeing (6½ km or 4 miles/hr) Horseback ("posting" to trot) Stream fishing (walking in light current in waders) Ice or roller skating (15 km or 9 miles/hr)
6–7 METs 21–25 ml O₂/min/kg 7–8 kcal/min (70 kg person)	Shoveling 10/min (22 kg or 10 lbs)	Walking (8 km or 5 miles/hr) Cycling (17½ km or 11 miles/hr) Badminton (competitive) Tennis (singles) Splitting wood Snow shoveling Hand lawn-mowing Folk (square) dancing Light downhill skiing Ski touring (4 km or 2½ miles/hr) (loose snow) Water skiing

Table 23.3—*continued*

	Occupational	Recreational
7–8 METs 25–28 ml O_2/min/kg 8–10 kcal/min (70 kg person)	Digging ditches Carrying 175 kg or 80 lbs Sawing hardwood	Jogging (8 km or 5 miles/hr) Cycling (19 km or 12 miles/hr) Horseback (gallop) Vigorous downhill skiing Basketball Mountain climbing Ice hockey Canoeing (8 km or 5 miles/hr) Touch football Paddleball
8–9 METs 28–32 ml O_2/min/kg 10–11 kcal/min (70 kg person)	Shoveling 10/min (31 kg or 14 lbs)	Running (9 km or 5½ miles/hr) Cycling (21 km or 13 miles/hr) Ski touring (6½ km or 4 miles/hr) (loose snow) Squash (social) Handball (social) Fencing Basketball (vigorous)

10 plus METs
32 plus ml O_2/min/kg
11 plus kcal/min (70 kg person)
	Shoveling 10/min (35 kg or 16 lbs)	Running
		  6 mph = 10 METs
		  7 mph = 11½ METs
		  8 mph = 13½ METs
		  9 mph = 15 METs
		  10 mph = 17 METs
		Ski touring (8 + km or 5 + miles/hr) (loose snow)
		Handball (competitive)
		Squash (competitive)

[a] Includes resting metabolic needs.
[b] Reprinted with permission from S. M. Fox *et al. Journal of the American Heart Association XLI* (4), 1972.
[c] 1 MET is the energy expenditure at rest, equivalent to approximately 3.5 ml O_2/kg body weight/minute.
[d] A major excess metabolic increase may occur due to excitement, anxiety, or impatience in some of these activities, and a physician must assess his patient's psychological reactivity.

Each risk factor increases the probability of developing coronary heart disease two to three times; if the person has more than one risk factor, the probability multiplies.[2] If hypertension and smoking are eliminated, the risk is substantially reduced. Hypertension is decreased by medication, low salt diet, weight loss, decreased life stress, relaxation, and conditioning exercise[2] within limits set by functional capacity.

The occupational therapist can help the patient to alter certain risk factors: smoking, reaction to life stresses, and coronary-prone behavior pattern or Type A personality[46] described by Rosenman and Friedman.

A behavior modification program in which the goals are clearly stated in small, achievable steps and positive reinforcement is offered for successes can be used to stop or decrease smoking. This program needs to be accompanied by education concerning the physiology of smoking presented using audiovisual materials. A group therapy approach in which the members of the group offer support to each other is useful.

Modern daily life consists of many stresses and strains on an individual due to frustrations. Group discussions can address alternate ways of reacting or handling situations. Putting the particular incident into perspective by asking "Is this worth dying for?"[47]

may help the person develop healthier habits of reacting. Drs. Eliot and Forker are reported to also suggest additional ways of coping with stress, some of which would provide topics for group discussion and individual reflection: (1) establish priorties; (2) identify objective, realistic, and obtainable goals; (3) try to modify a hard driving personality; (4) reduce frequency of stressful life change events; and (5) learn a relaxation technique and practice it daily.[47]

The Type A personality is characterized by free-floating hostility and a sense of time urgency.[45] It seems to be unmodifiable in persons who are at risk but who have not yet suffered an MI for several reasons, but primarily because it is a valued style and is seen as the basis for success.[45] Post-MI patients are ready to believe that the stress of trying to do too much in too little time was a risk factor and are ready for treatment.[45] The therapist needs to be a Type B personality or at least a Type A who is actively modifying her own behavior. The patient should trust and admire the therapist.[45]

Before treatment begins, it is necessary to determine if both components of the Type A personality are present and the degree of severity of each.[45] This is determined by a structured interview which provides the opportunity to observe the psychomotor manifestations, which are more reliable indicators than verbal responses.[45, 46, 48] The Behavior Pattern Interview relies on the interviewer's ability to make clinical judgments.[46] The interrater reliability of this test is $r = .85$ (content) and $r = .50$ (style).[46]

Those persons who are severely hostile and also exhibit time urgency, or whose general intelligence is so low that they cannot comprehend abstractions or symbolism are poor candidates for treatment.[45] Good candidates are older persons who exhibit more time urgency than hostility, who developed the behavior secondary to their milieu, who suspect their way of living needs to be changed, and who are nonegocentric.[45]

Treatment includes several facets, as described by Friedman.[45] The milieu is examined to learn to avoid or reinterpret the meaning, relevance, and significance of the stressful factors. The person learns to develop interests in things, events, and other persons outside of his own prime interests.

Change is motivated in several ways. The fact that neither time urgency nor free-floating hostility were responsible for success and may in fact have been the bases for failures is pointed out. The valuable facets of the personality that are lost in response to Type A behavior, such as leisurely participation and enjoyment of cultural and social activities, are also pointed out. The need to redevelop value for friendship, affection, and joy is paramount to successful treatment. The person needs to learn to restructure daily events so there is enough time to do the important tasks, to eliminate the others, and to value rest time without feelings of guilt. The person needs to learn to eliminate the free-floating hostility by recognizing it, avoiding circumstances which provoke it, and substituting acts of love and affection to fill the vacuum of emotion left by not getting angry. The new behaviors need to be practiced until learned.

Group therapy has been found helpful in modifying coronary-prone behavior, although other risk factors were not significantly altered.[44]

Vocational/Recreational Counseling

Return to work is psychologically helpful to decrease depression and anxiety concerning physical status, family role, and finances. Return to certain jobs may actually require less energy expenditure than many self-care activities.[16]

The MET level of a patient's work and recreational activities can be judged in general from MET charts. If doubt exists about the patient's ability or safety to do these activities, actual response should be measured. The occupational therapist should offer a simulated work situation to test for readiness to return to previous type of work, to determine the need for and usefulness of adapted methods and/or equipment to modify the energy demands, and to help the patient improve his work skill since increased skill results in decreased stress.[49]

Many factors other than intensity stress the heart.

One factor would be the need to use isometric contraction of small muscles, such as is required for grasp. Adapted methods that transfer the demand to larger muscles or utilize devices to provide stabilization should be used. The patient also needs to be helped to develop a work/rest schedule[49] that can be adhered to at his place of employment.

Other factors which may prevent the patient from returning to the particular job he held previously or doing the recreational activity of choice are competitive situations, environmental heat or humidity or very cold temperature, stressful relationships or situations, highly time-oriented schedules, lifting or pushing heavy loads, and lack of opportunity to relax after eating. He needs to be counseled regarding the risks these factors offer and directed toward less stressful work and/or play.

The self-employed individual is more likely to return to work sooner than workers.[50] There is not a good correlation between return to work and physical capability[50] across subjects studied. After 3 months, post-MI patients are usually capable of 8 to 9 METs yet only 50 to 75% return to work.[51] Psychotherapy and laboratory experiences in the occupational therapy clinic may help the patient overcome his fear of returning to work or point out secondary gains he is receiving from his condition.

MYOCARDIAL INFARCTION PROGRAM AT GRADY MEMORIAL HOSPITAL, ATLANTA, GEORGIA[28]

A 14-step program carried out under direct orders of the physician starts as the patient progresses through early recovery phases following a MI. There are four recovery phases described in this program as follows. The patient is progressed according to his particular response to activity at each step or phase.

Phase I—Coronary Care Unit

Low energy level physical activities are begun, such as those of steps 1 to 3 (see Table 23.2).

Phase II—Remainder of Hospitalization

The average hospitalization following uncomplicated MI is 21 days. Activity level is gradually increased with the goal of independent self-care, sitting, and graded rhythmic exercises progressing to walking and finally stair climbing. Patient and family education is an important part of the program. Steps 4 to 14 of the inpatient program (Table 23.2) are carried out.

Phase III—Convalescent Phase

The patient returns home and follows a program to progressively increase physical activity to a level which will permit return to work by the 8th to 12th week after a MI. Activities include light housework, desk work, and walking, which is graded in distance and speed to approximately 1 to 2 miles a day at a rate of 3 miles per hour.

Table 23.4
MINIMAL CARDIAC ACTIVITY[a]

Activity	Position	METS
Leather belt assembly	Sitting at table	1.25
Leather stamping	Sitting at table	1.35
Leather tooling	Sitting at table	1.30
Listening to radio	Sitting in easy chair	1.40
Bench assembly, light	Sitting at bench	1.40
Leather lacing	Sitting at table	1.45
Chip carving	Sitting at table	1.60

[a] Reprinted with permission from F. J. Kottke.[15]

Table 23.5
LIGHT CARDIAC ACTIVITY[a]

Activity	Position	METS
Eating	Sitting	1.50
Sewing	Sitting	1.60
Clerical work	Sitting	1.60
Setting type	Standing	1.60
Getting out of and into bed	Bed to chair	1.65
Leather carving	Sitting on chair	1.70
Weaving, table loom	Sitting on stool	1.70
Clerical work	Standing	1.80
Writing	Sitting	2.00
Typing	Sitting on chair	2.00
Bimanual activity test sanding, 50 strokes/min	Sitting on chair	2.00
Weaving, floor loom	Sitting on bench	2.10
Metal work, hammer	Standing	2.15
Printing, platen press	Standing	2.30
Bench assembly, moderate	Sitting	2.35
Hanging clothes on line	Standing—stooping	2.40

[a] Reprinted with permission from F. J. Kottke.[15]

Table 23.6
MODERATE CARDIAC ACTIVITY[a]

Activity	Position	METS
Playing piano		2.50
Dressing, undressing		2.50–3.50
Sawing, jeweler's saw	Sitting	1.90
Sawing, hack saw	Standing	2.55
Driving car		2.80
Bicycling, slowly		2.90
Preparing meals		3.00
Weight lifting, 10 lb lifted 15 in., 46/min	Sitting	2.80
Walking, 2.0 mph		3.20
Handsawing, wood	Standing	3.50
Warm shower		3.50

[a] Reprinted with permission from F. J. Kottke.[15]

Table 23.7
HEAVY AND SEVERE CARDIAC ACTIVITY[a]

Activity	Position	METS
Bowel movement	Toilet	3.60
Bowel movement	Bedpan	4.70
Making beds	Standing	3.90
Hot shower	Standing	4.20
Walking fast (3.5 mph)		5.00
Descending stairs		5.20
Scrubbing floor	Kneeling	5.30
Master, two-step climbing test		5.70
Weight lifting, 10–20 lb lifted 36 in., 15/min		6.50
Bicycling, fast		6.90
Running		7.40
Mowing lawn		7.70
Climbing stairs		9.00

[a] Reprinted with permission from F. J. Kottke.[15]

Phase IV—Recovery and Maintenance

The patient returns to work at a suitable occupational or activity level. Further increase in cardiac function is encouraged by participation in community physical fitness programs. The goals of this period are to enhance function, decrease risk factors, and prevent recurrence of the disease.

Reference

1. Oldridge, N. B. Compliance of post myocardial infarction patients to exercise programs. *Med. Sci. Sports*, *11*(4): 373–375, 1979.
2. Levy, R. L. *Heart Attacks*. Bethesda, Md.: National Institutes of Health publication no. 80-1803, 1980.
3. Thomas, C. L. (ed) *Taber's Cyclopedic Medical Dictionary*, 12th ed. Philadelphia: F.A. Davis, 1973.
4. Hartley, H. Lecture to seminar in Cardiac Rehabilitation, Boston University, June, 1978.
5. Dehn, M. M., and Mullins, C. B. Physiologic effects and importance of exercise in patients with coronary artery disease. *Cardiovasc. Med.*, (April): 365–385, 387, 1977.
6. Kattus, A. A., Chairman. The Committee on Exercise. *Exercise Testing and Training of Apparently Healthy Individuals: A Handbook for Physicians*. New York: American Heart Association, 1972.
7. New York Heart Association. *Diseases of the Heart and Blood Vessels—Nomenclature and Criteria for Diagnosis*, 6th ed. Boston: Little, Brown, 1964.
8. Kavanagh, T., and Shephard, R. J. Sexual activity after myocardial infarction. *Can. Med. J.*, *116*: 1250–1253, 1977.
9. Grant, A., and Cohen, B. S. Acute myocardial infarction: Effect of a rehabilitation program on length of hospitalization and functional status at discharge. *Arch. Phys. Med. Rehabil.*, *54*(5): 201–206, 1973.
10. Siegel, G. H. Informed consent in exercise testing and training programs (appendix A). In *Exercise Testing and Training of Individuals with Heart Disease or at High Risk for its Development: A Handbook for Physicians*, edited by A. A. Kattus. Dallas: American Heart Association, 1975.
11. Erb, B. D., Fletcher, G. F., and Sheffield, T. L. AHA committee report: Standards for cardiovascular exercise treatment programs. *Circulation*, *59*: 1084A–1090A, 1979.
12. Gordan, A. S., *et al.* American Heart Association committee on cardiopulmonary resuscitation and emergency cardiac care.

Standards for cardiopulmonary resuscitation (CPR) and emergency cardiac care (ECC). *J.A.M.A.*, 227(Suppl.)(7): 1974.

13. Committee on Emergency Cardiac Care. *CPR in Basic Life Support.* New York: American Heart Association, 1974.

14. Mead, W. F. Exercise rehabilitation after myocardial infarction. *Am. Fam. Phys.*, 15(March): 121–125, 1977.

15. Kottke, F. J. Common cardiovascular problems in rehabilitation. In *Handbook of Physical Medicine and Rehabilitation*, edited by F. H. Krusen, F. J. Kottke, and P. M. Ellwood. Philadelphia: W. B. Saunders, 1971.

16. Cohen, B. S. A program for rehabilitation after acute myocardial infarction. *South. Med. J.*, 68(2): 145–148, 1975.

17. Ellestad, M. H. *Stress Testing: Principles and Practice.* Philadelphia: F. A. Davis, 1976.

18. American College of Sports Medicine. *Guidelines for Graded Exercise Testing and Exercise Prescription.* Philadelphia: Lea & Febiger, 1976.

19. Erb, B. D. *Physician's Handbook for Evaluation of Cardiovascular and Physical Fitness*, 2nd ed. Nashville: Tennessee Heart Association, 1972.

20. Fletcher, G. F., and Cantwell, J. D. *Exercise and Coronary Heart Disease: Role in Prevention, Diagnosis and Treatment*, 2nd ed. Springfield, IL: Charles C Thomas, 1979.

21. Day, W. Lecture to seminar in Cardiac Rehabilitation, Boston University, June, 1978.

22. Lunsford, B. R. Heart rate: A clinical indicator of endurance. *Phys. Ther.*, 58(6): 705–709, 1978.

23. Menard, R. H. *Introduction to Arrhythmia Recognition.* San Francisco: California Heart Association, 1968.

24. Littmann, D. *Examination of the Heart. Part Five: The Electrocardiogram.* New York: American Heart Association, 1973.

25. Winsor, T. The electrocardiogram in myocardial infarction. In *Clinical Symposia.* Summit, N.J.: Ciba Pharmaceutical Company, Medical Education Division, 1968.

26. Dubin, D. *Rapid Interpretation of EKG's*, 3rd ed. Tampa, Fla. COVER Publishing Co., 1974.

27. Margolis, J. R., and Wagner, G. S. *Coronary Care: Arrhythmias in Acute Myocardial Infarction.* Dallas: American Heart Association, 1976.

28. Wenger, N. *Rehabilitation after Myocardial Infarction.* New York: American Heart Association, 1973.

29. Schang, S. J., and Pepine, C. J. Transient asymptomatic S-T segment depression during daily activity. *Am. J. Cardiol.*, 39(3): 396–402, 1977.

30. Siegal, G. H. Legal aspects of informed consent, stress testing, and exercise programs. In *Exercise Testing and Training in Coronary Heart Disease*, edited by J. Naughton and H. K. Hellerstein. New York: Academic Press, 1973.

31. Cumming, G. R. Comparison of treadmill and bicycle ergometer exercise in middle-aged males. *Am. Heart J.*, 93: 261, 1977.

32. Sutton, J. Exercise responses in post myocardial infarction patients. *Med. Sci. Sports*, 11(4): 366–367, 1979.

33. Ogden, L. D. Activity guidelines for early subacute and high-risk cardiac patients. *Am. J. Occup. Ther.*, 33(5): 291–298, 1979.

34. Ogden, L. D. Hands on: Cardiac rehabilitation. Guidelines for analysis and testing of activities of daily living with cardiac patients. *Physical Disabilities Specialty Section Newsletter* (of the American Occupational Therapy Association), 3(4): 1, 3, 1980.

35. Corcoran, P. J. Energy expenditure during ambulation. In *Physiological Basis of Rehabilitation Medicine*, edited by J. A. Downey and R. C. Darling. Philadelphia: W. B. Saunders, 1971.

36. Semmler, C., and Semmler, M. Counseling the coronary patient. *Am. J. Occup. Ther.*, 28(10): 609–614, 1974.

37. Ewing, D. J., Kerr, F., Irving, J. B., and Muir, A. L. Weight carrying after myocardial infarction. *Lancet*, 1(May 17): 1113–1114, 1975.

38. Ramos, M. U., et al. Cardiovascular effects of spread of excitation during prolonged isometric exercise. *Arch. Phys. Med. Rehabil.*, 54(11): 496–504, 1974.

39. Stein, R. A. The effect of exercise training on heart rate during coitus in the post myocardial infarction patient. *Circulation*, 55(5): 738–740, 1977.

40. Tobis, J. Sex counseling for postmyocardial infarction patients. *West. J. Med.*, 131(2): 133–134, 1979.

41. *Handbook for Participants*, Cardiac rehabilitation postgraduate course, University of Texas Medical Branch, 1977.

42. Hackett, T. P., and Cassem, N. H. Psychological adaptation to convalescence in myocardial infarction patients. In *Exercise Testing and Training in Coronary Heart Disease*, edited by J. Naughton and H. K. Hellerstein. New York: Academic Press, 1973.

43. Baile, W. F., and Engel, B. T. A behavioral strategy for promoting treatment compliance following myocardial infarction. *Psychosom. Med.*, 40(5): 413–419, 1978.

44. Rahe, R. H., Ward, H. W., and Hayes, V. Brief group therapy in myocardial infarction rehabilitation: Three- to four-year follow-up of a controlled trial. *Psychosom. Med.*, 41(3): 229–242, 1979.

45. Friedman, M. The modification of type A behavior in post-infarction patients. *Am. Heart. J.*, 97: 551–560, 1979.

46. Rowland, K. F., and Sokol, B. A review of research examining the coronary-prone behavior pattern. *J. Hum. Stress*, 3(September): 26–33, 1977.

47. Shearer, L. Stress and strain. *Parade*, December 19: 4, 1976.

48. Friedman, E. H., and Hellerstein, H. K. Influence of psychosocial factors on coronary risk adaptation to a physical fitness evaluation program. In *Exercise Testing and Training in Coronary Heart Disease*, edited by J. Naughton and H. K. Hellerstein. New York: Academic Press, 1973.

49. Brinkley, S. B. The use of exercise test results in vocational rehabilitation of cardiac clients. In *Exercise Testing and Training in Coronary Heart Disease*, edited by J. Naughton and H. K. Hellerstein. New York: Academic Press, 1973.

50. Krasemann, E. O., and Jungmann, H. Return to work after myocardial infarction. *Cardiology*, 64(3): 190–196, 1979.

51. Muir, J. R. The Rehabilitation of cardiac patients. *Proc. R. Soc. Med.*, 70(September): 655–656, 1977.

Supplementary Reading

Astrand, P-O, and Rodahl, K. *Textbook of Work Physiology*, New York: McGraw-Hill, 1970.

Dehn, M. M. Rehabilitation of the cardiac patient: The effects of exercise. *Am. J. Nurs.*, 80(March): 435–440, 1980.

Frank, K. A., Heller, S. S., and Kornfeld, D. S. Psychological intervention in coronary heart disease: A review. *Gen. Hosp. Psychiatry*, 1(1): 18–23, 1979.

Friedman, M., and Rosenman, R. H. *Type A Behavior and Your Heart.* Greenwich, Conn.: Fawcett Publications, 1974.

Gilbert, D. Energy expenditures for the disabled homemaker: Review of studies. *Am. J. Occup. Ther.*, 19(6): 321–328, 1965.

Hellerstein, H. K., Hirsch, E. Z., Ader, R., Greenblott, N., and Siegel, M. Principles of exercise prescription: For normals and cardiac subjects. In *Exercise Testing and Exercise Training in Coronary Heart Disease*, edited by J. P. Naughton and H. K. Hellerstein. New York: Academic Press, 1973.

Hendrickson, D., Anderson, J., and Gordon, E. A physiological approach to the regulation of activity in the cardiac convalescent. *Am. J. Occup. Ther.*, 14(6): 296, 1960.

Hollander, L. L. *Hypertension: Manual for Patients.* Boston: Massachusetts Rehabilitation Hospital, 1977.

Hollander, L. L. *Smoke Gets in Your Eyes!* Boston: Massachusetts Rehabilitation Hospital, 1977.

Hollander, L. L. *Take Heart!* Boston: Massachusetts Rehabilitation Hospital, 1977.

Huntley, N., and Mullvain, M. A. (eds.) *Basics of Cardiac Rehabilitation.* Minneapolis: Minnesota Occupational Therapy Association Cardiac Care Special Interest Group, 1978.

Mann, G. V. Diet-heart: End of an era. *N. Engl. J. Med.*, September 22: 644–649, 1977.

Mesenbourg, B., Daniewicz, C., and Schoening, H. Occupational therapy in coronary rehabilitation. *Am. J. Occup. Ther.*, 24(6): 428–431, 1970.

Passmore, R., et al. *Exercise Equivalents.* Denver: Colorado Heart

Association, Cardiac Reconditioning and Work Evaluation Unit.

Quiggle, A. B., Kottke, F. J., and Magney, J. Metabolic requirements of occupational therapy procedures. *Arch. Phys. Med. Rehabil.,* *35*(9): 567–572, 1954.

Scherlis, S., *et al.* Report of the Committee on Stress: Strain and heart disease, American Heart Association. *Circulation, 55*(5), 1977.

Weidman, W. H., *et al. Recreational and Occupational Recommendations for Use by Physicians Counseling Young Patients with Heart Disease.* Dallas: American Heart Association, 1971.

Zohman, L. R., and Tobis, J. S. *Cardiac Rehabilitation.* New York: Grune & Stratton, 1970.

chapter

24

Amputation and Prosthetics

Anne G. Fisher, M.S., OTR

Among the adult population can be found three groups of amputees: (1) individuals born with congenital limb deficiencies; (2) individuals with acquired amputations resulting from trauma; and (3) individuals with acquired amputations who have undergone secondary amputation surgery as part of the overall management of a primary disease or disorder.

The juvenile amputee (the child with a congenital limb deficiency or an acquired amputation sustained during childhood) is beyond the scope of this chapter. Juvenile amputees represent approximately 6% of the total amputee population. Because they are fitted and trained with prostheses and/or receive ADL training as children, their management is highly specialized and best carried out in one of the many regional juvenile amputee centers whose staff is trained and experienced in their care. By the time the juvenile amputee reaches adulthood, the need for services provided by the occupational therapist, beyond the occasional checkout of a new prosthesis, is rare.

Therefore, this chapter will be limited to a discussion of occupational therapy procedures for the individual with an acquired amputation sustained in adulthood. Principles of upper extremity preprosthetic treatment and prosthetic fitting and training will be emphasized. The role of occupational therapy in the treatment of lower extremity amputees and partial hand amputations will also be discussed.

LEVELS OF AMPUTATION[1-3]

Generally, diagnosis is descriptive and is based upon the level of amputation. An amputation which involves removal of part or all of the clavicle and scapula along with the upper limb is a forequarter amputation. When an amputation occurs at a joint, it is considered a

disarticulation; if the clavicle and scapula are left intact but the entire humerus is removed, the level of amputation is a shoulder disarticulation. When the amputation is through the humerus, the level is referred to as above-elbow. Amputation at the elbow is an elbow disarticulation, and if it is through the radius and ulna, the amputation is referred to as below-elbow. Above- and below-elbow amputations are further described as being very short, short, standard, or long, depending upon the relative length of the stump (residual limb). An amputation at the level of the wrist is a wrist disarticulation and, if through the metacarpals, the amputation is referred to as transmetacarpal. Transmetacarpal amputations as well as more distal amputations of the hand are generally referred to as partial hand amputations.

Some clinics do not adhere rigidly to the above criteria, especially when the amputation is near but not through the joint. In this instance, the diagnosis is based upon the type of prosthesis which is fitted. Hence, a very high above-elbow amputee whose stump is too short to be fitted with an above-elbow prosthesis may be diagnosed as a shoulder disarticulation. Even more commonly, the individual with an amputation just proximal to the elbow or the wrist and who is fitted with an elbow disarticulation or wrist disarticulation type prosthesis is diagnosed accordingly.

PROSTHETIC COMPONENTS[1, 3-5]

Terminal Devices

There are two categories of terminal devices: the hook and the hand. Dorrance voluntary opening split hooks are the most commonly fitted hook (Fig. 24.1). Adult hook sizes are 5, 6, and 7. The 5, 5X, and 5XA all have canted fingers which are designed to provide

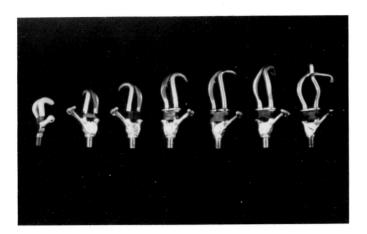

three-point prehension when grasping large, round objects. The A specifies that the hook is aluminum rather than steel, and the X specifies that the hook fingers are Neoprene lined. The 555 has lyre shaped fingers, is aluminum and is Neoprene lined. While the 555 is sometimes called the "housewife" hook, the 5XA is functionally superior because of the canted fingers (Fig. 24.2). Steel hooks and those without Neoprene lining are prescribed for heavy duty usage. As the aluminum hooks are lighter in weight, they are preferred by high level amputees. The 6, 7, and 7LO are different from other Dorrance hooks in that the fingers are straight and the hook is L-shaped. They are all stainless steel and are designed for heavy duty use. The 7 has two chucks, a nail holder, and a knife holder for holding objects of various shapes. The 7LO is identical, except that the opening between the hook fingers is larger to accommodate shovel or broom handles. The 6 is also like the 7, except that it has a locking mechanism which locks the fingers in the closed position.

The length of the hook from the base (wrist unit) to the tip of the hook fingers should be equal to or slightly longer than the distance from the wrist to the tip of the thumb on the sound hand (Fig. 24.3). While smaller hook sizes are available, they should not be fitted to adults, as their smaller size limits the size of the object which can be grasped.

Dorrance voluntary opening hands, like Dorrance voluntary opening hooks, are the type of hand most frequently fitted. As a voluntary opening device, tension on the control cable results in the index and middle fingers extending as the thumb abducts. (While voluntary closing devices, including the Sierra APRL hook and the APRL hand, had potential functional advantages, they were proven to be mechanically unreliable and are no longer fitted in most clinics.) The hand should be covered with a cosmetic glove of a color and style to match the characteristics of the patient's sound hand. The Dorrance hand comes in several sizes; the circumference of the hand at the metacarpophalangeal joints should be approximately ¼ inch less than the circumference of the sound hand (Fig. 24.4).

The hook is lighter in weight and more functional

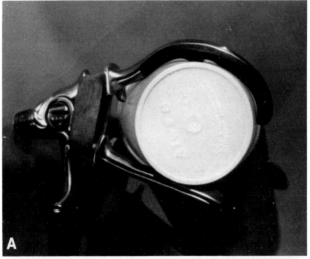

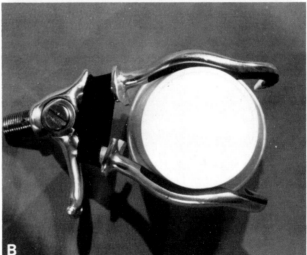

Figure 24.2 *A.* The canted fingers on the 5XA permit stable grasp of the inverted cup. *B.* The 555 only permits unstable two-point grasp.

than the hand and is recommended for all but social occasions when the amputee may prefer to wear the hand for cosmetic purposes. The fingers of the hand are too large for precision grasp, the size of objects

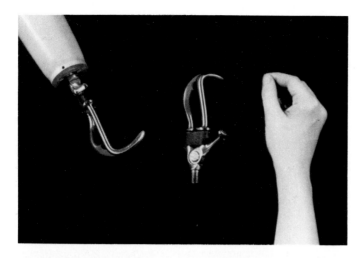

Figure 24.3 The hook correctly inserted into the wrist unit (*left*) and correct sizing of the hook when compared to the sound hand (*right*).

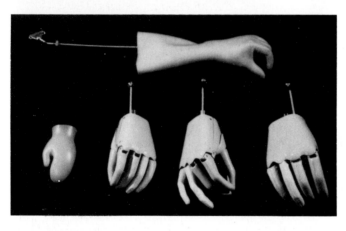

Figure 24.4 Infant passive mitt and voluntary opening hands, with and without cosmetic glove, in adult and child sizes.

which can be grasped is limited, and the fingers are oriented such that excessive internal rotation and abduction of the shoulder are required to grasp objects from the table surface. Furthermore, the cosmetic glove is subject to discoloration and staining from sunlight, clothing dyes, and foods and is easily cut or torn if the hand is allowed to bang against hard surfaces.

The Otto Bock voluntary opening hand is of endoskeletal design and as such seems to be less subject to damage to the glove. While functionally similar to the Dorrance hand, many patients prefer the appearance of the Otto Bock hand.

Otto Bock also manufactures an electric hand which is typically myoelectrically controlled, but can also be switch controlled. Also available is the United States Manufacturing/Fidelity Electronics/VANU electric hand. The advantages and disadvantages of electrically powered devices are discussed below.

Wrist Units

The wrist unit serves as a source of attachment for the terminal device; rotation of the terminal device in the wrist unit provides for pronation or supination of the terminal device. Wrist units are round or oval; the oval wrist unit is designed for use with wrist disarticulation type prostheses. Round units are preferred when a hand is worn, as the cosmetic glove is less

likely to bind when the hand is pronated or supinated. Otherwise, the shape is optional and varies from clinic to clinic.

Constant friction wrist units have set screws to adjust the amount of resistance to rotation of the terminal device. The amount of friction remains constant and can be adjusted by the amputee. Friction should be loose enough to allow the amputee to rotate the terminal device but tight enough to prevent terminal device rotation upon opening.

The friction on manual friction wrist units is determined by how far the terminal device is screwed into the wrist. The more the terminal device is screwed into the wrist, the more resistance is produced as a result of compression of a rubber washer. While satisfactory for some patients, most amputees dislike this type of unit, as rotation of the terminal device as little as 90° can reduce the friction so far as to result in the terminal device rotating when tension is applied to the control cable for opening.

Wrist units are also available which permit quicker interchange from hook to hand when the amputee frequently changes the type of terminal device worn. These units also provide locking of the terminal device to prevent rotation when lifting heavy objects; however, some amputees find that they do not withstand heavy duty usage.

Wrist units which permit flexion of the wrist are

useful for higher level bilateral amputees, as they allow the amputee to reach the midline of the body in order to manage front zippers and buttons during dressing and toileting. Those without levers which must be depressed to unlock the unit to change the amount of flexion are easier for the bilateral amputee to manage.

Forearm

The forearm component of the wrist disarticulation or below-elbow type prosthesis is the socket. The socket is of a standard type on the long below-elbow and wrist disarticulation type prostheses. The socket on the short below-elbow is either preflexed or self suspended (Muenster or NU supracondylar type). Myoelectric below-elbow prostheses have self-suspended sockets.

The forearm component of an elbow disarticulation, above-elbow, or shoulder disarticulation type prosthesis is the forearm shell.

Elbow

Standard wrist disarticulation, standard below-elbow, and preflexed below-elbow type prostheses have flexible, semirigid or rigid hinges which attach the forearm socket to the triceps pad and harness. Rigid hinges (metal) provide stability when the below-elbow stump is very short. Flexible hinges (Dacron tape or leather) are used with longer stumps, as they permit pronation and supination. Semirigid hinges are made of double-thickness Dacron tape or polyethylene and attach to the distal triceps pad and proximal socket. As they are very short, they function as rigid hinges.

The standard elbow unit on the elbow disarticulation type prosthesis is the outside locking elbow. As the lock is located outside on the medial aspect of the humeral socket, the axis of rotation of the elbow is at the same level as the sound arm. The positive locking (inside) elbow is incorporated into the prosthesis distal to the humeral socket. The turntable which is part of the unit permits the amputee to preposition the prosthesis in internal or external rotation. This elbow unit is better for heavy duty use. While it is standard on above-elbow and shoulder disarticulation type prostheses, its use on the elbow disarticulation or very long above-elbow type prostheses results in the prosthetic elbow center being lower than the sound elbow. In addition to being undesirable cosmetically, the longer than normal humeral length requires that the amputee abduct excessively to use the prosthesis in bilateral table top activities.

Commercially available electric elbows include the Liberty Mutual "Boston Arm" myoelectric elbow and the United States Manufacturing/Fidelity/VANU electric elbows. These are typically used in conjunction with electric hands; they are discussed in more detail below.

Upper Arm Component

The upper arm component of the standard below-elbow, preflexed below-elbow, and wrist disarticulation types of prostheses is the triceps pad. The triceps pad provides a source of attachment for the cable housing and the harness from which the prosthesis suspends.

The upper arm component of the elbow disarticulation and above-elbow type prostheses is the socket. The shoulder disarticulation type prosthesis upper arm component is the humeral section.

Shoulder

The inclusion of a shoulder joint is only necessary in shoulder disarticulation type prostheses. While some clinics still use rigid shoulder joints or abduction hinges, a shoulder joint which permits flexion or extension, as well as abduction or adduction, is a must if the amputee is going to realize any functional benefit from the prosthesis.

Harness/Suspension and Control System

The wrist disarticulation, standard, and preflexed below-elbow prostheses are suspended by standard below-elbow figure of eight harnesses (Fig. 24.5). The harness also provides a source of operation of the terminal device through the single control system. Single control system means that there is only one control cable, whose only purpose is to operate the terminal device.

Like other below-elbow type prostheses, self-suspended below-elbow type prostheses have single control systems. However, because the suspension is provided by the socket, a figure of nine harness is used as the source of operation of the terminal device.

Elbow disarticulation and above-elbow type prostheses are suspended by standard above-elbow figure of eight harnesses. The harness differs from the below-elbow type, as it must provide sources of control of both the elbow lock and the terminal device-forearm lift through a dual control system (Fig. 24.6).

The suspension of the shoulder disarticulation type prosthesis is provided by the shoulder cap (socket) and a chest strap. While a dual control system is conventional, the source of control varies. Usually, an axilla loop around the contralateral shoulder provides the source of control of the terminal device-forearm lift while the cable for control of the elbow lock is incorporated into the anterior portion of the chest strap.

A summary of prosthetic components according to amputation level is shown in Table 24.1.

REHABILITATION OF THE UPPER EXTREMITY AMPUTEE

The goal of rehabilitation of the amputee is independence in occupational performance tasks. Ideally, prosthetic fitting and training eliminates the need to modify the environment and enables the amputee to function more normally within it. Success, in terms of high levels of prosthetic skill and awareness, is dependent upon a comprehensive rehabilitation program which includes the fitting of a comfortable, mechanically sound prosthesis and thorough prosthetic train-

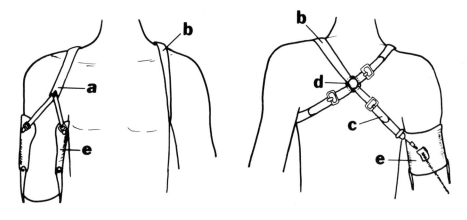

Figure 24.5 Anterior and posterior views of the standard below-elbow figure of eight harness: (*a*) anterior support strap and inverted "Y"; (*b*) axilla loop; (*c*) control attachment strap; (*d*) NU ring; and (*e*) triceps pad.

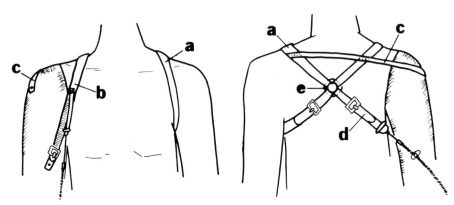

Figure 24.6 Anterior and posterior views of the standard above-elbow figure of eight harness. *a.* axilla loop; *b.* anterior suspensor and elbow lock control strap; *c.* lateral suspensor; *d.* control attachment strap; and *e.* NU ring.

ing. The stages of the rehabilitation process are illustrated in Fig. 24.7.

Preprosthetic Care and Early Postsurgical Fitting[1-4, 6, 7]

As soon as possible following surgery, the occupational therapist should initiate a program to regain and/or maintain muscle strength and range of motion of all remaining joints. If the amputation results in loss of the preferred hand, a program to increase one-handed skill and coordination of the nonpreferred hand is also necessary. At best, the prosthesis can only act as an assistive extremity; the remaining limb must assume the role of the preferred hand.

Bandaging the stump with elastic bandages will help to control edema and shape the stump in preparation for prosthetic fitting. Elastic bandages are applied so that the pressure is greatest distally and gradually decreases proximally. The bandages should not be fully stretched when applied, as this can result in wrapping too tightly or unevenly, such that the distal end of the stump swells. Bandaging too loosely results in the bandage not staying in place. The proper technique for upper extremity wrapping is shown in Figures 24.8 to 24.10. As wrapping continues until sufficient stump shrinkage has occurred for fitting with a definitive prosthesis (about 6 to 8 weeks), and the stump must be rewrapped three to four times daily, the amputee and family should be instructed in proper wrapping techniques.

In an attempt to (1) decrease the 50% or better rejection rate of upper extremity prostheses, (2) control edema and accelerate stump shaping, and (3) decrease the period of time the amputee is without a prosthesis to encourage the earlier development of new bilateral patterns using the prosthesis, some centers are trying early postsurgical fitting of upper extremity amputees. This technique involves the fitting of a rigid plaster dressing or temporary prosthesis worn over the surgical dressing which has incorporated into it all of the appropriate prosthetic components necessary to begin prosthetic training. Prosthetic training can thereby begin within days after surgery and does not have to wait until the definitive prosthesis has been fabricated. Prosthetic training with an early postsurgical fitting is carried out in the same manner as with a definitive prosthesis. However, the usual preprosthetic program described above may need to be modified. The temporary prosthesis provides a source of exercise which may be sufficient to maintain and/or increase range of motion and strength. Furthermore, because the temporary prosthesis controls edema, the need for stump bandaging may be reduced or eliminated.

Whether the amputee has conventional preprosthetic care or has an early postsurgical fitting, the program goals and techniques regarding range of motion, strength, coordination, and one-handed skill are based upon the evaluations and treatment techniques discussed in Chapters 7, 8, and 26.

Table 24.1
SUMMARY OF CONVENTIONAL PROSTHETIC COMPONENTS ACCORDING TO AMPUTATION LEVEL

Component		Wrist Disarticulation	Standard Below-Elbow	Short Below-Elbow (Conventional)	Short Below-Elbow (Self-Suspended)	Elbow Disarticulation	Above-Elbow	Shoulder Disarticulation and Forequarter
Terminal device		Hook	→					→
		Hand	→					→
Wrist	Shape	Oval	→					→
		Round	→					→
	Type	Constant friction	Constant friction / Manual friction / Quick disconnect					→
Forearm		Wrist disarticulation type socket	Standard below-elbow socket	Pre-flexed below-elbow socket	Muenster or NU supracondylar below-elbow socket	Forearm shell	→	→
Elbow		Flexible hinges	Flexible or semirigid hinges	Rigid or semi-rigid hinges	None	Outside locking elbow	Inside locking elbow	→
Upper arm component		Triceps pad	→	→	None	Elbow disarticulation type socket	Above-elbow type socket	Humeral section
Shoulder		None	→	→			→	Allows flexion/extension and abduction/adduction
Harness/Suspension		Standard below-elbow figure of eight harness	→	→	Figure of nine harness	Standard above-elbow figure of eight harness	→	Shoulder cap and chest strap
Control system		Single	→	→	↑	Dual	→	→

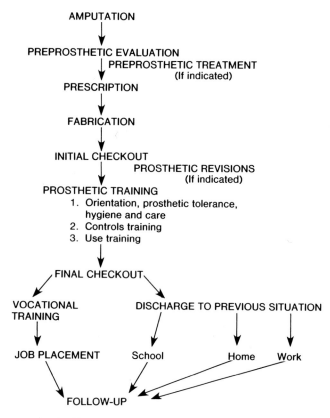

AMPUTATION

↓

PREPROSTHETIC EVALUATION

PREPROSTHETIC TREATMENT
(If indicated)

PRESCRIPTION

↓

FABRICATION

↓

INITIAL CHECKOUT

PROSTHETIC REVISIONS
(If indicated)

PROSTHETIC TRAINING
1. Orientation, prosthetic tolerance, hygiene and care
2. Controls training
3. Use training

↓

FINAL CHECKOUT

VOCATIONAL TRAINING   DISCHARGE TO PREVIOUS SITUATION

JOB PLACEMENT   School   Home   Work

FOLLOW-UP

Figure 24.7   Upper extremity rehabilitation process.

Prosthetic Checkout[1, 8]

As soon as the amputee is fitted with a prosthesis, whether it is temporary or definitive, the occupational therapist performs a prosthetic checkout. The prosthetic checkout determines whether or not the prosthesis fits properly, appears satisfactory, and is mechanically sound. It is an evaluation of the appearance, comfort, and function of a prosthesis. Good fit and alignment are especially important with the initial fitting, as discomfort or difficulty in operation of the first prosthesis may result in the ultimate rejection of the prosthetic limb. The initial checkout is completed before the amputee begins prosthetic training; the final checkout cannot be completed until all necessary revisions to the prosthesis are made and training is initiated or completed.

The prosthetic checkout form, based upon the *Manual of Upper Extremity Prosthetics*,[8] is shown in Table 24.2 and should be referred to in the following discussion.

Sizing

The overall length and the length of the terminal device, forearm, and humeral component of the prosthesis should be the same as the length of the comparable part of the sound limb. The overall length is evaluated by having the amputee stand erect with the uninvolved limb and the prosthesis extended and against the side of the body. The uninvolved limb is

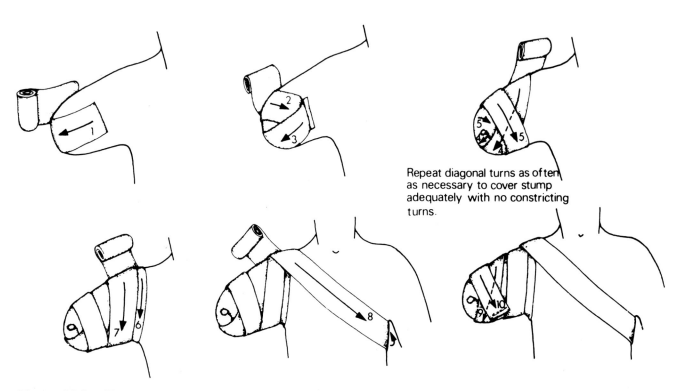

Figure 24.8   The important turns of a short above-elbow stump bandage. (Reproduced with permission from M. Vitali, M. *et al.*[3])

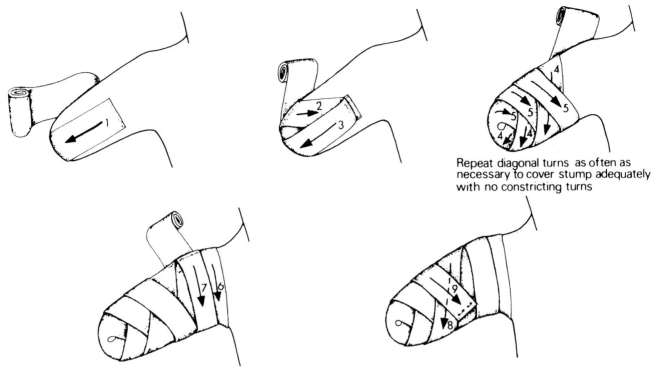

Figure 24.9 The important turns of a long above-elbow stump bandage. (Reproduced with permission from M. Vitali *et al.*[3])

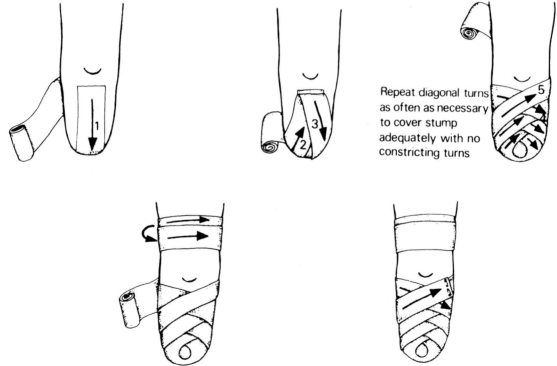

Figure 24.10 The important turns of a below-elbow stump bandage. (Reproduced with permission from M. Vitali, *et al.*[3])

measured from the acromion process to the tip of the thumb. This distance should equal the distance from the acromion process or shoulder joint to the tip of the hook or thumb of the cosmetic hand. Similarly,

the distance from the acromion to the lateral epicondyle and the distance from the lateral epicondyle to the tip of the thumb is compared to the distance from the acromion or shoulder joint to the lateral center of

Table 24.2
UPPER EXTREMITY PROSTHETIC CHECKOUT FORM

Upper Extremity Prosthetic Checkout

Name _____ Age _____ Amputee Type _____ R L

Description of Prosthesis _____

Evaluation of:	Sizing: 1. Uninvolved extremity	

_____ Old Limb

_____ New Limb—initial

_____ New Limb—final

	Acromion to epicondyle	_____ inches
	Epicondyle to thumb tip	_____ inches
	2. Prosthesis	

Weight (to nearest $\frac{1}{4}$ pound):

| | Acromion to hinge (elbow) | _____ inches |
| | Hinge to thumb or hook tip | _____ inches |

_____ pounds

Appearance

A. Terminal Device: Hook and/or cosmetic hand and glove
    1. Hook:
        _____ a. Does the hook function properly in all respects?
            _____ Are fingers sprung or worn?
            _____ Is Neoprene worn?
            _____ Does it stick or grate when passively opened or closed?
            _____ Is it noisy?
        _____ b. If Plastisol covering is used, is it undamaged and good color (not discolored or stained)?
        _____ c. Is hook the proper size?
    2. Cosmetic hand and glove:
        _____ a. Is the hand matching (proper) size?
        _____ b. Are the springs controlling prehension too strong, preventing the amputee optimal ease in operation (opening and closing)?
        _____ c. Is the cosmetic glove satisfactory in all respects?
            _____ Proper fit?
            _____ Undamaged or stained?
            _____ Properly matched color?
            _____ Pulled completely onto hand and forearm without wrinkling?
            _____ Without gapping in palm?
            _____ Doesn't bind when hand is rotated?

B. Wrist Unit
    1. _____ Does the wrist unit operate properly in all respects?
        _____ a. Friction too loose—hook rotates when opened in pronated position?
        _____ b. Friction too tight—amputee cannot preposition terminal device (TD)?
        _____ c. Friction cannot be adjusted?
        _____ d. Wrist sticks or grates when TD prepositioned?
        _____ e. Wrist disconnect unit does not operate smoothly?
    2. _____ If wrist flexion unit is used, does it operate?
        _____ a. Will it maintain extended position when TD is pronated or
        _____ b. Does it automatically pop into flexion when TD is opened?
        _____ c. Can amputee position it in flexion and extension?
        _____ d. If wrist flexion unit has one, can amputee depress lever and position unit into different positions of flexion?

C. Control System
    1. _____ Are all active operating controls so placed as to be satisfactorily operated by the amputee?
    2. _____ Is the control cable free from sharp bends which decrease efficiency and cause rapid cable wear?
    3. _____ Are the control cables arranged so that they do not pinch amputee's skin?
    4. _____ If a hook is to be interchanged with a hand, is the hook-to-hand adapter the correct length and do the ball and socket connections work properly? (If complete interchangeable cable system is used, it should be evaluated as a total control system.)

Table 24.2—*Continued*

	5._____	Is the cable long enough to allow full forearm extension with full pronation of the terminal device?
	6._____	Is the cable housing tipped with ferrules to prevent fraying?
	7._____	Is the cable housing sprung?
	8._____	If the cable housing is lined, is the lining properly in place and not showing any signs of wear?
*BE	9._____	Is the cable housing the proper length between the distal and proximal retainers? (If too long, housing will bulge out in a large loop; if too short, limits flexion or catches on hinge and damages system.)
†AE ‡SD	10._____	Does cable housing adequately cover cable without restricting forearm flexion?
†AE ‡SD	11._____	Is the lift loop short enough to allow adequate terminal device operation after full forearm flexion and is it heavy enough to prevent buckling?
†AE ‡SD	12._____	Does the lift loop pivot on screw and grip cable housing tightly enough to prevent slipping?

D. Elbow Hinges and Elbow Units

	1._____	Does elbow function properly and smoothly without excessive force to operate?
	_____	a. Does elbow joint bind?
	_____	b. Is there play in joint?
	_____	c. Is mechanism noisy?
	_____	d. Are there screws missing at joint?
†AE/‡SD	_____	e. Is the turntable too loose, or too tight to permit the amputee to operate?
†AE/‡SD	_____	f. Does the elbow lock phase properly?
†AE ‡SD	2._____	Is forearm set in adequate amount (10 to 15°) of initial flexion?
*BE	3._____	If flexible or semirigid hinges are used, are they short enough to provide necessary stability, or long enough to allow forearm rotation?

E. Shoulder Joint

‡SD	1._____	Can friction be adjusted so amputee can preposition?
‡SD	2._____	Is friction tight enough so that the prosthesis remains in the desired position, but loose enough to permit prepositioning?

F. Harness

	1._____	Is axilla loop and/or perineal straps and/or waist belt of such size, and so positioned as to afford adequate support and operation?
	2._____	Is the axilla loop, waist belt, or perineal strap comfortable to the amputee, and if necessary, is the axilla loop or perineal strap covered with felt or plastic?
	3._____	Is control attachment strap below midscapular level, and does it remain low enough to give adequate cable travel?
	4._____	Is harness adjusted properly for suspension and cable operation, but comfortable to amputee?
*BE †AE	5._____	Is the NU ring below C-7 and centered or resting toward the nonamputated side?
*BE	6._____	Does anterior support strap pass along the deltopectoral line?
†AE	7._____	Is elastic anterior suspensor adequate length and properly located?
*BE	8._____	Does triceps pad fit snugly without undue gapping during forearm flexion and TD operation?
*BE	9._____	Does triceps pad pinch patient's flesh?
	10._____	Can any additional straps be justified (beyond conventional harness)?

G. Fit

	1._____	Is the prosthesis the correct length?
*BE	2._____	Do the epicondyles have sufficient space?
	3._____	Does the socket trim line fulfill requirements of prescription and function?
	4._____	Is socket comfortable under weight stress?

H. General Workmanship

	1._____	Have all trimmed edges, rough spots, or uncured areas been sealed?
	2._____	Are all rivets properly peened and all screws securely fastened?
	3._____	Is arm color satisfactory?

Table 24.2—*Continued*

4._____ Are all soldered joints strong and neat?
5._____ Are all strap ends sealed to prevent fraying?
6._____ Is the interior of the socket absolutely smooth?

Range of Motion: (Active, A; Passive, P)

Prosthesis On			Prosthesis Off		
*BE Forearm flexion	_____	°A	*BE Forearm flexion	_____	°A
Forearm supination	_____	°A	Forearm supination	_____	°A
Forearm pronation	_____	°A	Forearm pronation	_____	°A
†AE					
‡SD Forearm flexion	_____	°A			
	_____	°P			
†AE Humeral flexion	_____	°A	†AE Humeral flexion	_____	°A
Humeral abduction	_____	°A	Humeral abduction	_____	°A
Humeral adduction	_____	°A	Humeral adduction	_____	°A

Terminal Device Opening (record in percentages):

_____ TD Opening—complete forearm flexion
_____ TD Opening—90° forearm flexion
_____ TD Opening—full forearm extension

Number of rubber bands _____
Prehension force _____

Forces

†AE
‡SD Force required to flex forearm from 90° _____

Tension stability (adult, 50 lbs; child, 1/3 body weight)
_____ inches at _____ lbs

Control system efficiency
_____ lbs to open TD
_____ lbs at cable hanger

$$\frac{\text{lbs to open TD}}{\text{lbs at cable hanger}} \times 100 = \_\_\_\_ \text{ \% of control system efficiency}$$

Recommended Standards:
BE, above 80%
AE, above 70%
SD, above 60%

Recommendations

Note:
*BE applies only to below-elbow or wrist disarticulation prostheses.
†AE applies only to elbow disarticulation or above-elbow prostheses.
‡SD applies only to forequarter or shoulder disarticulation prostheses.

_____ Date   _____ Therapist

8/2/81

rotation of the elbow hinge or lock and the distance from the elbow hinge or lock center of rotation to the tip of the hook or the thumb of the cosmetic hand, respectively.

Weight

The weight of the prosthesis is evaluated using a spring scale. The weight of the prosthesis should be

kept to a minimum; however, standards for weight are not available.

Terminal Device and Wrist Unit

The hook and/or hand are carefully examined for unnecessary wear, malfunction, and inappropriate sizing. If any of the listed problems are found, repair or replacement is recommended. The amputee's ability to operate the terminal device or wrist unit cannot be evaluated until the necessary training has been completed.

Control System

The basic principle for active (cable) operation of the prosthesis is that the amputee must move his body or a body part (body control motion) such that tension is applied to the control cable, and the distance between the most proximal attachment of the cable to the prosthesis and the point of attachment of the cable to the harness is lengthened. As shown in Figures 24.11 and 24.12, the body control motions for opening the terminal device are humeral flexion of the prosthetic arm and/or biscapular abduction. This applies to all but shoulder disarticulation or forequarter prostheses where the motion is humeral flexion and/or unilateral scapular abduction of the uninvolved limb. In the dual control system, the same cable and body motions which open the terminal device are used for active forearm lift (elbow flexion). The elbow lock on above-elbow or elbow disarticulation type prostheses is effected by a combination of downward rotation of the scapula with simultaneous shoulder abduction and hyperextension (Fig. 24.13). The body control motion to operate the elbow lock on shoulder disarticulation type prostheses is usually chest expansion. When the elbow lock is unlocked, pull on the terminal device control cable results in forearm lift. When the elbow lock is locked, the terminal device opens (Fig. 24.14 and 24.15). When checking out the prosthesis, it is important to determine if the controls are located such that the amputee can operate them, which can only be determined after training is initiated. The cable housing is also inspected to ensure that there are no problems which would cause increased friction in the control system. Increased friction reduces the efficiency and thereby increases the amount of effort which must be exerted to operate the prosthesis.

Elbow Hinges/Units and Shoulder Joint

The forearm on prostheses with dual control systems should maximally extend to 10 to 15° of initial flexion so that the amputee can more readily actively initiate forearm lift. The other items are self-explanatory.

Harness

Most amputees are fitted with prostheses which have an axilla loop as part of the harness. The axilla loop provides a stable point against which the amputee

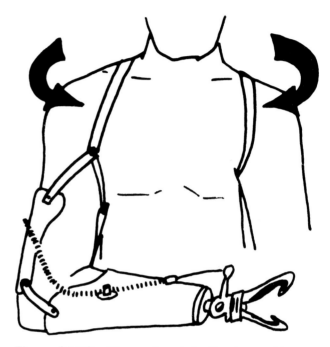

Figure 24.12 Biscapular abduction is used to supplement humeral flexion to produce terminal device opening.

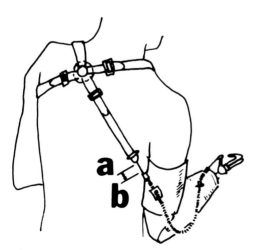
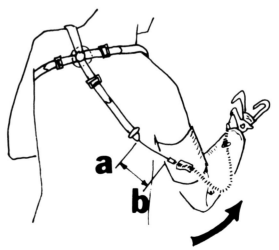

Figure 24.11 The basic body control motion of the below-elbow type prosthesis is humeral flexion which increases the distance between the distal attachment of the cable to the harness at the cable hanger (*a*) and the proximal attachment of the cable to the prosthesis (*b*).

Amputation and Prosthetics **439**

rigid standards with regard to alignment of the control system and/or the use of Dacron cable with Rulon-lined housings can increase the control system efficiency as much as 30%. It is well to remember ease in operation is a prerequisite for smooth and skillful use of the terminal device.

Prosthetic Training[1]

At the initiation of prosthetic training, the amputee is oriented to the prosthesis, and a program to increase prosthetic tolerance is begun. Orientation to the prosthesis includes instruction in prosthetic hygiene and care, how to put on and remove the prosthesis, the parts of the prosthesis, and how to carry out routine maintenance such as changing cables and rubber bands, adjusting friction at joints, and adjusting the harness.

The prosthesis is cleaned with a damp washcloth using mild soap and water. The socket is wiped clean daily. Detergent is avoided, as it may cause skin irritation; do not use abrasive cleansers, as they damage the plastic lamination. Acetone (nail polish remover) or alcohol can be used to remove heavy stains on the outside of the prosthesis, but avoid prolonged contact, as they may soften the lamination.

The harness can be removed or left on the prosthesis and hand washed using mild soap, water, and a nail brush. If the harness is removed, the buckle locations are marked with indelible marker so that the harness can be correctly adjusted when reapplied.

Stump socks and a t-shirt are worn under most prostheses and harnesses to help protect the skin from irritation and to absorb perspiration. A stump sock is not worn if the amputee is fitted with a self-suspending socket; a t-shirt is not necessary. The stump sock and t-shirt are changed daily. The stump socks are washed in soap, rather than detergent, to prevent skin irritation.

The stump is washed twice daily with mild soap and water and dried thoroughly. If heavy perspiration is a problem, a small amount of unscented baby powder or cornstarch can be applied to the stump before the prosthesis is applied in the morning.

The above- and below-elbow type prosthesis is put on and removed in a manner similar to putting on a (1) front opening or (2) slipover shirt: (1) The stump is inserted into the socket, which is held in the sound hand, and under the anteriorly fastening straps of the harness. The axilla loop is then swung behind the back as the prosthesis is raised overhead, and the sound arm inserted through the axilla loop. (2) The prosthesis is positioned in front of the amputee, and the sound arm and stump are inserted into the axilla loop and socket, respectively. Both arms are then raised to lift the prosthesis and harness up and over the head. With either method, the harness is set with the NU ring below C7 by using scapular retraction and depression. To remove the prosthesis, the amputee grasps the prosthesis with the sound hand and lifts the prosthesis overhead. The shoulder disarticulation prosthesis is put on using the sound hand and held in place with

the chin or by leaning against the wall as the chest strap is fastened.

Prosthetic tolerance is defined as the amputee's ability to adjust to the wearing of a prosthesis. Tolerance involves the amputee's attitude toward the prosthesis, as well as the physiological acceptance of it. To develop prosthetic tolerance, the amputee beings wearing the prosthesis for ½ hour. The stump is checked before and after each application for areas of irritation. If there is no sign of irritation when the prosthesis is removed, the prosthesis is immediately reapplied for an additional ½ hour. If irritation occurs, the prosthesis is not reapplied until after the redness clears. The wearing time is increased in this manner until the amputee is able to wear the prosthesis for 2 hours without irritation. Once the prosthesis can be worn for 2 hours, wearing time can be increased to fulltime wear, provided that the amputee is aware of the importance of removing the prosthesis should irritation or discomfort develop. If at any time the prosthesis persists in causing redness or irritation which lasts for more than ½ hour after removal, revision or relief is recommended.

Prosthetic training in the operation of the prosthesis begins with teaching the amputee to actively operate the control cables using the appropriate body control motions. This stage is known as controls training, but because it overlaps or is continuous with use training (training to develop skill in the use of prosthesis in activity), it is not a clearly defined period. In most instances, controls training is completed within one treatment session. The body control motions are first demonstrated by passively moving the amputated limb through the correct motion. The body control motion for terminal device operation is taught first. Once the amputee can actively open and close the terminal device, the amputee practices grasping objects of various sizes, densities, textures, and shapes. If the prosthesis has a dual control system, the elbow lock remains locked while terminal device operation is learned. Then, the elbow lock is unlocked by passively moving the prosthesis through the appropriate motion, thereby demonstrating the correct body control motion to the amputee. With the elbow lock unlocked, the amputee is asked to perform the same body control motion which opens the terminal device and is shown that this motion now results in forearm lift. The amputee's face should initially be protected by the therapist's hand in the event that the forearm is flexed so far as to cause the terminal device to hit the face. The amputee should practice elbow lock and unlock and the forearm lift separately until they are smoothly accomplished. The ability to combine forearm lift and elbow lock and unlock is then taught by asking the amputee to flex the forearm to varying degrees of elbow flexion and to hold the position while the elbow is locked. The elbow of above-elbow and elbow disarticulation type prostheses are more easily locked and unlocked when the forearm is flexed if only scapular depression and humeral abduction are used. This prevents the forearm from extending because of release on the tension of the terminal device control cable which would result if the amputee also extended to operate the elbow lock.

As the amputee develops skill in control of the terminal device, elbow lock, and forearm lift operation, manual controls, which include prepositioning the terminal device, shoulder joint, or humeral turntable using the sound hand, are taught. The amputee is then ready to begin learning to preposition the prosthesis in various positions, as appropriate for the activity. For example, to hold paper when cutting with scissors, the fingers of the hook must be parallel to the table, or horizontal. To grasp a jar, the hook fingers must be perpendicular to the table, or vertical.

By this time, the amputee has begun use training; prosthetic skill and awareness are more readily learned through the use of the prosthesis in bilateral activities of daily living appropriate for the needs and interests of the amputee. While there are many so-called "prosthetic techniques," the best approach to use in training is based upon skill in activity analysis and knowledge in prosthetic function and limitations. For example, the therapist working with an amputee for the first time might ask the patient to write his name on a piece of paper while seated at a table, without knowing how this task is accomplished using a prosthesis. The therapist should first analyze how the activity is normally accomplished. The nonpreferred extremity is positioned in approximately 45° of shoulder flexion and abduction, the elbow is flexed approximately 45°, and the forearm and hand lay flat across the paper to stabilize it while the individual writes with the writing implement in the preferred hand. This is then translated into prosthetic terms. As appropriate to the type of prosthesis, the shoulder joint is prepositioned into 45° of shoulder flexion and abduction, the elbow is flexed and locked at 45° of flexion and the terminal device is slightly pronated such that the forearm and terminal device will lay flat across the paper and hold it securely. The prosthesis always functions as the nonpreferred extremity does—as a stabilizer.

There are a few techniques which should be mentioned. When cutting meat, the fork is placed between the hook fingers and behind the prosthetic thumb (Fig. 24.18). The knife, as with the normal individual, is held in the sound (preferred) hand. The principles of dressing are the same as for the stroke patient: the prosthesis is dressed first and undressed last. Shoe laces can be tied in the usual manner, but if slippage of the lace in the hook fingers occurs when pulling on the lace, the hook can be opened, the lace wrapped around one of the hook fingers, and the hook closed for more secure grasp (Fig. 24.19).

With the bilateral amputee, the training procedures are the same for each limb; however, separation of controls must also be accomplished. Separation of controls involves keeping one terminal device closed to maintain grasp of an object while simultaneously opening the other terminal device. When two cable systems (one for operation of each terminal device) are attached to one harness, as they are for the bilateral amputee, the patient must learn to relax one control system while operating the other. If the amputee does not do this, any attempt to open one terminal device will also open the other. The point of stability from which the amputee pulls is no longer the harness (as it should be) but rather the opposite terminal device. This ability to separate controls enables the bilateral amputee to cut with scissors with one hook while holding paper securely in the other. When the amputee is first learning to separate controls, the occupational therapist can help the amputee by placing an additional amount of rubber band on the hook used to hold or stabilize and/or loosen the control attachment strap on the same side. Both of these procedures make it more difficult for the amputee to open the nonpreferred hook; the ability to keep the hook closed improves, but the ability to use it will lessen. In order to prevent this loss of skill, the amputee must eventually learn to maintain the stabilizing side extended at the shoulder to relax the tension on the control cable.

Throughout use training, the therapist tries to involve the amputee in the activity analysis process. This enables the amputee to determine how to use the prosthesis in new activities learned after discharge. It may also promote higher levels of prosthetic skill and awareness and encourage continued prosthetic use. The rejection rate among upper extremity amputees is high.[4] The reason for rejection can be physical or medical (weakness, incoordination, associated disability, pain, unsuitable stump for prosthetic fitting, etc.), or prosthetic (poor fit, mechanical unreliability).[3, 9] The prosthesis may also be rejected because the amputee develops one-handed activity patterns which permit independence in occupational performance tasks prior to prosthetic fitting and training and/or the amputee is required to use the prosthesis when the demands of the activity exceed the functional capabilities of the prosthesis.[3, 7, 10] The skillful use of a prosthesis may have less of an effect on independence in daily living tasks than on enabling the amputee to function more normally utilizing two-handed activity patterns. However, the therapist and the amputee must also realize the limitations of the prosthesis. Requiring the amputee to use the prosthesis when it is unrealistic results in imposing behavior on the amputee which is awkward and time consuming. Whenever it is more realistic, the principles of loss of use of one upper extremity (Chapters 26 and 27) are followed.

In preparation for discharge, consideration is given to the amputee's vocational and avocational interests. A community visit with follow-up training is indicated. Perhaps because of the limited number of commercially available components for that purpose, recreation is of special concern to upper extremity amputees.[9] Therefore, the development of special devices or techniques which enable the amputee to participate in recreational activities is an additional occupational therapy goal. Several devices which are not commercially available have been described in the literature.

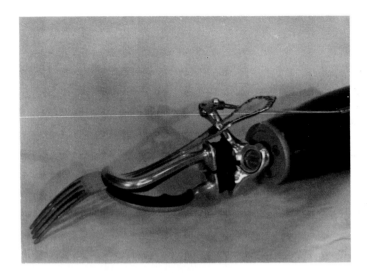

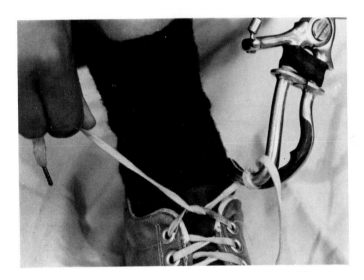

Figure 24.19 Stabilization of the shoe lace in the hook.

Adaptations of the bow for archery were described by Bender[1] and Zduriencik.[11] The bow can also be ordered directly from the factory with the hand grip still in block form. Pins can be added to the hand grip which insert into a female adaptor designed to attach to the wrist unit. The adaptor must be designed so that the bow can be aligned for direct pull on the bowstring to permit accurate aim.

A commercially available device for bowling is available through the amputee's prosthetist.[1] Redford[12] described a modification made to a Dorrance hook for holding a hockey stick, whereby metal pieces were welded to the hook fingers to make a closed loop. Sabolich[13] developed an adaptor for holding a fishing rod, and Bender[1] reported an adaptor for holding a golf club.

Most of these devices were designed to meet the special needs of the amputees who used them. Because they are not commercially available, the occupational therapist, prosthetist, and the amputee must work as a team to design and fabricate devices on an individual basis.

PARTIAL HAND AMPUTATION[14-16]

Partial hand amputations are usually the result of trauma and management and should be considered in the context of hand injuries in general. Therefore, the reader is referred to Chapter 18. This chapter will be limited to a discussion of prosthetic devices for partial hand amputations.

As with all levels of amputation, cosmesis and function are both given consideration. Passive cosmetic hands or fingers are of limited cosmetic and functional benefit. Cosmetic hands are worn like a glove; the part of the hand which is missing is filled with foam, rigid, or flexible material (Fig. 24.20A and B). While often requested initially, they are frequently rejected by the amputee. The role of the occupational therapist is generally limited to check out of the cosmetic device and instructing the patient in prosthetic hygiene and care appropriate to the device fitted.

In contrast, because of the special skills of the occupational therapist with regard to activity analysis, fabrication of orthotic devices, and design of adaptive

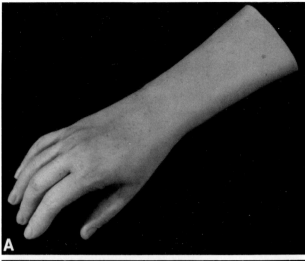

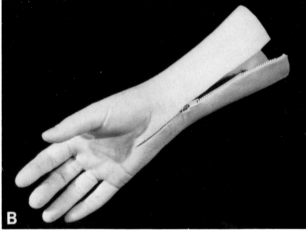

Figure 24.20 *A.* Dorsal view of a cosmetic hand. *B.* Volar view of a cosmetic hand.

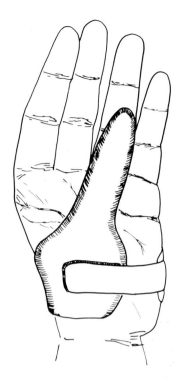

Figure 24.21 Partial hand prosthesis: plastic laminate thumb post.

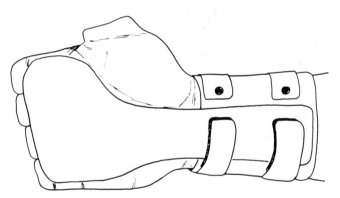

Figure 24.22 Partial hand prosthesis: opposition plate for loss of all digits (volar view).

equipment, the occupational therapist can play a major role in designing functional partial hand prostheses. A thorough interview to determine the client's needs and a complete evaluation of residual hand function to identify functional needs can provide the basis for the design of a partial hand prosthesis.

Partial hand prostheses are usually designed to meet a specific functional need of the patient. Lack of opposition, strength of opposition, and stability are the most common functional problems to be overcome. Following the interview and hand evaluation, the therapist can use metal (stainless steel rods or aluminum strips) and thermoplastic splinting material to design a prototype prosthesis or opposition post. By using these materials, the device can be easily modified until the optimal design is determined. Consideration must be given to the length, strength and range of motion of the residual digits and to the size, shape, and weight of the objects to be picked up. Most definitive partial hand prostheses are comprised of either a plastic laminate thumb post (Fig. 24.21) or some type of stainless steel opposition plate covered with rubber or another nonfriction material (Fig. 24.22) and are therefore fabricated by the prosthetist or orthotist.

PHANTOM LIMB[17-19]

While phantom sensation is present in all persons with amputations acquired in adulthood, the so-called painful phantom or phantom limb is experienced by 3 to 35% of the acquired adult amputee population and depends upon the type of population studied (*i.e.*, surgical, traumatic, war injuries, etc.). The phenomena of painful phantom is poorly understood. While it is often considered a medical or surgical problem, psychological factors may contribute.

The occupational therapist may become involved in the direct treatment of painful phantom. Melzack[17] found that increasing somatic input to the stump frequently reduced or abolished painful sensation. Percussion of the stump is often used but is of limited benefit to most patients. Berger[18] recommends the use of high frequency vibration for the treatment of painful phantom. Berger applied vibration two to three times a week for 15 to 20 minutes. If relief occurred, the patients were given a vibrator for home use. Most patients initially used the vibrator daily, but after 2 or 3 weeks, the patients were able to decrease the frequency of vibration to as little as 1 to 2 times/month. Further evaluation of this technique is needed.

Little research has been done to evaluate the effectiveness of biofeedback in reducing phantom limb. However, Pasnau and Pfefferbaum[19] indicated that the use of biofeedback for muscle relaxation of the ipsilateral or contralateral limb may be of some benefit and should be investigated.

ELECTRICALLY POWERED UPPER EXTREMITY PROSTHESES[4, 10, 20–25]

Electrically powered upper extremity prostheses or components are either switch or myoelectrically controlled. Switch control can be of two types. Switches which the amputee depresses by movement of the stump or scapula can be mounted in the socket, or pull switches which are activated by the conventional body control motions used to operate the terminal device or elbow lock can be incorporated into the harness. Simply stated, the electrical potential generated by a contracting muscle functions as a switch to activate myoelectrically powered prostheses. Whether the "switch" is a push button, pull switch, or myoelectric potential, the "switch" controls the flow of electric current from the battery to the motor.

Switch control is usually "on-off." When the switch is off, the battery is not connected to the motor, and the elbow or terminal device does not move. When the switch is on, the component moves in one direction only. Hence, one switch is needed for flexion of the elbow, and another switch is needed for elbow extension. Similarly, one switch opens the terminal device, and another closes the terminal device. The VANU pull switch has five positions. No movement occurs when the switch is in positions one, three, or five. The component moves in one direction (i.e., extends) when the switch is in position 2, and movement reverses (i.e., flexes) when the switch is in position 4.

Switch control of electrically powered prostheses is readily taught, provided that the switches are located in an optimal position for ease in operation. An amputee fitted with pull switches who has previously undergone training with a conventional prosthesis may not require controls training. Use training is approached in the same manner as described for conventional prostheses.

Myoelectric control systems are more complex and more expensive, as the myoelectric signal must be amplified and smoothed by more sophisticated electronics. Most common is the myoelectric below-elbow prosthesis (Fig. 24.23). Either one or two electrode sites and a reference electrode are necessary to control each component. When there are two electrode sites, they are usually located over antagonistic muscle pairs; contraction of one group of muscles opens the terminal device or flexes the elbow, and contraction of the antagonist results in the reverse motion. When there is only one electrode site, the amount or level of contraction determines which movement will occur. For example, a midrange or slow rate of contraction results in the hand closing, and a high level or fast rate of contraction results in the hand opening. When the muscle is relaxed, no movement occurs.

Occupational therapy for patients with myoelectric prostheses begins with preprosthetic controls training. Depending upon the system to be fitted, one or two pairs of electrodes are applied to the stump. A myotrainer, which is a specialized biofeedback unit, is used to determine the optimum electrode placement. Using trial and error, electrodes are located over superficial muscles which are capable of contracting but which do not contract during normal activity (i.e., elbow flexion and extension in the case of the below-elbow amputee). As soon as the optimum location is determined, the patient practices using the myotrainer to develop isolated control and the ability (if necessary) to control rate or force of contraction. The electric hand may be connected to the myotrainer at this stage, and the amputee practices controlling the amount of opening and closing of the hand. Use training begins as soon as the definitive prosthesis is completed and is carried out in the same manner as with a conventional prosthesis.

Amputees fitted with electrically powered prostheses are also given instruction in the specialized care and maintenance of their prosthesis, which includes procedures for recharging batteries and what to do if the prosthesis requires repair.

An increasing number of electrically powered devices are being fitted, and the acceptance rate is higher than with conventional prostheses.[10, 24] As far as is feasible, the prostheses are self-suspended and self-contained. Therefore, they require little or no harnessing and are more cosmetic, making them more acceptable to patients. However, because they are expensive, and are only fitted in centers which are able to provide specialized fitting, training, and maintenance, Lyttle et al.[23] recommend that they be fitted only to patients who are dissatisfied with the comfort, function, or appearance of their conventional prosthesis.

While electrically powered prostheses are more cosmetic, eliminate the need for uncomfortable harnessing, and require less energy and excursion to operate, they are not without disadvantages. Reliability remains a problem; the availability of a back-up prosthesis, spare parts, and/or the ability to interchange between body-powered and electrically powered components is necessary if the amputee is going to be a regular prosthetic wearer. Herberts et al.[10] state that inadequate repair service can lead to rejection even in a potential prosthetic user.

Whether or not the electrically powered hand is more functional than the hook remains controversial.[4, 24] The greater pinch force (up to 25 pounds)

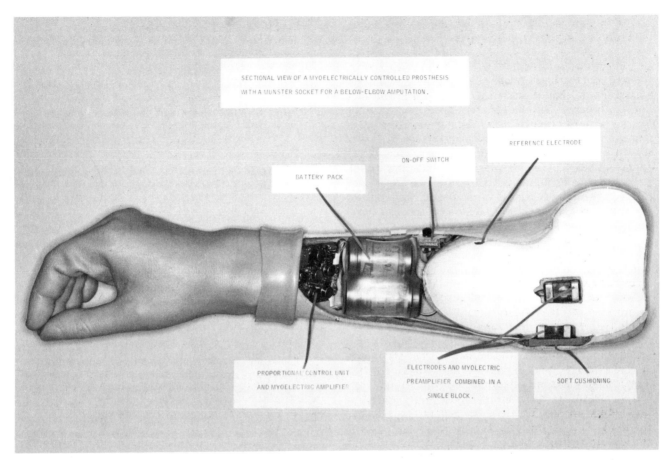

Figure 24.23 Below-elbow myoelectrically controlled prosthesis with Muenster-type socket. (Reproduced with permission from the *Inter-Clinic Information Bulletin, 11* (8): 1972.)

and wider opening makes them functionally superior to the body-powered hand.[25] For high level amputees, the use of an electrically powered elbow with a body-powered hook permits the use of a single cable housing for terminal device operation. As less excursion is needed to open the terminal device when the elbow is flexed, the amount of terminal device opening and/or pinch force increases.[21, 22]

LOWER EXTREMITY AMPUTEES[26–28]

Approximately 70% of acquired amputations involve the lower extremity. Most are necessary because of peripheral arterial disease or diabetes mellitus and involve individuals who are over 60 years of age. Many of these patients have the added problems of peripheral neuropathy, decreased resistance to bacterial and fungal infection, and visual impairment. Katrak and Baggott[27] found that approximately 85% of unilateral geriatric amputees were successfully fitted with prostheses and almost half of the patients who were not fitted attained wheelchair independence in activities of daily living tasks. These results were attained in a rehabilitation center which provided a comprehensive rehabilitation program, including occupational therapy.

Physical therapy assumes major responsibility for prosthetic checkout and gait training. The occupational therapist works closely with the physical therapist and provides a program which enhances the physical therapy goals and facilitates the rehabilitation process. Specific goals of occupational therapy are to maintain and/or increase upper extremity strength, increase standing balance and tolerance (with and without the prosthesis), achieve independence in daily living tasks (with and without the prosthesis), and to facilitate reintegration into the community. The program goals are based upon an interview to determine the amputee's needs and interests and a thorough evaluation of physical and mental status.

Upper Extremity Strengthening

Emphasis is placed on strengthening muscle groups needed for gait training and transfers. Strengthening of distal as well as proximal muscle groups is indicated, particularly if weakness is the result of a long hospitalization and/or if peripheral neuropathy is present.

Standing Balance and Tolerance

Prior to prosthetic fitting, the ability to balance on one leg and to bear weight for increasing periods of time is developed in conjunction with group, kitchen, and self-care activities. After prosthetic fitting, the amputee increases prosthetic tolerance while weight bearing in similar activities. Safety awareness is also developed.

Daily Living Tasks

Prior to prosthetic fitting, the patient is evaluated with regard to independence in dressing, toileting, bathing, kitchen, and transfer activities, and training is provided if indicated. Evaluation and treatment principles are based upon those described for loss of use of one side of the body (Chapters 26 and 27). Independence at this stage is particularly important, even for those amputees who are to be fitted and trained with prostheses. There are times for all prosthetic wearers when the prosthesis is not worn (*i.e.*, at night, when repairs are needed, if stump complications develop, etc.). Therefore, the amputee needs to be safe and independent in some secondary mode of ambulation (*i.e.*, wheelchair). Prior to and following prosthetic fitting, the development of functional mobility in conjunction with daily living tasks enables the amputee to improve self-confidence and to feel safe and comfortable during functional ambulation.

Stump hygiene and bandaging and the ability to put on and remove the prosthesis, once fitted, are taught and reinforced by all members of the rehabilitation team. There are many types of lower extremity prostheses, and the correct method for donning and doffing the prosthesis should be learned from the physical therapist. Dressing the prosthesis is accomplished in the same manner as with an upper extremity prosthesis: the prosthesis is dressed first and undressed last. Many amputees find it easier to put the shoe and sock on the prosthesis before putting the prosthesis on.

Home and community visits help to identify necessary modifications to the home and/or any additional training needed in preparation for discharge. Avocational and vocational exploration and driving evaluations are also provided, if indicated.

References

1. Bender, L. F. *Prostheses and Rehabilitation after Arm Amputation*. Springfield, Ill.: Charles C Thomas, 1974.
2. Steinbach, T. Upper limb amputation. *Prog. Surg.*, 16: 224–248, 1978.
3. Vitali, M., Robinson, K. P., Andrews, B. G., and Harris, E. E. *Amputations and Prostheses*. London: Baillière Tindall, 1978.
4. Malone, J. H., Childers, S. J., Underwood, J., and Leal, J. H. Immediate postsurgical management of upper-extremity amputation: Conventional electric and myoelectric prosthesis. *Orthot. Prosthet.*, 35 (2): 1–9, 1981.
5. Radocy, R., and Dick, R. E. A terminal question. *Orthot. Prosthet.*, 35 (1): 1–6, 1981.
6. Jones, R. F. The rehabilitation of surgical patients with particular reference to traumatic upper limb disability. *Aust. NZ J. Surg.*, 47 (3): 402–407, 1977.
7. Burkhalter, W. E., Mayfield, G., and Carmona, L. S. The upper-extremity amputee: Early and immediate post-surgical prosthetic fitting. *J. Bone Joint Surg.*, 58A (1): 46–51, 1976.
8. Santschi, W. R. (ed.) *Manual of Upper Extremity Prosthetics*, 2nd ed. Los Angeles: University of California at Los Angeles, 1958.
9. Chadderton, H. C. Prostheses, pain and sequelae of amputation, as seen by the amputee. *Prosthet. Orthot. Int.*, 1: 2–14, 1978.
10. Herberts, P., Körner, L., Caine, K., and Wensby, L. Rehabilitation of unilateral below-elbow amputees with myoelectric prostheses. *Scand. J. Rehabil. Med.*, 12: 123–128, 1980.
11. Zduriencik, S. Bow adapter. *Am. J. Ocup. Ther.*, 20 (2): 99–100, 1966.
12. Redford, J. B. Prostheses for hockey-playing upper-limb amputees. *Inter-Clinic Inform. Bull.*, 14 (6): 11–15, 1975.
13. Sabolich, L. J. An adapted fishing rod for arm amputees. *Inter-Clinic Inform. Bull.*, 12 (2): 13–15, 1972.
14. Bender, L. F. Prostheses for partial hand amputations. *Prosthet. Orthot. Int.*, 2: 8–11, 1978.
15. Kramer, S. Partial hand amputation. *Orthop.*, 1 (4): 314, 1978.
16. Tomaszewska, A., Kapczyńska, D., Konieczna, D., Dembinska, J., and Miedzyblocki, W. Solving individual problems with partial hand prostheses. *Inter-Clinic Inform. Bull.*, 13 (5): 7–14, 1974.
17. Melzack, R. *The Puzzle of Pain*. New York: Basic Books, 1973.
18. Berger, S. M. Conservative management of phantom-limb and amputation-stump pain. *Ann. R. Coll. Surg. Engl.*, 62 (2): 102–105, 1980.
19. Pasnau, R. O., and Pfefferbaum, B. Psychologic aspects of post-amputation pain. *Nurs. Clin. North Am.*, 11 (4): 679–685, 1976.
20. Childress, D. S., Holmes, D. W., and Billock, J. N. Ideas on myoelectric prosthetic systems for upper-extremity amputees. In: *The Control of Upper-Extremity Prostheses and Orthoses*, P. Herberts, R. Kadefors, R. Magnusson, and Petersén, I. Springfield, Ill.: Charles C Thomas, 1974.
21. Fisher, A. G. Functional results with electrically powered devices for children. In: *Workshop on Children's Prosthetics*, Washington, D. C.: National Academy of Sciences, 1976.
22. Fisher, A. G., and Childress, D. S. The Michigan electric hook: A preliminary report on a new electrically powered hook for children. *Inter-Clinic Inform. Bull.*, 12 (9): 1–10, 1973.
23. Lyttle, D., Sweitzer, R., Steinke, T., Trefler, E., and Hobson, D. Experiences with myoelectric below-elbow fittings in teenagers. *Inter-Clinic Inform Bull.*, 13 (6): 11–20, 1974.
24. Northmore-Ball, M. D., Heger, H., and Hunter, G. A. The below-elbow myo-electric prosthesis: A comparison of the Otto Bock myo-electric prosthesis with the hook and functional hand. *J. Bone Joint. Surg.*, 62B (3): 363–367, 1980.
25. Northwestern University Prosthetics-Orthotics Center. *Powered Upper-Limb Prosthetics for Prosthetists* (manual compiled by J.N. Billock for Course 691, 1974).
26. Humm, W. *Rehabilitation of the Lower Limb Amputee for Nurses and Therapists*, 3rd ed. London: Baillière Tindall, 1977.
27. Katrak, P. H., and Baggott, J. B. Rehabilitation of elderly lower-extremity amputees. *Med. J. Aust.*, 1: 651–653, 1980.
28. Schafer, R. Occupational therapy for lower extremity problems. *Am. J. Occup. Ther.*, 27 (3): 132–137, 1973.

Supplementary Reading and Courses

American Academy of Orthopedic Surgeons. *Atlas of Limb Prosthetics: Surgical and Prosthetic Principles*. St. Louis: C. V. Mosby, 1981.

American Orthotic and Prosthetic Association, Washington, D.C., *Orthotics and Prosthetics*.

Courses and manuals available from New York University, Prosthetics and Orthotics, NYU Post-Graduate Medical School, New York, N.Y.: *Upper-Extremity Prosthetics* and *Lower-Extremity Prosthetics*.

Courses and manuals available from Northwestern University, The Medical School, Prosthetic-Orthotic Center, Chicago, Ill.: *Lower Limb Prosthetics for Physicians, Surgeons, and Therapists; Upper Limb Prosthetics and Orthotics for Physicians, Surgeons, and Therapists; Management of the Juvenile Amputee for Physicians, Surgeons, and Therapists*.

Prosthetics and Orthotics, New York University Post-Graduate Medical School, New York, N.Y., *Inter-Clinic Information Bulletin*.

International Committee on Prosthetics and Orthotics of the International Society for the Rehabilitation of the Disabled, Copenhagen, *Prosthetics and Orthotics International*.

Murphy, E. F., and Horn, L. W. Myoelectric control systems: A selected bibliography. *Orthot. Prosthet.*, 35 (1): 34–45, 1981.

Taylor, C. L. The biomechanics of control in upper-extremity prostheses. *Orthot. Prosthet.*, 35 (1): 7–28, 1981.

PART NINE

Rehabilitative Approach

The goal of rehabilitation is return to family, job, and community. Some patients achieve this goal while others never do, or only partially do, because of the severity of their medical problems. Part Nine deals with evaluation and treatment related to a patient's ability to do activities of daily living, vocational and recreational activities, and to access the environment.

The rehabilitative approach is a compensatory approach appropriate for patients who will need to live with a disability on a temporary or permanent basis. The theory of this approach focuses on the use of a person's remaining abilities to achieve the highest level of independence possible for that individual in occupational performance tasks. Anything a person does related to his duties, roles, or life satisfactions is an occupational performance task. These may include self-care, homemaking, recreation, school, civic involvement, and work. When a person with a disability is unable to accomplish daily life tasks in the usual way, adapted techniques or equipment may enable him to be independent. Adapted techniques are preferred to equipment because they make the person's life more flexible and independent. If independence is not possible without equipment, many assistive devices are commercially available. When equipment is needed but is not a commercially manufactured item, the therapist must use ingenuity to devise specialized equipment. It may be false economy for the therapist to take the time to devise and/or make equipment which can be purchased. *Aids to Independent Living* by Lowman and Klinger is one comprehensive compilation of techniques and equipment for all aspects of daily life tasks.

Principles of compensation for each type of problem are stated and will serve as a basis for the therapist's and/or patient's creative problem solving when procedures or pieces of equipment listed are inadequate for a particular patient. There may be no technique or equipment to compensate for some problems; therefore, the patient will need to decide whether to eliminate the task from his daily life or to be dependent on someone else for performance of that task.

In this section we will present some standard adapted techniques and equipment used to achieve independence for patients with different types of disabilities. Some patients present several disability problems at once, *e.g.*, the arthritic patient has limited range of motion *and* limited strength. When more than one problem exists, the therapist will need to consult the subsections of the chapter applicable to a particular patient's problems.

chapter
25

Evaluation of Occupational Performance Tasks

Catherine A. Trombly, M.A., OTR

Independence in occupational performance tasks is the goal of rehabilitation in general and occupational therapy in particular. Whenever a person suffers a trauma or disease that results in a physical impairment, independence in these tasks is jeopardized. The occupational therapist must determine the patient's abilities and limitations. Evaluation of occupational performance tasks consists of systematic observation and/or interview to determine what tasks cannot be performed and what the limiting factors are. If the limiting factors can be improved or eliminated by direct restorative treatment, the therapist chooses one of the other two treatment approaches that is appropriate to the problem. If, however, the limiting factors are not amenable to change, the therapist teaches the patient to compensate for these limitations.

Except for self-care, no standardized evaluations of occupational performance tasks exist. The standardized self-care evaluations are also used in research and/or to measure the outcome of a rehabilitative program in terms of level of independence achieved during hospitalization. The most frequently cited tests are the Katz Index,[1] the Revised Kenny Self Care Evaluation,[2] and the Barthel Index.[3] These evaluations yield a numerical score. The Barthel Index and the Kenny Evaluation are more sensitive to change than the Katz Index.[4] The Barthel is more inclusive than the Kenny or the Katz.[4]

The Katz Index evaluates six functions, and scoring is based on ontogenetic development of self-care skills.[1,4] The Barthel Index looks at 10 functions. Total score can range from 0 to 100 (total independence) in increments of 5. Functions are weighted according to importance to independence.[3,4] A score of 60 seems to

be the transition from dependency to assisted independence.[5] The Revised Kenny Self-Care Evaluation looks at seven categories of self-care, each of which are broken down into specific tasks that define the activity. The patient scores either independent (I), dependent (D), needs assistance (A), or needs supervision (S) on each task. The activity is given a number score depending on the number of I, D, A, or S's earned. The category score is an average of the activity scores. The total self-care score is a total of category scores.[2]

All evaluation tools used should be valid, reliable, and sensitive enough to detect important changes. A valid test is one that measures what it purports to measure. Most evaluations of each task are valid on their face, *i.e.*, have logical validity.[6] The overall evaluation needs to weigh each item that defines the activity fairly in order to have content validity. The items are samples of a universe of behavior, but some are more important than others,[6] *e.g.*, "can use the stove safely" is a more important item than "can stir batter" in the universe of "meal preparation." If each were weighted equally, then the score would not really define the patient's "meal preparation" ability. A reliable test is one that measures the parameter under study consistently no matter who is scoring (interrater reliability) or when the scoring occurs (test-retest reliability). Reliability has rarely been established for the evaluations of occupational performance tasks in use. The tasks listed in departmentally composed tests are rarely even operationally defined, the initial step in establishing reliability. To operationally define something is to describe it so that another person could duplicate the process and arrive at the same conclusion or score. Sensitivity, the third characteristic of a good test, refers to the ability to detect the smallest increment of change that would be considered a significant change for the purpose of the test. As an example, for a therapist working on a day to day basis with a patient to increase ability to dress, the test should be sensitive enough to allow progress to be noted when different areas of the body can be dressed or different articles of clothing applied. However, for program evaluation the crucial piece of information is whether or not the patient is or is not independent in dressing, and therefore the tool used to measure is preferably less discriminating.

The level of measurement of most evaluations of occupational performance tasks is ordinal, that is, the score can be located on a ranking from dependent/is unable to independent/is able.

Evaluation of all occupational performance tasks is not done at the same time. Ability to do self-care, personal mobility, and to do leisure time activities within the current limits of the disability are usually done early and form the basis for the whole occupational therapy treatment plan that includes restorative therapy to enable independence. As recovery plateaus and discharge planning decisions are being considered, evaluations concerned with access to home and community, transportation, care of the home and children, hobbies, sports and family recreation, and job/educational abilities are done as applicable. In addition to the physical requirements of these tasks, soundness of judgment and perceptual/cognitive skills must be assessed to determine if these tasks can be safely and effectively accomplished.

Observation and interview are the methods of evaluation. Observation is preferred for accuracy, detection of faulty or unsafe methods, and for determination of the underlying reason that a particular task cannot be performed. Interview is used when observation is not permitted by the patient or when observation is not needed because the patient is a reliable reporter and the experienced therapist can validate the patient's description and understand the nature of the problems that may exist. If a patient reports questionable data and does not permit observation the therapist should verify the information by checking with others who have knowledge of the patient's performance. False information does not reflect a conscious intent to deceive, but probably reflects a denial of the problem, a carry over of the premorbid self-concept of being independent, or a strong wish to be independent that seems real.

In the area of activities of daily living (ADL), which includes self-care, mobility, and communication, observation of the various activities should be done at the time of day when these activities are normally done and in the location where the patient usually performs the tasks. Remember that people may have strong feelings of modesty regarding personal care which should be respected. The entire evaluation is not done at one time because it is fatiguing. The therapist should discontinue the evaluation if fatigue occurs. Items which would be unsafe or obviously unsuccessful are postponed until the patient's physical status improves; these are marked X (not indicated for testing at present) or some equivalent designation. The format for the evaluation form is usually a check list on which the therapist indicates whether each item can be done independently, with equipment, with supervision, with assistance, or not at all. Items which are not applicable are marked NA.

There is often space allowed on the form for periodic reevaluation using the same form. It is important to at least record the level of performance at admission and at discharge, since these records may be used in program evaluation, justification for service to third party payors, or in legal actions. If the patient is not independent in some required task at the time of discharge, plans must be developed to ensure that this task is done by others or that additional training is received.

Examples of nonstandardized Activites of Daily Living and Homemaking evaluation forms are included here. Other sample evaluation forms are given in other chapters of this part.

Table 25.1
EVALUATION OF DAILY LIVING ACTIVITIES[a]

Name: _____ Diagnosis: _____

Key to Grading:

Independence Grades:

    4 Normal performance

    3 Adequate performance, but dependent on special apparatus or environmental condition (specify in comment section)

Dependence Grades:

    2 Supervision needed to complete

    1 Assistance needed to complete

    0 Activity impossible

    X Not indicated for testing at present time

    NA Not applicable

Date:						
Rater:						
Mobility and locomotion						
1. Turn over in bed						
2. Sit up in bed						
3. Procure object from table beside bed						
4. Transfer from bed to w/c						
5. Transfer from w/c to toilet						
6. Transfer from w/c to tub/shower						
7. Get in and out of chairs						
8. Get in and out of car						
9. Wheelchair turning						
10. Wheelchair forward 30 ft						
11. Wheelchair up ramp						
12. Wheelchair down ramp						
13. Wheelchair forward 100 ft						
14. Get down and up from floor						
15. Move on floor not in upright position						
16. Pick up object from floor						
17. Operate automatic elevator						
18. Open and go through door with sills						
19. Do 7 in. steps with rails						
20. Do 7 in. steps without rails						
21. Cross street with traffic light						
22. Get wheelchair in and out of car						
23. Walk forward 30 ft						
24. Walk backward 10 ft						
25. Walk sidewards						
26. Walk carrying object						
27. Walk forward 100 ft						
28. Do bus steps						
Eating						
29. Eat with fingers						
30. Eat with fork						
31. Eat with spoon						
32. Cut with knife						
33. Drink from glass						

Table 25.1—*continued*

34. Drink from cup						
Hygiene						
35. Use handkerchief						
36. Wash hands						
37. Wash face						
38. Brush teeth						
39. Comb hair						
40. Care for nails						
41. Shave or make-up						
42. Arrange clothes at toilet						
43. Use toilet paper						
44. Bathe self						
45. Shampoo hair						
46. Care for menstrual period						
47. Manage catheter						
Dressing						
48. Put on/remove cardigan garment						
49. Put on/remove slipover garment						
50. Put on/remove outer coat						
51. Put on/remove trousers						
52. Put on/remove socks						
53. Put on/remove shoes						
54. Put on/remove underwear						
55. Tie shoes						
56. Tie bow or tie						
57. Lock and unlock braces						
58. Put on/remove braces						
59. Put on/remove slings or MAS						
60. Put on/remove handsplints						
Utilities						
61. Operate light switches (all types)						
62. Operate faucets (all types)						
63. Flush toilet						
64. Operate locks						
65. Plug in cord						
66. Wind watch or clock						
67. Open and close drawers						
68. Open and close windows						
69. Use scissors						
Communication						
70. Write name						
71. Handle own mail						
72. Handle money						
73. Use phone						

[a] Evaluation adapted from: University of Illinois, College of Medicine, School of Associated Medical Sciences, Curriculum in Occupational Therapy.

Table 25.2
HOMEMAKING EVALUATION

Name _____
Diagnosis _____ Onset _____
Disability _____
Precautions _____
Expected ambulation _____ Present level _____ Dominant hand _____
Visual limitations _____ Type of diet _____
1. Expected homemaker status: Assistive _____ Full-time _____
2. Description of home: Owned_____Rented_____Steps_____Elevator _____
    Floors_____No. of rooms_____Special problems _____
    _____
3. Diagram house interior (use reverse side of sheet)
4. Patient's expected responsibilities:
    Meal preparation_____Meal service_____Washing dishes_____Marketing _____
    Clothes washing: machine_____by hand_____. Drying clothes: _____
    machine_____hanging_____. Ironing_____Mending_____Washing windows _____
    Floor care: sweep_____, vacuum_____, wash_____. Cleaning: dusting _____,
    tidy up_____, heavy (walls, closets, cupboard, oven, refrigerator) _____.
5. Does the patient appear motivated toward homemaking activities? _____
6. Available help for household chores: _____
7. Available equipment
    Range: _____microwave_____electric_____gas_____automatic pilot _____
    Location of controls_____location oven_____self-cleaning? _____
    Description:
    Food preparation tools: Can opener: electric or manual _____.
    Knives: electric_____standard_____. Are knives sharp? _____
    Coffeepot: percolator or drip?_____electric_____standard _____.
    Fry pan: electric_____standard _____
    Refrigerator: Door opens: right_____left_____Freezer location: top _____
    bottom_____side_____Shelves: rotary_____pullout_____stable _____
    Self defrosting? yes_____no_____partially _____ Description:
    Sink: one well_____two well_____drainboard on right_____left _____
    Height_____standard_____deep_____shallow_____space under sink? _____
    Garbage disposal: yes_____no_____switch located? _____
    Dishwasher: top loading_____front loading_____location of controls: front_____back__
    description: _____
    Washer: automatic_____top loading_____front loading _____
    Location:__Controls: front_____back _____
    Dryer: electric_____gas_____. Location: _____.
    Controls: front_____back_____clothesline location _____.
    Height_____. Can it be lowered? _____ Method of transporting
    clothes and pins: _____.
    Ironing board: Adjustable?_____Location:_____Iron: standard _____
    steam_____Location of table or rack for finished clothes? _____
    Vacuum cleaner: upright_____tank_____built-in attachments _____

    Method of emptying _____
Electric mixer: portable _____ standard _____ Blender: _____
Electric roaster: _____ Hot plate: _____ Tea cart: _____
Knife sharpener: _____ Toaster: _____ Toaster oven: _____
Kitchen chair: no. _____ mobile _____ stationary _____
Cookbook: shortcut recipes _____ special diet _____

Table 25.3
EVALUATION[a, b]

	Initial	Discharge	Methods or person to be responsible for:
Cleaning activities			
Pick up objects from floor			
Wipe up spills (counter/floor)			
Make beds			
Change bed linens			
Use dust mop/shake			
Use broom			
Use dust pan			
Dust high and low surfaces			
Use vacuum cleaner			
Tidy up			
Transport cleaning materials			
Use wet mop/wring out			
Meal preparation			
Turn on water			
Light match and gas oven or burner			
Pour hot liquids			
Serve hot foods			
Open packaged foods			
Open ½ gallon milk carton			
Pour from milk carton			
Carry hot foods or pans			
Open screw top jars			
Use can opener			
Remove food from refrigerator			
Remove articles from cupboards			
Peel vegetables			
Use knives safely			
Break an egg			
Stir batter			
Use measuring spoons			
Use egg beater			
Pour batter			
Grease pan			
Open oven safely			
Use oven mitts			
Put pan in oven			
Use electric mixer/blender			
Use scissors			
Butter bread			
Baste meat			

Table 25.3—*Continued*

Use microwave oven			
Plan week's menu			
Meal service			
Set table			
Carry food to table			
Serve food at table			
Fold napkins			
Put on and remove table covering			
Sweep crumbs			
Scrape dishes			
Clear table			
Wash dishes and/or load dishwasher			
Dry dishes			
Dry silverware			
Scrub pots			
Wipe stove and table			
Laundry			
Sort clothes			
Hand laundry			
Use clothes pins			
Use clothes line/rack			
Plug in cord			
Iron shirt or dress			
Fold ironed clothes			
Set up ironing board			
Use washer			
Use dryer			
Fold clothes			
Sewing			
Thread needle			
Tie knot			
Sew on button			
Cut thread			
Mend rips			
Use sewing machine			
Heavy cleaning			
Cleaning stove/oven			
Clean and defrost refrigerator			
Wax floors			
Washing windows			
Cleaning tub			
Turn mattress			
Change storm windows/screens			

Table 25.3—*Continued*

Marketing In person			
Order by phone			
Receive and put away			

9. Summarize patient's capabilities following Evaluation:
10. Summarize patient's capabilities following Training:
11. Special equipment needed: (Check if recommended and list source and estimated cost.)

  _____ 1. Lapboard
  _____ 2. Spike board
  _____ 3. Suction cups
  _____ 4. Reaching tongs
  _____ 5. Wheeled cart
  _____ 6. Rocker knife
  _____ 7. Clip-on apron
  _____ 8.
  _____ 9.
  _____ 10.

12. Summarize plans for tasks not within patient's capability:

a Adapted with permission from a form devised by the Occupational Therapy Department of Highland View Cuyahoga County Hospital, Cleveland, Ohio, 44122.
b Key: 0, unable; 1, with assistance; 2, with supervision; 3, with adapted equipment; 4, independent.

References

1. Katz, S., *et al.* Studies of illness in the aged. The index of ADL: A standardized measure of biological and psychosocial function. *J.A.M.A.*, *185*(12): 914–919, 1963.
2. Iversen, I. A., *et al. The Revised Kenny Self Care Evaluation.* Publication 722 Sister Kenny Institute. Minneapolis: Abbott-Northwestern Hospital.
3. Mahoney, F. I., and Barthel, D. W. Functional evaluation: The Barthel index. *Md. State Med. J.*, *14*(2): 61–65, 1965.
4. Gresham, G. E., Phillips, T. F., and Labi, M. L. C. ADL status in stroke: Relative merits of three standard indexes. *Arch. Phys. Med. Rehabil.*, *61*(8): 355–358, 1980.
5. Granger, C. V., *et al.*, Stroke rehabilitation: Analysis of repeated Barthel index measures. *Arch. Phys. Med. Rehabil.*, *60*(1): 14–17, 1979.
6. Hasselkus, B. R., and Safrit, M. J. Measurements in occupational therapy. *Am. J. Occup. Ther.*, *30*(7): 429–436, 1976.

Supplementary Reading

Casanova, J. S., and Ferber, J. Comprehensive evaluation of basic living skills. *Am. J. Occup. Ther.*, *30*(2): 101–105, 1976.
Matsutsuyu, J. S. The interest check list. *Am. J. Occup. Ther.*, *23*: 323–328, 1960.

chapter
26

Activities of Daily Living

Catherine A. Trombly, M.A., OTR

Activities of daily living (ADL) are those occupational performance tasks that a person does each day to prepare for, or as an adjunct to, role tasks. The term, activities of daily living, is not exactly synonymous with self-care. Self-care is a more limited term which refers to the ability to dress, feed, toilet, bathe, and groom oneself, as well as miscellaneous common skills, such as using the telephone, communicating by writing, handling mail, paper money, coins, books, or newspapers. ADL also includes mobility which refers to being able to turn over in bed, come to a sitting position, move, and transfer from place to place. Driving is included in this chapter since it is considered an adjunctive daily task by many.

The occupational therapist is the rehabilitation specialist responsible for increasing the patient's independence in activities of daily living. All other therapy is supportive of that goal. Using the biomechanical or neurodevelopmental approaches, the therapist attempts to increase the patient's capabilities. If restorative therapy is able to return the patient to normalcy, no special therapy will be needed to increase independence in ADL; the patient will be doing the tasks as he is able. However, in many cases restorative therapy improves the patient's capabilities, but these remain less than normal. In these cases, the occupational therapist teaches the person new methods of doing these tasks or introduces or devises adapted equipment that will enable the person to be independent of another person for the task. Teaching the adapted method is preferred to using equipment so that the person can become truly independent. Issuing adapted equipment to make the person partially independent is sometimes justified, but depends on the investment

the patient has and the sense of satisfaction he receives in doing that particular task for himself.

The actual process of teaching the person the new techniques or how to use the adapted device depends on the patient's capacity for learning. For those patients without brain damage and of average intelligence, the teaching methods can be discussion, demonstration, or simply describing methods that others have found helpful. The patient may have suggestions about how a task might be accomplished, and his ideas should be respected and encouraged. Many techniques commonly in use have been developed by therapist-patient collaboration. Nonbrain-damaged persons should be taught in such a way that they become independent problem solvers. They need to learn to identify the problem, to understand the principle involved, and to be able to match a solution from a repertoire of solutions that have been found helpful in the past or that others have used. Practice will improve speed and ease of performance.

Patients with brain damage require more attention to the actual teaching process, which will be guided by the patient's particular learning problem. If the patient is unable to automatically do the task using old habit programs, he will be relearning a skill; therefore, much repetition is necessary. The learning may or may not transfer to other familiar tasks; therefore, he may need to practice each task until it is learned. Brain-damaged patients will probably not become problem solvers, and their prognosis for independence outside of a sheltered or familiar environment is limited. Some ADL tasks are not even attempted if judgment is impaired.

Patients who suffer damage to their dominant hemispheres usually have difficulty processing verbal or written language but are able to benefit from demonstrated or pictorial instruction. Those who suffer damage to their nondominant hemispheres may have difficulty with spatial relationships; therefore step-by-step verbal instruction is usually processed better than demonstration. Brain-damaged patients often have difficulty processing abstract information or large "chunks" of information at a time and need the instructions reduced to one- or two-word concrete cues. Given consistently over the course of practice sessions, these key word cues help the patient chain the task from beginning to end. It may be necessary to practice one step at a time; steps may be combined as learning progresses. Some patients however can only do the task if the whole chain is completed.[1]

Some profoundly, yet teachable, brain-damaged patients benefit from backward chaining. Backward chaining is an adaptation of Skinner's Law of Chaining, which he describes in this way: "The response of one reflex may produce the eliciting or discriminative stimulus of another."[2] In backward chaining of dressing skills, for example, assistance is given to do the task until the last step of the process is reached; the patient performs this one step independently with the satisfaction of having completed the task. Once the patient has mastered the final step, the therapist assists only to the next to the last step and the patient completes the two remaining steps. This process continues until the patient can do the entire task from start to finish independently.

There are some patients who are unable to learn, and their therapy must be deferred until their mental condition clears. Learning is prevented by loss of recent (or short-term) memory, severe receptive aphasia, disorientation to person or place, ideational apraxia, and the inability to identify or know the use of common objects. High anxiety also blocks learning, and therapy to reduce anxiety would be necessary if the patient exhibits this condition.

Since the rehabilitation approach involves teaching as its method of implementation, those patients who speak a language not known to the therapist and who do not understand demonstration will need to be taught through the help of an interpreter.

In order to plan treatment, results of the ADL evaluation must be considered with knowledge of the disability and with the results of sensorimotor evaluations so that reasonable expectations concerning the level of independence to be achieved can be estimated. In order to ensure success, the patient must have the prerequisite strength, mobility, endurance, balance, and coordination required by each task before it is attempted. Lack of sensation must be compensated for.

MOBILITY AND TRANSFERS

Mobility refers to movements on one surface involving change of position or location. Turning over in bed or pushing the wheelchair are examples of mobility.

Transfers refer to movement from one surface to another. For example, movements from the bed to the wheelchair or from the wheelchair to the car seat are transfers.

The type of transfer used depends on the degree of disability. If the patient is unable to move at all, a lift is required to carry him from one surface to another. If the patient is unable to bear weight on his lower extremities, and has weak upper extremities, an assisted or independent sliding transfer is taught. If the patient is unable to bear weight on his lower extremities but has strong upper extremities enabling him to depress his scapulae to lift his buttocks off of the surface, a depression transfer is the appropriate choice. If weight-bearing on the lower extremities is possible and permitted, a pivot transfer is used. When standing balance is a problem, this transfer is assisted.

Transfers will be described going in one direction. Reversing the process will accomplish the transfer in the other direction. *Note that the wheelchair must be locked for all transfers.* Transfers are most easily accomplished when the heights of the two surfaces involved in the transfer are the same.

When lifting or assisting a patient to transfer, the therapist must protect her own back by using proper body mechanics. The stronger leg muscles are used for the lifting by keeping the back straight and bending the knees whenever the patient is lifted up or lowered. The therapist evaluates her size and strength relative to the size and weight of the patient. Do not attempt a lift that seems unmanageable. Should you overestimate your strength or underestimate the weight of the patient and feel the patient slipping from your support, ease him to the floor and cushion the fall as well as you can.

Limited Range of Motion

Mobility and transfers can be done by persons with limited range. The important factor in these activities is the correct use of joints and avoidance of deforming forces (see Chapter 20). Some special devices to protect certain joints during crutch ambulation are crutches with forearm platforms or troughs to protect the distal upper extremity joints of rheumatoid arthritics from the joint deforming stresses of weight-bearing and resisted grasp. Enlarged or padded hand grips on crutches or canes can be used for patients with limited grasp or to protect small joints of the rheumatoid arthritic hand. Rubber or foam rubber hand grips are commercially available, or a customized hand grip can be fabricated using poly (methyl methacrylate) resin.[3]

For those with limited range of motion of the hips and knees combined with muscle weakness, coming to a standing position is facilitated by use of raised seating. Some examples are: (1) a raised toilet seat which can be attached to the rim of the toilet; (2) high or adjustable-height chairs such as executive office chairs; (3) a portable or electric or spring-loaded lift for existing chairs which tilts the chair seat forward to assist standing; (4) an additional cushion placed in existing chairs to raise the seat height to the required level; (5) a wheelchair fitted with an hydraulically controlled elevating seat which raises the seat when the patient is preparing to transfer.

A mobility aid available for those with weakness combined with the limited range of hip motion is a glider chair which has wheels on each leg. The chair is propelled by the feet. It can also be used for locomotion by patients limited by pain.

If the person is unable to bear weight on the legs and has weak arms, a sliding depression transfer is chosen. This transfer can be assisted or independent, depending on the extent of the person's disability.

Assisted Sliding Transfer

A sliding or transfer board is used to bridge the space between the transfer surfaces. A plastic sliding board is commercially available which has a very slippery surface. If a transfer board is made, it should be made from a 22- to 25-cm-wide piece of 1.5-cm-thick hard wood approximately 60 cm long, with tapered ends, sanded very smooth, and finished with varnish to provide a slippery gliding surface. The transfer board is positioned with one end well under the patient's hips and the other end on the surface to which the patient is transferring. Assistance is provided by holding the patient around the rib cage, waist, or waistband of trousers and sliding him along the board. The patient can place his arms around the therapist's neck or waist during the transfer. After the patient is safely onto the new surface, the legs are carried into place by the patient if possible or by the therapist if necessary.

Independent Sliding Transfer

A sliding transfer can be done independently by the person who does a series of minidepression transfers as he slides along the transfer board from one surface to the next (Fig. 26.1). A board may not be needed if the surfaces are contiguous.

Decreased Strength

The ability to roll over and to sit up in bed are necessary prerequisites to being able to dress and transfer. To roll over, the person with decreased strength in all four extremities holds the bedside rail or the arm of the wheelchair, which has been placed beside the bed and locked. He holds by grasping with the hand closest to that side of the bed or, if he lacks grasp, by hooking the distal forearm or extended wrist around the rail or the wheelchair handle. To gain the momentum necessary for rolling the upper trunk over, he then flings the other arm across the body using proximal musculature. He may then need to reach down and hook his extended wrist under his distal thigh to pull the leg over.

There are several methods a weak person can use to sit up. One is to use the vertical bars on the bedside rail to pull up using first a near bar and then each next bar to pull up to sitting. A sitting position beyond 90°

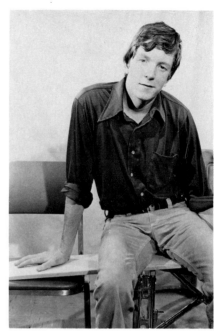

Figure 26.1 Transferring using a sliding board.

of hip flexion must be achieved to maintain balance. Another method is to use a rope ladder, which is tied to the foot of the bed. It has webbing bars attached between two webbing strips to form the ladder. The process is the same as used with the bedside rail: the arms are looped through successive bars to progressively achieve a sitting position.

To avoid the necessity for equipment, the patient can learn to come to a sitting position as follows: (1) roll to one side, for example, the right; (2) fling the top arm (left) backward to rest the elbow on the bed; (3) roll onto the left elbow and quickly fling the right arm back to rest the palm of the hand or fist on the bed; (4) roll to the right and quickly move the left arm to rest the hand on the bed; (5) having achieved a semi-sitting position resting on both hands, with the elbows extended or locked, the hands are "walked" forward to come to a forward-leaning position of greater than 90° of hip flexion to maintain balance.

Dependent Transfers

If the person is so weak that he is unable to roll over and come to a sitting position in bed, he is transferred by lifting.

A *three-person carry* is used to transfer a person who is lying down and must remain in a supported recumbent position. The three lifters position themselves on the same side of the individual to be transferred. They bend their knees and keep their backs straight. The person near the head puts one hand under the patient's neck and the other hand under the patient's scapulae; the person in the middle puts one hand under the patient's scapulae and the other hand under the patient's hips; the third person puts one hand under the patient's hips and the other hand under the patient's knees. On signal from the person supporting the head, all three lifters pull and roll the patient toward themselves to hold him against their chests as they rise to a standing position using their legs to lift. The person at the head continues to direct the transfer by leading the turn toward the transfer surface.

A *two-person carry* is used to transfer a person who can be placed in a sitting position. One lifter is positioned at the patient's head. After pulling the patient toward the edge of the bed and into a partial sitting position, the lifter flexes the patient's elbows so that the patient's forearms rest across his body. The lifter pushes his hands in under the axillae from back to front to grasp both of the patient's forearms just distal to the elbows. The other lifter assists by moving the patient's hips over to the edge of the bed by holding the patient securely under the knees. On signal from the person supporting the upper body, both lifters move the patient from the bed.

A *log roll transfer* can be done by one person. The wheelchair is locked in position, facing the foot of the bed, with the seat near the patient's hips, detachable arm removed, and a pillow over the wheel. The patient is rolled onto his side with his back toward the chair, his hips toward the chair seat at the edge of the bed, and with arms and legs flexed which distributes the weight to prevent rolling out of bed. The hips are moved onto the chair seat while the upper trunk and legs remain on the bed. Then the upper trunk is moved to an upright position in the chair and, finally, the feet are moved from the bed to the foot pedals of the wheelchair.

Mechanically Assisted Transfer. If the person who is to do the lift is weak compared to the size of the patient, and the patient is allowed to sit, a *mechanical lifter* can be used. One device (Hoyer lift)[4] has a seat and back support made of nylon material which is positioned under the patient. This support is then hooked to the hydraulic lifting mechanism which, when pumped, will lift the patient off the surface. The device is wheeled to the other surface, and slow release of the hydraulic mechanism lowers the patient to the surface. Another device has been adapted from a garage door opener which allows independent "dependent" transfer from one specific place to the other, e.g., bed to commode.[5] The use of a mechanical lift may mean the difference between discharge home or discharge to nursing home.[5]

Assisted Transfers

A variety of styles of assisted transfer are available. The *assisted sliding transfer* has already been described. Other types are listed here.

A *swivel trapeze bar* attached to an orthopedic frame at the head of the bed can be used to help lift the patient if he has upper extremity strength equal to lifting half his body weight. The wheelchair is positioned next to the bed, with the armrest removed and the brakes locked. The patient holds onto the trapeze by hooking his extended wrists around the bar to pull to sitting and then puts both forearms across the bar, assisted, if needed. The patient then contracts his elbow flexors to support the weight of his upper trunk. The therapist holds the patient's legs and pulls him off of the bed surface toward the foot of the bed and swings his lower body over to the chair. The trapeze swivels with the motion. Once seated, the patient releases his arms from the trapeze and positions his trunk in the chair.

The patient may also need assistance positioning himself in the wheelchair. A position change may be accomplished by one person standing behind the wheelchair. The wheelchair is locked and tipped backwards to its point of balance on the large back wheels. Shaking the chair assists gravity in sliding the patient's hips back into the chair. *Caution: Do not shake the chair if the patient has spasticity.* If the patient needs more assistance than this, his elbows are flexed so that his forearms rest across his body. The therapist pushes her arms in between the patient's arms and chest wall under the axillae to grasp each forearm just distal to the elbow. Force is applied upward to pull the patient into an upright posture. While lifting, the therapist guards the balance of the wheelchair with one knee to prevent it from toppling over backward.

Independent Transfers

Patients with weak upper and lower extremities may be able to do an *independent sliding transfer* (see Fig. 26.1), described previously. The *swivel trapeze bar transfer*, also previously described, can be done independently if upper extremity strength permits. The patient would lift his legs from the bed to the wheelchair foot pedals himself after he was in the wheelchair.

Independent Depression Transfer. For patients with paralyzed lower extremities but strong scapula depression and elbow extension, an independent depression transfer is done in this way: the wheelchair is positioned as close to the surface being transferred to as possible, and the brakes are locked. The feet are lifted off the foot pedals and placed on the floor one by one. Each foot pedal is raised out of the way. If the patient has poor trunk balance, he can hook one of his arms around the wheelchair upright while leaning to pull up the foot pedals with the other. The arm of the wheelchair on the side to which the transfer is to be done is removed. The patient slides forward on the seat of the wheelchair. He places one hand at a distance onto the surface he is transferring to and the other under his hip. He pushes down using scapular depression and elbow extension to lift the buttocks clear of the wheelchair and swings over to the other surface in one quick, smooth motion.

Sometimes, it is not possible to get the wheelchair close enough to the transfer surface. This most often occurs in relation to toilet or bathtub transfers. In this case, a sturdy straight-backed chair can be used to bridge the gap between the wheelchair and the toilet or tub seat.[6] A zipper back on the wheelchair may be needed to allow the patient to transfer directly backward when space near the toilet is severely limited or due to a particular patient's limitations.

For the patient who is confined to a wheelchair but has adequate upper extremity strength to propel a standard wheelchair, mobility training is important. A graded program toward independent wheelchair mobility proceeds as follows: from level, smooth surfaces to inclined, rough surfaces which are very difficult to manage in a wheelchair.

The patient also needs to learn to conquer curbs. Curbs require assistance at first. Explain to the patient what you plan to do before you do it. To assist a wheelchair up a curb, approach the curb with the front of the wheelchair and depress the foot projection on the back of the wheelchair frame while pulling back on the handles to put the casters over the curb. To assist a wheelchair down a curb, approach the curb backwards; let the large back wheels down first and then the casters. An alternative method of assisting a wheelchair down a curb uses a forward approach: tip the wheelchair back onto the large back wheels to the point of balance where the center of gravity is over the rear axle and then let the large wheels gently down the curb.

Good upper extremity strength and the ability to do a "wheelie" are needed to maneuver curbs independently.

A wheelie is done by giving a quick forward push on the handrims while simultaneously throwing the trunk back against the seat back[7]; this tips the chair backward and raises the casters off the floor. The patient then has to balance the wheelchair on its point of balance over the rear axle. Learning to do a wheelie takes much practice and some courage. A Wheelie Training Aid has been developed to allow the patient to practice without the need for a staff member present to guard.[7] Two nylon webbing straps are suspended from the ceiling and attached by way of pipe clamps to the handles of the wheelchair. The straps catch the patient and prevent him from going over backward when he fails to catch the balance point.[7]

To go up a curb the patient approaches the curb forwards. As the casters near the curb, he does a wheelie or pulls back quickly on the handrims to raise the front of the chair, which lifts the casters onto the curb. Then, while leaning forward, he propels the large back wheels onto the curb. To go down a curb the patient approaches the curb backwards, leans forward in the chair, and rolls down the curb. An alternative method for going down a curb uses a forward approach: the patient does a wheelie and rolls off the curb (Fig. 26.2).

Ascending and descending several stairs requires the assistance of two people. To take a person in a wheelchair up a flight of stairs, approach the stairs backwards. One person stands behind the chair and tips it backwards into its balanced position. The second person stands in front of the chair and holds the leg rest upright. While maintaining the chair at its point of balance on the back wheel, the person behind the chair pulls it up each step in succession while the

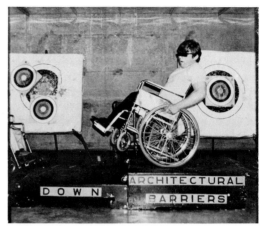

Figure 26.2 A "wheelie" demonstrated by a student at the University of Illinois.

person at the foot assists in lifting and maintains the point of balance. To take a person in a wheelchair down a flight of stairs, approach the stairs forward and with the wheelchair in a balanced position. The two people reverse the process for ascending stairs to lower the chair down each step in succession.

For those too weak to propel the wheelchair, an electric wheelchair is required (see Chapter 14). Batteries for wheelchairs should be of the deep-cycle type such as designed for powering fishing motors, golf carts, electric lawnmowers, etc. rather than the starting-lighting-ignition (SLI) type used in automobiles. The latter are not meant to be deep-cycled (discharged so that it cannot deliver the voltage needed) and recharged repeatedly as is required for wheelchair use.[8]

Incoordination

No special techniques are used to enable persons with incoordination to move in bed or to transfer. Unless they have concomitant weakness, in which case the techniques listed under the previous section would be used, they are able to do these activities. The problem of safety arises, and these patients must pay particular attention to safety factors. If judgment is poor, the patient will be dependent on others for supervision during transfer.

Wheelchair Mobility

Some incoordinated persons find it easier to propel a standard wheelchair by using their feet. Pushing backwards is easiest, but a rear view mirror is needed to prevent accidents!

The Loss of the Use of One Side of the Body

The person who has suffered a stroke and lost the use of one side of the body must relearn how to roll over and come to a sitting position in bed. In one method of rolling over from a supine position, the hemiplegic patient puts his unaffected foot under the affected ankle, carries his affected arm across his body, and then pulls himself over onto his unaffected side by holding the side of the bed. Another method is for the patient to clasp his hands, extend his elbows, and flex his shoulders to 90° so that he is reaching upward. Then he swings the arms toward one side first, then quickly swings them over to the other side. The momentum carries him onto his side.[9]

One method of coming to sitting on the edge of the bed is to put the unaffected foot under the affected ankle and carry the legs to the edge of the bed. Next, carry the affected arm across the body, simultaneously pull the head forward, and push against the bed with the uninvolved arm to come to a sitting position. The patient continues the upward thrust of his upper body while swinging his legs over the side of the bed. He should be guarded until the therapist is satisfied that he can do this procedure independently and safely. A hard mattress reduces the danger of falling. If the mattress at home is soft, a bed board can be suggested.

Another method of coming to sitting is advocated by Bobath.[9] At first the patient starts by clasping his hands and rolling over into the sound side as described above. With the arms still clasped together, he bends his sound elbow and pushes the upper trunk off the bed. He brings his sound leg over the edge of the bed, which brings him to a semisitting position. He then pushes with both arms (still clasped) while flexing the head toward the affected side, to bring himself upright. The affected leg is simultaneously lowered as he pushes upright. The therapist may need to assist with the head lateral flexion and swinging the affected leg off the bed until the patient learns the technique and gains sufficient strength.

Assisted Transfers

The hemiplegic person is able to accept weight on one or both lower extremities and is therefore a candidate for a pivot transfer. The patient always transfers with his strong side leading, or toward, the non-involved side.

Assisted 90° Pivot Transfer. For a pivot transfer from wheelchair to chair, the locked wheelchair is positioned at an acute angle to the side of the chair placed on the patient's noninvolved side. The therapist faces the patient, who is sitting with his feet on the floor, approximately 20 to 30 cm apart, and directly under his knees. The therapist bends her knees to meet and support the patient's knees. She reaches under the patient's arm to position her hands on the scapula of the involved side or takes hold of the waistband of the patient's trousers. As the patient leans forward and pushes down on the wheelchair armrest with the noninvolved arm to assist standing, the therapist supports one of the patient's knees and assists it into extension while lifting from the scapula or trousers (Fig. 26.3).

After the patient is standing and balanced, the therapist pivots with the patient to turn so that the patient now stands in front of the chair. The therapist helps to lower the patient into the chair slowly by bending her knees as the patient sits. The patient puts his noninvolved hand on the armrest to assist in lowering

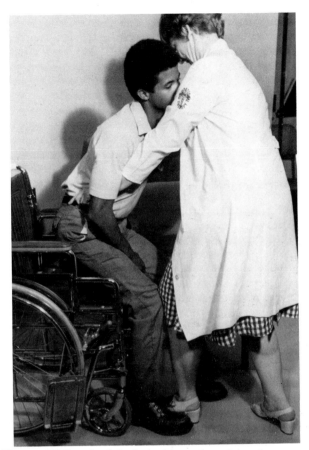

Figure 26.3 Assisted pivot transfer: rising from one surface.

himself slowly into the chair (Fig. 26.4). Before the student therapist does the transfer with a patient, she needs to experiment and practice to determine how to place her feet in relation to the patient's feet to offer the best stability to the patient's knee and to prevent tripping each other.

Independent Transfer

Independent 90° Pivot Transfer. In this transfer, the process is the same as noted above, except that it is done without help. To review, the wheelchair is locked in position next to the surface to be transferred to, which is located on the patient's noninvolved side. The front of the wheelchair seat should be perpendicular to, or at an acute angle to, the front of the seating surface to be transferred to. The patient lifts the foot pedals and slides forward in the wheelchair. The feet are flat and slightly apart on the floor, directly under the knees.

Using a rocking motion to gain momentum, the patient then presses with the noninvolved foot to extend that leg while pushing down on the arm of the wheelchair with the noninvolved arm to come to a standing position. Once balanced in a fully standing position, the patient reaches to the surface to which he is transferring, pivots, and lowers himself to the surface.

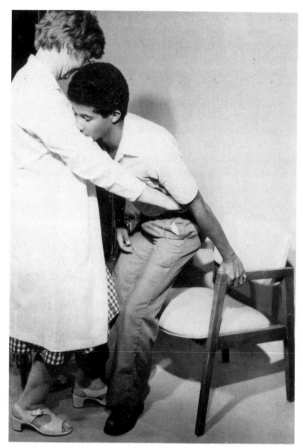

Figure 26.4 Assisted pivot transfer: lowering onto the other surface.

Independent 180° Pivot Transfer. The 180° independent pivot transfer is done similarly to the 90° pivot but requires the patient to turn much more after standing in order to reach the surface to which he is transferring. This transfer is chosen when required by the circumstances such as in a bathroom or other areas where the wheelchair cannot be positioned for a 90° pivot. Wall bars assist in doing a 180° pivot safely.

Wheelchair Mobility

If the patient is confined to a wheelchair either temporarily or permanently, he can learn to propel a standard wheelchair. To do so, the hemiplegic uses both the unaffected arm and leg. The leg provides both power and compensatory steering. A one-arm drive wheelchair, which is commercially available, is confusing to hemiplegics but would be appropriate for patients who have a disability that leaves one arm as the only functional extremity and who have the cognitive and perceptual abilities to learn to operate the chair.

Blindness

This disability of course does not interfere with bed mobility or transfers. Ambulatory mobility is limited, however.

Mobility is taught by a peripatologist, a specialist in blind mobility. Through extensive special training, a blind person can become independently mobile. The long cane method is preferred. The technique of using a dog guide requires specialized training for the person and the dog. Seeing eye dogs, in harness, are working and should never be diverted by someone else or petted without permission of the owner. When leading a blind person, in lieu of independent mobility, the blind person holds the leader's upper arm and walks about one-half step behind the leader. The leader holds his arm close to his body so that the blind person gets sensory input from the leader's arm and body. In that way, the blind person can sense unevenness in the terrain, steps, turning corners, etc. Verbal cautioning is unnecessary unless there is an overhanging object, such as a branch of a tree, in the path.

SELF-CARE

In studies of independence in self-care, Katz *et al.*[10] found that patients with chronic illness regained independence in the following order: feeding, continence, transferring, going to toilet (social and cultural aspects), dressing, and bathing. They hypothesized from observations that loss of these functions would occur in reverse order. Comparison of their conclusions concerning the sequence of the development of self-care independence with child developmental and anthropological observations revealed an ontogenetic consistency. Based on their findings it would seem appropriate for treatment planning to follow this sequence. Some additions can be made, such as the insertion of grooming after feeding and undressing before dressing. Conversely, some diagnostic conditions may require modifications of this sequence. For example, a spinal cord-injured patient may transfer before he develops continence and, in fact, may never regain continence.

Not all patients achieve total independence in self-care. It may be necessary for the occupational therapist to train family members in proper methods of supervising or assisting the patient to perform tasks in the most efficient and safe manner for both patient and family member.

All tasks which the patient will be required to perform independently once discharged must be practiced in a manner similar to the way they will be done. For example, if a patient will bathe in a tub at home, it is inadequate to only practice sponge bathing while hospitalized. It is also inadequate to eliminate from practice the details of self care such as nail care, ear care, menstrual care, handling catheter, hair setting, contact lens care and use, etc. or to assume that all self-care tasks which a particular person may need to learn are listed on the evaluation checklist.

As each task is taught, all potentially needed equipment should be close at hand. For early training in dressing, clothing that is a size too large should be used since it can be managed more easily. Attention should also be placed on the design details of clothing as some designs are more easily donned by persons with certain disabilities. The details to be considered are the cut of the garment, the sleeve style, type of closure or fasteners, and fabric.[11] Clothing design for the handicapped is just beginning to be attended to by designers and pattern makers. Methods to adapt clothing for wheelchair users, and other disabled persons, have been published by the Sister Kenny Institute.[12]

If the patient must learn to feed himself using adapted utensils, one training sequence is to start with sticky foods that will not easily slide off of the spoon. Skill and endurance in the use of the equipment is sought through practice. Once skilled in basic use of the utensil, the patient is ready to feed himself an entire meal. The therapist should ensure that the meal will be easy to eat, *i.e.*, not spaghetti for dinner and sliced peaches for dessert! The first independent meal should be a pleasant, successful experience, not one spent adjusting the equipment.

Communication devices have burgeoned with the development of rehabilitation engineering. There are three types of devices: (1) direct selection devices which print, out of a fairly large array, the one item that the person points to or activates by some control transducer; (2) scanning devices in which the device points to the item or groups of items in an array one at a time and may or may not print it; and (3) encoding devices which accept codes and translate them into whole messages.[13, 14] These devices are used by those too incoordinated to speak clearly or by those too paralyzed to write or use a standard typewriter for written communication. It is necessary to evaluate the patient and choose the best type of equipment for him.[13, 14] The cost may be prohibitive[14] for the ideal solution, but less sophisticated devices, such as language boards that simply have the alphabet or phrases written on them to which the patient points, may increase the person's abilities. Because the more sophisticated instruments may enable an otherwise unemployable person to be employed, the cost may be justified, and financial help may be available from the Vocational Rehabilitation Services.

Techniques and equipment for self care presented in this chapter are not the only methods of accomplishing these particular tasks. This presentation is not meant to be exhaustive but rather to provide the student therapist with a repertoire of basic skills with which she can approach her patient with confidence. Many tasks not mentioned here either do not require adaptation, or the adaptation can be extrapolated from the examples cited. Sources of equipment are rehabilitation supply stores. The annual *Accent on Living Buyer's Guide* lists sources for all types of equipment.[15] The Independence Factory will make devices requested to meet a particular need; they will also provide directions for self construction of devices.[16]

Limited Range of Motion

The principles of compensation for limited range of motion are to increase the person's reach by means of extended handles and to substitute for limited range by use of adaptations.

Feeding

The problem may be one of inability to close the hand enough to grasp the utensil or the inability to bring the hand to the mouth.

Enlarged or elongated handles can be added to spoons or forks. The elongated handle may need to be angled to enable the patient to reach his mouth. Remember that the longer the handle, the heavier and less stable is the device; therefore, the handle should be only as long as is absolutely necessary. Handles may be temporarily enlarged by wrapping a washcloth, foam rubber, or other material around the handle and securing it with a rubber band. Commercially available utensils with handles of plastic or adjustable aluminum can be used more permanently. Also, Polyform can be used to mold and enlarge handles for permanent use.[17]

A universal cuff, or utensil holder, can be used when grasp is not possible. This cuff fits around the palm and has a pocket for insertion of the handle of a utensil (Fig. 26.5).

Grooming

The problems are the same as for feeding. Enlarged or extended handles can be attached to a comb (Fig. 26.6), brush, toothbrush, shampoo brush, lipstick tube, or safety razor.

Aerosol deodorant, hair spray, powder, and perfume can be used by those with limited range.

Another person may be needed to thoroughly wash and curl a woman's hair; a simple hair style is recommended.

Toileting

The problem is the inability to reach. The patient may not be able to sit on a low commode; therefore, a raised toilet seat would be necessary. The toilet tissue dispenser should be located within reach.

Gravity will assist in pulling clothes down; larger clothes slide off more easily. Wiping tongs can extend

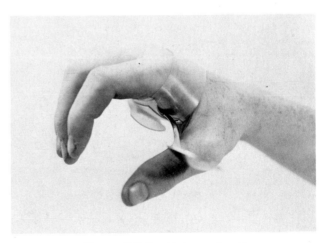

Figure 26.5 Universal cuff.

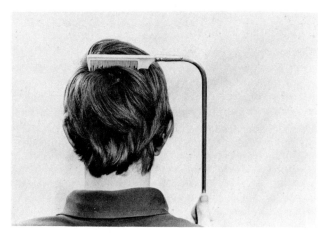

Figure 26.6 Long handled comb.

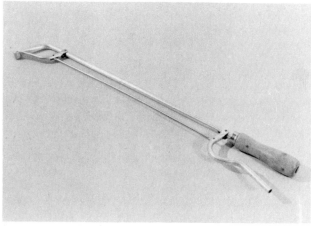

Figure 26.7 Voluntary opening reacher which remains closed to hold objects without exertion of the patient.

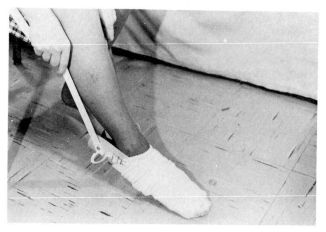

Figure 26.8 One type of stocking aid.

reach when using toilet tissue. If grasp is poor, the tissue can be wrapped around the hand to eliminate the need for grasping it. A bidet eliminates the need for wiping by hand. A dressing stick (a long rod with a hook attached to one end) can be used to pull up the clothing. Sanitary napkins with adhesive strips can be used easier than tampons; the protective paper can be removed using the teeth.

Dressing

Lack of reach and grasp and the inability to raise the arms at the shoulders or to bend the legs at the hips or knees are possible problems encountered in dressing.

A dressing stick can be used to pull clothing over the feet or to reach hangers in the closet. Reaching tongs can be used to remove clothes from shelves, to start clothes over parts of the body, or to pick up objects from floor (Fig. 26.7). A reacher can be made by adding a spring clip to a yardstick.[18]

Putting on socks or stockings is a major problem. A sock or *stocking aid* for people who are unable to reach their feet can be made to hold the stocking open while putting the foot in (Fig. 26.8). This may be purchased or made from x-ray film or thermoplastic splinting material by cutting a triangle with rounded corners out of the film, and attaching three straps or strings to the base of the triangle. To use, the triangular film is folded, and the cone is inserted into the foot of the stocking; the top of the stocking is pushed down below the top edge of the cone. While the strings are held, the stocking is tossed over the toes, and the person's foot is moved into the foot of the stocking. The cone is then removed by pulling the strings, bringing it out of the stocking behind the heel. The stocking will now be within reach and can be pulled up onto the leg.

An alternative method is to place a piece of foam rubber on the floor to help get the stocking onto the foot after it is placed on the toe with a reacher. This method consists of pushing the foot forward across the foam rubber, which provides friction and holds the stocking as the foot slides in.[6] As this method can be

done standing up or sitting on a high stool, it may be particularly helpful to post-hip replacement patients who are not allowed to flex the hip.

Another solution is to sew a garter to each end of a long piece of webbing. The garters are attached to either side of a sock or stocking to pull them up to a point on the leg where they may be reached.

A long shoehorn assists in putting on shoes when the feet cannot be reached. Some long shoehorns have a hook on the opposite end which may be used as a dressing stick. Loafer style shoes or elastic shoelacers avoid the need to tie shoelaces.

Garters attached to webbing straps may be used to pull up slacks. Cardigan shirts are used instead of slipover garments. The dressing stick or reacher is used to bring the garment around the shoulders.

Velcro tabs can replace buttons or hooks if limited mobility in the fingers prevents buttoning or fastening. To preserve the look of a buttoned garment, the buttonhole is sewn closed, and the button is attached over the hole. Then hook and pile Velcro tabs are sewn to replace the button.[19] Velcro is sold in small circles or in strips. Strips can be cut into small squares for tabs.

Bathing

The same problems encountered in dressing are seen to interfere with this task.

The transfer into the tub is facilitated by safety rails *securely* mounted to the studs in the wall beside the bathtub or attached to the side of the bathtub. A securely fastened rubber mat should be placed in the tub, even if the tub has nonskid surface, and one outside the tub, unless the bathroom is carpeted.

A tub seat is used when the patient is unable to get down into the bottom of the tub or get up from there. Different heights and styles are available and need to be evaluated for each patient in terms of stability and ease of transfer.

A hand-held shower spray is used for rinsing if a tub seat is required. Flat handles on faucets do not require grasp and allow better leverage for turning them on.

It is helpful if the soap is on a string. It can be purchased that way or made by drilling a hole through a cake of soap and attaching a cord. The soap is either worn around the neck or hung within easy reach. When grasp is limited, a sponge or a terrycloth bath mitt may be preferred. A long-handled bath sponge may be needed to reach the feet or back; some are designed to hold the soap inside of the sponge.

A terrycloth bathrobe is effective for drying.

Miscellaneous

Writing and telephoning may be problem areas. If pinch is limited, the size of the writing instrument can be increased by using sponge rubber or a foam hair curler,[6] or the pencil can be passed through the holes in a practice golf ball. If the person cannot raise the telephone receiver to the ear and hold it there, an extended arm which clamps on the table permanently holds the receiver at a convenient height. If the extended arm is of the gooseneck type the receiver can be put in different positions. A lever is attached to the phone to depress the activator buttons, and the phone is answered by raising this lever.

Decreased Strength

The principles of compensation for weakness or decreased strength are to use gravity to assist, to change body mechanics or leverage, to use lightweight devices, and to use electrical appliances. When muscle weakness involves all four extremities, the techniques and devices are extensive and, therefore, this section will focus on compensation for involvement of all four extremities. If the patient is weak in his lower extremities with normal upper extremities, many of the techniques or devices will be unnecessary. Other equipment suggestions have been listed in the chapter on spinal cord injury.

Feeding

The problem is the inability to grasp or to bring the hand to the mouth.

Mobile arm supports or suspension slings may be required for proximal weakness, or a table or lapboard at axilla height may be used to offer support for the arm and to eliminate gravity. As strength increases, the surface can be lowered.

Some splints provide pinch to hold the utensils. Lightweight untensils are used. If the patient has weak grasp without the splint, lightweight, enlarged handles can be used. A universal cuff can be used to hold the utensil if grasp is absent. A "spork," a utensil which combines the bowl of a spoon with the tines of a fork, is used with the cuff to eliminate the need to change utensils. Some of these have a swivel feature to substitute for the inability to supinate. Gravity and weight of the food keep the bowl level on the way to the mouth (see Fig. 26.9). For cutting, a sharp, serrated knife is used since less force is needed and it is less likely to slip.

Sandwich holders that hold a sandwich in a trough and have a handle which the patient can manage are available.

An attachable, open-bottomed handle can be added to a glass or beer can to permit picking them up in the absence of grasp. A mug with a T-shaped handle or a handle that allows all four fingers to be inserted provides leverage and stabilizes the fingers around the mug, allowing pick up when only tenodesis grasp is present. A stretch terrycloth coaster placed around a glass can provide friction to assist a weak grasp.[6]

Grooming

The inability to grasp and pinch need to be dealt with to enable the patient to groom himself.

A universal cuff or a splint can be used to hold a rattail comb, toothbrush, lipstick tube, or safety razor if grasp is absent. If grasp is weak, lightweight, enlarged handles may be enough.

Electric razor holders that have a handcuff provide a safer method of shaving than use of a safety razor.

A small round plastic brush with or without a cuff attachment may be used to assist in shampooing hair.[6]

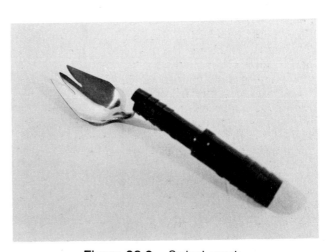

Figure 26.9 Swivel spork.

Toileting

In addition to the transfer, the handling of the body to lower and raise the clothing and the lack of pinch and grasp are the problems.

Pants can be gradually pulled down while the patient is in the wheelchair by leaning to one side and then the other. If the patient uses an indwelling catheter or external drainage device, the collection bag can be emptied into the toilet without the need to transfer or remove the clothing.

A raised toilet seat is used by quadriplegic individuals to create a space between the seat and toilet bowl rim to allow for insertion of a suppository.

A suppository inserter is commercially available for those with weak or absent pinch. It is attached to a handcuff for use by quadriplegic patients and has a spring ejector which releases the suppository after it is properly positioned in the rectum. An inspection mirror may be needed if the patient lacks anal sensation.

Tissue can be wrapped around the hand for use. If the patient has precarious balance, it may be necessary to transfer back to the wheelchair before raising the clothing. Menstrual needs can be met by use of adhesive-backed sanitary pads.

Dressing

The problems are the need to learn new ways of using the stronger limbs to move the paralyzed limbs to dress them and also the lack of pinch and grasp.

While in bed and by using the wrist extensors and elbow flexors, patients with spinal cord injury at C_6 and below can pull the knees up to dress the lower extremities.

A dressing stick with a loop attached to the end opposite the hook can help quadriplegics. They pull against the loop, using wrist extension, in order to stabilize tenodesis grasp of the stick.

The sock aid and long-handled shoehorn previously mentioned may be useful. Loops of twill tape can be added to the cuffs of socks to facilitate pulling them on by hooking the thumb in the loop.

A buttonhook, attached to a cuff or with a built-up handle, is used when fingers are unable to manipulate a button to fasten it. The hook is inserted through the buttonhole to hook the button and pull it through the buttonhole. The other hand is used to hold the garment near the buttonhole (Fig. 26.10).

A loop of string or leather lacing may be attached to the zipper pull of trousers or other garments, so that in the absence of pinch, the thumb can be hooked in the zipper pull to close the zipper. A hook can also be used.

Primarily, the following methods of quadriplegic dressing were described by Margaret Runge, OTR, in an article, "Self Dressing Techniques for Patients with Spinal Cord Injury" in the *American Journal of Occupational Therapy*.[20]

Trousers (and Undershorts). Sitting in bed with side rails up, the trousers are positioned with the front up and legs over the bottom of the bed. The trousers

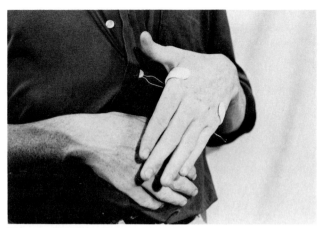

Figure 26.10 Button hook on a cuff. Note zipper pull hook on other end.

are tossed or a dressing stick with wrist loop is used to position them.

One leg is lifted by hooking the opposite wrist or forearm under the knee, and the foot is put into pants leg. The thumb of the other hand hooks a belt loop or pocket to hold the trousers open. Working in a cross-body position aids stability for those with poor balance. The other foot is inserted. The palms of the hands are used to pat and slide trousers onto the calves, attempting to get the trouser cuffs over the feet. The wrist(s) is hooked under the waistband or in the pockets to pull the trousers up over the knees. The patient continues to pull on the waistband or pockets while returning to supine position to pull the trousers up on the thighs. This may need to be repeated. Hooking the wrist or thumbs in the crotch helps pull up the trousers. In a side-lying position, the thumb of the top arm is hooked in the back belt loop, and the pants are pulled over the buttocks. Then the patient rolls to the other side and repeats the process until the trousers are on. In a supine position, the trousers can be fastened using a zipper pull loop and Velcro tab closing or buttonhook. Removing the trousers is accomplished essentially by reversing the procedures and pushing the pants off.

Socks. While sitting in the wheelchair, the patient crosses one leg over the other and uses tenodesis pinch to put on the sock and the palms of the hands to help pull it on. If the patient is unable to cross his legs, the foot can be placed on a stool or chair. If trunk balance is poor, one arm can be hooked around the wheelchair upright while reaching with the other hand, or the socks can be put on in a sitting position in bed by crossing first one leg and then the other. A sock cone or aid may be helpful in getting the sock over the toes if the patient is unable to reach his feet. Socks are removed by pushing them off with a dressing stick, long shoehorn, or the thumb hooked in the sock edge.

Long Leg Braces (Knee-Ankle-Foot Orthoses) for Paraplegics. While the patient is sitting in bed, the brace is positioned beside the leg, and then the patient lifts his leg over into the brace. If the shoe is attached to the brace, the foot is first put into the shoe. It is helpful to unlock and flex the knee of the brace to press the shoe against the bed and pull on the uprights to get the heel into the shoe. Then, with the knee still flexed, the shoe can be tied. Next, the knee is straightened, and the knee pad is fastened, and then the thigh band.

In order for a brace to be worn under trousers the brace must be attached to the shoe with removable calipers. In this instance the patient first puts on his socks, the brace, his trousers, then his shoes, and then attaches the brace to the shoe.

Once the patient is in the wheelchair, other garments are put on.

Shoes. Loafer-type shoes are most practical for nonambulatory patients. Shoes are put on by crossing one leg at a time as for putting on socks. The shoe is pulled onto the foot by holding the sole of the shoe in the palm of the hand. With the foot on the floor, or on the foot pedal of the wheelchair, the foot is pushed down into the shoe by pushing on the knee. A long shoehorn may be helpful for getting the heel into the shoe.

Shoes can be removed by pushing them off with the shoehorn.

Cardigan Garments (Shirts or Blouses). The shirt is positioned with the brand label of the shirt facing down and the collar toward the knees. The arms are put under the shirt and into the sleeves. The shirt is pushed on until the sleeves are over the elbows. The shirt is gathered up by using wrist extension and by hooking the thumbs under the shirt back. Then the shirt is placed over the head. The shoulders are shrugged to get the shirt down across the shoulders. The wrists are hooked into the sleeves to free the axillae. The patient then leans forward and reaches back with one hand to rub the shirt back in order to pull it down. The shirt fronts are lined up, and buttoning begins from the bottom button up, using a buttonhook. With the exception of buttons, an overhead garment is put on in a similar manner.

A cardigan garment is removed by pushing first one side and then the other off the shoulders and then alternately elevating and depressing the shoulders to allow gravity to assist in lowering the shirt down the arms. Then one thumb is hooked into the opposite sleeve to pull the shirt over the elbow, and the arm is removed from the shirt.

Bra. Either a front or back closure style can be used. Velcro can replace hooks for fastening, but many patients can manage the standard hook fastener if it is hooked in front at waist level. After the bra is hooked it is positioned with the cups in front, and the arms are placed through the shoulder straps. Then, by hooking the opposite thumb under a strap, one strap at a time is pulled over the shoulder.

Bathing.

The problems are the transfer, sitting equilibrium, lack of lower extremity movement, and lack of pinch and grasp.

A padded board placed across one end of the tub provides a level transfer surface. The padding helps to prevent decubiti. The back of the wall of the tub enclosure can be used for trunk support. A padded straight chair can be used either in the tub or in a shower stall. Suction cups or "skis" on the bottom of the chair provide stability for transfers. Other bath seats are available with and without back support or padding. Each patient's requirements need to be evaluated and a seat selected to fit them.

Grab bars secured to the studs of the wall help during the transfer and while seated. A suction cup-backed bath mat is used in the bottom of the tub.

The faucets must be placed within reach and must have flat handles for ease in tapping them off and on using the fist. A hand held shower is used. Water temperature is adjusted by turning on the cold water first and then adding the hot to prevent scalding desensitized skin. Soap on a string is helpful. A bath mitt is used if grasp is weak or absent. A large towel is used for drying off before transferring back to the chair.

A custom-made shower stall installed in a person's home provides the best solution for bathing. The shower area has a raised slope to prevent the water from running out, but allows the passage of a special shower wheelchair. Such a chair is meant to be wet without being damaged.

Miscellaneous.

The quadriplegic patient will encounter problems with holding a book and turning the pages, with writing or recording notes in business or school, and possibly telephoning.

If a person is unable to hold a book, racks are available. Some support a book on a table while others are designed to hold a book overhead for reading supine in bed. If a person is reading supine, prism glasses are needed to direct the vision to a 90° angle so that the book may be seen.

If page turning is difficult, some of the following ways of increasing friction might be of assistance: (1) tacky fingers, which is a sticky substance available in stationary stores, can be applied to a patient's weak fingers; (2) a rubber thimble or finger cot that can be put on a posted thumb when the patient wears a splint; (3) a pencil with the eraser end down, used in a universal cuff or hand splint; and (4) a mouthstick with a friction tip end. Electric page turners for the severely disabled are available. They automatically turn pages when activated by microswitch or other means of control.

An alternative for the severely paralyzed is "talking books." These are records that were originally only made available to the blind, but are now by law available to the physically handicapped. The Library of Congress has a large collection of records, including many current issues of magazines. The records are free and can be ordered by mail or through the hospitals division of the local library. Particular books needed by students or professionals will be recorded on request.

For writing, splints that provide pinch can hold the writing instrument. Felt tip pens mark with little pressure and are therefore easier to use. If pinch is absent, and the patient does not use a splint, a pencil holder (Fig. 26.11) which encircles the pencil as well as the thumb and index finger can be made of thermoplastic materials.

If the arms cannot be used, a mouthstick with pencil attached can become an effective writing tool with practice.

If writing is not possible or speed of recording is important, as in taking notes in the classroom, a tape recorder can be used. If necessary, the mechanical controls can be adapted.[19] If the recorder has electronic controls, it can be adapted by use of microswitches or other transducers.

Electric typewriters with automatic carriage return can be used by paralyzed persons who type using either typing sticks or a mouthstick. A mouthstick is preferably made by a dentist who molds a mouthpiece of dental acrylic to conform to the patient's dentition and to which is added a lightweight wooden, plastic, or aluminum rod with an eraser or other type of end piece. Self-correcting ribbon may be useful, depending on the manner in which it is activated by the particular typewriter. The IBM machine can be fitted with paper roll dispenser which feeds 20-cm (8-inch) paper into the typewriter for persons unable to pick up sheets of paper and start them into the machine.

The POSSUM typewriter can be used by totally paralyzed persons. POSSUM stands for Patient Operated Selector Mechanisms and refers to the Latin word meaning "I am able."[21] It was developed in England. A pneumatic control tube is attached to a mouthpiece and secured in a position convenient to the mouth; control is by sip and puff. When the patient sips or puffs, solenoids (electrical switching devices) depress the keys. Letters are arranged on a grid according to frequency of use. Starting position is at the bottom left corner. Suction on the tube advances a light across the columns; when the correct column is reached, blowing on the tube starts the light advancing up the column, and when the correct letter is reached,

release of pressure causes the letter to be typed and the control to be returned to start. The rate at which the light moves can be adjusted to eight different speeds as skill increases (Fig. 26.12).

Two severely disabled quadriplegics unable to use mechanical controls of a typewriter key board have been successful in using a newly developed voice-controlled computer terminal which types out the spoken message. Further development and study of the use of this device to provide employment opportunities for the severely disabled is ongoing.[22]

C_6 level quadriplegics can pick up the receiver and bring it to the ear. An executive shoulder rest attached to the receiver holds it there until the conversation is finished. Using a flexor hinge hand splint or a universal cuff, a dialing stick can be one with a knob that fits into a hole of the rotary dial, or simply a pencil used eraser end down.

For patients with greater paralysis of the upper extremities, automatic telephone dialers are available.[13, 16]

Incoordination

The principles of compensation for problems of incoordination are to provide stability and to substitute for lack of fine skill. The patient is taught to use his body in as stable a posture as is possible, to sit when possible, to stabilize the upper extremities by bearing weight on them against a surface or by holding the upper arms close to the body, or both. Stabilizing the head may improve a person's ability to control his upper extremities. Friction surfaces, weighted utensils, weighted cuffs added to the distal segments of the extremities, and the use of larger and/or less precise fasteners all contribute to increasing independence of an incoordinate person by lessening the effects of the incoordination.

Feeding

The plate is stabilized on a friction surface (wet towel, wet sponge cloth, no-skid mat, etc.). A plate

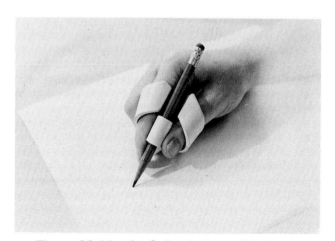

Figure 26.11 An Orthoplast pencil holder.

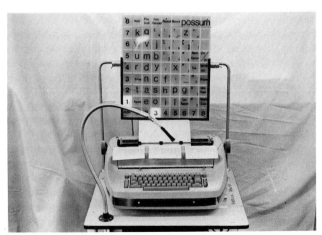

Figure 26.12 POSSUM typewriter operated electronically by sip and puff signals to select and type characters.

guard is attached to the left of the plate for a right-handed person, or vice versa, to prevent the food from being pushed off when scooped. The utensil may be weighted for stability, may have an enlarged handle to facilitate grasp, and may be plastisol-coated to protect the person's teeth. Sharp utensils are to be avoided. A weight cuff on the wrist is often chosen rather than a weighted utensil because the cuff can be heavier and negates the necessity to weight each item the patient will use. The person may successfully drink from a covered glass or cup that has a sipping spout. A cup can be adapted by using plastic food wrap as a cover, with a straw poked through it.[6] Some may use a long plastic straw which is held in place by a straw holder attachment; the patient moves his head to the straw, but he does not touch it with his hand. A severely incoordinated person with good strength and endurance may use an upper extremity control brace, or friction feeder,[23] which supports the arm and dampens the patient's motion through the use of friction discs at each joint. The amount of friction can be adjusted.

Grooming

Weighted cuffs on the wrists may help some patients gain greater accuracy while grooming. Large lipstick tubes are easier to use than small ones. The arms will need to be stabilized to use lipstick. A simple hair style that does not need setting or arrangement is the best choice. For a patient who has difficulty holding a large comb, a military-style brush with a strap can be used.

Roll on or stick deodorant is preferred to aerosol since they eliminate the risk of accidentally spraying the substance into the eyes. An electric razor is preferred to a safety razor both because it is more easily held and because a safety razor can cause a cut if it is involuntarily moved sideways over the skin. Patients with fairly good head control improve their accuracy by holding the electric razor steady and moving their face over the cutting surface. An electric toothbrush is also useful both because it is heavier and because it can be held steady and the head moved. This same principle can be employed when filing the nails: fasten the emery board to a flat surface and move each nail over it. Cutting the nails may be an unsafe procedure for incoordinate patients and, therefore, filing is recommended. Sanitary napkins with the adhesive strips that hold them in place are a preferred solution, although the sanitary belt holders designed to just slip the ends of the pad in without the need to thread them may also be managed.

Dressing

Clothes that facilitate independent dressing are front opening, loosely fitting garments with large buttons, Velcro tape closures, or zippers. The wrinkle-resistant and stain-shedding materials enable the person to look well-groomed throughout the day. To overcome difficulty with buttoning, a buttonhook with an enlarged and/or weighted handle, if necessary, can be used. A loop of ribbon, leather, or metal chain can be attached to the zipper pull so that the person can hook it with a finger instead of pinching the zipper pull. To eliminate the need to fasten hooks on a bra, these can be replaced with Velcro. To don the bra, it is easier for the patient to put it around her waist, which is thinner and puts less tension on the garment, then fasten it in front where she can see what she is doing, turn it around, put her arms in, and pull it up into place. Elastic straps make this a relatively easy procedure. Some persons prefer to use an all elastic slipover-type bra with no hooks. Shoes can be of the loafer style or can have flip closures to eliminate tying. Tie shoes can be adapted using zipper shoelaces or elastic shoelaces. Patients who ambulate may need to wear tie shoes for stability and support. If a man wears a tie, he may choose to slide the knot down and pull the tie off over his head without undoing the knot or to use clip ties if his degree or coordination allows that.

Bathing

The patient may independently bathe, but must adhere closely to safety precautions. A rubber suction cup bath mat is placed outside the tub to stand on while transferring and another is placed in the tub. It is important to be certain that the mats are securely stuck before trusting one's safety to them. Safety bars should be placed where they would be most useful to the particular person's needs: one mounted into the studs of the wall at the side of the tub and one mounted on the rim of the tub may be necessary. A bath chair or seat can eliminate the difficulty of trying to stand up from a sitting position at the bottom of the tub. If a seat is used, a hand-held shower spray needs to be available. If the patient chooses to shower instead of bathe, the mats, safety bars, and seat must also be provided. In either case, water should be drawn once the patient has transferred in and is seated; a mixer tap is ideal but, if unavailable, the cool water should be turned on first and the hot water added to prevent scalding.

Soap on a string keeps the soap retrievable, or a bath mitt with a pocket to hold the soap can be used. The water should be drained before the person attempts to stand to transfer out of the tub. An extra large towel or large terry wraparound robe facilitates the drying process.

Miscellaneous

Communication is a problem to some incoordinated persons. For typing, a shield which covers the keyboard and has holes cut out over the keys prevents misstrikes. Such shields are available from IBM and from Royal, but if a shield is not available for a particular typewriter, one can easily be made from acrylic. A board placed in front of the typewriter on which the forearms can be stabilized would offer support for the arms while typing. IBM distributes a wooden armrest which attaches to the front of the keyboard.

For the severely incoordinated person, computer

operated typing (or communication) systems have been developed. One such is the *Auto Con*, developed at the University of Wisconsin in Madison. It has a large board with the letters alphabetically arranged and numbers and other characters similar to a typewriter. The letters selected are transferred to a TV monitor. Corrections are more easily made than on a conventional typewriter. The unit has been reported as an aid to classroom communication for a severely involved cerebral palsied child at Kennedy Memorial Hospital in Boston.[24]

Manual Communications Module, which is a portable, frequency-selective communication device, has been used successfully by severely involved cerebral-palsied adults to substitute for verbal communication in social situations.[25] It is operated by a keyboard and has a LED (light emitting diode) display. It can also be used to communicate over the telephone to someone who has a compatible unit for decoding and was, in fact, originally designed for that purpose for the deaf.[25]

Loss of the Use of One Upper Extremity or One Side of the Body

The methods described below will pertain to the hemiplegic patient who has lost the use of one side of his body. The methods and equipment may also be used by the unilateral upper extremity amputee if necessary. However, the amputee will need less adaptation because he has normal trunk and lower extremity function, as well as normal perception and cognition. Persons with temporary casts or restrictions of use of one upper extremity can also benefit from these ideas.

The principles of compensation for loss of use of one upper extremity or one side of the body are to provide substitution for the stabilizing or holding function of the involved upper extremity and to adapt the few truly bilateral activites so they can be done unilaterally.

Feeding

This task is essentially a one-handed task, except for cutting meat and spreading bread. These tasks can be done by use of adapted equipment.

Meat can be simultaneously stabilized and cut by use of a rocker knife, a knife with a sharp curved blade that cuts when rocked over the meat (Fig. 26.13). The tool that combines a rocker knife and a fork is dangerous and is to be avoided.

Bread can be spread if stabilized on a nonslip surface or trapped in the corner of a spikeboard and spread toward the corner (Fig. 26.14). Soft spreads facilitate this process.

Grooming

The problem here is the need to attend to the unaffected extremity and to find substitutions for two-handed activities.

Applying deodorant to the unaffected arm is more easily done using an aerosol spray unless the person

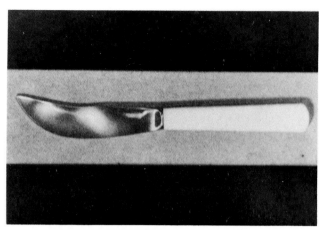

Figure 26.13   Rocker knife for one-handed cutting.

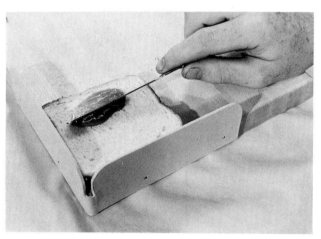

Figure 26.14   Spreading one-handed by trapping bread in the corner of a spike board.

has excellent range and can reach the axilla and thereby use other types of applicators. To allow application of deodorant to the affected axilla, that arm is passively placed away from the body.

Fingernails of the unaffected hand are cleaned by rubbing them on a small suction cup brush attached to the basin; they are filed by rubbing the nails over an emery board secured to a table or other flat surface. The nails of the affected hand can be cleaned and trimmed using the person's habitual methods.

Using a different brush but of the same design, the person can scrub his dentures by rubbing them over the brush, which is fastened to the inside of the basin. Partially filling the basin with water and laying a facecloth in the bottom cushions the dentures if they are dropped accidentally.

An electric razor is recommended if judgment is impaired; accidents are possible with a safety razor.

Toileting

The problem is arranging the clothing, which is a two-handed activity normally.

There should be a grab bar mounted on the wall beside the toilet to assist transfer. Once standing, anyone wearing trousers unfastens them, and gravity takes them down. If the patient's balance is precarious and will interfere with retrieving them after using the toilet, the person can put the affected hand in the pocket, which prevents the trousers from sliding below the knees. A woman can lean her affected side against the adjacent wall, if available, for balance; she can then raise her dress on the affected side and tuck it between her body and the affected arm. Then she lowers her underpants to knee level and pulls the dress up on the unaffected side. A dress or skirt that wraps around facilitates this process by allowing the woman to reach across the front of herself and pull the material forward to anchor it between her body and the affected arm; then she lowers her underpants and holds the remaining material aside while seating herself using the grab bar. The toilet tissue has to be mounted conveniently to the unaffected side. The patient will be able to manage menstrual needs by use of tampons or adhesive type sanitary napkins.

Dressing

The following methods are taken from material prepared by the occupational therapy staff of Highland View Cuyahoga County Hospital in Cleveland, Ohio, and from an article in the *American Journal of Occupational Therapy* by Gladys Brett, OTR[26] As a general rule, the affected limb is dressed first and undressed last.

Shirt or Cardigan Garment. *A. Overhead Method to Put on and Remove.* This method is least confusing for a patient with sensory and perceptual impairment, but is cumbersome for dresses and is not used for coats.

1. To keep the shirt from twisting, hold the collar and shake.
2. Put the shirt on the lap, label facing up, and the collar next to the abdomen; shirt tail draped over knees.
3. Open the sleeve for the affected arm from the armhole to the cuff.
4. Pick up the affected hand and put into the sleeve.
5. Pull the sleeve up over the elbow.
6. Put the unaffected hand into the armhole. Raise the arm out and push it through the sleeve.
7. Gather the back of the shirt from tail to collar.
8. Hold the gathered shirt up, lean forward, duck the head, and put the shirt over the head.
9. To straighten the shirt, lean forward, work the shirt down over the shoulders, and reach back and pull the tail down.
10. To button, line up the shirt fronts, match each button with correct button hole, starting with bottom button.

To remove the shirt, the patient unbuttons it, leans forward, and uses the unaffected hand to gather the shirt up in back of the neck. He ducks the head, pulls the shirt over the head, then takes the shirt off the unaffected arm first.

B. Over the Shoulder Method to Put on and Remove. The more aware patient may prefer this method, especially if he has some voluntary control of his affected extremity and can place his extremity into the garment, because it is similar to the customary method. This method is also used for coats.

1. To keep the shirt from twisting, hold the collar and shake.
2. Put the shirt on the lap, label facing up and collar next to the abdomen; shirt tail draped over knees. Patient may prefer to hold the shirt out in front of him.
3. Put the affected hand into one sleeve.
4. Pull the sleeve up over the elbow.
5. Grasp the collar at the point closest to the unaffected side.
6. Hold tightly to the collar, lean forward, and bring the collar and shirt around the affected side and behind the neck to the unaffected side.
7. Put the unaffected hand into the other armhole. Raise the arm out and up to push it through the sleeve.
8. To straighten the shirt, lean forward, work the shirt down over the shoulders, reach back and pull the tail down, and then straighten the sleeve under the affected axilla.
9. To button, line up shirt fronts, match each button with the correct buttonhole, starting with the bottom button.

To remove the shirt, unbutton it and use the unaffected hand to throw the shirt back off the unaffected shoulder. Work the shirt sleeve off the unaffected arm. Press the shirt cuff against the leg and pull the arm out. Lean forward. Use the unaffected hand to pull the shirt across the back. Take the shirt off of the affected arm.

Pullover Garment. *Putting on:*

1. Garment is positioned on the lap, bottom toward chest and label facing down.
2. Using the unaffected hand, roll up the bottom edge of the shirt back, all the way up to the sleeve on the affected side.
3. Spread the armhole opening as large as possible. Using the unaffected hand, place the affected arm into the armhole and pull the sleeve up onto the arm past the elbow.
4. Insert the unaffected arm into the other sleeve.
5. Gather the shirt back from bottom edge to neck, lean forward, duck head, and pass the shirt over the head.
6. Adjust the shirt on the involved side up and onto the shoulder and remove twists.

Removing. 1. Starting at top back, gather the shirt up, lean forward, duck head, and pull the shirt forward over the head.
2. Remove the unaffected arm, then the affected arm.

Trousers. Modifications of these methods are used for men's and women's underclothing and pantyhose.

Putting on Trousers:

1. Sit. *Note:* If wheelchair is used it is locked. Move the unaffected leg beyond the midline of the body for balance.

2. Grasp the ankle or calf of the affected leg. Lift and cross the affected leg over the unaffected leg.

3. Pull the trousers onto the affected leg up to, but not above, the knee.

4. Uncross the legs.

5. Put the unaffected leg into the other pant leg.

6. Remain sitting. Pull the pants up above the knees. If the wheelchair is used, place footrests in "up" position.

7. To prevent the pants from dropping when standing, put the affected hand into the pant pocket, or the thumb into a belt loop.

8. Stand up. Pull the pants up over the hips. Persons with *poor balance:* remain seated and pull the pants up over the hips by shifting from side to side. Persons with *good balance:* button and zip pants while standing. Persons with *poor balance:* button and zip pants from a seated position.

Removing Trousers. Sit. *Note:* If sitting in wheelchair be sure wheelchair is locked. Unfasten the pants. Work the trousers down on the hips as far as possible. Stand. Let the trousers drop past knees. Sit. Remove the trousers from the unaffected leg. Cross the affected leg over the unaffected leg. Remove the trousers from the affected leg. Uncross the legs.

Alternate method for persons with *poor balance:* place locked wheelchair or chair against a wall. Sit. Unfasten the trousers. Work the trousers down on the hips as far as possible. Put the wheelchair foot rests in "up" position. Lean back against the chair and press down with the unaffected leg to raise the buttocks slightly. Lean from side to side in the chair. Use the noninvolved arm to work the trousers down past the hips. Remove the trousers from the unaffected leg. Cross the affected leg over the unaffected leg. Remove the trousers from the affected leg. Uncross the legs.

Socks or Stocking. *Putting on:*

1. The person sits in a straight chair (with arms if balance is questionable) or in a locked wheelchair with foot pedals in up position.

2. The unaffected leg is placed slightly beyond midline of body toward the affected side, and the affected leg is crossed over it by grasping the ankle. If the person has difficulty in maintaining the leg in this position, a small stool under the unaffected leg will increase hip flexion angle and hold the affected leg more securely. If the patient cannot cross his legs, the heel is rested on a small stool, and a reacher is used to put the sock onto the toe and pull it up.

3. The top of the sock is opened by inserting the fist into the cuff area and then opening the fist and spreading the fingers.

4. The sock is put on the foot by slipping the toes into the cuff opening made under the spread hand. The sock is then pulled into place, and wrinkles are eliminated.

Removing. The leg is positioned as when putting the sock on. The sock is then pushed off with the unaffected hand.

Shoes. A loafer type shoe is put on the unaffected foot with the shoe on the floor. The foot is started into the shoe, and a shoehorn is used to help ease the foot into the shoe. A tie shoe is put onto the foot after the leg is crossed over the affected one to bring the foot closer. Sometimes, it is necessary to insert a shoehorn in this position and then carefully lower the foot with the shoe half on and finish getting it on the foot by repeatedly pushing down on the knee and adjusting the shoehorn. A long shoehorn is helpful if the patient is not able to safely bend over to use a conventional one.

Tying the shoes is a problem. It is possible to tie a conventional bow one-handed, but it requires fine dexterity and normal perception. The amputee may prefer to do this or use loafer style shoes. The hemiplegic patient can use flip closure shoes, zipper or Velcro adaptations, or Kno-bows on tie shoes. Or, he can learn a simplified, effective one-hand shoe tie as illustrated (Fig. 26.15). This method can be improved by putting the lace through the last hole from the outside of the shoe toward the tongue of the shoe. If done this way, the tension of the foot against the shoe holds the lace tight while the bow is being tied.

Short Leg Brace (Ankle-Foot Orthosis). If the patient uses a metal brace, it is usually designed so that the fastener is on the side toward the unaffected hand. Velcro closures are used primarily.

Putting on:

1. Pull the tongue of the shoe up through the laces so it does not push down into the shoe as the brace is put on.

2. Sit. Use a straight chair with arms or a locked wheelchair with the footrests up. Bring the unaffected leg past midline in front of the body. Cross the affected leg over the unaffected leg.

3. Use the unaffected hand to hold the brace by the calf band. Swing the brace back, then forward so that the heel is between the side bars and the leg is in front of the calf band. Continue to swing the shoe forward until the toes are at the shoe opening.

4. Turn the shoe inward and insert the toes at a slight angle. This keeps the toes from catching at the sides of the shoe.

5. Pull the brace on as far as possible. Hold the brace in place by pressing on the calf band with the unaffected leg.

6. Use a shoehorn; insert it flat and directly under the heel of the foot in the back.

7. Leave the shoehorn in place. Grasp the calf band.

8. Pulling up on the calf band, uncross the leg.

9. Position the affected foot on the floor so that the heel is at a point just ahead of the knee. Push the heel forward while moving the shoehorn into an upright positon with the unaffected hand.

10. Work the foot into the shoe by pushing downward on the knee and moving the shoehorn back and forth.

11. Grasp the brace upright and pull up until the foot slips into place in the shoe. Remove the shoehorn.

12. Fasten the strap, being careful not to snag stockings. Fasten the shoes.

Removing. Sit. Cross the affected leg over the un-

1. Tie a knot in one end of the shoelace.

   Thread the unknotted end up through the hole nearest the toe of the shoe, on the left side.

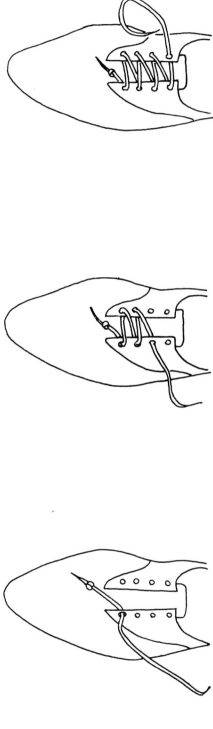

2. Take the lace across the tongue of the shoe and up under the flap on the opposite side of the shoe.

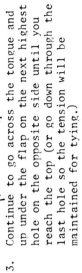

3. Continue to go across the tongue and up under the flap on the next highest hole on the opposite side until you reach the top (or go down through the last hole so the tension will be maintained for tying.)

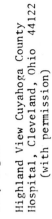

4. Circle around toward the toe of the shoe and go under the part of the lace that is going across the tongue to the last hole.

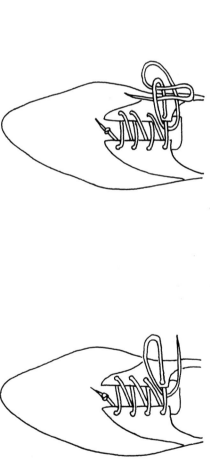

5. Circle around toward the top of the shoe. Pull free lace through the loop down toward the ankle and out to the left side.

6. Pull loop tight

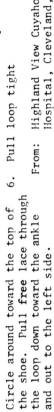

From: Highland View Cuyahoga County Hospital, Cleveland, Ohio 44122 (with permission)

Figure 26.15 One-handed shoe tie method—right hemiplegic.

affected leg. Unfasten the straps and the laces. Push down on the calf band of the brace until the shoe is off the foot.

If the patient uses a posterior shell, the brace is put on the leg and the strap is fastened before the shoe is put on. It may be necessary to add another strap near the ankle to hold the brace onto the foot while attempting to put on the shoe.[27] The shoe is put on as mentioned above for the unaffected foot. It is difficult to put the shoe on with the posterior shell in place.

Bra. To put on a bra, it is placed around the back at waist level and turned to hook in front where the patient can see what she is doing. It is then rotated to proper position, the affected arm is placed through the shoulder strap, and then the unaffected arm is placed through the other shoulder strap. The bra is pulled up into place. It is removed by reversing the process.

The above processes apply to ready-made brassieres. A plump patient may need an adapted front closing bra if she cannot approximate the two edges of the bra to fasten it. Two flat metal belt keepers are sewn on the side of the bra opening that is on the involved side. Two cotton twill straps are sewn opposite these keepers on the other side of the bra opening. The hook part of Velcro is sewn as tabs on the ends of the twill straps near the bra. The pile part of the Velcro is sewn at the distal ends of these straps. After the bra is on, fastening is done by threading these straps from the noninvolved side, through the keepers on the involved side. They are pulled to bring the two ends of the bra together, and then are secured with the Velcro closures.

Bathing

The bathing arrangements described for patients with incoordination apply to hemiplegic persons also. In addition, these patients find a long-handled bath sponge that has a pocket to hold the soap useful to allow bathing of the unaffected upper arm and the back. The lower arm of the unaffected side is bathed by putting the soapy washcloth across the knees and rubbing the arm back and forth over it unless the patient has some return of function and can use a bath mitt on the affected hand.

If sensory impairment exists, extra precautions should be taken to be certain of water temperature.

The hemiplegic patient should dry himself as much as possible while still seated on the bath chair before transferring out of the tub. The water is completely drained from the tub before the transfer is attempted. The patient may need assistance with the transfer if there is not enough room near the tub to position the wheelchair so that his noninvolved side leads.

A unilateral amputee can bathe as usual, but a rubber mat or nonskid strips in the tub, a grab bar, and letting the water drain before exiting are worthwhile safety measures.

Miscellaneous

There has been a one-handed typing method developed for persons with the use of only one upper extremity.[6] Persons with only one functional arm need to stabilize the paper when writing in longhand. The paper can be secured using masking tape, a clipboard, a weight, the affected extremity acting as a weight, or other similar means.

Blindness

Organization and consistency in the placement of objects is necessary in order for the blind person to be able to efficiently locate things. Memory training may be necessary for the newly blinded individual. He will need to develop increased awareness of the information that he receives from his senses of smell, touch, hearing, and taste. This awareness does not automatically occur but must be developed through training. Orientation to the environment is achieved through these senses, although a verbal description of the surroundings by someone else is extremely valuable.

Feeding

The patient explores the placement of dishes, glasses, and utensils at his place. If dining alone, he explores the location and identifies the food by feel, using fork and taste. If dining with a companion, he can be instructed verbally using a clock method of description, *e.g.*, meat is located at 3 o'clock. Pouring liquid is done without spilling by touching the rim of the cup or glass with the container from which he is pouring and by putting a finger tip of the hand that is holding the glass over the edge to determine when the glass is full enough. Salt is distinguished from pepper by taste or use of differently shaped shakers. Food is cut by finding the edge of the food with the fork, the fork is then moved onto the meat a bite-sized amount, and the food is cut, keeping the knife in contact with the fork.

Grooming

A major problem is identification of objects. This can be done through the use of taste, touch (size, shape, texture), location, or braille labels. The application of cosmetics or toiletries is another problem; fingers of the assistive hand can be guides, *e.g.*, when shaving sideburns or applying eyebrow pencil. Aerosol sprays may not be preferred because the blind person cannot determine the extent of the spray although, as in the case of perfume, this does not matter.

Dressing

The blind person has no difficulty with the physical aspects of dressing. The only problems that arise relate to appearance. The blind person needs a system to coordinate colors of clothes and compatibility of style. One system of identification is to use French knots in certain patterns to designate color or identify all components of a total costume. Another system is to store clothes of like color together. Hems, buttons, seams, and socks should be checked for mending. Colorless wax polishes can be used to shine shoes. Clothes should always be hung properly to prevent wrinkles. Wrinkle-free, stain-resistant, no-iron fabrics are preferred. Listening to the weather report guides the person's selection of appropriate clothing, as for anyone. Clothing selection should be done with the assistance of a sighted person who can describe colors and style. Purchase of a garment of the same style in different colors should be avoided because color identification is often done by remembering which style is a certain color.

Miscellaneous

The blind person can use a signature or writing guide to stay within boundaries while writing in longhand. Braille can be written by hand using a stylus and plate or on a machine similar to a courtroom stenotype. Braille writing is done mirror image to the way it is read.

Besides braille and talking books, new technological advances are providing new means for the blind to "read" regular print. One such device is the *Optacon*.[28]

The Telesensory Systems' *Optacon* converts printed letters into direct tactual representations of the letters for use by the blind. The Optacon is $2 \times 6 \times 8$ inches and can be carried around for use in reading posted messages, signs, or library materials not available in braille. A miniature camera, attached to the device by a cord, receives the printed word, and phototransistors send signals which are converted by the Optacon into a pattern on vibrating reeds where the fingers interpret the pattern. Speed of reading is slower than braille, but when braille translations or readers are unavailable or impractical, it is a valuable tool. Its price limits general use.

Other computer devices change the printed word into spoken language.

Telephoning is no problem for the blind person as soon as he memorizes the dial.

The patient can tell time using a braille watch. Sounds of the day, the radio, or TV can provide a general orientation to time.

Tactile discrimination enables the person to identify coins; paper money is discriminated by the way it is folded after its denomination has been identified previously by someone else. Consistency is important here as in all aspects of the blind person's life. Some countries use paper money of different sizes for different denominations, but unfortunately that is not so in the United States yet.

DRIVING

The ability to drive provides the greatest freedom of mobility for the physically disabled. Those with limited range of motion may require special seating, but may otherwise be able to drive. Those with severely limited lower extremity range can use hand-controlled automobiles as developed for spinal cord-injured patients. Those with severely limited upper extremity range may not be able to be independent drivers.

Many persons with decreased strength can be safe drivers with the proper selection of the car, necessary adaptations, and training in the use of hand or foot controls as appropriate to the disability. Quadriplegic patients with a level of injury at C_6 or below are considered potential candidates for driver training.

Car Selection

If a wheelchair-bound person is to use a sedan type car independently, it must be a two-door sedan which is large enough to allow access for the wheelchair to be stored behind the front seat, with a high enough door opening space to accommodate the wheelchair handles, and with a large enough door to allow space in front for ease of transfer. The person may choose to use a van with a ramp or hydraulic lift and wheelchair stabilizers which allow him to sit in the wheelchair while driving.

An automatic transmission is needed if hand or foot controls are used.

Hand controls can be attached to the brake and accelerator. There are many different types of hand controls. Most require at least moderate strength (4 to 6 kg) to push or pull the levers, but some "less effort" or "zero effort" models which require about 1 kg for acceleration, braking, and steering are now being produced.[29] However, they are very expensive since they must have an emergency backup system to keep the controls "less effort" in the event of engine failure.[29]

In an effort to control for equipment-dependent accidents, the Veteran's Administration (VA) now requires that drive controls meet quality requirements before they are purchased by the VA for disabled veterans.[30, 31] When choosing hand controls, all disabled drivers would be wise to adhere to the VA requirements.

Foot controls can be used to steer by those with no upper extremity function.[32] Finger controls are similar to hand controls but are more sensitive to smaller movements and can be operated by finger motion only.

Power seats, power steering, power brakes, and power windows are needed. The car may have a hand-operated dimmer switch on the turn signal, or one can be added.

Other adapted equipment needed include the following.

1. A swivel steering wheel knob or cuff allows the steering wheel to be operated with one hand while the other controls the hand-operated accelerator and brake.

2. A handle can be attached to the windshield wiper knob to give leverage for operating the windshield washer.

3. A piece of wood secured to the keys for the door and ignition provides leverage for turning the key.

4. A seat belt and shoulder harness are essential.

5. A two-way radio receiver is useful to call for assistance if needed.

One method the person could use to transfer into a two-door car and bring the wheelchair in is as follows. He would approach the car on the passenger side, move the power seat all the way back, and transfer into the car using either a depression transfer, a sliding board transfer, or a gutter hook-assisted transfer. This latter transfer utilizes a loop suspended from a flat wide metal hook that fits in the rain gutter of the car above the door. The loop is used to pull against, similarly to using a trapeze when transferring from bed. Once transferred into the car, the person secures his trunk balance, and then leans to remove the wheelchair cushion. He folds the chair and puts the casters on the edge of the car near the entrance to the back seat. He moves to the driver's seat and then moves the entire seat forward. He tips the passenger seat back forward and leans to reach the front casters of the wheelchair to pull it into the space behind the passenger seat. A board which levels the back floor makes transfer of the wheelchair easier. Then he tips the passenger seat back into place and adjusts the entire seat to a comfortable driving position. He reaches across to close the passenger door. A stick with a hook may be helpful to extend the reach. If spasm is a problem or a possibility, the legs are positioned so that a spasm would not send the feet against the brake or accelerator.

If it is not possible for the patient to get the wheelchair into the car independently, hydraulic lifts are available which attach across the roof of the car and lift the wheelchair up and into the car.[6]

When parking the car, it is important to remember that a 1.3 meter (4 ft) space on the passenger side is required for transfer. It is wisest to park on a flat area and at the right of a line of cars. Parking spaces designated for handicapped drivers are marked to allow for transfer space.

Incoordinated persons may or may not be able to drive safely, depending on the severity of their disability.

The *Aetna Drivo-Trainer Simulator* (Fig. 26.16) can be used preliminarily to driver training to test the reaction speed and judgment of the patient. The patient sits in a mock-up car module with standard (or adapted) driving devices mounted as in a car. He watches a movie, steers, and reacts to the driving situations as they appear on the screen. His timing and responses are electronically recorded. If these aspects of driving are all right, a handicapped driver training course is then appropriate for the disabled driver. Such a course is similar to the training course for all new drivers, except that it teaches the person to use necessary adapted equipment safely. Occupational therapists often direct these programs. Most states require disabled drivers to be reeducated prior to examining them for a license.

Persons with the loss of use of one side of the body due to stroke may, with medical clearance, drive with few adaptations. Medical clearance is needed not so much for physical health problems, but rather the sequellae of the stroke. Whether or not the patient has hemianopsia; impaired perception, thought processes, or judgment; or slow automatic reactions must be taken into account before the patient is cleared for driving training. The Aetna Drivo-Trainer Simulator provides the opportunity to test whether these deficits exist without actually jeopardizing others by testing the patient in traffic. An evaluation with this simulator is recommended for all patients with brain damage because judgment deficits and slow reactions are sometimes not apparent during other evaluations but would definitely interfere with safe driving abilities. If he passes this simulated test, driving retraining or license tests are allowed.

The car of a person with loss of one upper extremity ought to have automatic transmission and power steering. A swivel steering wheel knob is needed to steer safely. If the patient has lost the use of his right arm, the gear shift lever and turn indicator will need to be remounted on the left of the steering column. A left-footed accelerator may also be indicated; these can be ordered as accessories on a new car.

References

1. Brodal, A. Self-observations and neuro-anatomical considerations after a stroke. *Brain,* 96: 675–694, 1973.
2. Skinner, B. F. *The Behavior of Organisms.* New York: Appleton-Century-Crofts, 1938.
3. Yeakel, M., and Margetis, P. A customized crutch hand grip. *Am. J. Occup. Ther., 23* (5): 410–412, 1969.
4. Ted Hoyer & Company, Inc., 2222 Minnesota Street, Oshkosh, Wisc. 54901.
5. Alexander, L. Bed to commode lift increases independence. *Accent on Living, 23* (4): 108–109, 1979.
6. Lowman, E., and Klinger, J. *Aids to Independent Living.* New York: McGraw-Hill (Blakiston Division), 1969.
7. Dutton, N., Davis, K., Lupo, S., and Wepman, S. "Wheelie" aide. *Phys. Ther., 59* (1): 35–36, 1979.
8. Wise, E. H. The best battery for your wheelchair or for your van lift. *Accent on Living, 23* (3): 98–103, 1978.
9. Bobath, B. *Adult Hemiplegia: Evaluation and Treatment,* 2nd ed. London: William Heinemann Medical Books, 1978.
10. Katz, S., *et al.* Studies of Illness in the aged. The index of ADL: A standardized measure of biological and psychosocial function. *J.A.M.A., 185* (12): 914–919, 1963.
11. Levitan-Rheingold, N., Hotte, E. B., and Mandel, D. R. Learning to dress: A fundamental skill toward independence for the disabled. *Rehabil. Lit., 41* (3-4): 72–75, 1980.
12. Bowar, M. T. *Clothing for the Handicapped: Fashion Adaptations for Adults and Children.* Minneapolis: Sister Kenny Institute, 1978.

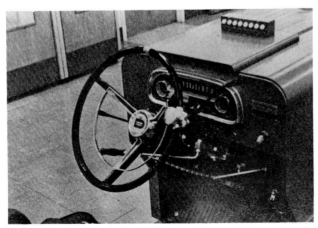

Figure 26.16 Aetna driver trainer at Highland View Hospital, Cleveland, Ohio.

13. Vanderheiden, G. C. Augmentative modes of communication for severely speech- and motor-impaired. *Clin. Orthop. Related Res., 148:* 70–86, 1980.
14. Communication devices available but are out of reach to many. *Accent on Living, 25* (4): 26–35, 1981.
15. Garee, B. (ed.) *Accent on Living: Buyer's Guide,* 1982-83 edition. P.O. Box 700, Bloomington, Ill. 61701.
16. Gadgets galore: Buy 'em or make 'em cheap. *Accent on Living, 25* (4): 37, 1981.
17. Hansen, A. M. W. *Making Adaptive Equipment with Polyform* (Technical Bulletin #2-128-R1). Rolyan Medical Products, P.O. Box 555, Menominee Falls, Wisc 53051.
18. Lowry, B. Reacher. *Am. J. Occup. Ther., 31* (4): 259, 1977.
19. Reich, N., and Otten, P. Are buttons and zippers confidence trippers? *Accent on Living, 25* (3): 98–99, 1980.
20. Runge, M. Self dressing techniques for patients with spinal cord injury. *Am. J. Occup. Ther., 21* (6): 367–375, 1967.
21. Parish, J. G. A study of the use of electronic environmental control systems by severely paralysed patients. *Paraplegia, 17:* 157–160, 1979-1980.
22. Glenn, J. W., Miller, K. H., and Broman, M. T. Voice terminal: May offer opportunities for employment to the disabled. *Am. J. Occup. Ther., 30* (5): 308–312, 1976.
23. Holser, P., Jones, M., and Ilanit, T. A study of the upper extremity control brace. *Am. J. Occup. Ther., 16* (4): 170–175, 1962.
24. Bullock, A., *et al.* Communication and the nonverbal multihandicapped child. *Am. J. Occup. Ther., 29* (3): 150–152, 1975.
25. Workman, A. A. Communication system for the nonverbal severely disabled. *Am. J. Occup. Ther., 33* (3): 194–195, 1979.
26. Brett, G. Dressing techniques for the severely involved hemiplegic patient. *Am. J. Occup. Ther., 14* (5): 262–264, 1960.
27. Quintana, L. A. Braintree Hospital, personal communication, 1981.
28. Goldish, L., and Taylor, H. The Optacon: A valuable device for blind persons. In: *The New Outlook for the Blind,* 49–56, 1974.
29. Risk, H. F. Pros and cons of the "less effort" steering and braking systems for the severely handicapped driver. *Am. Corr. Ther. J., 34* (5): 154–155, 1980.
30. VA evaluates car hand controls. *Accent on Living, 21* (2): 46, 1976.
31. Alarming statistics? Disabled drivers have more accidents. N.Y. study. *Accent on Living, 23* (4): 44–45, 1979.
32. Rosenkoetter, R. Valerie drives with her bare feet. *Accent on Living, 25* (1): 100–102, 1980.

Supplementary Reading

Communication

Andrews, B., Miller, S., Horrocks, D., Jibowu, J. O. N., and Chawla, J. C. Electronic Communications and Environmental control systems for the severely disabled. *Paraplegia, 17:* 153–156, 1979-1980.

Beukelman, D. R., and Yorkston, K. N. Nonvocal communication: Performance evaluation. *Arch. Phys. Med. Rehabil., 61:* 272–275, 1980.

Joubert, Z. F. Fingercom—An Electronic communicator for the disabled. *Med. Biol. Eng. Comput., 17* (4): 489–491, 1979.

Ross, J. A. A study of the application of Blissymbolics as a means of communication for a young brain damaged adult. *Br. J. Disord. Comm., 14* (2): 103–109, 1980.

Steadman, J. W., Ferris, C. D., and Rhodine, C. N. Prosthetic communication device. *Arch. Phys. Med. Rehabil., 61* (2): 93–97, 1980.

Mobility

Flaherty, P., and Jurkovich, S. *Transfer for Patients with Acute and Chronic Conditions.* Minneapolis: American Rehabilitation Foundation, 1970.

McGee, M., and Hertling, D. Equipment and transfer techniques used by C_6 quadriplegic patients. *Phys. Ther., 57*(12): 1372–1375, 1977.

Self Care

American Heart Association. *Do It Yourself Again.* 7320 Greenville Ave. Dallas, Tex. 75231, 1969.

American Heart Association. *Up and Around.* 7320 Greenville Ave., Dallas, Tex. 75231.

Asenjo, A. *A Step-by-Step Guide to Personal Management for Blind Persons.* New York: American Foundation for Blind, 1970.

Ford, J. R., and Duckworth, B. *Physical Management for the Quadriplegic Patient.* Philadelphia: F. A. Davis, 1974.

Fred Sammons, Inc. *Be OK Self-Help Aids,* catalogue, Box 32, Brookfield, Ill. 60513.

Functionally Designed Clothing and Aids, catalogue. Vocational Guidance and Rehabilitation Services. 2239 East 55th Street, Cleveland, Ohio 44103.

J. A. Preston Corporation, catalogue. 71 Fifth Avenue, New York, N.Y. 10003.

The Left Hand, catalogue. 140 W. 22nd Street, New York, N.Y. 10011.

Newton, A. Clothing: A positive part of the rehabilitation process. *J. Rehabil., 42*(5): 18–22, 1976.

Occupational Therapy and Nursing Education Staff at Kenny Rehabilitation Institute. *Self-care for the Hemiplegic.* Minneapolis: American Rehabilitation Foundation, 1970.

Poole, J., and Parkinson, M. M. Bilateral shoulder disarticulation: Equipment used to facilitate independence. *Am. J. Occup. Ther., 34*(6): 397–399, 1980.

Rehab Aids, catalogue. Box 612, Tamiami Station, Miami, Fla. 33144.

Sears, Roebuck & Co., *Home Health Care Catalogue.* Sears Tower, Chicago, Ill. 60684, 1981.

Yep, J. O. Tools for aiding physically disabled individuals to increase independence in dressing. *J. Rehabil., 43*(5): 39–41, 1977.

chapter

27

Homemaking and Child Care

Catherine A. Trombly, M.A., OTR

Training in adapted methods of homemaking and child care begins when the patient's function has been restored to the expected near maximal level. This training, therefore, usually takes place close to the time of discharge. Some homemaking activities may be appropriate therapeutic activities and can be incorporated into program planning earlier.

WORK SIMPLIFICATION

Homemaking and child care are energy-consuming for anyone, but for disabled persons who must use adapted methods these activities require an even greater expenditure of energy and, unless modified, may consume a disproportionate amount of the person's remaining energy.[1] Techniques to conserve personal energy become indispensable for these individuals. The principles and some suggestions are listed here. Other suggestions that can be used are frequently being published these days in magazine and newspaper columns aimed at the able bodied working wife and mother.

The principles of energy conservation or work simplification listed here apply in general to all the disability categories presented.

Limit the Amount of Work

Eliminate steps of a job or whole jobs that are not essential to one's life-style. The patient should determine for herself what is necessary by asking herself why it is necessary, if the job is worth expenditure of energy required, and what would happen if the job were left undone.

Some short cuts to suggest include the following. Permanent press and jersey materials eliminate the need for ironing. Making a bed entirely from under-sheet to spread at one corner before moving to do the same at the next corners eliminates much walking. Teaching family members to put their belongings and laundry in the proper place eliminates the need to tidy-up the house. Soaking dishes eliminates the need to scrub them. Allowing the dishes to air dry eliminates drying. The step of returning clean dishes to the cupboard can be eliminated by reusing them directly from the dish drainer or dishwasher. The use of plastic tablecloths or paper placemats instead of cloth ones eliminates laundry. The use of casserole dishes for cooking and serving eliminates an extra set of dishes to wash. Frozen entrees and other prepared foods eliminate preparation and the need to wash the cooking dishes. Shopping by telephone and by mail order eliminate work that requires tremendous amounts of energy; this method of shopping may be the only way the person can do this task. The use of the freezer eliminates the need to do frequent marketing. The use of paper diapers eliminates this aspect of laundering.

Plan Ahead

Plan the week's activities so that heavy tasks can be distributed over the days. The full day's activities should be carefully planned to incorporate periods of rest between bouts of work and to alternate active jobs with quiet ones. A flexible, written plan improves the homemaker's efficiency. The tasks should be prioritized so that those that must be done are done before the person runs out of time and energy. If a task doesn't seem to be getting done day after day because of its low priority, perhaps it is not important and can be eliminated. Each activity should be thought out ahead of time and all necessary supplies and equipment gathered prior to doing the job. The equipment should be put away before starting the next task so that if energy fails, the home is still tidy. A plan for the family's contribution to running the household is needed also.

Organize Storage

Supplies and equipment should be stored where first used and within easy reach. Duplicate sets of equipment in different locations are useful; for example, floor care equipment located on both the first and second floors of a two-story house. Extraneous, seldom used equipment should be stored out of the way. If possible, things should not be stored behind other things nor under other things because of the energy consumed in trying to reach them. Vertical storage of dishes, baking pans, etc. is ideal. Narrow shelf storage or easily gliding pull-out shelves solve some storage problems; peg boards, lazy susans, and back of the counter storage solve others.

Sit to Work

Arrange work areas so that implements are within easy reach of the posture normally assumed for each task. Reaching is energy-consuming.

Use Correct Equipment

Energy is conserved if the tools fit the job and are in good condition. Personal energy is also conserved if electrically powered equipment is used and indeed may be the only method by which a disabled person can accomplish a task. A dishwasher that does not require prior rinsing of the dishes, a self-cleaning electric stove, a self-defrosting refrigerator with an easily accessible freezer, a garbage disposal, a microwave oven (not for patients with pacemakers), crock pots, and an electric can opener are valuable energy-saving tools and are recommended for the disabled homemaker. As many of these as can be afforded should be purchased according to the priority established by each homemaker's needs and requirements. The specific features that each appliance must have in order to be used should be discussed with the patient.

Use Efficient Methods

Use the two arms in symmetrical, smooth motions when possible. Use the force available from muscles at proximal joints rather than the smaller more distal joints and muscles. Slide objects; do not lift. Contiguous counter space, especially between the sink, stove, and refrigerator is very important. Use a wheeled service cart and laundry basket when possible to transport items. Avoid prolonged holding by using stabilization when possible. Suction cup bases, heavy pots and pans, nonskid mats, wet towels, and wet sponge cloths are all ways to stabilize. Locate switches and controls within easy, safe reach; appliance controls ought to be located in the front for accessibility. Be sure lighting is good.

Rest

Fatigue leads to poor body mechanics and safety awareness. Regular rest periods should be incorporated into the day's work plan. Mothers of young children are advised to rest when the child sleeps, even though it is tempting to use that time for doing a task uninterrupted.

It is strongly recommended for conservation of energy and for safety of all disabled homemakers that oven cleaning, defrosting the refrigerator, hanging curtains, yard work, etc. be assigned to other family members, to temporary hired household help, or to a commercial cleaning service. Most of these tasks need to be done once a year; therefore, they can be done in a staggered fashion over the whole year to balance out payments to a service.

HOMEMAKER TRAINING

Homemaking takes place on two levels: managerial and participative performance of tasks. The severely disabled homemaker may be an effective home manager, directing the efforts of other family members or paid household help. She can manage the finances and oversee the shopping. Training for this level may not be necessary for the experienced homemaker; some discussions about how this could be done might suffice. An inexperienced homemaker may need practice in hypothetical financial management and in directing others effectively by words alone.

Homemaker services, Home Health Aides, and Meals-on-Wheels are all programs available in many communities that enable a patient with limited abilities to remain in her home by providing essential services which the homemaker is unable to do. Each program offers different types and levels of services. For the homemaker who can afford it, commercial housekeeping services are increasing in availability and can be hired for weekly or seasonal cleaning chores.

The activities which the homemaker can reasonably expect to do should be discussed in detail and practiced. The therapist should suggest adapted methods or adapted equipment that will make the task possible if the homemaker is unable to do it in a standard way. To train the participative homemaker in tasks for which she needs to learn new methods, the therapist should be skilled in demonstrating the technique in a way that is as close as possible to the manner the disabled person will be expected to do it. The therapist should sit or stand beside the person while demonstrating to eliminate right-left confusion. The patient performs the activity in imitation of the therapist while the therapist cues the patient about the key points. Practice increases skill and should not be bypassed.

For mothers of infants, a flexible baby doll that is life-sized and weighted to simulate a baby may be used for practice of child care methods. To be realistic, the weight must be distributed throughout the doll, not just in the hollow head and limbs. A mother who is questionably safe in caring for the lifeless doll would be advised to have help in the care of her lively youngster.

Child care is complicated by the nature of the disability, the particular demands of children at various developmental stages, and by environmental conditions.[2] The child aged 8 months to 2½ years is the greatest challenge because he is mobile and can't be reasoned with.[2] He needs to be contained in a safe area.[2] All energy-saving suggestions that put controls of appliances and supplies and equipment within each reach of the mother do so for the child also!

The handicapped mother will need to be a consistent disciplinarian in so far as she must rely on the child's obedience for his own safety. A toddler must come when called and must stop doing things when told. A disabled mother must teach her child to accommodate to her disability.[3] Even a toddler is helpful in picking things up off the floor for mother and in running to get something. The toddler can also be taught to climb safely in and out of his crib and can learn to assist in dressing himself. Older children are even more helpful and learn important personal skills and values in the process of helping mother.[3]

Mothering involves more than physical care of the child, and the disabled mother is encouraged to allow time in her daily routine to play with and counsel her child.

In addition to the suggestions listed above that apply generally to homemakers, the following sections note some other specific suggestions for types of disability. Given the principles, and learning some examples of applying the principle, the clever housewife will devise methods that suit her best to solve household problems. Training must emphasize the problem-solving method so that the housewife develops true independence.

Compensation for Limited Range of Motion

The principles are to extend the person's reach via extended handles and to confine the work to a compact area.

Marketing

Since the patient may need assistance because many items are placed out of reach, marketing by phone or mail is recommended.

Food Preparation, Service, and Cleanup

Reacher tongs can be used to get lightweight objects from high or low places. A wall oven or countertop microwave oven eliminates bending. Small electrical appliances can be placed within easy reach. If ambulatory aids are used, a wheeled cart may be needed, unless dishes can be slid along a counter to a point near the table. A sponge cloth mitt, commercially available, or one made from terry cloth[4] will be useful for arthritic persons for washing dishes. Joint protection methods specific to persons with rheumatoid arthritis can be found in Chapter 20.

Housecleaning

Articles that extend the person's reach such as reacher tongs for picking up objects from the floor or holding a dust rag to reach distant places, a feather duster, a long-handled sponge to clean the bathtub, and a long-handled dustpan are often necessary. A child's broom and mop are handy for wiping up spills.[5] Vacuum cleaner wand attachments can be used for cleaning out-of-reach places. The duster attachment of the vacuum cleaner is also helpful. Beds should be placed so the patient can work from both sides without leaning while making them. A self-wringing sponge mop and a flexible-handled dry mop are useful for patients with limited range of motion.

Laundry

If the patient is ambulatory, a top-loading automatic washer and raised dryer would eliminate bending; however, if the patient is wheelchair-bound, a front-loading washer and dryer would be best. If the patient is wheelchair-bound and must use a top-loading machine, a mirror mounted over it at an angle to enable the person to see into the tub and a reacher stick or tongs will be necessary. Maytag washer and dryer controls can be optionally fitted with large four-pronged knobs.[6]

Mending would be best accomplished with a sewing machine. The patient may need assistance with threading the needle or need to use a needle-threading device.

Child Care

To eliminate the need for bending, a raised playpen could be used, and the crib mattress could be raised. A crib that accommodates the mother's wheelchair, has storage and a sliding railing to allow access to the baby was designed for a wheelchair-bound mother (Fig. 27.1).[3] The baby could be bathed in the kitchen sink or a bathinet.

Compensation for Weakness

The principles are to use lightweight and/or powered equipment and to allow gravity to assist.

Marketing

It is advisable to purchase small containers and pieces of meat because they are more easily handled and are lightweight. Forethought concerning opening of the packages should direct the patient toward zipper-pull boxes and plastic bags that can be cut with scissors, etc.

Food Preparation, Service, and Cleanup

Lightweight utensils, pots, and pans are necessary. Electric equipment, such as a can opener, counter top mixer, knife, small broiler oven, microwave oven, fry pan, and blender with a lightweight container conserve energy and/or allow the patient to work seated at convenient tabletop height. Knives and peelers should be very sharp so the tool does its job easily. A French chef's knife allows the patient to use leverage rather than a back and forth sawing motion for chopping. Built-up handles on cooking utensils may be needed for patients who use splints. A spike board to stabilize the vegetable or meat being cut may be necessary (Fig. 27.2). A spike board is a hardwood cutting board

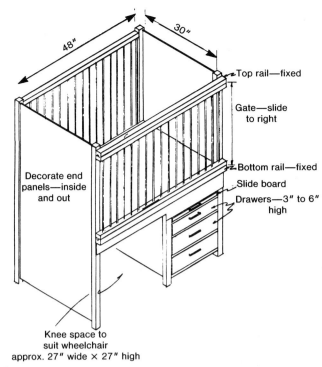

Figure 27.1 Crib with knee space to accommodate a wheelchair, handy storage, and sliding gate side rails. Designed by Lee and Gordon Heintzman. (Reproduced with permission from V. M. Dunn.[3])

48″

30″

Top rail—fixed

Gate—slide to right

Bottom rail—fixed

Slide board

Drawers—3″ to 6″ high

Decorate end panels—inside and out

Knee space to suit wheelchair approx. 27″ wide × 27″ high

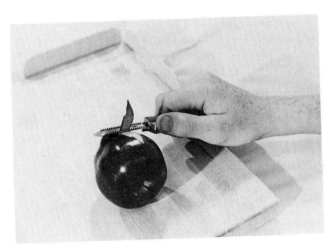

Figure 27.2 One-handed peeling of an apple stabilized on stainless steel nails of a spike board.

which has three aluminum, or preferably stainless steel, nails hammered through the middle of the board so that the pointed ends protrude about 2 inches to hold the food. It usually has suction cup legs to stabilize the board on the counter. The spike board should be finished using vegetable oil, not varnish. When not in use the spikes on the board should be covered by wedges of cork.

Loop handles of various types can be added to cooking utensils, such as spatulas,[7] or to dishes to be used in microwave ovens[8] to aid a patient with little

or no grasp to use them. It is important to remember when building adapted equipment for use in microwave ovens that metal or glue may not be used.

Scissors, if they can be used, are useful to open packages or to cut vegetables and some meats. Resting the side of the container that a person is pouring from onto the edge of the container that is being poured to (which must be stabilized) utilizes leverage rather than energy. An egg can be cracked by someone with weak hands, such as a C_6 quadriplegic, by grossly grasping it and throwing it sharply into the bottom of an empty bowl where it will split in two and the shell can be removed. If the egg must be separated it can be poured into a commercial egg separator.

The stove should have push-button controls located in the front. If the patient is confined to a wheelchair, a mirror mounted over the back of the stove and angled to reflect what is cooking in the pots may be necessary.

An automatic ice maker in the refrigerator alleviates the dependency on someone else to get ice or the need to warm the ice tray to release the ice. If the patient is confined to a wheelchair, the freezer of the refrigerator is best located beside the cold storage area rather than on the top or bottom.

The wheelchair homemaker will need to have a convenient work area that accommodates the wheelchair and allows her to be comfortable while working. The sink will need modification so that the wheelchair can fit under it. A lap apron is useful for the wheelchair homemaker because it provides a firm surface to place things on and has a lip to prevent their being knocked off in transit (Fig. 27.3). It does not interfere with pushing the wheelchair. However, it is dangerous to carry hot items, especially liquids, using this.

Housecleaning

The use of a self-propelled vacuum cleaner allows some weak persons to do this job; maintenance of balance against the pull of the vacuum cleaner is a consideration, however. Use of lightweight tools, such as dry mops, brooms, sponge mops, etc., may enable floor care. Aerosol cleanser for tub and basin dissolves grime with little rubbing.

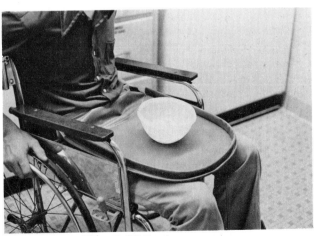

Figure 27.3 Lap apron.

If fitted sheets are used on a bed, they should be loose-fitting. Fitted sheets can be adapted by opening the two fitted corners at the bottom edge and sewing Velcro strips, so that when the bed is made the corners can be snugged up using the Velcro.[9] When making a bed, weak patients usually do not tuck the bed clothing in. Lightweight blankets and spreads are used. The idea of enclosing blankets or a quilt inside of a large pillowcase-like covering that is common in Europe makes a neat bed without the need to tuck sheets in. The covering acts like the sheet and spread and is laundered as frequently as sheets would be. These cases open entirely on one side which aids in putting the quilt inside. They can be purchased in specialty stores or made by sewing together sheets cut to the correct size. Velcro would be a better fastener than buttons.

If the patient works from a wheelchair, the bed must be placed so the wheelchair can get around it. The patient completes the bedmaking at each corner before moving to the next.

Laundry

Choice of a front- or top-loading washer depends upon whether the patient is wheelchair-bound or ambulatory. If wheelchair-bound, the patient can transport the clothes by putting them in a drawstring duffle bag, hooking the string over a wheelchair handle,[10] and dragging the bag.

Push-button controls on the washer and dryer are easier to use than knobs. If knobs are used they may need to be adapted to allow the patient to use them. Premeasured packages of soap and bleach avoid the need to handle large containers. It would be economical if these supplies were purchased in larger containers and then measured into individual packets by someone able to do it. A table for folding clothes should be convenient to the dryer and of the correct height. Hangers should be nearby for immediate hanging of permanent press items as they are removed from the dryer. If the patient chooses to iron, the iron should be set so that it is a little cooler than usual. An asbestos pad can be used on the end of the ironing board so the iron can be placed there to eliminate the need of standing the iron up each time while preparing the clothes for the next ironing stroke.

Child Care

A weak mother may not be able to participate fully in the care of her child; she should reserve the most fun things for herself if possible and delegate the more mechanical tasks to the helper. The safest place for a weak mother to handle her baby is on the floor, if she is able to get up and down from the floor. The baby can be sponge-bathed, dressed, fed, and played with there. Of course, the floor should be clean, carpeted, and draft-free. If the mother is unable to get to the floor, a crib with a swing-open side will allow the mother to wheel her wheelchair close to the baby or allow the ambulatory mother to sit on the crib mattress while with the baby. Crib mattress heights are adjustable.

Feeding the baby can best be done with the child in an infant seat or propped up on pillows. Premeasured formula is ideal but expensive. Formula prepared by another family member can be stored in the refrigerator for the day; the nipple covers should be on loosely. Breast feeding eliminates the work of formula preparation and bottle sterilization. An electric baby dish that warms the solid food can be placed in a convenient position and keeps the food warm throughout the mealtime.

Clothing for baby should be large, made of stretchy material, and have closures the mother can handle. Commerically available disposable diapers with tape tab closures eliminate pins, plastic pants, and laundry.

Emergency help should be easily, quickly, and consistently available. The child will learn to accommodate to the mother's disability as he grows older. Older children can be very helpful; the mother can learn to direct their activities verbally for the benefit of all and in such a way that increases the children's self-esteem and does not make them feel imposed upon.

Compensation for Incoordination

Principles that are useful are the use of techniques to stabilize the proximal segments of the limbs, to damp the movement of distal segments using weight, and to provide an environment in which the person feels safe and competent. Unless severely disabled, the incoordinated homemaker is likely to be independent.

Marketing

Depending upon the severity of the disability, the patient may need help.

Food Preparation, Service, and Cleanup

The major problem facing the incoordinated person in the kitchen is the need for stability to prevent spillage, breakage, or accidents with sharp utensils or hot equipment, food, or beverages. In addition to the stabilizing methods mentioned in the chapter on self-care, heavy equipment or utensils offer stability. Cast iron pots, ironstone dishes, and heavy bowls serve these patients best because they aid in stabilizing the distal part of the extremities. Casseroles and pots and pans with double handles offer greater stability by anchoring the distal parts of both upper extremities. Weighted wrist cuffs may also be used to dampen tremors or provide anchoring.

Nonslip mats and sponge cloths can be used under most items to provide friction and stability. A spike board to anchor meat, fruit, and vegetables while cutting them is useful (Fig. 27.2). A serrated knife is less likely to slip than a straight-edged one.[11] When cutting or peeling, the patient must stabilize her arms proximally and direct the stroke away from herself. A French fry basket may be placed in a saucepan before vegetables are put in for cooking; this allows draining the vegetables by lifting out the basket to lessen the chance for scald burns. Prepared foods are especially useful for this homemaker.

A counter top mixer should be used rather than a hand-held mixer. An electric skillet used at the table eliminates the need for transferring items from the oven or stove. A milk carton holder with a handle helps in pouring milk.

The stove should have front controls. The patient must avoid reaching over hot pots to the back of the stove. Starting the oven after the food has been placed in seems safest. Lighting a gas stove would be unsafe.

Sliding the food and dishes along contiguous counter surfaces is safest. A wheeled cart that is weighted at its base may also be used safely with training. Double handled or large handled serving dishes are best.

When washing dishes, a dish towel or sponge cloth could be put on the bottom of the sink to cushion the fall of dishes and glassware and/or the sink could be filled with water before putting in the dishes. Dishes of chip-resistant material will look best the longest. Soaking dishes, rinsing by hand spray, and drip drying eliminate some handling when breakage could occur.

Disposable nonslip placemats would be helpful in table setting.

Housecleaning

Heavier work tools provide stability. A duster mitten may be more useful than trying to maintain grasp of a duster. Bric-a-brac ought to be eliminated or stored where dusting will be unnecessary. Fitted sheets for the bed are helpful.

Laundry

Premeasured soap and bleach packages avoid measuring-type spills. Ironing should be eliminated by the use of no-iron materials.

Child Care

A mildly incoordinate person can care for an infant using such stabilizing measures as holding her proximal extremities close to her body and sitting to work. She can hold the baby safely in the tub by using a bath seat (Fig. 27.4). She can use a wide safety strap on the dressing table. It is also safer for this mother to work with her child on the floor. Disposable, tape-tab diapers and Velcro-closing clothing are recommended. Feeding an infant with a spoon may not be safe unless the incoordination is truly minimal.

A more severely incoordinate mother would be unsafe in the care of an infant, but may be able to assist her toddler to dress if clothing is selected properly. *Suggestions for Physically Handicapped Mothers on Clothing for Pre-School Children* by Eleanor Boettke[12] is an old reference (1957) but the principles apply. Ideas from *Self-Help Clothing for Handicapped Children*[13] can be adapted to enable the child to dress independently.

Compensation for the Loss of Use of One Upper Extremity or One Side of the Body

The two problems for the one-handed homemaker are to find a way to stabilize the object being worked on, which is usually done by a person's assistor hand, and to accomplish the few truly bilateral activities.

The principles that apply here are to find methods or equipment to substitute for the lost functions.

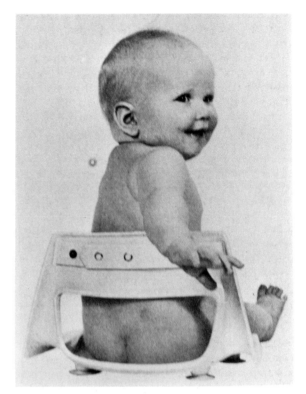

Figure 27.4 Infant bath seat with suction cup base and waist strap. (Reproduced with permission from E. Lowman and J. Klinger.[14])

Marketing

A heavy marketing cart may be used for support by an ambulatory independent hemiplegic person while walking in the supermarket, but he must not rely on it for support when bending to reach items. A lightweight cart is unsafe to lean on while walking. The hemiplegic person should give a light cart a push, then use his cane or walker to walk to meet the cart. Some hemiplegic persons have visual perceptual problems that may interfere with the efficiency of their shopping, *e.g.*, hemianopsia, impairment of figure-ground discrimination, and discrimination of depth perception. A wheelchair-bound hemiplegic person may find phone and mail shopping more suitable; actual visits to the shops will require assistance.

The upper extremity unilateral amputee will rarely need assistance while shopping. The bilateral amputee may need assistance, depending upon his skill with his prostheses.

Food Preparation, Service, and Cleanup

The unilateral upper extremity amputee can be totally independent using methods and equipment outlined below and in other references. The hemiplegic patient may be less independent due to lower extremity involvement and concomitant cognitive and perceptual disabilities. Compensatory techniques for minimizing the effects of the cognitive and perceptual deficits are mentioned in the chapter on hemiplegia.

To stabilize dishes, bowls, pots, etc., a suction cup

base, a wet towel or sponge cloth, a nonslip rubber pad or placemat can be placed under them. For more secure holding of a bowl, a cut out in a slide-out board which fits the size of bowls usually used is useful. Heavy pans will stay in place during stirring. An anchoring device is commercially available; it holds the handle of the pot in one place while the pot is on the stove. A spike board holds meat, vegetables, and fruit while cutting or peeling. Some spike boards have metal lips at two edges to form a raised corner against which a slice of bread can be snugged while spreading butter etc. on it (see Fig. 26.14). A jar, box, or flip-top can can be opened by stabilizing the item between the knees, or holding it against the counter edge with the patient's body, or putting it in a shallow drawer which is held as closed as possible by the person's body. A Zim jar opener is a solution for screw-on lids (see Fig. 20.2). Items can be "cornered" to stabilize them when working on them; for example, a dish can be cornered in the sink while washing it.

Bilateral activities can be made unilateral by use of adaptations. Beating batter or eggs can be done using one-handed egg beaters, which are commercially available, or an electric mixer. Cans can be opened using a one handed can opener[14] (Fig. 27.5) or by placing the can on sponges stacked high enough to put the can in contact with the cutting teeth of a regular electric can opener (Fig. 27.6). These are the preferred methods; however, an alert, dexterous person may use an ordinary, sharp Ecko brand "miracle roll" turnkey-type hand can opener. The person applies and locks the can opener onto the stabilized can; once locked, he can turn the key to cut the can (Fig. 27.7). Zip-open packages are easiest to open and should be purchased when possible. Other packages can be opened by stabilizing the package on its long edge and cutting the top with a sharp knife. Scissors, especially lightweight cushioned grip scissors, are very useful for many tasks in the kitchen, such as opening plastic or cellophane bags. Milk bottles with caps are easier to open than milk cartons, although the latter are possible by prying the edges apart with a table knife. The carton must be

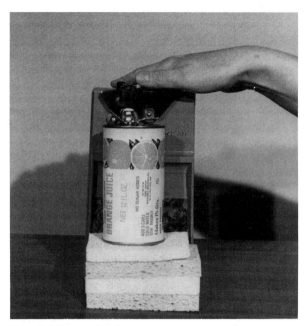

Figure 27.6 Opening a can one handed by supporting the can on sponges while activating a standard electric can opener.

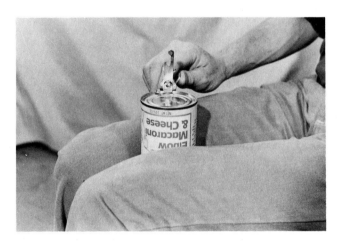

Figure 27.7 Opening a can one-handed using a key-type can opener.

stabilized, of course. To drain vegetables, put a French fry basket in the pot before putting the vegetables in, then lift to drain or use a slotted spoon.

Putting casseroles in the oven is very difficult; lightweight ones with one handle long enough so the patient can grasp it safely or ones with two swing-over-the-top handles that can be held by one hand are possibilities. Sliding the casserole from a pushcart to the pulled out oven shelf is safest but possible only if the heights of these are equal.

To sift flour, one handed sifters are available. To roll dough, hold the rolling pin in the center. To crack and separate an egg, use the chef's egg crack: hold the egg in the palm using the four fingers and thumb. There should be a separation between the index and middle fingers. Crack the egg sharply on the side of

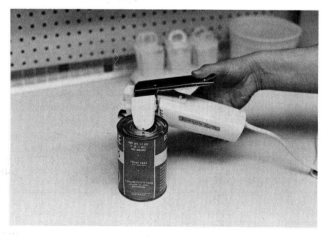

Figure 27.5 Ronson electric can opener which can be used one-handed.

the bowl at the point between the index and middle fingers, then, as in one motion, pull the two halves of the egg apart by further separating the fingers. Commercial egg separators are available to separate the yolk from the white.

The pans, dishes, etc. should be stored vertically to alleviate the need to lift off items stored on top of other items, put them down, get the needed one, then put the others back.

For cutting, a sharp knife can be used on a stabilized object. A rocker knife or meat-cutting wheel (wallpaper casing wheel)[15] can be used on nonstabilized objects because the push force is downward. To meet specific needs, there are many gadgets available, such as an egg slicer, grapefruit sectioner, garlic press, one-handed food chopper, etc. Serving salad can be done using commercially available "salad scissors" in which two salad servers are joined with a scissor grip.

Transporting items can be done by using a wheeled cart, a basket, an apron with large pockets, or similar solutions.

Dishwashing is facilitated by soaking and air drying the dishes. For loss of use of one hand, the soiled dishes should all be placed on one side of the sink and the dish drainer on the other side, so the flow of work is energy conserving. A hand-held spray is helpful for rinsing. A restaurant style suction based brush is used for glassware. A sponge cloth or rubber mat in the bottom of the sink reduces breakage and provides a friction surface to hold the utensil against for scrubbing. Cleaning up as one prepares meals reduces the likelihood of stuck-on soil. If spills do become stuck on the stove or counter, a wet sponge can be put on the spills and eventually they will soften and wipe off.

Housecleaning

Bedmaking is facilitated for the hemiplegic person with figure-ground deficit if the top sheet is a contrasting color to the bottom sheet. Again, the bed could be made completely at each corner before going on to the next to conserve energy.

A long-handled dustpan that balances open when placed on the floor is useful. Floor spills must be cleaned up immediately to prevent falls. There are sponge mops that can be squeezed one-handed by sliding the squeezer mechanism up the handle. A string mop can be wrung by the use of a self-wringing type pail by which the water is extracted when a lever is pushed. An electric floor scrubber may be useful. The new no-wax floors are easiest to maintain.

A tank-type vacuum cleaner permits the patient to sit and reach areas to be cleaned using the long hose.

Sewing

The one-handed homemaker can sew by using an electric machine with foot or knee controls or sew by hand by stabilizing the material with weights or in an embroidery hoop mounted in a convenient place. The needle can be threaded while it is held in a pin cushion or a bar of soap. Material can be cut if it is weighted to prevent slipping.

Child Care

For feeding, the infant should be propped up on pillows, rested against the arm of an upholstered chair, or be in an infant seat. There are highchairs with one-handed tray release mechanisms. The screw top nursing bottles are easier to manage than the plastic liner type. An electric baby dish heats the food in a safe manner and keeps the food warm during the meal. Tongs could be used to take hot baby food jars out of the warming water if this method is used.

To bathe the baby, before drawing the water into the tub or kitchen sink, strap the baby into a suction-based bath seat (see Fig. 27.4) to secure him. Turn the cold water on before the hot. Let the water out and dry the baby as well as possible before lifting him out onto another dry towel.

For dressing the baby, disposable diapers with tab closures are easiest. It is not impossible to use regular pinned diapers but requires much practice. Zippers are difficult to fasten unless the mother can devise a method to hold the bottom taut. Dressing the baby on a dressing table that has a wide Velcro closure strap to secure the baby is convenient because it reduces the amount of squirming possible, but dressing can be done most safely on the floor. To put the baby on the floor, the mother can first sit on a chair and then slide the baby gently down her legs to the floor. Playing with the baby on the floor is more worry-free.

Compensation for Blindness

The principles are to substitute senses of smell, touch, and hearing and to adhere to an established routine and order.

There are many books written on the details of methods used by blind persons. A few of the more common methods are mentioned here.

Marketing

Although the person may order by telephone, help will be needed to label the items with braille tags[16] when the order is delivered. The blind person must organize storage in a consistent, noncluttered manner because she relies on her memory to find things.

Food Preparation, Service, and Cleanup

Frozen dinners are useful. The oven dial must be marked in braille to indicate "off," "broil," and every 50 degrees. Push-button burner controls are best, but braille indicators or raised dots can be used for the dial type. The timer or accessory timer needs to be marked in braille, also. Long oven mitts should be used when using the oven. The organization of the refrigerator must be consistent; pull-out shelves reduce the likelihood of knocking over items and spills. Contiguous counter space also reduces accidental dropping and spilling. The American Foundation for the Blind[17] has a catalogue of useful items for the blind including a dispenser for sugar in one-teaspoon amounts (cubes or packages are an alternative), a pot for pouring off water without removing the lid (the French fry basket idea already mentioned is an alternative), a knife with a thickness guide for slicing meats, cheese, tomatoes, etc.

The blind person relies heavily on his memory and senses of hearing, smell, and touch to work in the kitchen. Hot and cold water, in some houses, sound differently running from the tap; boiling water makes noise; spices and foods smell differently; ripe fruit and vegetables smell and feel differently from unripe. The fingertips of the assistive hand guide the working hand when peeling, slicing, etc.

Housecleaning

Bedmaking is no problem after the bedclothing is centered on the bed by matching the centerfold to the center of the bedframe and discriminating the top from the bottom of the sheets by feeling the hems. Dusting is facilitated by getting rid of clutter. Spray waxes are less desirable than liquids because the person cannot see the extent of the sprayed liquids. Liquid cleansers should be applied to the cloth, not directly to the furniture. Tidying and cleaning the bathroom as it is used keeps that room ready for use of visitors as well as reducing the need for frequent all-over cleaning. Vacuuming, mopping, etc. is done systematically by devising a system to remember what has and has not been done. Furniture is placed consistently. Animals should be taught to lie in out-of-the-way places.

Laundry

Fasten paired items together when they are taken off, using sock holders, pins, etc. Prepacked, individual measures of detergent and/or bleach are convenient. Ironing, if not eliminated, can be done by using a cooler iron (Braille markings) than usual for the fabric type (determined by touch) and by smoothing the material with one hand while ironing with the other. If a person lacks skill in this bilateral activity, the smoothing hand can wear an oven mitt or glove.

References

1. Gilbert, D. W. Energy expenditures for the disabled homemaker: Review of studies. *Am. J. Occup. Ther.* 19(6): 321–328, 1965.
2. Chamberlain, M. A. Social implications of rheumatoid arthritis in young mothers. *Rheumatol. Rehabil.* (Suppl.): 70–73, 1979.
3. Dunn, V. M. Tips on raising children from a wheelchair. *Accent on Living*, 22(4) 78–83, 1978.
4. Vorburger, L. Wash up. *Accent on Living*, Fall: 125, 1980.
5. Lunsk, A. S. Clean sweep. *Accent on Living*, Summer: 62, 1980.
6. New Products and Services. *Accent on Living*, Spring: 93–98, 1978.
7. Burkhardt, B. Loop-handled utensils. *Am. J. Occup. Ther.*, 29(7): 423, 1975.
8. Collins, A. D. Adapted plate for use in a microwave oven. *Am. J. Occup. Ther.*, 32(9): 586–587, 1978.
9. Fastow, K. Adapted fitted bed sheets. *Am. J. Occup. Ther.*, 31(6): 393, 1977.
10. Compton, A. E. Handy tote bag. *Accent on Living*, Summer: 63, 1980.
11. Klinger, J., Frieden, F., and Sullivan, R. *Mealtime Manual for the Aged and Handicapped.* New York: Simon & Schuster (Essandess Special Edition), 1970.
12. Boettke, E. M. *Suggestions for Physically Handicapped Mothers on Clothing for Pre-School Children.* Storrs, Conn.: School of Home Economics, University of Connecticut, 1957.
13. Bare, C., Boettke, E., and Waggoner, N. *Self-Help Clothing for Handicapped Children.* Chicago: National Society for Crippled Children and Adults, 1962.
14. Lowman, E., and Klinger, J. *Aids to Independent Living.* New York: McGraw-Hill, 1969.
15. Souga, C. Meat cutting wheel for one-handed patients. *Am. J. Occup. Ther.*, 22(3): 211, 1968.
16. (AID) for blind seen in new alphabet. *Accent on Living*, Spring: 42–44, 1975.
17. *Aids and Appliances.* American Foundation for the Blind, Inc., 15 West 16th St., New York, N.Y. 10011.

Supplementary Reading

American Heart Association. *Do It Yourself Again: Self-Help Devices for the Stroke Patient.* New York: American Heart Association, 1965.

Asenjo, A. *A Step-by-Step Guide to Personal Management for Blind Persons.* New York: American Foundation for the Blind, 1970.

Buyer's guide (yearly publication). *Accent on Living*, P. O. Box 700, Bloomington, Il. 61701.

Frederick, B., Clark, V. L., Brown, B. E., Nelsen-Allen, C. E., and Amble, D. S. *Body Mechanics: Instruction Manual. A Guide for Therapists.* Redmond, Wash.: Express Publications, 1979.

Oppliger, H. R., and Brunner, E. Electronic measuring cup for the blind. *IEEE Trans. Biomed. Eng.*, 24(4): 386–388, 1977.

Payne, K. Doing the impossible—it's all in learning how. *Accent on Living*, Spring: 38–49, 1980.

Rusk, H., *et al. Rehabilitation Monograph VIII: A Manual for Training the Disabled Homemaker*, 3rd ed. New York: Institute of Rehabilitation Medicine, New York University Medical Center, 1967.

Schafer, R. Occupational therapy for lower extremity problems. *Am. J. Occup. Ther.*, 27(3): 132–137, 1973.

Strebel, M. B. *Adaptations and Techniques for the Disabled Homemaker*, publication 710. Minneapolis: Sister Kenny Institute, Dept. of Research & Education, 1980.

Wright, S. B. Being independent—mobility aids can help. *Accent on Living*, 24(3): 46–48, 1979.

chapter

28

Leisure Time Activities for the Physically Disabled

Catherine A. Trombly, M.A., OTR

Leisure time activities can add zest to the life of physically disabled persons, just as they do to the life of the nondisabled. Play is intrinsically motivated and self-regulated by the individual[1] and thereby contributes to a person's feeling of being in control of his own life. Recreational activities can provide opportunities to redevelop social relationships,[2] to redevelop competency and self-esteem, and to maintain or increase strength and endurance and other physical gains made in the rehabilitation program.[3, 4] For these reasons, development of avocational interests and skills should be included as part of the rehabilitation process. The patient who had no hobbies or interests other than work prior to disability can be encouraged to develop hobbies by experiencing their benefits while in the rehabilitation center.

The newly disabled person may need guidance in choosing and initiating activities which are both interesting and useful to his growth and development as a person as well as possible within his capabilities. One study indicated that the depression following a major disabling accident (spinal cord injury) reduced the person's motivation to participate or be interested in recreational interests previously enjoyed.[3] Another study tested and found support for the hypothesis that increasing the level of physical fitness of poststroke patients would also improve their self concept.[5] Too often the all-consuming interest becomes the disability and the limitations it imposes; interest in recreational activities can put the focus on achievement.

The occupational therapist's role in this aspect of the patient's life is based on the assumption that "play is a need-fulfilling and appropriate occupation in the life of every person."[1] Knowledge of motor and psy-

chosocial activity analyses enables the occupational therapist to suggest recreational pursuits that are within the capabilities of the person and that will contribute to the goals the disabled person has for his life. The occupational therapist can devise or suggest adapted methods or specialized equipment needed by the disabled person to accomplish the particular activity of his choice. The adaptations are made using the same principles as cited in the chapters on self-care and homemaking. Sometimes, the specific solution needs to be collaboratively worked out by an expert in the sport or activity, the patient, and the occupational therapist, all contributing their knowledge of the particular situation.

If a therapeutic recreation specialist is part of the rehabilitation team, the occupational therapist may be less involved in selecting and adapting activities to meet the patient's goals, but may be more active in helping the patient discover what physical and mental abilities he has to capitalize on and what life goals and values may be met through avocational pursuits.

Some examples of activities and suggestions for adaptations of equipment or method are included here. This is by no means an exhaustive survey; the reader is referred to the literature and to special societies cited in the references.

ARTS AND CRAFTS

Involvement in the arts can be passive or active. Music, art, drama, literature, dance or rhythmic movement can all be enjoyed on several levels. They offer the participant refreshment from daily work and a sense of achievement if participation is active.

Musical instruments can be adapted to enable some disabled musicians to continue their interest. For example, a person with weak forearms and elbows can use a piano if a smooth wooden shelf is attached to the piano in front of the keys to rest the arms on while playing.[6]

Paintbrush handles can be enlarged for easier grasp or adapted to be held in the mouth.[6] Paint cups can be secured in a cutout board to stabilize them to prevent spilling for a person with incoordination. Easels can be readily adjusted to a suitable angle.[6]

Wheelchair square dancing is an organized recreation in a number of communities.

Involvement in crafts not only gives one a sense of accomplishment, but also may help maintain physical gains of the rehabilitation process and may even result in limited earnings if the product is clever and the workmanship good. One popular craft is needlework. Sewing aids are available to hold, mark, or cut material. Self-threading needles allow threading by pushing the thread into the eye of the needle while the needle is held in a cake of soap, beeswax, a pin cushion, etc. Needlework can be held in place on a pillow or on hoops or other frames that attach to the table (Fig. 28.1) or clamp on a person's knee to allow one-handed persons to enjoy this activity.[6] For patients with lower extremity weakness, adapted microswitch controls for the sewing machine can be mounted so the patient can operate the machine using his chin or any other part of his body over which he has voluntary motor control and sensation while freeing both hands to guide the material.[6]

GAMES

Games are competitive and, as such, absorb the person's attention even if the person is an observer. If

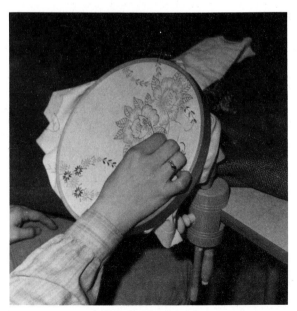

Figure 28.1 Frame which permits a person with use of one hand to do needlework.

a participant, they activate a person's perceptual and intellectual abilities to the level needed to meet the challenge. Usually games are social interactions, especially if a club is organized. Board games such as checkers, chess, monopoly, and scrabble can be modified by enlarging or reducing the size of the board or the pieces. The pieces can also be weighted, altered in shape, magnetized, or held in place with Velcro to allow persons with limited range, strength, or coordination to play.[6] Supine patients can use magnetized or Velcroed pieces which allow the playing board to be fastened in an upright or upside down position. Prism glasses which allow viewing of something held perpendicular to the person may be needed. The glasses allow the patient whose eyes look directly ahead to see what is at or towards his waist or feet. Card games are popular and can bridge generations and bring together people of various backgrounds who share equal enthusiasm. Playing cards can be large, small, marked in braille, magnetized, shuffled by machines, or held in card holders.[6] Card holders hold the hand of cards so each card is visible to the card player; they can be purchased commercially or made by cutting slots in a piece of wood, by using an upended scrub brush, or by using the edges of a book held closed by an elastic band.

Electronic games can be used by those with limited upper extremity function. They offer a fine opportunity for interaction and friendly competition between the disabled person and his nondisabled friends.

HOBBIES

A hobby pursued with enthusiasm can put the person in contact with other people, disabled and nondisabled, who share the same interest through magazines, clubs, and organizations that spring up related to a certain hobby. Hobbies can range from the usual solitary interests such as reading, collecting, or calligraphy to those that involve other people such as ham radio, camping, or travel, to the more daring interests for those with adventurous spirits. Camping for handicapped adults and children is becoming more possible with the greater emphasis and awareness of the need to reduce architectural barriers in all types of environments.[7] Travel is also becoming easier for the wheelchair bound.[8, 9] Planning the trip and reliving it afterwards with friends via photographs are part of the pleasure of travel. Photography is possible for persons with limited hand use with care in selection of equipment and by adaptive methods of holding the camera and releasing the shutter.[6, 10]

For those with determination, nothing seems impossible. One man, who is a high level paraplegic from birth, pilots his own plane while lying on a special gurney and using hand controls.[11] Another paraplegic pilots a helicopter and does ariel photography.[12] Equally implausible, however less daring, was the development of an authors group among young severely disabled persons with articulation problems so severe they were not easily understood. It resulted in their learning to produce creative writing pieces which were published and sold and in becoming better listeners and speakers through the discussions.[13]

Gardens can be adapted for enjoyment by the blind by marking the exhibits in braille, by raising the flower beds to near hand level, and by clearly demarcating the walkways by raised edging. Fragrant flowers and herbs would be a great pleasure. Raised garden beds or flower pots or planters enable a wheelchair patient to garden comfortably.[6] Involvement in garden clubs and competitions can add another dimension to the pleasure of gardening.

SPORTS

Both team and individual sports are engaged in by disabled persons of all types. Some become champions, some do it for fitness, and others do it for the challenge. The sports have rules and equipment suitable to the players.

Those with physical disabilities have the need for exercise to maintain good cardiovascular health just as the nondisabled do. Basketball, swimming, and long-distance wheelchair races fulfill the requirements needed for good cardiovascular training because they are dynamic exercises, use many muscle groups, require intensity of over 50% maximum capacity, and are performed over a relatively long performance time.[4]

Basketball,[14] softball,[15] track and field,[2] swimming,[2] table tennis, fencing,[6] weight lifting, archery,[16] dartchery, and marathoning[17] are all sports for which there are organized competitions. College- and industry-sponsored wheelchair teams engage in competition with each other. Also there are games with "normal" teams who use wheelchairs for the event. Both teams use special sports chairs which are designed for maximum maneuverability.

The ParaOlympics are held every 4 years following the Olympic games.[18] As in any competition, categories of player abilities ensure that the competition is among persons of equal ability and are, therefore, fair, *i.e.*, a paraplegic does not compete against a quadriplegic. There are national competitions for the various ParaOlympic sports to select the best representatives from the U.S.A. to compete with the best wheelchair athletes from other countries.

Kayaking, roller skating, and skate boarding are all possible by some daring amputees or spinal cord-injured persons.[15] Horseback riding has been found physically and psychologically beneficial as part of the rehabilitation program of patients diagnosed with cerebral palsy, poliomyelitis, arthritis, stroke, trauma, or blindness.[19, 20] Contraindications to this sport that were cited include epilepsy with uncontrolled seizures, severe mental retardation, susceptibility to decubitus ulcers, or progressive neuromuscular disease that affects the upper extremities needed to control the horse.[20]

Adaptations have been devised to enable persons with certain handicaps to fish (pole holders for an upper extremity amputee[6] or a stroke patient[21]); and hunt (gun mount for a quadriplegic)[22]; to do boating (open-ended sailboat with swivel seat and window shade type sail for lower extremity disabled persons)[23]; ride motorcycles (hand controls and side car for wheelchair for paraplegic)[24]; ski (adapted ski poles for lower extremity amputees, tandem skiing for the blind, and others)[25, 26]; bowl (device to propel the ball for person with upper extremity weakness)[27]; play baseball or do archery (special terminal devices used in place of a hook or hand for an upper extremity amputee).[6]

References

1. Gunn, S. L. Play as an occupation: Implications for the handicapped. *Am. J. Occup. Ther.*, 29 (4): 222–225, 1975.
2. Wheelchair Sports. One avenue to a happy, healthy life. *Accent on Living*, 25 (2): 36–41, 1980.
3. Rogers, J. C., and Figone, J. J. The avocational pursuits of rehabilitants with traumatic quadriplegia. *Am. J. Occup. Ther.*, 32 (9): 571–576, 1978.
4. Jochheim, K. A., and Strohkendle, H. The value of particular sports of the wheelchair-disabled in maintaining health of the paraplegic. *Paraplegia, 11:* 173–178, 1973.
5. Brinkmann, J. R., and Hoskins, T. A. Physical conditioning and altered self-concept in rehabilitated hemiplegic patients. *Phys. Ther.*, 59 (7): 859–865, 1979.
6. Lowman, E., and Klinger, J. *Aids to Independent Living*, Chapters 56–60. New York: McGraw-Hill, 1969.
7. Scouting, Camping Opening up for Disabled Youths and Adults. *Accent on Living*, 21 (2): 88–92, 1976.
8. Annand, D. Sail away on the Love Boat. *Accent on Living*, 25 (4): 50–54, 1980.
9. Pietkiewicz, P. Seeing America. *Accent on Living*, 25 (1): 78–86, 1980.
10. Have Fun with Photography. *Accent on Living*, 21 (3): 68–73, 1976.
11. Miller, H. L. How this paraplegic flies an airplane. *Accent on Living*, 25 (2): 74–75, 1980.
12. Powers, J. M. How this paraplegic flies a helicopter. *Accent on Living*, 25 (2): 76–78, 1980.
13. Fearing, V. G. An authors group for extended care patients. *Am. J. Occup. Ther.*, 32 (8): 526–527, 1978.
14. Pykare, J. 30th wheelchair basketball games. *Accent on Living*, 23 (1): 82–83, 1978.
15. Accent on Pictures. *Accent on Living*, 25 (4): 58–59, 1981.
16. Kenoyer, M., and Kenoyer, N. Bullseye! *Accent on Living*, 25 (1): 22–25, 1980.
17. Marathon for fast and fit. *Accent on Living*, 25 (2): 42–46, 1980.
18. Lipton, B. The role of wheelchair sports in rehabilitation. *Int. Rehabil. Rev.*, 21 (2): 1970.
19. Disabled on Horseback? *Accent on Living*, 23 (1): 88–93, 1978.
20. Woods, D. Horseriding catching on as therapy for the disabled. *Can. Med. Assoc. J.*, 121 (5): 631–634, 650, 1979.
21. Crewe, R. A. Fishing for the hemiplegic. *Br. J. Occup. Ther.*, 38 (9): 195, 1975.
22. Szeto, A. Y. J. Hunting rifle for quadriplegic patients. *Arch. Phys. Med. Rehabil.*, 60 (9): 425–427, 1979.
23. Lundberg, Lasse. personal communication, Goteburg, Sweden.
24. World champion paraplegic motorcyclist talks about 8,000 mile ride to speed cure of spinal cord injury. *Accent on Living*, 21 (3): 88–92, 1976.
25. Skiing on one leg! *Accent on Living*, 21 (3): 56–63, 1976.
26. Thrills and spills on the downhill run. *Accent on Living*, 25 (3): 38–39, 1980.
27. Bowl with your feet. *Accent on Living*, 22 (1): 94–95, 1977.

Supplementary Reading

Corcoran, P. J. *et al.* Sports medicine and the physiology of wheelchair marathon racing. *Orthop. Clin. North, Am.*, 11 (4): 697–716, 1980.

Mouthstick handles small, light items. *Accent on Living, 24* (3): 86–87, 1979.

Overs, R. P. Avocational evaluation and work adjustment: A deterrent to dependency. *J. Rehabil., 42* (6): 21–24, 40, 48, 1976.

Selected Resources

The National Wheelchair Athletic Association, 40-24 62nd St., Woodside, N.Y. 11377.

The United States Association for Blind Athletes, 55 W. California Ave., Beach Haven Park, N.J. 08008.

Senior Olympics, 5670 Wilshire Blvd., Los Angeles, Calif. 90036.

The National Association of Sports for Cerebral Palsy, PO Box 3874 Amity Station, New Haven, Conn. 06525.

Blind Outdoor Leisure Development (BOLD), 533 East Main St., Aspen, Colo 81611.

National Inconvenienced Sportsmen's Association (NISA), 3738 Walnut Ave., Carmichael, Calif. 95608.

New England Handicapped Sportmen's Association, 18 Tremont St., Boston, Mass.

North American Riding for the Handicapped Association (NARHA), Thistlecroft, Park St., Mendon, Mass. 01756.

Therapeutic Horsemanship, Inc., Mrs. Sandy Rafferty, M. A., OTR, Director, Route 1, Valley Road, Pacific, Mo. 63069.

Breckenridge Outdoor Education Center, P.O. Box 697, Breckenridge, Colo. 80424.

Boating for the Handicapped, Guidelines for the Physically Disabled, by Eugene Hedley, Ph. D. Available from: Products Manager, Human Resources Center, I. U. Willets Rd., Albertson, N.Y. 11507.

Riding for Rehabilitation, a Guide for Handicapped Riders and Their Instructors, by Joseph Bauer. Available from: Can Ride, 209 Deloraine Ave., Toronto, Canada M5M 2B2.

Handicapped Boater's Association Magazine, P.O. Box 1134, Ansonia Station, N.Y. 10023.

chapter

29

Environmental Evaluation and Community Reintegration

Catherine A. Trombly, M.A., OTR

Persons who have acquired a disability need to learn new skills and attitudes so that they may live the rest of their lives in ways that are satisfying to them. Rehabilitation is this learning process. Discharge to the community is the goal. However, life does not automatically start anew when the disabled person "graduates" from the rehabilitation center. At the center, they experience an ideal environment both architecturally and attitudinally. However, "many handicapped (persons) feel frustrated and helpless in public places with the countless stairs and endless stares".[1] Part of rehabilitation must be a transitional process in which problem solving and coping skills are learned and self esteem heightened so that the disabled person who expects to be active in the community can act confidently and take charge. Therefore, a reintegration program should include knowledge of architectural barriers; solutions and problem solving skills to facilitate correction or bypassing of barriers in order to enable the person to live and work independently; and development of coping skills to allow the person to act confidently.

ARCHITECTURAL BARRIERS

Persons who are paralyzed and must use wheelchairs or ambulatory aids, who are blind and need orienting aids, or who are old, have low endurance, or are unable to move quickly or negotiate rough terrain or many stairs are prevented from use of public buildings, parks and other facilities unless architectural

barriers are eliminated. The international sign of access (Fig. 29.1) displayed on a building indicates its accessibility for wheelchair users. The Rehabilitation Act of 1973 provided that all federally owned, financed, or leased buildings and transportation facilities constructed[2] since 1968 be fully accessible to the handicapped.[2] The Architectural and Transportation Barriers Compliance Board is a Federal board charged with enforcing this legislation. Unfortunately, because of politics and poor organization, this board failed to function at its expected level. Federally funded institutions were slow to comply.[2] The Comprehensive Rehabilitation Services Amendments (P.L. 95-602), passed in 1978, expanded the responsibilities and clout of this board.[3]

The 1978 Amendments made quality of life of the physically disabled a priority. It established, and funded through 1981, a program of services for independent living by the severely disabled, in which the disabled persons were to be "substantially involved."[3] One service is the Independent Living Centers now being established across the country which provide referral and direct services relating to housing, attendant care, transportation, and social-vocational counseling. These centers are important in light of the fact that modern family life is changing. Families are smaller and more mobile; both spouses work; old folks live longer and may live a distance from their grown children; the divorce rate is high. The family is ill-equipped to deal with members with permanent handicaps.[4] Therefore, many handicapped persons must

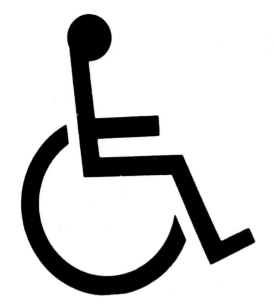

Figure 29.1 International symbol of wheelchair accessibility.

rely on their own resources or be institutionalized. The Independent Living Centers are meant to enhance their resources.

Architectural barriers have been identified and, in response, the American National Standards Institute has published specifications for making buildings and facilities accessible to, and usable by, the physically disabled.[5] The common barriers encountered in public buildings and private homes and their solutions are listed here. Most barriers are against the use of a wheelchair, with curbs and stairs the most common ones. Elevators eliminate this barrier inside buildings. Outside entrances can be ramped. To enable a wheelchair-bound person to negotiate a ramp independently there must be a ratio of 12 inches of ramp length for each inch of rise.[5] For example, if a door entrance is 24 inches from the ground, the ramp must extend 24 feet. The ramp may need to zigzag if the required length would extend it into the street or extend it longer than 30 feet. Any ramp must have one, preferably two, railings, a nonskid surface, fireproof construction, and platforms 5 ft. square at the beginning, end, and at each turn in a zigzagging ramp.[5] A canopy or automatic snow-melting equipment should be provided for outdoor ramps in snowy location.

Curbs are eliminated at crosswalks by curb cuts using the 12:1 ratio for proper rise. A cut that is set back into the sidewalk and ends at the street is safer for wheelchair users than a ramp which starts at the curb and continues into the street.

Thresholds should be as flush as possible. Stairs for the ambulatory disabled should have bilateral railings and flat risers of 7 inches maximum height.

Heavy doors are barriers to the disabled as they are to many nondisabled persons. Revolving doors and doors that open out are difficult or impossible to manage for wheelchair-bound persons. The timed elec-

tric eye doors are excellent for the handicapped as well as the ladened shopper.

The space required for a wheelchair to turn around is 360 square inches (60 inches × 60 inches).[5] All doors should be 32 inches wide to accommodate wheelchairs.[5] In public bathrooms the stall doors must open out to allow the door to be closed after the wheelchair is in. Adequate turning radius is also necessary for access to the toilet stall. The stall must be wide enough (3 ft) and long enough (5 ft) to accommodate the chair.[5] It is helpful if safety grab bars are available and the toilet is wall-mounted so the seat is 22 inches from the floor. The faucets of the basin should be the lever or push-on type with a mixer spout. The soap dispenser should be operable by either pushing or tipping it. Water fountains, or at least cups near the fountain, should be easily accessible. The water fountain should be both hand- and foot-operated. Telephones should be mounted low and in modern sound barriers rather than booths. Push buttons are easier to use than rotary dial. The phone should have an amplifier device for the hard of hearing.

Room identification, elevator buttons, building, or shopping mall layouts should be in braille to be accessible to the blind. Doors that open to dangerous areas, such as to the boiler room, should be identified for the blind by special signals such as knurled doorknobs.

Parking spaces for the handicapped driver must be wide enough for the car and for the transfer, an additional 4 feet. Street-crossing lights should be set slow enough to allow safe crossing. They should be equipped with sound alarms for the blind. Fire and police alarm boxes should be set low enough for wheelchair persons to use; a design change could make them inaccessible to children.

Public recreation areas, campgrounds, YMCAs, community recreation facilities, and schools should have a shower with padded seat for use by paraplegics, quadriplegics, and others of similar disability.

Supermarkets are not currently designed for the handicapped; the checkout areas are barriers, some of the food is displayed out of reach, assistance is scarce, and the narrow fence openings that some stores have to prevent theft of shopping wagons also prevent access to wheelchairs.

Some theaters have accommodated to the handicapped by designating areas where they can sit in their wheelchairs while viewing the show; others, however, still require the person to transfer to a theater seat, and the wheelchair is stored in the back of the theater where exit in case of fire would be impossible.

A survey form based on the standards, originally developed to use in preparing city guides for the handicapped, can be helpful for individuals to use during the reintegration educational process. It is published here (Table 29.1). Others are available to suit particular needs such as to select accommodations for meetings at which disabled persons will participate.[6]

Since most public transportation systems were built before 1968, the law does not apply and, therefore, making transportation accessible to the ambulatory

Table 29.1
BUILDING SURVEY TO DEVELOP GUIDES FOR THE HANDICAPPED

National Society for Crippled Children and Adults, 2023 W. Ogden Ave., Chicago, Ill. 60612

Name and Type of Building _____ Phone Number _____

Street Address _____City _____State _____

Person Interviewed _____ Title _____

1. Offstreet Parking

   a. Is an offstreet parking area available adjacent to building? .... Yes No
   b. If adjacent offstreet parking is not available, identify and give location of nearest and most convenient parking area.

   _____

   c. Are parking area and building separated by a street? .... Yes No
   d. Is the surface of the parking area smooth and hard (no sand, gravel, etc.)? .... Yes No

2. Passenger Loading Zone

   a. Is there a passenger loading zone? .... Yes No
   b. If yes, where is it located in relation to selected entrance? _____

   _____

3. Approach to Selected Entrance

   a. Which entrance was selected as most accessible? _____
   b. Is the approach to the entrance door ground level? .... Yes No
   c. Is there a ramp in the approach to or at the entrance door? .... Yes No
   d. If there are any steps in the approach to or at the entrance, give total number of steps ......
   e. If there are steps, is there a sturdy handrail on at least one side or in the center? .... Yes No

4. Entrance Door

   a. What is the width of the entrance doorway (with door open)? ....
   b. Is the door automatic? .... Yes No
   c. Are there steps between entrance and main areas or corridor? .... Yes No
   d. If yes, what is the total number of steps? ....
   e. If there are steps, is there a sturdy handrail in the center or on at least one side? .... Yes No

5. Elevator

   a. Is there a passenger elevator? .... Yes No
   b. Does it serve all essential areas? .... Yes No

6. Essential Areas (areas to which access is essential if building is to be used)

   Area 1 _____ Area 2 _____

   Area 3 _____

7. Access from Entry to Essential Areas

	(1)	(2)	(3)
a. Is the usable width of corridors and aisles at least 32 inches? ..	Yes No	Yes No	Yes No
b. Is the narrowest clear doorway with door open 28 inches wide or more?	Yes No	Yes No	Yes No
c. If not, what is the width?			

Table 29.1—*continued*

8. Interior of Essential Areas

   a. Are there any steps between essential areas not served by elevators? .... Yes No   Yes No   Yes No

   b. Does each flight of steps have a sturdy handrail on at least one side or in the center? .... Yes No   Yes No   Yes No

9. Public Toilet Rooms

   a. Where are toilet rooms located? .... Men _____
                                       Women _____

   b. Would one need to go up or down steps to get to toilet room? .... Yes No   Yes No

   c. If so, how many? ....

   d. If there are steps, does each flight of steps have a sturdy handrail on at least one side or in the center? ....

	Men	Women
	Yes No	Yes No

   e. What is the width of toilet room entrance doorway (with door open)? ......

   f. Is there a free space in the room to permit a wheelchair to turn? .... Yes No   Yes No

   g. What is width of widest toilet stall door?

   h. Does this stall have handrails or grab bars? .... Yes No   Yes No

10. Public Telephone

   a. Where is the most accessible phone located? _____

   b. What type (booth, wall, desk)? _____

   c. If phone is in a booth, what is width of booth door (with door open)? ....

   d. Is the handset 48 inches or less from the floor? .... Yes No

   e. Does the phone have amplifying controls for the hard of hearing? .... Yes No

11. Interior (auditorium, church, restaurant, etc.)

   a. What is the distance from floor to edge of restaurant table? ....

   b. If there are booths, can a wheelchair be placed at the open end of the booth? .... Yes No

   c. In theaters, public halls, churches, etc. can persons remain in wheelchairs? .... Yes No

   d. If yes, where? _____

   e. Can arrangements be made to reserve wheelchair space? .... Yes No

12. Assistance and Aids Available

   a. Is there an attendant who will take cars? .... Yes No

   b. Is there help available for those needing assistance in entering (doorman, porter)? .... Yes No

   c. If not, is help available for those needing assistance if arranged for in advance? .... Yes No

   d. Who to call in advance for assistance _____

   e. Telephone number _____

   f. Are wheelchairs available? (at airports, hotels, museums, etc.)? .... Yes No

13. Motel or Hotel Guest Rooms

   a. What is width of the entrance door to guest room (with door open)? ....

   b. What is width of entrance door to bathroom (with door open)? ....

   c. Are there handrails or grab bars near the toilet? ....

   d. Are there handrails or grab bars for the bath and shower? ....

---

handicapped has lagged behind remedying barriers in buildings in the U.S.A. However, the National Mass Transportation Assistance Act of 1974 amended Section 16(a) of the Urban Mass Transportation Administration Act of 1964 to state in part that it is "national policy that elderly and handicapped persons have the same right as others to utilize mass transportation facilities and services."[7]

Bus steps can be eliminated by use of a hydraulic lift in place of the stair; this change would make buses accessible to wheelchairs (Fig. 29.2).

The rapid transit or subway can be designed so that

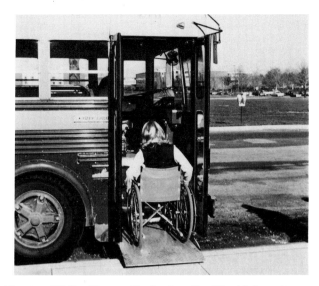

Figure 29.2 Bus with hydraulic lift, University of Illinois.

the floor of the vehicle is flush with the loading platform. Access to the platform can be gained by use of elevators.

One system that has made an attempt to comply is the Bay Area Rapid Transit in San Francisco. It is accessible to wheelchairs and allows realistic commuting by the wheelchair-bound.[8] It is not perfect but better than in most places. Some inconveniences experienced by the handicapped are due to the indifference of the able-bodied who are unhelpful, especially during rush hour[8]—every commuter's lament.

Home Evaluation

The living quarters to which the patient will be discharged may also have architectural or safety barriers. A home evaluation is necessary for every patient returning home with a residual disability and expectations of independent functioning on some level. It is done at about the time of discharge when the patient has reached his peak in rehabilitation skills. Sometimes the evaluation can be done by interview with the patient and family, preferably after a home visit. If the problems are complex, the evaluation is done by visit. For a patient who has had to learn adapted methods of self care and mobility, the visit is usually done by the occupational and physical therapist together. The patient and responsible family members are present in the home during the visit. The patient has all ambulation aids which he customarily uses. Whether by visit or interview, preparation for the evaluation requires the therapist to list the disabilities and probable areas of difficulty for this particular patient. For example, a post-stroke patient who uses a cane and has not regained use of the upper extremity may have difficulty with ambulation, stairs, using the kitchen and other home care chores, carrying things, and getting in and out of the bathtub. The therapists would need to be alert to check these tasks specifically. By using a form such as the one developed by Rita

Lefkovitz, M.O.T., and published here (Table 29.2), the evaluation proceeds by reenacting the patient's daily routine and noting what cannot be done and why. The problems are solved or noted as they arise during the course of the visit.

The most common changes that need to be made in the home are: installation of a ramp or railings to enter and exit the home, removal of scatter rugs and extraneous furniture, removal of thresholds, addition of tub or toilet safety grab bars, rearrangement of furniture, raising the bed height, moving the telephone near to the bed, putting a center pull on dresser drawers, rearrangement of kitchen storage, and lowering the clothes in the closet by use of a suction spring rod or a dowel hung by rope from the bar above.[9] Arrangements for summoning aid in the case of an emergency or the availability of a network of concerned others who regularly check on the patient who lives alone are also evaluated.

Suggested specifications for an ideal wheelchair kitchen are listed here[10] since this is one room that needs major modifications if the homemaker is wheelchair-bound. Sometimes, funding for remodeling is available from the Rehabilitation Services Administration. If not, the changes must be prioritized and implemented when the budget permits. A U-shaped or corridor type layout is better than a large square kitchen which requires much moving around from appliance to appliance. Some counters should be lowered to 30 inches in height and should have a space underneath to accommodate the wheelchair. The top cabinets should be lowered to 12 inches above the counter. An eye-level oven with a drop front and self-cleaning feature is better than a traditional stove. Westinghouse produces a built-in oven that has a swing open door. A counter top cook stove should be installed in one of the 30 inch counters with roll space beneath. Alternatively to the conventional cook stove configuration, four burners can be installed in a row if reaching to the back of a stove would be a problem. In either case, controls should be front mounted. A shallow sink is ideal for the person who must sit to use it. If there is a basement, the garbage disposal can be installed below floor level so that it will not interfere with rolling under the sink. A side-by-side refrigerator-freezer is the best choice for a wheelchair homemaker.

The therapist must explain why each recommendation is made. Sometimes, families are reluctant about making changes in the home. When the therapists sense this, they must remember that they are guests in the home and should refrain from actually rearranging. The therapists should teach the person to be as independent as possible within the limitations or make clear how the patient would be limited with the present arrangements. If the patient needs assistance, the family member is taught how to assist him safely using the proper body mechanics.

At the end of the evaluation, a report is written to the patient and his family. It is worded for understanding and acceptance of the ideas presented. The report contains a list and description of every important

Table 29.2
HOME EVALUATION
_____

Type of Home
_____ Apartment: What floor does patient live on? _____

Is elevator available? _____

_____ Single family home: Number of floors_____ Which are used by the patient?

Entrances to Building or Home

1. *Location*—Front, Back, or Side (Circle One)

    a. Which entrance is used most frequently or easily?_____
    b. Can patient get to entrance?_____

2. *Stairs*—Does patient manage outside stairs?_____

    a. Width of stairway_____
    b. Number of steps_____Height of steps_____
    c. Railing present as you go up. R_____ L_____ Both_____
    d. Is ramp available for wheelchair patient?_____ length_____ height of rise_____.

3. *Door*

    a. Can patient unlock, open, close, lock door? (Circle for yes)
    b. Is doorsill present, give height_____ and material_____
    c. Width of doorway_____
    d. Can patient enter_____ leave_____ via door?

4. *Hallway*

    a. Width of hallway_____
    b. Are any objects obstructing the way?_____

Approach to Apartment or Living Area (Omit if not applicable)

1. *Hallway*

    a. Width_____
    b. Obstructions?_____

2. *Steps*

    a. Does patient manage?_____
    b. Width of stairway_____
    c. Number of steps_____Height of steps_____
    d. Railing present as you go up. R_____ L_____ Both_____
    e. Is ramp available?_____Length_____Height of rise_____

3. *Door*

    a. Can patient unlock, open, close, lock door? (Circle one)
    b. Doorsill? Give height_____ Material_____
    c. Width of doorway_____
    d. Can patient enter_____ leave_____via door?

Table 29.2—*continued*

4. *Elevator*

    a. Is elevator present_____Does it land flush with floor?_____
    b. Width of door opening_____
    c. Height of control buttons_____
    d. Can patient manage elevator alone?_____

Inside Home

Note width of hallway and of door entrances.
Note presence of doorsills and height.
Note if must climb stairs to reach room.

1. Can patient move from one part of house to another?
    a. Hallways
    b. Bedroom
    c. Kitchen
    d. Bathroom
    e. Living room
    f. Others

2. Can patient move safely?_____

    a. Note loose rugs   d. Highly waxed floors
    b. Electrical cords   e. Sharp-edged furniture
    c. Faulty floors   f. Animals

3. Note areas of potential danger for patient.

Bedroom

1. *Light Switch*—Accessible?_____Can patient open and close windows?

2. *Bed*

    a. Height_____Width_____
    b. Both sides of bed accessible?_____Headboard present?_____Footboard?_____
    c. Is bed on wheels?_____Is it stable?_____
    d. Can patient transfer wheelchair/bed_____and bed/wheelchair?_____

3. Is *night table* within patient's reach from bed?_____Is telephone on it?_____

4. *Clothing*—Are patient's clothes located in bedroom?_____
                Can patient get clothes from dresser?_____
                Closet?_____Elsewhere?_____

Bathroom

1. Does patient use wheelchair_____walker_____in bathroom?

2. Does wheelchair_____walker_____fit into bathroom?

3. Light switch accessible?_____Can patient open and close window?_____

4. What materials are bathroom walls made of?_____

    a. If tile, how many inches does it extend from the floor beside the toilet?
    b. How many inches from the top of the rim of the bathtub?_____

Table 29.2—*continued*

    5. Does patient use toilet?_____

        a. Can patient transfer independently to and from toilet?_____
        b. Does wheelchair wheel directly to toilet for transfers?_____
        c. What is height of toilet seat from floor?_____
        d. Are there bars or *sturdy* supports near toilet?_____
        e. Is there room for grab bars to be installed?_____

    6. Can patient use sink?_____What is height of sink?_____

        a. Able to reach and turn faucets?_____
        b. Is there knee space beneath sink?_____
        c. Is patient able to reach necessary articles?_____

    7. *Bathing*

        a. Does patient take tub bath?_____Shower?_____Sponge bath?_____
        b. If uses tub, can patient transfer safely without assistance?_____
        c. Bars or sturdy supports present beside tub?_____
        d. Is equipment necessary? (tub seat, handspray attachment, tub rail, no-skid strips, grab rails, other_____)
        e. Can patient manage faucets and drain plug?_____
        f. Height of tub from floor to rim_____
        g. Is tub built-in_____or on legs_____?
        h. Width of tub from the inside_____
        i. If uses separate shower stall, can patient transfer independently and manage faucets?_____
        j. If patient takes sponge bath, describe method.

Living Room Area

    1. Light switch accessible?_____Can patient open and close window?_____

    2. Can furniture be rearranged to allow passage of wheelchair?_____

    3. Can patient transfer from wheelchair to and from sturdy chair?_____Height of chair seat_____.

    4. Can ambulatory patient sit and rise from chair?_____Sofa?_____

    5. Can patient manage TV, radio or other devices?_____

Dining Room

    1. Light switch accessible?_____

    2. Is patient able to use table?_____Height of table_____

Kitchen

    1. What is the table height?_____Can wheelchair fit under?_____

    2. Can patient open refrigerator door and take food?_____

    3. Can patient open freezer door and take food?_____

    3. *Sink*

        a. Can patient be seated at sink?_____
        b. Can patient reach faucets?_____turn them on and off?_____
        c. Can patient reach bottom of basin?_____

Table 29.2—*continued*

4. *Shelves and cabinets*

    a. Can patient open and close?_____
    b. Can patient reach dishes, pots, silver, and food?_____
Comments:

5. *Transport*

    a. Can patient carry utensils from one part of kitchen to another?_____

6. *Stove*

    a. Can patient reach and manipulate controls?_____
    b. Light pilot on oven?_____
    c. Manage oven door?_____
    d. Place food in oven and remove?_____
    e. Manage broiler door?_____
    f. Put food in and remove?_____

7. *Other Appliances*

    a. Can patient reach and turn on appliances?_____
    b. Can patient use outlets?_____

8. *Counter space*—Is there enough for storage and work area?_____

9. *Diagram:*

    (Include stove, refrigerator, sink, table, counters, others if applicable)

Laundry

1. If patient has no facilities, how will laundry be managed:

2. Location of facilities in home or apartment, and description of facilities present:

3. Can patient reach laundry area?_____

4. Can patient use washing machine and dryer?_____

    a. Load and empty?_____
    b. Manage doors and controls?_____

5. Can patient use sink?_____

    a. What is height of sink?_____
    b. Able to reach and turn on faucets?_____
    c. Knee space beneath sink?_____
    d. Able to reach necessary articles?_____

6. Is laundry cart available?_____

7. Can patient hang clothing on line?_____

8. Ironing board

    a. Location:
    b. Is it kept open?_____
    c. If not kept open, can patient set up and take down ironing board?_____
    d. Can patient reach outlet?_____

Table 29.2—*continued*

Cleaning

1. Can patient remove mop, broom, vacuum, pail from storage?_____

2. Use equipment? (Mop, broom, vacuum, etc.)_____

Emergency

1. Location of telephones in house:

2. Could patient use fire escape or back door in a hurry if alone?_____

3. Does patient have neighbors, police, fire and M.D. phone numbers?_____

suggestion made. Source, cost, and description of equipment that is needed are specified. The cost of this equipment must be within the family's budget, or sources of financing must be sought; usually, the social service department of a rehabilitation facility assumes this responsibility. If modifications are necessary, they are listed with specifications. If the family agrees to these, help may be appreciated in locating a tradesman to do the work. Therapists can develop knowledge of such resources by talking to former patients who made modifications in their homes.

A summary report of the recommendations, including the therapists' judgment of the wisdom of discharging the person home, is sent to the referring physician and included in the medical record. If the patient is returning to work, a similar environmental evaluation may be necessary at the place of employment.

ATTITUDINAL BARRIERS

Due to laws which have enabled greater visibility of the handicapped and the initiative of the disabled to speak out for their rights and to educate the able-bodied about their abilities, attitudes of condescension and pity are changing to acceptance, admiration, and expectation. However, as familiarity increases, it also seems that the indifferent attitude of the general public is extending to the handicapped. This is unfortunate because the occasional helping hand needed to bypass an architectural barrier may be less readily offered. The handicapped person needs to learn how to ask for help.

REINTEGRATION PROGRAMS

Programs that prepare the patient for discharge allow the person to practice overcoming architectural and transportation barriers and understanding the attitudes of the general public with the opportunity to discuss the successes, failures, and frustrations with peers and rehabilitation personnel. The program may include informational sessions, group discussions of the experiences of those members who have ventured out of the rehabilitation center, and actual practice in arranging and carrying out outings typical of the patient's expected needs postdischarge. In the practice sessions, the patient is put into situations which are within his capabilities but present problems so that he can learn to anticipate and solve problems. He assumes as much responsibility as he can at the time in arranging and conducting the outing. The therapist takes up the slack in responsibility if necessary and is there to provide assistance in unexpected situations. The patient learns to plan ahead by inquiring by phone about the accessibility of buildings and by arranging with building superintendents for special parking and entrance help if necessary.

Guidebooks for the larger cities and some turnpikes have been developed by organizations such as the Junior League or the National Society for Crippled Children and Adults (Easter Seals) and are usually available from the Chamber of Commerce of the particular city. The guidebooks include information about what architectural barriers or special adaptations exist at churches, theaters, restaurants, transportation depots, historical sights, museums, hotels, and some stores. Colleges and universities often also have guidebooks to their campuses. These guidebooks are helpful and can be used by the patient when planning outings to help him focus on what problems to anticipate and inquire about before visiting any building not included in the guide. Through the group discussions and outings, he learns how to interact with the nondisabled who do not always know how to interact with him. He can learn ways to put the able-bodied at ease and to ask for, or refuse, help.

The need for a reintegration program is supported by a survey that was conducted among disabled and nondisabled college students.[11] It was found that there was a significant difference in feelings of confidence between these groups in these areas: cognitive-problem solving skills of managing money, conserving physical energy, finding a place to live, making decisions; school-vocational skills of going on a job interview, filling out forms, finding a job, planning a school program, talking to employers or teachers; home skills; and community mobility skills. There was no difference in feelings of confidence regarding abilities to manage activities of daily living, which would indicate that traditional rehabilitation is effective; however it is "clear that provision of traditional rehabilitation services alone does not guarantee life satisfaction".[11]

A group therapy program that provided both information and experiences to psychiatric patients attempting to transition to the community was reported.[12] The information given included community resources, nature of the environment out of hospital, housing, budgeting, and job information. Emphasis was also placed on leisure time interests and problem-solving experiences.

One method devised to teach spinal cord-injured patients to foresee what barriers to full accessibility might exist in homes was tested on 10 subjects randomly assigned to experimental and control groups. The method was an audiovisual presentation of wheelchair mobility requirements, standards of accessibility, and common problems encountered by wheelchair-bound persons in homes. There was a statistically significant difference in scores between experimental and control subjects in their ability to notice environmental problems in an actual test home.[13]

Practical experiences to prepare the patient for actual outings are of course required. One program that is reported in the literature is a remedial gym class for a group of 8 to 10 patients of mixed diagnoses.[14] The goals were to increase independence and confidence in one's ability. The minimum criterion for membership was the ability to stand independently. Some of the exercises were: practice on all types of stairs, getting on and off a simulated bus platform in a crowd and within time limits, games to prepare for walking on uneven surfaces with the noise and hubbub of traffic and people introduced, obstacle courses, and practice in getting up from the floor.

A program of community outings was rated as very useful by rheumatoid arthritic patients in increasing their self confidence.[15] The program was designed to evaluate a patient's functional abilities to do skills that are required out of hospital and to assess each patient's problem-solving skills in relation to his own disability regarding architectural barriers, joint protection techniques, the avoidance of decubiti, etc. Minimum criteria for participation included mobility and activities of daily living (ADL) independence to the level expected. A COTA (certified occupational therapy assistant) planned the outing with the patient, based on the patient's needs. If the patient was going to be active, the outings were to markets, banks, restaurants, and sometimes to the job. If the patient were going to be limited, less ambitious outings were planned. A checklist was used to evaluate the experience.

Studies such as these suggest ideas for development of community reintegration programs.

References

1. MacElman, R. M. Society vs. the wheelchair. Pediatrics, 63 (4): 576–579, 1979.
2. Silver, M. Federal compliance board under fire. Accent on Living, 22 (1): 24–31, 1977.
3. Ross, E. C. New rehabilitation law. Accent on Living, 23 (3): 23, 1978.
4. Zisserman, L. The modern family and rehabilitation of the handicapped. Am. J. Occup. Ther., 35 (1): 13–20, 1981.
5. American National Standards Institute. Specifications for Making Buildings and Facilities Accessible to, and Usable by the Physically Handicapped. 1430 Broadway, New York, N.Y. 10018, 1971.
6. What makes a meeting site accessible? Accent on Living, 21 (3): 28–34, 1976.
7. Transportation for the Disabled. Accent on Living, 20 (1): 36, 1975.
8. Tanaka, T. BART: How accessible? Accent on Living, 25 (1): 58–61, 1980.
9. Lowman, E., and Klinger, J. Aids to Independent Living: Self Help for the Handicapped. New York: McGraw-Hill (Blakiston Division), 1969.
10. Webb, C. Tips on making your kitchen accessible. Accent on Living, 23 (3): 104–109, 1978.
11. Burnett, S. E., and Yerxa, E. J. Community-based and college-based needs assessment of physically disabled persons. Am. J. Occup. Ther., 34 (3): 201–207, 1980.
12. Heine, D. B. Daily living group: Focus on transition from hospital to community. Am. J. Occup. Ther., 29 (10): 628–630, 1975.
13. Wittmeyer, M. B., and Stolov, W. C. Educating wheelchair patients on home architectural barriers. Am. J. Occup. Ther., 32 (9): 557–564, 1978.
14. Whycherley, J. Group therapy in the treatment of the hemiplegic patient. Nursing Mirror, 73–76, 1974.
15. Kales-Rogoff, L. Community skills experience for rheumatic disease patients. Am. J. Occup. Ther., 33 (6): 394–395, 1979.

Supplementary Reading

Adaptive Environments. Design and Construction of Settings that Meet Each Person's Special Needs. Massachusetts College of Art, 26 Overland St., Boston, Mass. 02215.
Baum, C. M. Nationally speaking: Independent living—A Critical Role for Occupational Therapy. Am. J. Occup. Ther., 34(12): 773–774, 1980.
Block, J. Income tax deductions for home improvements. Accent on Living, 21(3): 36–37, 1976.
Cary, J. R. How to Create Interiors for the Disabled: A Guidebook for Family and Friends. New York: Pantheon Books (Division of Random House), 1978.
Dolan, E., and Dolan, F. How we made our home accessible. Accent on Living, 22(3): 24–30, 1977.
El-Ghatit, A. Z., Melvin, J. L., and Poole, M. A. Training apartment in community for spinal cord injured patients: A model. Arch. Phys. Med. Rehabil., 61(2): 90–92, 1980.
Frieden, L. Independent living models. Rehabil. Lit., 41(7–8): 169–173, 1980.
Heard, C. Occupational role acquisition: A perspective on the chronically disabled. Am. J. Occup. Ther., 31(4): 243, 247, 1977.
Housing Designs for the Handicapped. Access Chicago. Rehabilitation Institute of Chicago, 345 East Superior, Chicago, Ill. 60611, 1974.
Lewis, L. How to win the parking space battle: A practical guide for the handicapped driver. Accent on Living, 25(3): 92–94, 1980.
Rehabilitation Gazette: International Journal of Independent Living for the Disabled. 4502 Maryland Avenue, St. Louis, Mo. 63108.
Wittmeyer, M. B., and Peszczynski, M. Housing for the disabled. In: Orthotics Etcetera, edited by J. B. Redford. Baltimore: Williams & Wilkins, 1980.
Wolff, R. Center for independent living opening new frontiers for disabled. Accent on Living, 24(2): 34–40, 1979.

chapter

30

Employment for the Physically Disabled

Catherine A. Trombly, M.A., OTR

For some persons, return to work following a physical disability is a prime concern; for others, it is not. People value work differently. It may be the major focus of one person's life and may even define him as a person in his own eyes, but for another person work may simply be the means to the end of participating in other, more pleasurable, aspects of life. There are also those who find no value in work and actually see it as an interruption to their "true life." People in this latter category easily accept the limitations of the disability relative to work and prefer to receive compensation from insurance companies or social welfare agencies.

With advancing technology and changes in societal attitude regarding the value of the disabled person, the level of motivation of the individual is probably the greatest determining factor concerning return to work postinjury. Motivation refers to a person's determination or persistence in pursuing a goal. When no motivation exists, or can be generated, the rehabilitation specialists must realize that vocational planning-evaluation-training will be unsuccessful. For those patients motivated by earning power and/or personal satisfaction, more opportunities than ever exist for employment. Electronic technology, for example, makes available more sedentary jobs in the design, assembly, repair, and operation of computers, information systems, appliances, and games. The physically disabled are often limited to sedentary jobs. The job market is very competitive for the disabled.[1] However, based on predictions of the types of jobs that will be most available in the future, it seems that the qualified disabled will have opportunities. The ex-

pected rise in demand is seen for technical, professional, and clerical jobs.[1]

Whereas in past generations a person learned a trade or profession which he and society expected him to pursue for his lifetime; now, and increasingly in the future, it is expected that people will make several career changes in their lifetimes. Vocational counseling for both able-bodied and disabled is more common and imaginative. Enough good arguments have been offered concerning the economics of investing in the retraining and placement of the disabled in tax-paying jobs vs. relegating them to tax-absorbing status that this issue is no longer germane to decision-making regarding vocational planning for the disabled.

Laws currently are in force which prohibit discrimination against hiring the handicapped for a job he can be judged capable and safe to perform (qualified). This is section 504 of the Rehabilitation Act of 1973. Section 503 provides for affirmative action in hiring the handicapped. Both of these laws apply only to companies or contractors which do more than $2500 worth of business for the U.S. government or receive Federal grants.[2]

One problem that arises in returning the physically disabled to work in small private industries is the refusal of the employer's insurance company to cover such employees for job-related injuries or to allow such an uninsurable person to be employed there.

Some persons who do value work are not ready at the time of discharge from the rehabilitation center to consider return to work or to work through the process of determining abilities for work because they are still in a period of mourning for their loss. Therefore, these persons need to know where to go for these services when they are ready.

There are some disabled persons for whom work postdisability is not possible, despite its positive value to the person. Persons close to retirement age would be unlikely to be hired, as is true for the older unemployed able-bodied person. Those with frequent concurrent illnesses that would result in absenteeism are not good candidates unless their illnesses can be controlled. For example, a spinal cord-injured patient prone to urinary tract infections needs to have that condition corrected before seeking employment. Persons with brain damage which severely interferes with learning or appropriate social behavior would also not be candidates. These persons need to be taught satisfying avocational pursuits, if possible, to enhance the quality of their lives.

For those that are employable, prevocational evaluation and vocational training become rehabilitation goals.

PREVOCATIONAL EVALUATION AND VOCATIONAL PLANNING

Residual physical disability requires the person to either change his type of employment or to resume previous employment using adapted tools or methods. In either case, the person's ability to work safely and efficiently must be determined. In most rehabilitation centers, many rehabilitation specialists contribute to this decision. The role of each varies from center to center, depending on who is on the team, but in general the roles are the following. The physician determines that the patient's medical status permits work. The physical therapist contributes information concerning strength, endurance, whole body control, mobility, and locomotion skills of the patient. The psychologist determines the person's intellectual capacities and abilities; he may also do interest inventories, personality tests, and academic placement tests. The vocational counselor contributes information concerning the patient's aptitude and skill based on testing either using job sample methods or testing within a work situation.[3] Testing by use of concrete functional tasks may result in more accurate knowledge of a brain-damaged patient's abilities than use of standardized tests which require him to cope with complex, abstract concepts.[3] The vocational counselor is also a major source of information concerning the demands of particular jobs. The occupational therapist contributes information about the patient's abilities relative to job-related tasks. The abilities evaluated may include coordination, endurance, cognitive-perceptual abilities related to following instructions or handling objects, manual skill, work habits, self care status, and the need for adapted techniques, tools, or environment. The occupational therapist, after analyzing the person's former job using activity and environmental analysis methods and knowing the patient's ability to work outside of the home, offers an estimate of whether the person can succeed at the former occupation.

How the individual values work in general and the type of work in particular needs to be determined by some member of the team. A person who once held a managerial position may not be able to emotionally accept employment at a job which he views as less prestigious. A manual laborer who has a limited view of his abilities to do other types of work may be too emotionally insecure to accept a more intellectually, but less physically, demanding job. Each type of reaction needs careful therapy to facilitate acceptance of this new aspect of the self concept.

Personal skills that are prerequisite to employment need to be evaluated for those who were never employed, have a poor work history, or have suffered brain damage. Personal skills refer to the ability to behave appropriately, a sense of time and responsibility, the ability to read, write, and handle money, acceptable personal hygiene, the ability to accept and use supervision, the ability to make friends and get along with others, and other such developmental tasks.[4] The occupational therapist would probably be the source of much of this information.

Prevocational Testing

All the information mentioned above contributes to the prevocational evaluation of an individual. In addition, commercially available prevocational tests which test a person's ability to do competitive manual work have been devised to help in counseling, training decisions, and placement of patients. These tests are usually administered by the vocational counselor or work evaluator, but some occupational therapists who specialize in prevocational evaluation and training also use them. The types of tasks and opportunities for behavioral observation under work conditions that these tests afford are similar to other occupational therapy evaluations. Three of fourteen tests which have been thoroughly reviewed and compared by Botterbusch[5] will be mentioned here. The reader is referred to the original source for greater detail of these and for information on the other tests. Botterbusch states that most work sample systems are technically inadequate in that validity, reliability, and norms are poorly established, if at all.[5] The COATS (Comprehensive Occupational Assessment and Training System) and Micro-TOWER Systems seem to be the only ones with reliability, validity, and a data base completed. The TOWER System, developed by the Institute for Crippled and Disabled (ICD) in New York, is the oldest complete work evaluation system.[5]

The COATS system consists of four sections, each with three program levels: the Job Matching System, which matches the person's preferences, experiences, and abilities to employment and/or training opportunities based on the *Dictionary of Occupational Titles* (DOT); the Employability Attitudes System, which allows the client to evaluate his attitudes and compare them to the attitudes seen as important by employers for hiring, promoting, and firing of employees; the Work Sample System, which contains 26 work samples that are representative of tasks common to types of trades; the Living Skills System, which tests those skills needed to be a functional literate in contemporary society. The instruction is given by way of audiovisual cartridges.[5]

The Micro-TOWER System was devised by ICD to be used for general rehabilitation patients of average intelligence. The system contains 13 work samples which measure 8 specific aptitudes, plus general learning ability. The samples are organized into five major groups: motor, spatial, clerical perception, numerical, and verbal. The results are related to specific jobs in the 4th edition of the DOT. The cost depends on how many people are being tested at a time; each person needs a set of equipment, as does the evaluator.[5]

The TOWER System was originally developed by ICD for use with physically disabled persons, but it is now also used with other types of clients, such as the emotionally disabled. The system contains 93 work samples organized into 14 job training areas: clerical, drafting, drawing, electronics assembly, jewelry manufacturing, leathergoods, machine shop, lettering, mail clerk, optical mechanics, pantograph engraving, sewing machine operation, welding, workshop assembly. Within each major area, the work samples are graded in complexity. The recommendations that can be derived from the results are limited to jobs that relate to the work samples and do not relate to DOT classifications. The system was normed on disabled persons, and no industrial norms are available. It is a useful system for thorough evaluation in limited areas. Each facility must build its own work samples; ICD estimates the initial cost to be approximately $5000.[5]

There are no prevocational tests for evaluating professional or executive-type business skills. Special testing situations would need to be devised to determine if the person were able to do all essential physical components of the job safely. Evidence of good judgment and normal intellectual and perceptual abilities would be gathered from psychological and occupational therapy testing and observation of the patient. If these minimal requirements were met, then the patient's ability to do the more subtle aspects of the job would need to be evaluated in actual work situations by persons knowledgeable about the performance standards.

For those just entering a profession, college education is required. Testing to meet the usual university and departmental entrance requirements would have to be done. If the profession required the person to handle instruments or other people, the applicant would have to show evidence that he could do this with or without adaptation.

The process of vocational planning begins with the various evaluations and continues through the phase of prevocational training. Following evaluation, certain types of jobs can be eliminated from consideration by virtue of their physical demands and the patient's expected maximum ability in that area. Others can be eliminated by virtue of their intellectual demands in light of the patient's capacities. Selection will continue to be narrowed, based on interest, aptitude, realistic appraisal of the training required, and the person's willingness to invest time and effort.

The vocational counselor is responsible for vocational planning with the client. Group discussions among current and former patients of similar disability are also helpful in this regard.

PREVOCATIONAL TRAINING

Prevocational training refers to the teaching-learning of work habits and job-related skills that are prerequisite to actually training for a particular trade or profession. The ability to achieve a certain strength of grasp or the ability to move objects from one place to another quickly and accurately are examples of job-related skills. Care to finish projects neatly and being prompt for appointments are examples of good work habits.

Psychotherapy to address the emotional issues of return to work with a physical disability may be considered a part of prevocational training also.

The occupational therapist contributes to prevocational training by (1) facilitating the client's emotional adjustment to the change in self concept or need to change careers; (2) remediating the cognitive-perceptual-motor deficits which limit job opportunity; and (3) treating developmental deficits that would interfere with the person's ability to work or to seek employment in a competitive market. The training that the occupational therapist does with the patient to prepare him to live as independently as possible also contributes to the likelihood of his employability.

To facilitate the client's emotional adjustment, group therapy, as suggested in Chapter 2, is used. Goals are to assist the patient to accept himself as a worthy person, though changed; to value his working ability, although skills that may have been a source of pride to him are now impossible; to develop realistic expectations of himself and the working community; to redevelop his former level of motivation for work; and to explore new career possibilities. The group discussions could be organized around information presented by former patients with similar diagnoses, by group interviews of experts in the fields of interest to find out what the job requirements actually are, or by discussion of published information. The group discussions should help the person realize that work for the disabled is no longer stereotyped, for example, watchmaking for paraplegics and broom-making for the blind, but that there are a large variety of jobs that are being done successfully by even the most severely disabled, limited only by drive and imagination.

Because there needs to be greater awareness of the possible job opportunities that some disabled persons have found, a compilation is published here. One homebound worker operates a service agency which rents out specialized labor; money earned comes from charging the customers one-third more than each worker's hourly salary.[6] Disabled persons who are experienced actors are being sought for TV and films.[7, 8] Experience can be gained from community or college theater, just as it is by the nondisabled. There is a demand for micrographic technicians to microfilm documents and other material produced by the information explosion; severely disabled are doing this work.[9] The American Association for the Advancement of Science (AAAS) has established an Office of Opportunities in Science to study the needs and contributions of disabled scientists and science students.[10] Other jobs done by severely disabled persons include: parking code enforcement personnel of the police department ("Quad Squad"),[11] vocational counselor,[12, 13] comedian,[14, 15] disc jockey,[16] dentist,[17, 18] anaesthesiologist,[19] medical student,[20] computer programmer,[21, 22] accountant,[23] owner-manager of bed and bath boutique and decorator service,[24] owner-inventor of medical products,[25] orthotist, and farmer.[26]

The new job should fit a person's realistic self image and values regarding work. Discussions of issues concerning work values, *e.g.*, job *vs.* career, pay *vs.* personal satisfaction, office work *vs.* physical work, small company or large, etc., will help the person not only to clarify his values but also to develop realistic attitudes and self perceptions.

Remediation of the cognitive-perceptual-motor deficits has been the concern of the previous chapters of this book. The preparation for work starts from the beginning of the rehabilitation process with training to improve function. Independence in self care and mobility are generally prerequisites to being able to work outside of the home. Therapy to improve strength, range of motion, coordination, perception, etc. that is done to improve the person's independence in self care and mobility also improves the person's work-related skills. Ability to manipulate objects in the environment and/or problem solve are other prerequisite skills addressed in occupational therapy.

Treating the developmental deficits is a goal for the occupational therapist, who usually becomes aware of these in the course of treating the patient for other reasons. Self care training, therapeutic activity and sports, group discussions, or group projects all generate pieces of information concerning the person's readiness for employment. Special situations may need to be devised, however, to gather information or to allow the patient to practice basic skills such as promptness, thoroughness, neatness, safety, accuracy, use of supervision without dependency or resentfulness, acceptance of responsibility, and tolerance for working 8 hours. The nature of occupational therapy provides an ideal laboratory experience for such learning to take place.

The patient who has never worked before may need assistance in learning job acquisition skills. All persons seeking a job for the first time after disability need to learn that in addition to the usual behavior of any job applicant (good grooming, knowledge about the particular business, a definite job goal, evidence of dependability, and a well-composed resumé or reference list), he needs to take the initiative to put the interviewer at ease regarding the disability and how it relates to the job sought.[27] This would prevent a naive interviewer from refusing the job on the basis of preconceived ideas. The person needs to act confidently and let the interviewer know what skills he expects to bring to the company.[27] Role playing in occupational therapy can provide the opportunity to learn good job interview skills.

VOCATIONAL TRAINING

Vocational training refers to the actual training program that the worker will undergo to learn the trade or profession that he has decided on. The training prepares the person for competitive job seeking. Whereas the disabled will not be blatantly discriminated against, they will not be preferentially hired either. They must be qualified. Training for some is done in a few special rehabilitation centers in the U.S.A., such as the Woodrow Wilson Rehabilitation Center in Virginia, or in sheltered workshops throughout the country, such as Goodwill Industries or the Society for the Blind Workshops. Many patients do not need to be trained in these special settings and can be mainstreamed into community vocational-technical high schools and colleges, especially since these are being made more accessible.[28] The training is done by persons expert in the trade or profession. The cost of training may be funded by the Rehabilitation Services Administration, as finances permit.

The vocational counselor finds the training program to suit the patient's needs and may help place the patient in a job, once trained.

The only role the occupational therapist would have at this stage of vocational rehabilitation is to evaluate the patient's need or design for the necessary adaptations that the person will need to do the job for which he is training.

The physical and/or occupational therapist may need to go to the work or training place to do an environmental evaluation similar to the home evaluation described in Chapter 29 if the patient is unable to do it for himself.

References

1. Job market for disabled: Good and bad news! *Accent on Living*, 21(2): 63, 1976.
2. Turned down because of your handicap? *Accent on Living*, 23(1): 34–39, 1978.
3. Weiss, L. Vocational evaluation: An individualized program. *Arch. Phys. Med. Rehabil.*, 61(10): 453–454, 1980.
4. Ryan, P. A. Widening their horizons: A model career development program for severely physically disabled youth. *Rehabil. Lit.*, 40(3): 72–74, 1979.
5. Botterbusch, K. F. *A Comparison of Commercial Vocational Evaluation Systems*. Materials Development Center, Stout Vocational Rehabilitation Institute, University of Wisconsin-Stout, 1980.
6. Lamb, S. Is good service hard to find? *Accent on Living*, 25(1): 20–21, 1980.
7. Vallero, S. Talent agency promotes experienced disabled actors. *Accent on Living*, 25(1): 57, 1980.
8. Two-time Oscar winner makes a comeback. *Accent on Living*, 25(3): 64, 1980.
9. Disabled learn microfilming techniques in special class. *Accent on Living*, 23(4): 84–85, 1979.

10. Disabled scientists getting it together. *Accent on Living*, 23(4): 92–93, 1979.

11. Heilpern, N. Quad squad. *Accent on Living*, 24(3): 26–28, 1979.

12. Kasper, R. An overnight success—In only 23 years. *Accent on Living*, 25(3): 20–21, 1980.

13. Quad named Massachusetts Rehab Commissioner. *Accent on Living*, 22(1): 43, 1977.

14. Haffner, T. E. More than show 'n tell. *Accent on Living*, 25(3): 76–78, 1980.

15. Higgins, M. Comedy routines: Stand-up and sit-down style. *Accent on Living*, 25(4): 84–85, 1981.

16. Lynn, R. Disc jockey by braille. *Accent on Living*, 25(3): 87–90, 1980.

17. Olive, R. Disabled dentist back in practice. *Accent on Living*, 25(3): 100, 1980.

18. Bosco, A. They practice the healing arts from wheelchairs: Wheelchair dentist. *Accent on Living*, 22(2): 58–59, 1977.

19. Alsofrom, J. They practice the healing arts from wheelchairs: Wheelchair doctor. *Accent on Living*, 22(2): 59–61, 1977.

20. Rosenkoetter, R. Quad accepted by medical school. *Accent on Living*, 24(2): 24–26, 1979.

21. Good salaries available to disabled who qualify. *Accent on Living*, 23(1): 44–47, 1978.

22. Linthicum, S. Technical training for the severely disabled: A model. *Rehabil. Lit.*, 38(11–12): 373–375, 1977.

23. Hanna, J. Business booming thanks to computer. *Accent on Living*, 25(4): 93–95, 1981.

24. Guthertz, A. T. Quad runs bed and bath boutique. *Accent on Living*, 23(3): 24–27, 1978.

25. Butcher, L. Paralyzed from the waist down, Wayne Nelson runs a $100,000 a Year Business. *Accent on Living*, 22(1): 63–65, 1977.

26. Brinkman, G. Double amputee makes successful farmer. *Accent on Living*, 25(2): 66–70, 1980.

27. Your job interview. *Accent on Living*, 23(1): 40–43, 1978.

28. Improved opportunities for disabled college students goal of new national group. *Accent on Living*, 24(2): 29, 1979.

Supplementary Reading

Bailey, D. M. Vocational theories and work habits related to childhood development. *Am. J. Occup. Ther.*, 25(6): 298–302, 1971.

Can totally blind find jobs? *Accent on Living*, 22(1): 66–74, 1977.

Cromwell, F. S. *Occupational Therapist's Manual for Basic Skills Assessment: Primary Prevocational Evaluation.* Pasadena, Calif.: Fair Oaks Printing, 1960.

Dictionary of Occupational Titles. U.S. Government Printing Office, Washington, D.C. 20402.

Disabled in many different occupations. *Accent on Living*, 24(4): 80–81, 1980.

How to get a civil service job. *Accent on Living*, 21(2): 59–61, 1976.

Kester, D. L. Prevocational Training. In: *Willard and Spackman's Occupational Therapy*, 5th ed., edited by H. L. Hopkins and H. D. Smith. Philadelphia: J. B. Lippincott, 1978.

Kohring, C., and Tracht, V. S. A new approach to a vocational program for severely handicapped high school students. *Rehabil. Lit.*, 39(5): 138–146, 1978.

Maki, D. R., McCracken, N., Pope, D. A., and Schofield. A systems approach to vocational assessment. *J. Rehabil.*, 45(1): 48–51, 1979.

Maurer, P. Antecedents of work behavior. *Am. J. Occup. Ther.*, 25(6): 295–297, 1971.

The President's Committee on Employment of the Handicapped. *Accent on Living*, 25(2): 50–53, 1980.

Wallace, A., and Woodring, R. Basic Prevocational evaluation in an acute general hospital. *Am. J. Occup. Ther.*, 18(6): 250–254, 1964.

Index